EXERCISE
AND DIABETES

A Clinician's Guide to Prescribing Physical Activity

Sheri R. Colberg, PhD, FACSM

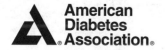
American Diabetes Association®

Director, Book Publishing, Abe Ogden; *Managing Editor*, Greg Guthrie; *Acquisitions Editor*, Victor Van Beuren; *Production Manager*, Melissa Sprott; *Copyediting*, Cenveo; *Composition*, ADA; *Cover Design*, Kim Woody; *Printer*, Versa Press, Inc.

Printed in the United States of America
1 3 5 7 9 10 8 6 4 2

The suggestions and information contained in this publication are generally consistent with the *Clinical Practice Recommendations* and other policies of the American Diabetes Association, but they do not represent the policy or position of the Association or any of its boards or committees. Reasonable steps have been taken to ensure the accuracy of the information presented. However, the American Diabetes Association cannot ensure the safety or efficacy of any product or service described in this publication. Individuals are advised to consult a physician or other appropriate health care professional before undertaking any diet or exercise program or taking any medication referred to in this publication. Professionals must use and apply their own professional judgment, experience, and training and should not rely solely on the information contained in this publication before prescribing any diet, exercise, or medication. The American Diabetes Association—its officers, directors, employees, volunteers, and members—assumes no responsibility or liability for personal or other injury, loss, or damage that may result from the suggestions or information in this publication.

♾ The paper in this publication meets the requirements of the ANSI Standard Z39.48-1992 (permanence of paper).

ADA titles may be purchased for business or promotional use or for special sales. To purchase more than 50 copies of this book at a discount, or for custom editions of this book with your logo, contact the American Diabetes Association at the address below, at booksales@diabetes.org, or by calling 703-299-2046.

American Diabetes Association
1701 North Beauregard Street
Alexandria, Virginia 22311

DOI: 10.2337/9781580404853

Library of Congress Cataloging-in-Publication Data
Colberg, Sheri, 1963-
  Exercise and diabetes : a clinician's guide to prescribing physical activity / Sheri R. Colberg, PhD, FACSM.
    pages cm
  Includes bibliographical references and index.
  ISBN 978-1-58040-485-3 (alk. paper)
  1. Diabetes--Exercise therapy. 2. Diabetics--Rehabilitation. I. Title.
  RC661.E94C652 2012
  616.4'620642--dc23
                          2012038644

For my loving husband, Ray,
and my three wonderful sons, Alex, Anton, and RayJ.
Thanks for your nonstop support and boundless love.

Contents

Why This Book?

Myriad types of physical movement have a positive impact on physical fitness, morbidity, and mortality in individuals with diabetes, and although exercise has long been considered a cornerstone of diabetes management, many health-care providers fail to prescribe it. Many fitness professionals may be unaware of the complexities of including physical activity in the management of all types of the disease. Giving patients or clients a full exercise prescription that takes comorbid conditions into account may be too time-consuming for or beyond the expertise of many health-care and fitness professionals.

The purpose of this book, therefore, is to cover the recommended types and quantities of physical activities that can and should be undertaken by all individuals with any type of diabetes, along with precautions related to medication use and diabetes-related health complications. Medications used to control diabetes should augment, rather than replace, lifestyle improvements like increased daily physical activity.

Until now, professional books with exercise information and prescriptions were not timely or sufficiently interactive to easily provide busy professionals with access to the latest recommendations for each unique patient. Simply instructing patients to "exercise more" is not motivating or informative enough to get them regularly or safely active. *Exercise and Diabetes* is changing all that with its up-to-date and easy-to-prescribe exercise and physical activity recommendations and relevant case studies.

Read, learn, and quickly be ready to effortlessly prescribe effective and appropriate exercise to everyone. Your reward will be a collective increase in the health and fitness of all people with diabetes.

Key Terms

Aerobic exercise: Physical movement that results from rhythmic muscular contractions that are primarily fueled by the aerobic metabolism of energy in the body; oxygen-based generation of energy is usually the main source for any activity lasting longer than 2 min continuously.

Autonomic neuropathy: Disease affecting the nerves innervating the heart, gastrointestinal, and genitourinary tract; cardiovascular autonomic neuropathy (CAN) is the most common, studied, and clinically important type of this neuropathy.

Cardiorespiratory (aerobic) fitness: The ability of the circulatory and respiratory systems to supply oxygen to skeletal muscles during sustained (aerobic) physical activity.

Continuous glucose monitoring (CGM): Newer technologies that allow for subcutaneous monitoring of glucose levels with frequent readings (usually every 5 min).

Daily lifestyle activity: All physical activities done during the course of a day involved with self-care, basic locomotion, and other movement other than planned exercise sessions (also called activities of daily living [ADL]).

Diabetic ketoacidosis (DKA): High level of blood ketones (e.g., β-hydroxybutyrate, acetoacetate, acetone), accompanied by hyperglycemia, that can result in coma or death if not treated in a timely manner.

Estimated average glucose (eAG): Alternate method to report hemoglobin A1C levels, as an estimated average glucose in mg/dl instead of percent (e.g., A1C value of 6.0% equates to an eAG of 126 mg/dl); the relationship between A1C and eAG is described by the formula $(28.7 \times A1C) - 46.7 = eAG$. An online calculator is available at professional.diabetes.org/GlucoseCalculator.aspx.

Gestational diabetes mellitus (GDM): A hyperglycemic condition developing most often during the third trimester of pregnancy (when placental hormones decrease insulin action); although it usually resolves postpartum, it is associated with a greater risk for the mother of developing type 2 diabetes later in life.

Hemoglobin A1C (or A1C): Test to assess glycemic control that reflects a time-averaged blood glucose concentration (as a percent) over the previous 2–3 months; a normal value is ~4.0–6.0%.

Hyperglycemia: An elevated blood glucose level (i.e., blood glucose ≥126 mg/dl).

Hypoglycemia: An abnormally low blood glucose level (i.e., blood glucose <70 mg/dl).

Insulin resistance: A condition in which there is a relative lack of insulin action in insulin-sensitive tissues (primarily skeletal muscle) needed to maintain normal glucose levels.

Latent autoimmune diabetes of the adult (LADA): A form of type 1 diabetes that is often slower in onset and diagnosed in adults.

Metabolic syndrome: A syndrome characterized by a constellation of disorders, including insulin resistance, obesity, central adiposity, glucose intolerance or diabetes, dyslipidemia, and hypertension.

Muscular endurance: The ability of muscles to contract using submaximal force over a period of time, based on criteria such as the number of pushups that can be done in a minute.

Muscular strength: The maximal ability of a muscle to exert force, often measured as the amount of resistance that can be moved one time (one-repetition maximum).

Nephropathy: A microvascular disease affecting the kidneys, resulting in excessive urinary protein (microalbuminuria, followed by gross proteinuria) as a marker of end-stage renal disease.

Peripheral neuropathy: Disease affecting the nerves in the extremities, especially the lower legs and feet, resulting in pain or loss of sensation and increased risk of amputation.

Resistance (strength) exercise: Physical activity aimed at increasing muscular strength or muscular endurance through the use of resistance or weights.

Retinopathy: A disease caused by long-term damage to blood vessels of the retina caused by elevated blood glucose levels; the stages include nonproliferative (less severe) and proliferative (more advanced and severe form), the latter of which is the leading cause of new blindness in adults.

Self-monitoring of blood glucose (SMBG): The practice of using blood glucose monitoring devices outside of clinical settings to monitor changes in blood glucose levels.

Type 1 diabetes (T1D): Immune-mediated disease that selectively destroys the pancreatic β-cells, leading to a central defect in insulin release upon stimulation; although more commonly associated with youth, it can develop in individuals of any age and frequently occurs in adulthood as well as in latent autoimmune diabetes of the adult.

Type 2 diabetes (T2D): Disease directly related to insulin resistance, formerly thought to afflict persons older than the age of 40 years, which now has an increasing prevalence in younger children and adolescents; this type of diabetes accounts for 90–95% of all cases of the disease.

Chapter 1

Diabetes, Physical Activity, Exercise, and Fitness Overview

The burden associated with diabetes, prediabetes, and related metabolic disorders is undeniably growing. Federal government estimates released in 2011 placed the number of Americans with diabetes at nearly 26 million (with one-quarter of cases likely still undiagnosed)—or ~8.3% of the total population. Another 79 million American adults have prediabetes, which is an asymptomatic state characterized by moderate insulin resistance, impaired fasting glucose (IFG), or impaired glucose tolerance (IGT). People with prediabetes have glucose levels that are higher than normal but lower than those classified as diabetes. About 25% of individuals with prediabetes will develop type 2 diabetes (T2D) within 3 to 5 years (U.S. Department of Health and Human Services 2011). Moreover, it is now estimated that one in three Americans born in the year 2000 or later will develop diabetes during their lifetimes, with rates closer to 50% in high-risk, ethnic populations (Narayan 2003, 2006).

In spite of the salutary effects of achieving optimal blood glucose control, only slightly more than half of individuals with diabetes currently are reaching recognized treatment goals (Cheung 2009). Although physical activity has long been considered a cornerstone of diabetes management and a critical factor in optimizing treatment, prescribing specific exercise for individuals with various types of diabetes (or even prediabetes) can be a daunting task for the time-pressured health-care provider or the diabetes-naïve fitness professional. A fundamental need in facilitating such exercise prescription is an enhanced understanding of the types of diabetes and how physical activity requirements and abilities may differ among them.

Case in Point: Weight, Blood Pressure, and T2D

MJ, a 48-year-old woman diagnosed with T2D 4 years ago, is having trouble controlling her weight and blood pressure. She wants to discuss safe and appropriate ways to be more physically active to address these issues and improve her overall health and diabetes management. From her physician, she already has received medical clearance to start increasing her activity level with no specific restrictions. Her medications include a sulfonylurea (glipizide) and an antihypertensive agent. MJ reports testing her blood glucose usually just once a day in the morning before breakfast. She currently is not doing any planned exercise and has not been active for the past 10 years or so, although she claims to be motivated to start being more physically active now to increase her energy levels.

Resting Measurements

Height: 64 inches
Weight: 190 lb
BMI: 32.6 kg/m² (obese)
Heart rate: 85 beats per minute (bpm)
Blood pressure: 138/86 mmHg (on medication)

Fasting Labs

Plasma glucose: 148 mg/dl A1C: 7.4%
Total cholesterol: 190 mg/dl
Triglycerides: 200 mg/dl
High-density lipoprotein cholesterol: 38 mg/dl
Low-density lipoprotein cholesterol: 112 mg/dl

Questions to Consider

1. How should MJ go about increasing her physical activity level?
2. Does MJ need to take any precautions related to exercise participation?
3. What strategies will help motivate MJ and support her efforts to establish regular physical activity as a lifelong habit?

(Continued on page 9.)

BASICS OF DIABETES SELF-MANAGEMENT

Effective management of any type of diabetes involves use of self-monitoring of blood glucose (SMBG), administration of appropriate medications to regulate blood glucose levels, regular participation in physical activity and exercise, and body weight management, as well as dietary and other lifestyle improvements, for example, stress management (St John 2010, American Diabetes Association 2013b). Regular physical activity facilitates improved blood glucose control in T2D and may offer a similar benefit in gestational diabetes mellitus (GDM) (Dyck 1998, Davenport 2008, Colberg 2010). Although regular exercise does not uniformly improve glycemic management in those with type 1 diabetes (T1D) unless appropriate regimen changes are made, exercise is still considered a safe and effective adjunct therapy for diabetes management and complication prevention (American Diabetes Association 2013b). Exercise interventions for individuals with diabetes ideally should involve a multidisciplinary team of specialists that includes the diabetes (or other qualified) physician, certified diabetes educator, registered dietician, and exercise professional to facilitate individual education and lifestyle changes to manage this disease. Self-management skills are essential to success, and diabetes education is an important tool to improve glycemic control, regardless of the type of diabetes that an individual has (American Diabetes Association 2013b).

CLASSIFICATION AND ETIOLOGY OF DIABETES

Four classifications of diabetes are categorized based on etiology: T1D, T2D, GDM (diagnosed during pregnancy), and diabetes resulting from other specific origins (e.g., genetic defects, drugs and chemicals, pancreatic disease, surgery, and infections). The major types are T1D and T2D, with the latter type describing 90–95% of all cases, whereas T1D accounts for only 5–10% of the population with diabetes (American Diabetes Association 2013a). The major characteristics of these classifications are given in Table 1.1.

Table 1.1 Characteristics of T1D, T2D, and Gestational Diabetes

Factor	T1D	T2D	Gestational Diabetes
Age at onset	Often early in life, but may occur at any age	Usually older than age 30 years, but may occur at any age	Most often diagnosed at 24–28 weeks of gestation
Type of onset	Rapid to slower: generally short duration of symptoms in children and adolescents; slower progression in adults diagnosed later in life (as LADA)	Slow progression (may be undiagnosed for years)	Slow rise in blood glucose levels during pregnancy due to release of placental hormones; may be more rapid during third trimester
Genetic susceptibility	HLA-related DR3 and DR4, ICAs, IAAs; limited or no family history	Frequent genetic background (family history), but not HLA related	Some genetic and environmental influences; likely to recur in subsequent pregnancies; 40–60% will develop T2D within 5–10 years
Environ-mental factors	Virus, toxins, autoimmune stimulation	Obesity, poor nutrition, physical inactivity, POP exposure	Obesity, poor nutrition, physical inactivity
Islet cell antibodies	Present at onset	Usually not observed	Not observed
Endogenous insulin	Minimal or absent	Stimulated response either adequate with delayed secretion or reduced but not absent; insulin resistance present	Inadequate insulin responses, particularly to food intake; insulin resistance heightened by placental hormones
Nutritional status	Thin or overweight; catabolic state (recent weight loss)	Obese, overweight, or normal; little or no recent weight loss	Obese, overweight, or normal

Table 1.1 Characteristics of T1D, T2D, and Gestational Diabetes (*continued*)

Factor	T1D	T2D	Gestational Diabetes
Symptoms	Thirst, polyuria, polyphagia, fatigue	Mild or frequently none; acanthosis nigricans; PCOS in females	Mild or frequently none
Ketosis	Common at onset or during insulin deficiency	Unusual (resistant to ketosis except during infection or stress)	Unusual
Control of diabetes	Wide glucose fluctuation without effective management of insulin doses, food intake, and physical activity patterns	Variable, but usually greatly enhanced by lifestyle improvements (e.g., dietary adherence, weight loss, exercise, stress management)	Variable, but responsive to dietary changes, physical activity; may or may not require insulin during pregnancy
Dietary management	Essential, but must be balanced with insulin dosage	Essential; may suffice for blood glucose management	Essential; may suffice for blood glucose management
Insulin	Required for all (eventually)	Required for ~40%	Variable
Oral hypo-glycemic	Usually not effective (unless insulin resistant as well)	Effective	Effective, but only certain ones are advisable during pregnancy

LADA, latent autoimmune diabetes of the adult; HLA, human leukocyte antigen; DR, D-related antigen; ICA, islet cell antibodies; IAA, insulin autoantibodies; POP, persistent organic pollutants; PCOS, polycystic ovary syndrome.

T1D

T1D is caused by autoimmune destruction of pancreatic β-cells usually leading to an absolute deficiency of insulin secretion and likely triggered by environmental factors that remain poorly defined or predicted (American Diabetes Association 2013a). Formerly called juvenile-onset or insulin-dependent diabetes, T1D is commonly diagnosed in children and adolescents, but this immune-mediated type of diabetes can occur in individuals of any age. About half of the cases of T1D currently are being diagnosed in adults and frequently are diagnosed and classified as latent autoimmune diabetes of the adult (LADA). Rates of β-cell destruction involved in the onset of T1D generally are slower in older-onset cases than in youth—thus giving rise to the LADA category, which is still not clearly defined or universally used. In addition, many older individuals with this type of diabetes initially may be misdiagnosed with T2D instead.

T2D

Insulin resistance is the hallmark of T2D, and the risk of developing it increases with age, obesity, and physical inactivity. Genetic and environmental factors are strongly implicated in the development of T2D, but they are complex and not clearly defined. Some β-cell dysfunction or β-cell loss is evident at onset, leading to relative rather than absolute defects in insulin secretion (American Diabetes Association 2013a). This type of diabetes disproportionately affects ethnic minorities: its prevalence rates are about twofold greater in Hispanic and Latino, African American, Native American, Asian, and Pacific Islander populations than in non-Hispanic whites (U.S. Department of Health and Human Services 2011). It is also more common in individuals with hypertension or dyslipidemias and in women with a prior history of GDM (American Diabetes Association 2013a). Formerly called adult-onset or non–insulin-dependent diabetes and associated with older age, this type of diabetes leads many individuals to become insulin-requiring over the course of the disease. Moreover, its diagnosis in youth has risen dramatically over the past two decades. The initial diagnosis of T1D in children and adolescents can be complicated by the presence of insulin resistance and obesity, although recognition of T2D in youth may be delayed by the misconception that only adults can develop it.

GESTATIONAL DIABETES

GDM is also on the rise and is associated with a 40–60% chance of the mother developing T2D in the next 5 to 10 years (U.S. Department of Health and Human Services 2011, American Diabetes Association 2013a). Moreover, it is known to be potentially harmful to both mother and fetus if not controlled (Hapo Study Cooperative Research Group 2008, Metzger 2010). For example, larger or fatter infants have been shown to be more likely to develop both hypoglycemia and hyperinsulinemia in the few hours following birth, suggesting a strong relationship between maternal glycemia and fetal insulin production (Metzger 2010). It is generally diagnosed with a 75 g oral glucose tolerance test (OGTT) that is given to all women not known to have prior diabetes at 24–28 weeks of gestation. Given the rise in prevalence of undiagnosed T2D among women of childbearing age, however, it is now reasonable to screen women with diabetes risk factors at their initial prenatal visit. Women with GDM also should be screened for persistent diabetes 6–12 weeks postpartum (American Diabetes Association 2013a, 2013b).

DIAGNOSIS OF DIABETES

T1D AND T2D

Currently, the American Diabetes Association recommends the use of any of the following four criteria for diagnosing diabetes: 1) hemoglobin A1C value of 6.5% or higher; 2) fasting plasma glucose ≥126 mg/dl (7.0 mmol/l); 3) 2 h plasma glucose ≥200 mg/dl (11.1 mmol/l) during an OGTT using 75 g of glucose; or 4) classic symptoms of hyperglycemia (e.g., polyuria, polydipsia, and unexplained weight loss) or hyperglycemic crisis with a random plasma glucose of 200 mg/dl (11.1 mmol/l) or more (American Diabetes Association 2013a, 2013b) (Table 1.2). In the absence of unequivocal hyperglycemia, the first three criteria should be confirmed by repeat testing on a second occasion.

GESTATIONAL DIABETES

The International Association of Diabetes and Pregnancy Study Groups recently developed revised recommendations for the diagnosis of GDM (International Association of Diabetes 2010). After an overnight fast of at least 8 h, the pregnant woman ingests 75 g of glucose orally, with monitoring of fasting plasma glucose and 1 and 2 h postingestion glucose values. The diagnosis is made when any one of the following plasma glucose values is exceeded: fasting ≥92 mg/dl (5.1 mmol/l); 1 h ≥180 mg/dl (10.0 mmol/l); or 2 h ≥153 mg/dl (8.5 mmol/l) (American Diabetes Association 2013a, 2013b). It is expected that these new criteria will increase the prevalence of GDM because they require only that one abnormal value be recorded, whereas the former criteria required two to be met. Also, given that some cases diagnosed during pregnancy are actually cases of undiagnosed T2D, it is recommended that women with a history of GDM be screened for diabetes 6–12 weeks after delivery, using nonpregnant diagnostic criteria during an OGTT (American Diabetes Association 2013a).

PREDIABETES

Individuals with prediabetes have glucose levels that do not meet the criteria for diabetes, but that are higher than normal, putting them at risk for related metabolic disorders. They can meet one or both criteria for IFG and IGT to be classified as being at high risk for developing T2D, or their overall glucose levels can exceed normal (as determined with an A1C test). Currently, prediabetes is diagnosed with fasting plasma glucose of 100–125 mg/dl (6.1–6.9 mmol/l) (i.e., IFG), 2 h OGTT plasma glucose of 140–199 mg/dl (7.8–11.0 mmol/l) (i.e., IGT), or an A1C of 5.7%–6.4%.

PHYSICAL ACTIVITY VERSUS EXERCISE

Before the discussion moves from what type of diabetes an individual has to which type of activity he or she should be doing, the professional needs to understand the meaning of the terms physical activity and exercise, which are used interchangeably in this book. By definition, physical activity is any bodily movement produced by the contraction of skeletal muscle that substantially increases energy expenditure (above resting), whereas exercise training is the subset of planned, structured, and repetitive bodily movements done with the intention of developing or maintaining physical fitness, which includes cardiovascular, strength, and flexibility training options (Haskell 2007, Nelson 2007).

Although use of the broader "physical activity" in place of the narrower "exercise" has caused some confusion even among health-care and fitness professionals, the intent is simply to recognize that many types of movements can have a positive

Table 1.2 Diagnosis of Diabetes by Type

Diabetes Diagnosis	Fasting Plasma Glucose	Glucose Tolerance (Oral)	A1C	Symptoms
Type 1 (or LADA)	Plasma glucose ≥126 mg/dl (7.0 mmol/l)	2 h value ≥200 mg/dl (11.1 mmol/l) during OGTT	6.5% or higher	Classic symptoms of hyperglycemia or hyperglycemic crisis with a random plasma glucose ≥200 mg/dl (11.1 mmol/l)
Type 2	Plasma glucose ≥126 mg/dl (7.0 mmol/l)	2 h value ≥200 mg/dl (11.1 mmol/l) during OGTT	6.5% or higher	Classic symptoms of hyperglycemia or hyperglycemic crisis with a random plasma glucose ≥200 mg/dl (11.1 mmol/l)
Gestational	Plasma glucose ≥92 mg/dl (5.1 mmol/l)	1 h value ≥180 mg/dl (10.0 mmol/l), or 2 h ≥153 mg/dl (8.5 mmol/l) during OGTT		
Prediabetes	Plasma glucose 100–125 mg/dl (5.6–6.9 mmol/l)	2 h value 140–199 mg/dl (7.8–11.0 mmol/l) during OGTT	5.7–6.4%	

LADA, latent autoimmune diabetes of adults; OGTT, oral glucose tolerance test.

impact on health-related physical fitness without qualifying as a planned exercise. In fact, more than one type of physical activity (such as combined aerobic and resistance training programs, along with lifestyle movement) is frequently required to yield measurable improvements for each of the components in the health-related fitness category.

Exercise training programs for individuals with diabetes typically include activities to enhance cardiovascular capacity (aerobic fitness) and muscular fitness and strength in people of all ages, as well as flexibility and balance in older individuals. Each person's exercise program, however, should be modified according to his or her habitual physical activity, physical function, health status, exercise responses, and stated goals (Garber 2011). Adults who are unable or unwilling to meet the recommended minimal exercise targets can still benefit from engaging in amounts of exercise and other physical activities (like daily movement) that fail to meet those levels. Such strategies can be used when helping individuals with and at risk for diabetes make positive and lasting changes in their physical activity and exercise habits.

UNDERSTANDING AND DEFINING PHYSICAL FITNESS

It is imperative that health-care and fitness professionals use the same fitness terminology. Physical fitness has long been defined as "a set of attributes that people have or achieve relating to their ability to perform physical activity" (Caspersen 1985). What complicates physical fitness is that there are many different reasons to engage in a physically active lifestyle, including gaining positive health outcomes and optimizing sports and athletic performance. To simplify matters, the following table (Table 1.3) organizes the accepted terminology into four different categories of physical fitness: physiological fitness, health-related fitness, skill-related fitness, and sports.

The terminology of fitness is intended to be inclusive rather than athletic in nature when considering what affects an individual's fitness level and health outcomes. For instance, individuals with diabetes do not need to have skill-related talents, participate in sports, or work out at a fitness club to achieve physiological or health-related benefits from increased physical fitness. Thus, a primary goal of the diabetes health-care and fitness professionals should be to encourage individuals to engage in appropriate physical activities to help them achieve positive health- and fitness-related outcomes.

PHYSIOLOGICAL FITNESS

Physiological fitness in particular relates to how an individual performs a physical activity, given that physiological fitness is most influenced by the regular

Table 1.3 Fitness Categories and Related Terminology

Category	Related Terminology
Physiological	Metabolic Morphological Bone integrity Other
Health related	Cardiovascular fitness Musculoskeletal fitness (endurance and strength) Flexibility Body composition
Skill related	Agility Balance Coordination Power Speed Reaction time Other
Sports	Team Individual Lifetime Other

inclusion of habitual physical activity (or, conversely, physical inactivity). In particular, metabolic fitness refers to the status of metabolic systems and variables predictive of the risk for diabetes and cardiovascular disease; increases in fitness lower the risk of both diabetes and heart problems (Simmons 2008, Sui 2008, Look Ahead Research Group 2010, Seeger 2011). Similarly, morphological fitness focuses on improvement in body compositional factors, such as body circumference, body fat, and regional body fat distribution, all of which can affect metabolic health and diabetes management (Jacob 2006, Iqbal 2007, Wang 2008, Lee 2009). Finally, bone integrity refers to bone strength and the status of bone mineral density, which can be positively affected by regular participation in almost any type of physical activity (Gorman 2012).

HEALTH-RELATED PHYSICAL FITNESS

Although it is closely related to the aforementioned category of physiological fitness with regard to metabolic health, the health-related physical fitness category contains terms that are recognized for their direct relationship to good health: cardiovascular fitness, musculoskeletal fitness, body composition, and flexibility. All of these components of fitness are important for patients with diabetes for optimal health and performance. For the individual engaging in a fitness program, many of these components are measurable over time, such as changes in body composition with exercise training or body fatness during weight loss or regain. Success of interventions often is judged on the basis of such changes.

A frequently measured parameter associated with exercise training is cardiovascular fitness (also known as cardiorespiratory fitness or aerobic fitness), which is the ability of the circulatory and respiratory systems to supply oxygen during sustained physical activity (McGavock 2004, Church 2005, Sui 2008, Lee 2009, Williams 2011). Musculoskeletal fitness includes both muscular endurance and muscular strength, which reflect the ability to continue to perform without fatigue and maximal ability to exert force, respectively (American College of Sports Medicine 2009). Flexibility measures the range of motion available at a joint (Herriott 2004). Finally, body composition in this health-related category refers to the relative amounts of fat and fat-free mass that an individual has (which can affect overall health); the fat-free component includes muscle, bone, body water, organs, and other body parts that are not fat (Lee 2005, Iqbal 2007, Wang 2008, Chomentowski 2009, Bray 2012, de Souza 2012). Excess body fat can affect both physiological and health-related fitness, depending on its relative amount and regional distribution.

Case in Point: Continued

A thorough interview with MJ to discuss her personal beliefs, past experiences, preferences, and concerns about increasing her activity levels is required to assist the health-care or fitness professional working with her to gain a better understanding of MJ's view of physical activity. Any preprogram conversations also should include a discussion of the possibility of developing hypoglycemia during or after physical activity (given her use of a sulfonylurea), the best types of carbohydrates to keep handy during all activities (like glucose tablets or gels or hard candy), and the importance of monitoring blood glucose before and after exercise to establish typical response patterns. Once her exercise routine is established, she may need to talk with her health-care provider about possibly reducing her medication dose to prevent hypoglycemia.

(Continued on page 14.)

HEALTH EFFECTS OF PHYSICAL ACTIVITY AND FITNESS FOR DIABETES

Although many American adults are not physically active, just 39% of adults with diabetes in the U.S. are physically active—defined as engaging in moderate or vigorous activity for at least 30 min thrice weekly—compared with 58% of other adults (Kirk 2004, Morrato 2007). In spite of the fact that myriad studies have shown that physical activity has a positive impact on diabetes management and prevention of complications, many health-care providers still are hesitant to prescribe it, and fitness professionals may be ignorant of precautions needed to handle the complexities of the disease with exercise as an added variable. Moreover, giving diabetic individuals a full exercise prescription that takes comorbid conditions into account may be too time-consuming for or beyond the expertise of many health-care and fitness professionals.

Unfortunately, simply instructing diabetic individuals to "exercise more" is frequently not motivating or sufficiently informative to get them regularly and safely active enough to benefit their fitness levels, diabetes control, and overall health (Morrato 2006). Moreover, professional books with exercise information and prescriptions have not been up to date or interactive enough to provide busy professionals with access to the latest tools and recommendations for each individual's unique circumstances and requirements, and exercise remains woefully underprescribed for individuals with diabetes, almost all of whom can benefit from it immensely.

PREVENTION OF T2D WITH PHYSICAL ACTIVITY

The "exercise is medicine" dogma launched by the American College of Sports Medicine campaign in 2007 cites diabetes as one of its hallmark diseases. At this point, it has been well established that participation in regular physical activity as part of lifestyle improvements can prevent or delay the onset of T2D (Tuomilehto 2001, Knowler 2002, Duncan 2003, Laaksonen 2005, Hamman 2006, Li 2008). Early on, studies assessing physical activity via self-report showed that higher levels are associated with reduced risk for T2D, regardless of the method of physical activity assessment or types of activities (Helmrich 1991, Manson 1991, Hu 1999). Greater volumes of physical activity may provide more protection, although both moderate walking and vigorous activity are associated with a decreased risk, as is better cardiovascular fitness (Wei 1999, Sui 2008).

In three larger intervention studies, the role of physical activity in T2D prevention in high-risk individuals has been examined (Diabetes Prevention Program [DPP] Research Group 2002, Knowler 2002, Pan 1997). Amazingly, all their results were similar, showing that modest weight loss (~7% reduction in initial body weight) combined with increased physical activity and dietary improvements (a healthier low-calorie, low-fat diet) significantly reduces the incidence of developing T2D and that these lifestyle changes were more effective in older individuals. The first of these studies, the Chinese Da Qing study, included an exercise-only treatment arm that showed that even modest changes in exercise (i.e., 20 min of mild or moderate, 10 min of strenuous, or 5 min of very strenuous exercise 1–2 times a day) can reduce diabetes risk by 46% compared with 42% for diet plus exercise and 31% for diet alone (Pan 1997). Both the Finnish Diabetes Prevention Study (Eriksson 1999, Tuomilehto 2001) and the DPP (Knowler 2002) included intensive, lifestyle modifications targeting modest weight loss, dietary improvements, and an average of 30 min of daily, moderate physical activity (Eriksson 1999, Tuomilehto 2001). The DPP, which studied 3,234 high-risk men and women, consisted of medication (metformin), lifestyle modification, and control groups (Knowler 2002). In the DPP, intensive lifestyle modification resulted in a 58% risk reduction that was almost twice the impact of metformin use (31% reduction). Although weight loss was the dominant predictor of a lower incidence of diabetes, the DPP showed that regular participation in physical activity can reduce risk by 44% even when modest weight-loss goals are not achieved (Laaksonen 2005, Hamman 2006, Lindstrom 2006). In summary, physical activity does play a role in preventing T2D in high-risk individuals, across ethnic groups, and in both sexes (Kosaka 2005, Ramachandran 2006).

Moderate exercise like brisk walking reduces risk of T2D (Helmrich 1991, Hu 1999, Hu 2001, Kosaka 2005, Ramachandran 2006). A meta-analysis that assessed the preventive effects of moderate-intensity physical activity reported that walking on a regular basis, typically done for 2.5 h per week or more, significantly reduces diabetes risk (Jeon 2007). The preventive effects of resistance training have not been studied to date. Likewise, although T2D is increasing in prevalence in children and adolescents, no trials have been completed that address whether physical activity or exercise prevents T2D in youth.

Limited studies suggest that to prevent and manage T2D, goals for youth should include limiting daily screen time (television, computer, or video game) to <60 min per day and doing at least 60 min of daily physical activity (McGavock 2007). The Treatment Options for Type 2 Diabetes in Adolescents and Youth (TODAY) study (Zeitler 2012) assessed the importance of physical activity as part of a behavioral lifestyle intervention to prevent T2D in youth. The results suggested that metformin combined with lifestyle intervention (e.g., greater physical activity) was intermediate in their ability to manage blood glucose levels and not significantly different from the use of medications (either metformin alone or metformin plus rosiglitazone).

ACUTE EFFECTS OF PHYSICAL ACTIVITY ON INSULIN ACTION AND HORMONES

Insulin. Most benefits of physical activity on diabetes management and prevention of T2D are likely due to acute and chronic improvements in insulin action (Boulé 2001, O'Gorman 2006, Galbo 2007). The acute effects of a recent bout of exercise account for the majority of these improvements, but are short-lived, whereas regular exercise training generally results in a more lasting effect. Although responses can vary, most people with any type of diabetes experience a decrease in their blood glucose levels during mild- and moderate-intensity exercise and up to 2–72 h afterward, necessitating frequent participation to maintain enhanced insulin action (Cartee 1989, Boulé 2001, O'Gorman 2006, Galbo 2007).

Although exercise cannot prevent T1D, it can lessen the potential decrements in insulin action that can occur due to inactivity; even individuals with T1D can become similarly insulin resistant and require larger insulin doses to manage blood glucose levels when not engaging in regular physical activity (Okamoto 2011). Circulating insulin levels during exercise must usually be lowered with appropriate dosing and timing of doses of exogenous insulin, however, to replicate the most normal physiological responses possible to prevent hypoglycemia, along with ingestion of additional carbohydrates to maintain blood glucose levels during most exercise sessions (Chokkalingam 2007a, Gallen 2011, West 2011).

Glycogen stores in the liver and skeletal muscles need to be replenished following each bout of physical activity, which is accomplished via an increased rate of blood glucose uptake during recovery from exercise until the depleted glycogen stores are fully replaced. This activity may take 24 to 48 h to complete, during which time both insulin sensitivity and fat oxidation in skeletal muscles usually are enhanced (Cartee 1989, Goodpaster 2003, Boon 2007). Combined hyperinsulinemia and hyperglycemia during moderate exercise in individuals with T1D, however, does not suppress the release of hepatic glycogen to maintain blood glucose levels (Chokkalingam 2007b), although total body glucose uptake is increased by having higher insulin levels (Chokkalingam 2007a).

Glucose-raising hormones. Endogenous insulin secretion normally decreases during exercise in people without diabetes and in most people with T2D who still secrete insulin. Its suppression is an essential step in allowing hepatic glucose production to ramp up to maintain the balance of glucose in the blood (Galbo 2007, Szewieczek 2009). Exercise causes the release of glucose-raising hormones like epinephrine and norepinephrine in an intensity-dependent manner, with exponentially more being released in response to intense compared with moderate- or low-intensity activity (Manetta 2002, Kreisman 2003). Other hormones like glucagon, cortisol, and growth hormone significantly influence how the primary fuel substrates (i.e., carbohydrate, protein, and fat) are mobilized and used for energy production (Kreisman 2003). Exercise-induced changes to the secretion of key hormones, as shown in Table 1.4, allow alternate fuels to be made available as energy sources while maintaining glucose homeostasis. In individuals dependent on exogenous insulin, these counterregulatory hormone responses can be altered. For example, growth hormone secretion during exercise in T1D has been found to be normal as long as normal blood glucose levels are maintained, but it is suppressed during hyperglycemic conditions (Jenni 2011).

HEALTH BENEFITS OF CHRONIC EXERCISE TRAINING

The benefits of regular physical activity participation are numerous. Current evidence suggests physical activity improves insulin action, lowers blood glucose levels, improves BMI (commonly placing individuals into categories of normal,

Table 1.4 Metabolic and Exercise Responses of Hormones

Hormone	Exercise Response	Metabolic Effect of Hormonal Response
Insulin	Decreases (endogenous insulin only)	Facilitates hepatic glucose production and free fatty acid release from adipose tissue; allows for lesser additive effect on blood glucose levels of insulin and muscle contractions
Glucagon	Increases	Increases hepatic glucose production via glycogenolysis and gluconeogenesis, thereby increasing glucose supply available in the blood; high peripheral and portal insulin levels can prevent it from rising adequately
Epinephrine	Increases	Stimulates muscle glycogen breakdown and free fatty acid production, which provides glycerol as a substrate for gluconeogenesis; enhances hepatic glucose production during exercise; decreases insulin secretion
Norepinephrine	Increases	Stimulates hepatic glucose production; reduces muscular glucose uptake during physical activity; decreases insulin secretion
Growth hormone and cortisol	Increase	Increase lipolysis; decrease insulin-stimulated glucose uptake (i.e., heighten insulin resistance); increase supply of glycerol and amino acids to liver for gluconeogenesis; result primarily in delayed effects that are important to fuel availability during prolonged activities

overweight, or obese based on weight and stature), and reduces multiple risk factors for cardiovascular disease (Kang 1996, Cuff 2003, Goodpaster 2003, Kriska 2006, Zoppini 2006, Hordern 2008). These important metabolic changes demonstrate the significant role that physical activity and exercise have in the prevention and management of T2D, in particular. Blood glucose management with physical activity as an added variable in T1D can be more challenging, but most of the same metabolic and overall health benefits are possible for these individuals as well (as shown in Table 1.5).

Many research studies have found lower levels of cardiovascular fitness in individuals with prediabetes and T2D, in particular (Church 2005, Simmons 2008, Sui 2008, Lee 2009), but even in some children and adults with T1D (Williams 2011). Fitness gains are certainly possible for individuals undergoing training, but professionals should take this finding into account when prescribing appropriate exercise training regimens for anyone with diabetes. On the other hand, not everyone with diabetes has a lower fitness level to start. For example, a recent study examined whether glycemic status influences aerobic function in women with T1D and whether aerobic function is reduced relative to healthy women (Item 2011). There were no differences, however, between the two groups, either in the oxidative enzyme activity or in capillary-to-fiber ratio. Their mitochondrial capacity depended on the A1C level in untrained women with T1D, but it was not reduced relative to untrained healthy women. Exercise training in children with T1D has been shown to effectively reverse endothelial dysfunction and improve

Table 1.5 Health Benefits of Regular Physical Activity Participation

Health Parameter Changes with Exercise Training	T1D	T2D
Cardiovascular		
Aerobic capacity or fitness level	⇑	⇑ or ⇔
Resting pulse rate and rate-pressure product	⇓	⇓
Resting systolic BP (in mild-moderate hypertension)	⇓	⇓
HR at submaximal loads (aerobic only)	⇓	⇓
Lipid and lipoproteins		
HDL-C	⇑	⇑
LDL-C	⇓ or ⇔	⇓ or ⇔
VLDL-C	⇓	⇓
Total cholesterol	⇔	⇔
Total cholesterol/HDL (cardiovascular risk)	⇓	⇓
Metabolic		
Insulin sensitivity and glucose/fat metabolism	⇑	⇑
A1C (overall glycemic control over 2–3 months)	⇓ or ⇔	⇓
Postprandial thermogenesis (thermic effect of food)	⇑	⇑
Anthropometric measures		
Body mass (with aerobic exercise in particular)	⇓ or ⇔	⇓
Fat mass (including unhealthy visceral fat)	⇓	⇓
Fat-free mass (primarily from resistance exercise)	⇑	⇑ or ⇔
Psychological outcomes		
Self-concept and self-esteem	⇑	⇑
Depression and anxiety	⇓	⇓
Stress response to psychological stimuli	⇓	⇓

BP, blood pressure; HDL-C, high-density lipoprotein cholesterol; HR, heart rate; LDL-C, low-density lipoprotein cholesterol; VLDL-C, very low-density lipoprotein cholesterol; ⇑, increase; ⇓, decrease; ⇔, no change.

physical fitness, demonstrating that engaging in appropriate training is important for all individuals with any type of diabetes (Trigona 2010, Seeger 2011).

Case in Point: Wrap-Up

In MJ's case, because she has been sedentary and is obese, it is best to start with exercise done at a lower intensity and progress her slowly with structured activities to avoid the development of athletic injuries, exercise nonadherence, or lack of motivation, with a goal of increasing her amount of physical activity gradually over a period of weeks to months.

Exercise Program Goals

Activity: The initial focus will be on lifestyle physical activity that MJ enjoys doing and can easily fit into her lifestyle, such as daily walking.

Intensity, Frequency, and Duration: Because MJ is currently inactive, she should be encouraged to start with short activity bouts of low- to moderate-intensity forms of physical activity that can be incorporated into her daily routine, such as doing 5–10 min of slow walking several times daily, 5–6 days a week. The exercise duration then can be increased gradually to 10 min per session, three times a day, and the walking speed increased slowly. Short intervals interspersed into her normal walking will improve her fitness levels more quickly and assist in management of blood glucose levels and postactivity blood pressure as well.

Progression: Long-term exercise goals should focus on progressively increasing amounts and frequency of activity to reach the minimum recommended levels of 150 min of moderate or vigorous exercise spread throughout the week, and MJ should be advised to add in some resistance training at least 2 days a week as well.

Daily Movement: For weight management purposes, MJ's goal is to maximize her caloric expenditure each week with planned activities, but also by adding in greater daily movement during nonexercise times (i.e., more daily living activity). The professional working with her can help her to identify physical activities that she might be interested in trying to incorporate into her daily lifestyle, even if it is simply to stand more each day or take more daily steps (which can easily be measured by wearing a pedometer).

Behavioral Changes: MJ's self-efficacy in being active can be enhanced by helping her to set realistic and specific goals that she can successfully accomplish, such as making a list of five ways to be more active throughout the day and trying one of them each week. She should be encouraged to ask questions and come up with her own ideas and suggestions for overcoming her exercise barriers and becoming (and staying) more physically active.

For most people with any type of diabetes, exercise can be undertaken safely and blood glucose levels can be managed effectively to the overall benefit of their diabetes management and health. Professionals who interact with people with any type of diabetes have an important and challenging role in helping them become and stay more physically active to manage their diabetes and their health.

PROFESSIONAL PRACTICE PEARLS

- Although diabetes is categorized into four main types, most individuals have T2D (90–95% of cases), are overweight or obese, and have a sedentary lifestyle.
- T1D can occur at any age; when its onset is during adulthood, it can be classified as LADA and may (at least initially) be misdiagnosed as T2D.

- Although exercise is technically a planned activity that is a subset of the broader term physical activity, they both involve bodily movement and can be used interchangeably.
- The terminology of fitness is intended to be inclusive rather than athletic in nature when considering what affects an individual's fitness level and health outcomes.
- The potential health benefits of regular physical activity participation are numerous and include lowering the risk for development of T2D.
- Individuals with diabetes, particularly those with T2D, may be starting their exercise programs with cardiovascular fitness levels that are lower than normal for their age.
- Enhanced insulin sensitivity, which follows an acute bout of exercise, can lower insulin needs for a period of hours to days afterward and may increase the risk of hypoglycemia.
- Physical activity improves insulin action, lowers blood glucose levels, improves BMI, and reduces multiple risk factors for cardiovascular disease in diabetes.

REFERENCES

American College of Sports Medicine: American College of Sports Medicine position stand. Progression models in resistance training for healthy adults. *Med Sci Sports Exerc* 41:687–708, 2009

American Diabetes Association: Diagnosis and classification of diabetes mellitus. *Diabetes Care* 36 (Suppl.1):S67–S74, 2013a

American Diabetes Association: Standards of medical care in diabetes—2013. *Diabetes Care* 36 (Suppl. 1):S11–S66, 2013b

Boon H, Blaak EE, Saris WH, Keizer HA, Wagenmakers AJ, van Loon LJ: Substrate source utilisation in long-term diagnosed type 2 diabetes patients at rest, and during exercise and subsequent recovery. *Diabetologia* 50:103–112, 2007

Boulé NG, Haddad E, Kenny GP, Wells GA, Sigal RJ: Effects of exercise on glycemic control and body mass in type 2 diabetes mellitus: a meta-analysis of controlled clinical trials. *JAMA* 286:1218–1227, 2001

Bray GA, Smith SR, DeJonge L, de Souza R, Rood J, Champagne CM, Laranjo N, Carey V, Obarzanek E, Loria CM, Anton SD, Ryan DH, Greenway FL, Williamson D, Sacks FM: Effect of diet composition on energy expenditure during weight loss: the POUNDS LOST study. *Int J Obes* (Lond) 36:448–455, 2012

Cartee GD, Young DA, Sleeper MD, Zierath J, Wallberg-Henriksson H, Holloszy JO: Prolonged increase in insulin-stimulated glucose transport in muscle after exercise. *Am J Physiol* 256:E494–E499, 1989

Caspersen CJ, Powell KE, Christenson GM: Physical activity, exercise, and physical fitness: definitions and distinctions for health-related research. *Public Health Reports* 100:126–131, 1985

Cheung BM, Ong KL, Cherny SS, Sham PC, Tso AW, Lam KS: Diabetes prevalence and therapeutic target achievement in the United States, 1999 to 2006. *Am J Med* 122:443–453, 2009

Chokkalingam K, Tsintzas K, Norton L, Jewell K, Macdonald IA, Mansell PI: Exercise under hyperinsulinaemic conditions increases whole-body glucose disposal without affecting muscle glycogen utilisation in type 1 diabetes. *Diabetologia* 50:414–421, 2007a

Chokkalingam K, Tsintzas K, Snaar JE, Norton L, Solanky B, Leverton E, Morris P, Mansell P, Macdonald IA: Hyperinsulinaemia during exercise does not suppress hepatic glycogen concentrations in patients with type 1 diabetes: a magnetic resonance spectroscopy study. *Diabetologia* 50:1921–1929, 2007b

Chomentowski P, Dubé JJ, Amati F, Stefanovic-Racic M, Zhu S, Toledo FG, Goodpaster BH: Moderate exercise attenuates the loss of skeletal muscle mass that occurs with intentional caloric restriction-induced weight loss in older, overweight to obese adults. *J Gerontol A Biol Sci Med Sci* 64:575–580, 2009

Church TS, LaMonte MJ, Barlow CE, Blair SN: Cardiorespiratory fitness and body mass index as predictors of cardiovascular disease mortality among men with diabetes. *Arch Intern Med* 165:2114–2120, 2005

Colberg SR, Sigal RJ, Fernhall B, Regensteiner JG, Blissmer BJ, Rubin RR, Chasan-Taber L, Albright AL, Braun B, American College of Sports Medicine, American Diabetes Association: Exercise and type 2 diabetes: the American College of Sports Medicine and the American Diabetes Association: joint position statement. *Diabetes Care* 33:e147–e167, 2010

Cuff DJ, Meneilly GS, Martin A, Ignaszewski A, Tildesley HD, Frohlich JJ: Effective exercise modality to reduce insulin resistance in women with type 2 diabetes. *Diabetes Care* 26:2977–2982, 2003

Davenport MH, Mottola MF, McManus R, Gratton R: A walking intervention improves capillary glucose control in women with gestational diabetes mellitus: a pilot study. *Appl Physiol Nutr Metab* 33:511–517, 2008

de Souza RJ, Bray GA, Carey VJ, Hall KD, LeBoff MS, Loria CM, Laranjo NM, Sacks FM, Smith SR: Effects of 4 weight-loss diets differing in fat, protein, and carbohydrate on fat mass, lean mass, visceral adipose tissue, and hepatic fat: results from the POUNDS LOST trial. *Am J Clin Nutr* 95:614–625, 2012

Diabetes Prevention Program (DPP) Research Group: The Diabetes Prevention Program (DPP): description of lifestyle intervention. *Diabetes Care* 25:2165–2171, 2002

Duncan GE, Perri MG, Theriaque DW, Hutson AD, Eckel RH, Stacpoole PW: Exercise training, without weight loss, increases insulin sensitivity and postheparin plasma lipase activity in previously sedentary adults. *Diabetes Care* 26:557–562, 2003

Dyck RF, Sheppard MS, Cassidy H, Chad K, Tan L, Van Vliet SH: Preventing NIDDM among aboriginal people: is exercise the answer? Description of a pilot project using exercise to prevent gestational diabetes. *Int J Circumpolar Health* 57 (Suppl. 1):S375–S378, 1998

Eriksson J, Lindstrom J, Valle T, Aunola S, Hamalainen H, Ilanne-Parikka P, Keinanen-Kiukaanniemi S, Laakso M, Lauhkonen M, Lehto P, Lehtonen A, Louheranta A, Mannelin M, Martikkala V, Rastas M, Sundvall J, Turpeinen A, Viljanen T, Uusitupa M, Tuomilehto J: Prevention of type II diabetes in subjects with impaired glucose tolerance: the Diabetes Prevention Study (DPS) in Finland. Study design and 1-year interim report on the feasibility of the lifestyle intervention programme. *Diabetologia* 42:793–801, 1999

Galbo H, Tobin L, van Loon LJ: Responses to acute exercise in type 2 diabetes, with an emphasis on metabolism and interaction with oral hypoglycemic agents and food intake. *Appl Physiol Nutr Metab* 32:567–575, 2007

Gallen IW, Hume C, Lumb A: Fueling the athlete with type 1 diabetes. *Diabetes Obes Metab* 13:130–136, 2011

Garber CE, Blissmer B, Deschenes MR, Franklin BA, Lamonte MJ, Lee IM, Nieman DC, Swain DP, American College of Sports Medicine: American College of Sports Medicine position stand. Quantity and quality of exercise for developing and maintaining cardiorespiratory, musculoskeletal, and neuromotor fitness in apparently healthy adults: guidance for prescribing exercise. *Med Sci Sports Exerc* 43:1334–1359, 2011

Goodpaster BH, Katsiaras A, Kelley DE: Enhanced fat oxidation through physical activity is associated with improvements in insulin sensitivity in obesity. *Diabetes* 52:2191–2197, 2003

Gorman E, Chudyk AM, Madden KM, Ashe MC: Bone health and type 2 diabetes mellitus: a systematic review. *Physiother Can* 63:8–20, 2012

Hamman RF, Wing RR, Edelstein SL, Lachin JM, Bray GA, Delahanty L, Hoskin M, Kriska AM, Mayer-Davis EJ, Pi-Sunyer X, Regensteiner J, Venditti B, Wylie-Rosett J: Effect of weight loss with lifestyle intervention on risk of diabetes. *Diabetes Care* 29:2102–2107, 2006

Hapo Study Cooperative Research Group, Metzger BE, Lowe LP, Dyer AR, Trimble ER, Chaovarindr U, Coustan DR, Hadden DR, McCance DR, Hod M, McIntyre HD, Oats JJ, Persson B, Rogers MS, Sacks DA: Hyperglycemia and adverse pregnancy outcomes. *N Engl J Med* 358:1991–2002, 2008

Haskell WL, Lee IM, Pate RR, Powell KE, Blair SN, Franklin BA, Macera CA, Heath GW, Thompson PD, Bauman A: Physical activity and public health: updated recommendation for adults from the American College of Sports Medicine and the American Heart Association. *Med Sci Sports Exerc* 39:1423–1434, 2007

Helmrich SP, Ragland DR, Leung RW, Paffenbarger RS Jr: Physical activity and reduced occurrence of non-insulin-dependent diabetes mellitus. *N Engl J Med* 325:147–152, 1991

Herriott MT, Colberg SR, Parson HK, Nunnold T, Vinik AI: Effects of 8 weeks of flexibility and resistance training in older adults with type 2 diabetes. *Diabetes Care* 27:2988–2989, 2004

Hordern MD, Cooney LM, Beller EM, Prins JB, Marwick TH, Coombes JS: Determinants of changes in blood glucose response to short-term exercise training in patients with type 2 diabetes. *Clin Sci* (Lond) 115:273–281, 2008

Hu FB, Stampfer MJ, Solomon C, Liu S, Colditz GA, Speizer FE, Willett WC, Manson JE: Physical activity and risk for cardiovascular events in diabetic women. *Ann Intern Med* 134:96–105, 2001

Hu FB, Sigal RJ, Rich-Edwards JW, Colditz GA, Solomon CG, Willett WC, Speizer FE, Manson JE: Walking compared with vigorous physical activity and risk of type 2 diabetes in women: a prospective study. *JAMA* 282:1433–1439, 1999

International Association of Diabetes, Panel Pregnancy Study Groups Consensus, Metzger BE, Gabbe SG, Persson B, Buchanan TA, Catalano PA, Damm P, Dyer AR, Leiva A, Hod M, Kitzmiler JL, Lowe LP, McIntyre HD, Oats JJ, Omori Y, Schmidt MI: International Association of Diabetes and Pregnancy Study Groups recommendations on the diagnosis and classification of hyperglycemia in pregnancy. *Diabetes Care* 33:676–682, 2010

Iqbal R, Rafique G, Badruddin S, Qureshi R, Cue R, Gray-Donald K: Increased body fat percentage and physical inactivity are independent predictors of gestational diabetes mellitus in South Asian women. *Eur J Clin Nutr* 61:736–742, 2007

Item F, Heinzer-Schweizer S, Wyss M, Fontana P, Lehmann R, Henning A, Weber M, Boesiger P, Boutellier U, Toigo M: Mitochondrial capacity is affected by glycemic status in young untrained women with type 1 diabetes but is not impaired relative to healthy untrained women. *Am J Physiol Regul Integr Comp Physiol* 301:R60–R66, 2011

Jacob AN, Salinas K, Adams-Huet B, Raskin P: Potential causes of weight gain in type 1 diabetes mellitus. *Diabetes Obes Metab* 8:404–411, 2006

Jenni S, Christ ER, Stettler C: Exercise-induced growth hormone response in euglycaemia and hyperglycaemia in patients with type 1 diabetes mellitus. *Diabet Med* 27:230–233, 2011

Jeon CY, Lokken RP, Hu FB, van Dam RM: Physical activity of moderate intensity and risk of type 2 diabetes: a systematic review. *Diabetes Care* 30:744–752, 2007

Kang J, Robertson RJ, Hagberg JM, Kelley DE, Goss FL, DaSilva SG, Suminski RR, Utter AC: Effect of exercise intensity on glucose and insulin metabolism in obese individuals and obese NIDDM patients. *Diabetes Care* 19:341–349, 1996

Kirk AF, Mutrie N, Macintyre PD, Fisher MB: Promoting and maintaining physical activity in people with type 2 diabetes. *Am J Prev Med* 27:289–296, 2004

Knowler WC, Barrett-Connor E, Fowler SE, Hamman RF, Lachin JM, Walker EA, Nathan DM: Reduction in the incidence of type 2 diabetes with lifestyle intervention or metformin. *N Engl J Med* 346:393–403, 2002

Kosaka K, Noda M, Kuzuya T: Prevention of type 2 diabetes by lifestyle intervention: a Japanese trial in IGT males. *Diabetes Res Clin Pract* 67:152–162, 2005

Kreisman SH, Halter JB, Vranic M, Marliss EB: Combined infusion of epinephrine and norepinephrine during moderate exercise reproduces the glucoregulatory response of intense exercise. *Diabetes* 52:1347–1354, 2003

Kriska AM, Edelstein SL, Hamman RF, Otto A, Bray GA, Mayer-Davis EJ, Wing RR, Horton ES, Haffner SM, Regensteiner JG: Physical activity in individuals at risk for diabetes: Diabetes Prevention Program. *Med Sci Sports Exerc* 38:826–832, 2006

Laaksonen DE, Lindstrom J, Lakka TA, Eriksson JG, Niskanen L, Wikstrom K, Aunola S, Keinanen-Kiukaanniemi S, Laakso M, Valle TT, Ilanne-Parikka P, Louheranta A, Hamalainen H, Rastas M, Salminen V, Cepaitis Z, Hakumaki M, Kaikkonen H, Harkonen P, Sundvall J, Tuomilehto J, Uusitupa M: Physical activity in the prevention of type 2 diabetes: the Finnish Diabetes Prevention Study. *Diabetes* 54:158–165, 2005

Lee DC, Sui X, Church TS, Lee IM, Blair SN: Associations of cardiorespiratory fitness and obesity with risks of impaired fasting glucose and type 2 diabetes in men. *Diabetes Care* 32:257–262, 2009

Lee S, Kuk JL, Davidson LE, Hudson R, Kilpatrick K, Graham TE, Ross R: Exercise without weight loss is an effective strategy for obesity reduction in obese individuals with and without Type 2 diabetes. *J Appl Physiol* 99:1220–1225, 2005

Li G, Zhang P, Wang J, Gregg EW, Yang W, Gong Q, Li H, Jiang Y, An Y, Shuai Y, Zhang B, Zhang J, Thompson TJ, Gerzoff RB, Roglic G, Hu Y, Bennett PH: The long-term effect of lifestyle interventions to prevent diabetes in the China Da Qing Diabetes Prevention Study: a 20-year follow-up study. *Lancet* 371:1783–1789, 2008

Lindstrom J, Ilanne-Parikka P, Peltonen M, Aunola S, Eriksson JG, Hemio K, Hamalainen H, Harkonen P, Keinanen-Kiukaanniemi S, Laakso M, Louheranta A, Mannelin M, Paturi M, Sundvall J, Valle TT, Uusitupa M, Tuomilehto J: Sustained reduction in the incidence of type 2 diabetes by lifestyle intervention: follow-up of the Finnish Diabetes Prevention Study. *Lancet* 368:1673–1679, 2006

Look Ahead Research Group, Wing RR: Long-term effects of a lifestyle intervention on weight and cardiovascular risk factors in individuals with type 2 diabetes mellitus: four-year results of the Look AHEAD trial. *Arch Intern Med* 170:1566–1575, 2010

Manetta J, Brun JF, Perez-Martin A, Callis A, Prefaut C, Mercier J: Fuel oxidation during exercise in middle-aged men: role of training and glucose disposal. *Med Sci Sports Exerc* 34:423–429, 2002

Manson JE, Rimm EB, Stampfer MJ, Colditz GA, Willett WC, Krolewski AS, Rosner B, Hennekens CH, Speizer FE: Physical activity and incidence of non-insulin-dependent diabetes mellitus in women. *Lancet* 338:774–778, 1991

McGavock J, Sellers E, Dean H: Physical activity for the prevention and management of youth-onset type 2 diabetes mellitus: focus on cardiovascular complications. *Diab Vasc Dis Res* 4:305–310, 2007

McGavock J, Mandic S, Lewanczuk R, Koller M, Muhll IV, Quinney A, Taylor D, Welsh R, Haykowsky M: Cardiovascular adaptations to exercise training in postmenopausal women with type 2 diabetes mellitus. *Cardiovasc Diabetol* 3:3, 2004

Metzger BE, Persson B, Lowe LP, Dyer AR, Cruickshank JK, Deerochanawong C, Halliday HL, Hennis AJ, Liley H, Ng PC, Coustan DR, Hadden DR, Hod M, Oats JJ, Trimble ER, Hapo Study Cooperative Research Group: Hyperglycemia and adverse pregnancy outcome study: neonatal glycemia. *Pediatrics* 126:e1545–e1552, 2010

Morrato EH, Hill JO, Wyatt HR, Ghushchyan V, Sullivan PW: Physical activity in U.S. adults with diabetes and at risk for developing diabetes, 2003. *Diabetes Care* 30:203–209, 2007

Morrato EH, Hill JO, Wyatt HR, Ghushchyan V, Sullivan PW: Are health care professionals advising patients with diabetes or at risk for developing diabetes to exercise more? *Diabetes Care* 29:543–548, 2006

Narayan KM, Boyle JP, Geiss LS, Saaddine JB, Thompson TJ: Impact of recent increase in incidence on future diabetes burden: U.S., 2005–2050. *Diabetes Care* 29:2114–2116, 2006

Narayan KM, Boyle JP, Thompson TJ, Sorensen SW, Williamson DF: Lifetime risk for diabetes mellitus in the United States. *JAMA* 290:1884–1890, 2003

Nelson ME, Rejeski WJ, Blair SN, Duncan PW, Judge JO, King AC, Macera CA, Castaneda-Sceppa C: Physical activity and public health in older adults: recommendation from the American College of Sports Medicine and the American Heart Association. *Med Sci Sports Exerc* 39:1435–1445, 2007

O'Gorman DJ, Karlsson HK, McQuaid S, Yousif O, Rahman Y, Gasparro D, Glund S, Chibalin AV, Zierath JR, Nolan JJ: Exercise training increases insulin-stimulated glucose disposal and GLUT4 (SLC2A4) protein content in patients with type 2 diabetes. *Diabetologia* 49:2983–2992, 2006

Okamoto MM, Anhe GF, Sabino-Silva R, Marques MF, Freitas HS, Mori RC, Melo KF, Machado UF: Intensive insulin treatment induces insulin resistance in diabetic rats by impairing glucose metabolism-related mechanisms in muscle and liver. *J Endocrinol* 211:55–64, 2011

Pan XR, Li GW, Hu YH, Wang JX, Yang WY, An ZX, Hu ZX, Lin J, Xiao JZ, Cao HB, Liu PA, Jiang XG, Jiang YY, Wang JP, Zheng H, Zhang H, Bennett PH, Howard BV: Effects of diet and exercise in preventing NIDDM in people with impaired glucose tolerance. The Da Qing IGT and Diabetes Study. *Diabetes Care* 20:537–544, 1997

Ramachandran A, Snehalatha C, Mary S, Mukesh B, Bhaskar AD, Vijay V, Indian Diabetes Prevention Programme: The Indian Diabetes Prevention Programme shows that lifestyle modification and metformin prevent type 2 diabetes in Asian Indian subjects with impaired glucose tolerance (IDPP-1). *Diabetologia* 49:289–297, 2006

Seeger JP, Thijssen DH, Noordam K, Cranen ME, Hopman MT, Nijhuis-van der Sanden MW: Exercise training improves physical fitness and vascular function in children with type 1 diabetes. *Diabetes Obes Metab* 13:382–384, 2011

Simmons RK, Griffin SJ, Steele R, Wareham NJ, Ekelund U: Increasing overall physical activity and aerobic fitness is associated with improvements in metabolic risk: cohort analysis of the ProActive trial. *Diabetologia* 51:787–794, 2008

St John A, Davis WA, Price CP, Davis TM: The value of self-monitoring of blood glucose: a review of recent evidence. *J Diabetes Complications* 24:129–141, 2010

Sui X, Hooker SP, Lee IM, Church TS, Colabianchi N, Lee CD, Blair SN: A prospective study of cardiorespiratory fitness and risk of type 2 diabetes in women. *Diabetes Care* 31:550–555, 2008

Szewieczek J, Dulawa J, Strzalkowska D, Batko-Szwaczka A, Hornik B: Normal insulin response to short-term intense exercise is abolished in type 2 diabetic patients treated with gliclazide. *J Diabetes Complications* 23:380–386, 2009

Trigona B, Aggoun Y, Maggio A, Martin XE, Marchand LM, Beghetti M, Farpour-Lambert NJ: Preclinical noninvasive markers of atherosclerosis in children and adolescents with type 1 diabetes are influenced by physical activity. *J Pediatr* 157:533–539, 2010

Tuomilehto J, Lindstrom J, Eriksson JG, Valle TT, Hamalainen H, Ilanne-Parikka P, Keinanen-Kiukaanniemi S, Laakso M, Louheranta A, Rastas M, Salminen V, Uusitupa M: Prevention of type 2 diabetes mellitus by changes in lifestyle among subjects with impaired glucose tolerance. *N Engl J Med* 344:1343–1350, 2001

U.S. Department of Health and Human Services, Centers for Disease Control and Prevention: *National Diabetes Fact Sheet: National Estimates and General Information on Diabetes and Prediabetes in the United States, 2011.* Atlanta, GA, U.S. Department of Health and Human Services, Centers for Disease Control and Prevention, 2011

Wang X, Lyles MF, You T, Berry MJ, Rejeski WJ, Nicklas BJ: Weight regain is related to decreases in physical activity during weight loss. *Med Sci Sports Exerc* 40:1781–1788, 2008

Wei M, Gibbons LW, Mitchell TL, Kampert JB, Lee CD, Blair SN: The association between cardiorespiratory fitness and impaired fasting glucose and type 2 diabetes mellitus in men. *Ann Intern Med* 130:89–96, 1999

West DJ, Stephens JW, Bain SC, Kilduff LP, Luzio S, Still R, Bracken RM: A combined insulin reduction and carbohydrate feeding strategy 30 min before running best preserves blood glucose concentration after exercise through improved fuel oxidation in type 1 diabetes mellitus. *J Sports Sci* 29:279–289, 2011

Williams BK, Guelfi KJ, Jones TW, Davis EA: Lower cardiorespiratory fitness in children with type 1 diabetes. *Diabet Med* 28:1005–1007, 2011

Zeitler P, Hirst K, Pyle L, Linder B, Copeland K, Arslanian S, Cuttler L, Nathan DM, Tollefsen S, Wilfley D, Kaufman F: A clinical trial to maintain glycemic control in youth with type 2 diabetes. *N Engl J Med* 366:2247–2256, 2012

Zoppini G, Targher G, Zamboni C, Venturi C, Cacciatori V, Moghetti P, Muggeo M: Effects of moderate-intensity exercise training on plasma biomarkers of inflammation and endothelial dysfunction in older patients with type 2 diabetes. *Nutr Metab Cardiovasc Dis* 16:543–549, 2006

Chapter 2
Pre-Exercise Evaluation and Assessment

A safe and effective exercise program for people with diabetes minimizes the acute risks and long-term complications associated with physical activity while maximizing the benefits (Bernbaum 1989, Gilchrist 2000, Seeger 2011). As the benefits frequently outweigh the risks, regular participation in a variety of physical activities should be recommended and encouraged for almost all individuals with diabetes, keeping in mind that certain comorbidities (whether diagnosed or not) may carry a higher risk than others.

Case in Point: Pre-Exercise Screening, Cardiovascular Risk, and Disease Detection

AB is a 58-year-old man who has had type 2 diabetes (T2D) for ~10 years and is interested in starting a new exercise training program at a local community center. The exercise that he intends to do revolves around a program of aerobic exercise on a treadmill at an intensity equal to ~75% of his heart rate reserve (see chapter 4 for more information on prescribing exercise intensity), which is considered a vigorous physical activity—that is, more intense than his normal daily walking pace (i.e., brisk walking). Although he has engaged in several exercise training programs off and on over the past few years, his most consistent physical activity currently is playing golf on most weekends (which includes walking and carrying his clubs). His only medications are metformin (used to control morning hyperglycemia) and a lipid-lowering drug to reduce cholesterol levels.

Questions to Consider

1. Should AB schedule an appointment with his primary physician or other health-care provider for a pre-exercise medical evaluation and examination?
2. Does AB need to undergo a graded exercise stress test before participation in his planned exercise intensity?

(Continued on page 27.)

MEDICAL SCREENING AND EXAMINATION

Ideally, most individuals diagnosed with diabetes should consult a health-care provider before beginning an intense physical fitness program (Colberg 2010, 2011).

An absolute requirement to do so before participation in all types of physical activity should not be uniformly enforced, however, as it may prevent individuals from gaining any of the health and psychological benefits associated with being normally physically active, such as undertaking brisk walking as part of their activities of daily living.

SCREENING FOR DIABETES-RELATED COMPLICATIONS

Given that exercise participation can be complicated by the presence of diabetes-related health complications (Sigal 2004), before undertaking new higher-intensity physical activity, individuals are strongly advised to undergo a detailed medical evaluation and screening for acute and chronic blood glucose control, physical limitations, medications, and macrovascular and microvascular complications associated with the heart, blood vessels, eyes, kidneys, feet, and nervous system (Colberg 2010). A medical examination conducted before undertaking a new physical activity or fitness program can include determination of the presence of diabetes-related (or other) comorbidities (e.g., cardiovascular disease, neuropathy, nephropathy, and retinopathy) that can affect an individual's ability to undertake certain types of physical training, increase cardiovascular risk, or predispose them to injuries (Sigal 2004, 2006; Colberg 2010). Certain conditions may be contraindicated or predispose individuals to injury, such as uncontrolled hypertension, severe autonomic neuropathy, severe peripheral neuropathy or history of foot lesions, and unstable proliferative retinopathy. The individual's age and previous physical activity level also should be considered (American Diabetes Association [ADA] 2013). Such health considerations should be factored into an exercise prescription for it to be both safe and effective.

PHYSICAL EXAMINATION

Minimally, starting body weight, heart rate, and resting blood pressure ideally should be assessed before exercise participation. In addition, inspection of the lower extremities for edema and the presence of arterial pulses is recommended, along with tests of neurological function, especially if the individual has prescribing prior bouts of dizziness or faintness during or following physical exertion. Given that such symptoms could result from any number of conditions, including autonomic dysfunction, cardiovascular insufficiency, medication use, or dehydration, among others, a determination of the cause (if possible) is helpful in prescribing appropriate physical activity regimens. Likewise, a visual inspection of the feet and lower extremities can reveal any contraindications to weight-bearing exercise, including unhealed ulcerations. A history of falls is also clinically relevant, given that certain exercise interventions like balance training have been shown to lower the risk of falling in people with T2D (Morrison 2010). Finally, the health-care or fitness professional should be made aware of any orthopedic or other limitations (like prior joint surgery) that might affect exercise prescription for the individual.

Case in Point: Continued

Before starting his supervised aerobic exercise training, AB is advised by his personal trainer to have a checkup with his health-care provider to assess his overall health, diabetes control, and potential for cardiovascular and other diabetes-related complications. At that appointment, he obtains the following results:

Resting Measurements

Height: 70 inches
Weight: 196 lb
BMI: 28.1 (overweight)
Waist circumference: 41 inches
Heart rate: 74 beats per minute (bpm)
Blood pressure: 128/80 mmHg

Fasting Labs

Fasting plasma glucose: 120 mg/dl
A1C: 6.3%
Total cholesterol: 150 mg/dl (on medication)
Triglycerides: 100 mg/dl
High-density lipoprotein cholesterol: 45 mg/dl
Low-density lipoprotein cholesterol: 85 mg/dl

Even though his diabetes appears to be well controlled and despite not having any cardiovascular symptoms, AB's physician recommends that he undergo a graded exercise stress test before starting intense exercise, to rule out the possibility of coronary artery disease, given his elevated number of cardiovascular risk factors: older age, diabetes for >10 years, waist circumference, history of elevated cholesterol levels, and a family history of heart disease (AC's father died at age 54 years from a heart attack).

The results of AB's maximal treadmill test (with 12-lead electrocardiogram) are normal, with no evidence of coronary ischemia during the test and no arrhythmias noted. His maximal blood pressure reaches 220/85, and his maximal heart rate is 154 bpm (expected age-based maximal heart rate of 162 bpm). His maximal oxygen consumption (VO_2) is 21.2 ml/kg/min (milliliters of oxygen per kilogram of body weight per minute), which is low based on norms for his age (58 years) and sex (male).

Exercise Program Goals

Activity: AB starts his exercise training program with his personal trainer after all testing has been completed by undertaking treadmill walking, as desired. In addition, he plans to continue golfing as many weekends as possible for 3–4 h at a time to maintain a higher level of unstructured activities.

Intensity, Frequency, and Duration: On the advice of his personal trainer, AB initially undertakes only 20 min of moderate-intensity treadmill walking done at 50% of his heart rate reserve (HRR; which for him, is a target HR of 114 bpm;

see chapter 4 for details about how to prescribe exercise intensity using this method), 3 days per week. His goal is to work up to doing intense exercise (at 75% of his HRR, or a target HR of 134 bpm) for at least 30 min at a time.

Progression: For the first 2–3 weeks of training, AB progresses by first increasing the intensity of his training up to his target (by aiming for a HR that is 5–10 bpm higher each subsequent week), and after another 2 weeks he increases his exercise time by 5 min a week until he reaches 30 min of continuous, intense walking for each of his thrice-weekly exercise sessions. He continues this program for 12 weeks total, at which point he plans to add in twice-weekly sessions of resistance work.

Exercise Goals: His long-term exercise goal is to complete a minimum of 90 min of vigorous aerobic exercise weekly, along with another 90 min of moderate-to-intense resistance training.

(Continued on page 30.)

PRE-EXERCISE STRESS TESTING TO DETECT CARDIOVASCULAR DISEASE

LOW-INTENSITY TRAINING

For individuals who wish to participate in low-intensity activities like walking, physicians and other health-care providers should use clinical judgment in deciding whether to recommend pre-exercise testing (Colberg 2010). Conducting exercise stress testing before walking that does not exceed the cardiovascular demands of an individual's usual activities of daily living may not be routinely necessary as a diagnostic tool for cardiovascular disease, and requiring it may create barriers to participation in all physical activities. Moreover, current guidelines avoid automatic inclusion of lower-risk individuals in graded exercise testing requirements, given that their risk of a false-positive test is higher and may outweigh the benefits of detection of cardiovascular abnormalities (Colberg 2011).

HIGHER-INTENSITY TRAINING

For exercise more vigorous than brisk walking or exceeding the demands of everyday living, it remains unclear whether sedentary and older individuals with type 1 diabetes (T1D) or T2D will benefit from undergoing graded exercise testing or other types of routine cardiovascular testing (Bax 2007). Depending on the individual's age, diabetes duration, and presence of additional cardiovascular risk factors or diabetes-related complications, however, the risks associated with conducting such testing may be justified when it can reveal underlying pathologies that potentially affect either the safety or efficacy of more intense exercise participation.

The prevalence of symptomatic and asymptomatic coronary artery disease is greater in individuals with T2D (Kothari 2002, Eddy 2008), and maximal graded exercise testing can identify a small proportion of asymptomatic people with severe coronary artery obstruction (Curtis 2010). Although the latest ADA Standards of Medical Care state that the need for screening asymptomatic diabetic patients for coronary artery disease remains unclear (Bax 2007, ADA 2013), graded exercise stress test with electrocardiogram (ECG) may be indicated for diabetic individuals to detect cardiovascular disease based on the criteria in Table 2.1 (Colberg 2010). Providers should use clinical judgment in this area. Certainly, high-risk patients should at least be encouraged to start physical activity participation with short periods of low-intensity exercise and to increase the intensity and duration slowly.

RISK ASSESSMENT

The UKPDS Risk Engine (www.dtu.ox.ac.uk/riskengine/index.php) (Stevens 2001) may be used to calculate expected 10-year cardiovascular risk based on age, sex, smoking, A1C levels, diabetes duration, lipids, blood pressure, and race or ethnicity. Most young individuals with a low risk of coronary artery disease are not likely to benefit from pre-exercise stress testing done with the primary intent of detecting coronary artery disease, particularly given that the lower the coronary artery disease risk, the higher the chance of having a false-positive test (Stevens 2001, Fowler-Brown 2004). In the Look AHEAD (Action for Health in Diabetes) trial, although exercise-induced abnormalities were present in 22.5% of the >1,000 study participants, only greater age was associated with increased prevalence of all abnormalities during maximal exercise testing (Curtis 2010).

TESTING OF HIGHER-RISK INDIVIDUALS

Symptomatic individuals may benefit from diagnostic cardiac stress testing, both for diagnostic purposes and to assist in safe and effective exercise prescription that avoids exacerbating pre-existing cardiac limitations during exercise (such

Table 2.1 Criteria for Consideration of Graded Exercise Stress Testing

Age >40 years, with or without cardiovascular disease risk factors other than diabetes
Age >30 years and • T1D or T2D of >10 years' duration • Hypertension • Cigarette smoking • Dyslipidemia • Proliferative or preproliferative retinopathy • Nephropathy, including microalbuminuria
Any of the following, regardless of age • Known or suspected coronary artery disease, cerebrovascular disease, or peripheral vascular disease • Autonomic neuropathy • Advanced nephropathy with renal failure

as an ischemic threshold). For those with known or suspected coronary artery disease, the clinical value of a noninvasive exercise stress test may be better ascertained primarily by stratifying subjects into either low- or high-risk groups based on the number of cardiac risk factors, family history, and current symptoms (Curtis 2010). For asymptomatic patients with diabetes, however, identification of cardiovascular risk factors and risk stratification may assist health-care providers in justifying the use of graded exercise testing, but is not currently recommended (Bax 2007). In any case, all decisions regarding the necessity of such testing should attempt to more effectively target the select individuals at higher risk for underlying cardiovascular disease (Sigal 2004). For example, individuals with silent myocardial ischemia have a poorer prognosis than those with normal stress tests, and their risk is further accentuated if cardiac autonomic neuropathy coexists (ADA 2013).

USE OF STRESS TESTING TO DETECT ISCHEMIA

A systematic review for the U.S. Preventive Services Task Force (2004) concluded that stress testing should not be routinely recommended to detect ischemia in asymptomatic individuals with a low coronary risk (<10% risk of a cardiac event over 10 years) because the risks resulting from the invasive testing done after a false-positive test outweigh the benefits of detection (Fowler-Brown 2004). Individuals who exhibit nonspecific electrocardiograph changes in response to exercise or who have nonspecific ST- and T-wave changes at rest may need follow-up testing. The Detection of Ischemia in Asymptomatic Diabetics (DIAD) trial involving 1,123 individuals with T2D and no symptoms of coronary artery disease, however, found that screening with adenosine-stress radionuclide myocardial perfusion imaging for myocardial ischemia over 4.8 years did not alter rates of cardiac events (Young 2009). Therefore, the cost-effectiveness and diagnostic value of more-intensive testing remain in question (Sigal 2004, 2006; Colberg 2010).

Case in Point: Event Discussion

At the end of 12 weeks of intense aerobic training and just before starting his resistance workouts, AB is being instructed on the use of the resistance equipment by his personal trainer when he falls to the floor following a short cardio warm-up and goes into full cardiac arrest within 5 min. The community center houses an automated external defibrillator (AED), which his personal trainer brings to his side while a concerned onlooker calls 911 to summon emergency medical assistance. The AED indicates that AB needs cardioversion, and his trainer initiates the shock that restarts AB's heart before the paramedics arrive on the scene from a nearby fire station another 5 min later.

Following this event AB is hospitalized, but no myocardial damage is found. His cardiac arrest is determined to have been caused by a potentially fatal arrhythmia (ventricular fibrillation), which was found after later review of the rhythm recorded by the AED during the event. Upon further examination by a cardiologist, AB is found to have 100% blockage of one of his primary coronary vessels (left anterior descending) but appears to have developed collateral circulation there, likely as the result of the vigorous exercise training program that he undertook before having this event, which prevented any infarction of the myocardium in the area fed by that vessel. Thus, it is decided that his cardiac arrest was simply caused by the arrhythmia initiated by the agitated state of his heart as a result of the blockage. Following bypass surgery, he is released from the hospital and cleared to participate in cardiac rehabilitation after a few weeks.

Additional Questions to Consider

1. Should the pretraining medical and exercise stress testing have been able to detect AB's coronary artery disease before it became potentially fatal?
2. Is there another form of testing that AB should have undergone before starting his training?
3. Did the intense exercise training actually help or hurt AB, given his undiagnosed cardiovascular disease?

(Continued on page 32.)

TESTING OF LOW-RISK INDIVIDUALS FOR FITNESS ASSESSMENT

Although graded exercise testing currently is advised primarily for previously sedentary people with diabetes who want to undertake activity more intense than brisk walking to assess cardiovascular risk (Sigal 2006, Colberg 2010), in some cases, testing (with or without ECG monitoring of heart function) may be undertaken for other purposes. In addition to diagnosing or defining the prognosis of known cardiac disease, exercise stress testing is presently used to assess physical fitness, determine functional capacity, prescribe an exercise plan, and guide cardiac rehabilitation training. With these alternate assessments in mind, the aforementioned risk-based criteria do not exclude the possibility of conducting graded exercise stress testing on individuals with a low risk of cardiovascular disease or those who are planning to engage in less-intense exercise (Stevens 2001). In the absence of contraindications to maximal stress testing, it still can be considered for anyone with T1D or T2D who simply wants to assess his or her fitness level or use the maximal or peak results to determine appropriate exercise training intensities and other fitness goals. Although clinical evidence does not definitively determine who should never consider undergoing such testing, potential benefits should be weighed against the risk associated with unnecessary procedures for each individual, especially in individuals with a higher risk profile (Kothari 2002, Sigal 2004).

PRE–RESISTANCE TRAINING EXERCISE TESTING

As for resistance training, no studies have yet addressed whether pre-exercise stress testing is necessary or beneficial before participation in such activity. At present, most testing centers are equipped for maximal stress testing, but not for an alternate form of testing involving resistance exercise. Because coronary ischemia is less likely to occur during resistance compared with aerobic exercise eliciting the same heart rate, resistance exercise may not even induce ischemia in most individuals (Ghilarducci 1989, Featherstone 1993). A review of 12 studies of resistance exercise in men with known coronary artery disease reported no angina, ST-segment depression (indicative of coronary ischemia), abnormal hemodynamics, ventricular dysrhythmias, or other complications during such exercise (Wenger 1995).

Case in Point: Wrap-Up

AB was completely asymptomatic of coronary artery disease before this event, and it was not detected by a graded exercise test, which shows that this testing is not infallible and far from conclusive. Given his lack of any cardiac symptoms, it would not have been advisable—either from a medical standpoint or a financial one—to recommend or require additional, possibly more invasive, testing of his cardiovascular status before this event.

Finally, the intense exercise training that AB had completed before this event was completely appropriate under the circumstances and, in fact, it likely helped save his life by stimulating the growth of new, collateral vessels that prevented myocardial damage despite full blockage of a crucial coronary artery feeding the left ventricle. Effectually, his exercise participation saved his life twice: once by stimulating the growth of new collateral circulation to his heart and again by placing him in a facility that had an AED available to treat him during his event. AB later said to his personal trainer that had his event occurred on the golf course, where he had spent the whole day before, he likely would not have survived it.

For most people with diabetes, low-level physical activities can be undertaken without the need for a medical exam or graded exercise test that potentially could create barriers to participation. In some cases, however, higher-risk individuals desiring to undertake moderate- or vigorous-intensity exercise training may benefit from undergoing a medical evaluation and possible stress testing with ECG before participation to diagnose pre-existing cardiovascular problems that may make such training more risky.

PROFESSIONAL PRACTICE PEARLS

- Most individuals diagnosed with diabetes should consult a health-care provider before beginning an intense physical activity program, but an absolute requirement to do so in all cases would create unnecessary barriers to participation in low-level activities.
- Before undertaking new higher-intensity physical activity, providers may use their judgment in recommending whether individuals with any type of diabetes should undergo a detailed medical evaluation and screening.
- For individuals wishing to participate in low-intensity activities only, pre-exercise testing is likely not beneficial, and providers should use their clinical judgment in deciding whether to recommend it.
- Graded exercise testing should not be routinely recommended to detect ischemia in asymptomatic individuals with a low coronary risk because the

risks resulting from the invasive testing done after a false-positive test out-weigh the benefits of detection.

- Symptomatic individuals may benefit from diagnostic cardiac stress testing, both for diagnostic purposes and also to assist in safe and effective exercise.
- To date, no studies have addressed whether pre-exercise stress testing is necessary or beneficial before participation in resistance training (although likely it is not).
- Graded exercise testing may be undertaken in low-risk and other individuals to determine fitness levels or to obtain testing results for effective exercise prescription.

REFERENCES

American Diabetes Association: Standards of medical care in diabetes—2013. *Diabetes Care* 36 (Suppl. 1):S11–S66, 2013

Bax JJ, Young LH, Frye RL, Bonow RO, Steinberg HO, Barrett EJ: Screening for coronary artery disease in patients with diabetes. *Diabetes Care* 30:2729–2736, 2007

Bernbaum M, Albert SG, Cohen JD: Exercise training in individuals with diabetic retinopathy and blindness. *Arch Phys Med Rehabil* 70:605–611, 1989

Colberg SR, Sigal RJ: Prescribing exercise for individuals with type 2 diabetes: recommendations and precautions. *Phys Sportsmed* 39:13–26, 2011

Colberg SR, Sigal RJ, Fernhall B, Regensteiner JG, Blissmer BJ, Rubin RR, Chasan-Taber L, Albright AL, Braun B, American College of Sports Medicine, American Diabetes Association: Exercise and type 2 diabetes: the American College of Sports Medicine and the American Diabetes Association: joint position statement. *Diabetes Care* 33:e147–e167, 2010

Curtis JM, Horton ES, Bahnson J, Gregg EW, Jakicic JM, Regensteiner JG, Ribisl PM, Soberman JE, Stewart KJ, Espeland MA, Look Ahead Research Group: Prevalence and predictors of abnormal cardiovascular responses to exercise testing among individuals with type 2 diabetes: the Look AHEAD (Action for Health in Diabetes) study. *Diabetes Care* 33:901–907, 2010

Eddy DM, Schlessinger L, Heikes K: The metabolic syndrome and cardiovascular risk: implications for clinical practice. *Int J Obes* (Lond) 32 (Suppl. 2):S5–S10, 2008

Featherstone JF, Holly RG, Amsterdam EA: Physiologic responses to weight lift-ing in coronary artery disease. *Am J Cardiol* 71:287–292, 1993

Fowler-Brown A, Pignone M, Pletcher M, Tice JA, Sutton SF, Lohr KN: Exercise tolerance testing to screen for coronary heart disease: a systematic review for the technical support for the U.S. Preventive Services Task Force. *Ann Intern Med* 140:W9–W24, 2004

Ghilarducci LE, Holly RG, Amsterdam EA: Effects of high resistance training in coronary artery disease. *Am J Cardiol* 64:866–870, 1989

Gilchrist J, Jones BH, Sleet DA, Kimsey CD, Center for Disease Control: Exercise-related injuries among women: strategies for prevention from civilian and military studies. *MMWR Recomm Rep* 49:15–33, 2000

Kothari V, Stevens RJ, Adler AI, Stratton IM, Manley SE, Neil HA, Holman RR: UKPDS 60: risk of stroke in type 2 diabetes estimated by the UK Prospective Diabetes Study risk engine. *Stroke* 33:1776–1781, 2002

Morrison S, Colberg SR, Mariano M, Parson HK, Vinik AI: Balance training reduces falls risk in older individuals with type 2 diabetes. *Diabetes Care* 33:748–750, 2010

Seeger JP, Thijssen DH, Noordam K, Cranen ME, Hopman MT, Nijhuis-van der Sanden MW: Exercise training improves physical fitness and vascular function in children with type 1 diabetes. *Diabetes Obes Metab* 13:382–384, 2011

Sigal RJ, Kenny GP, Wasserman DH, Castaneda-Sceppa C, White RD: Physical activity/exercise and type 2 diabetes: a consensus statement from the American Diabetes Association. *Diabetes Care* 29:1433–1438, 2006

Sigal RJ, Kenny GP, Wasserman DH, Castaneda-Sceppa C: Physical activity/exercise and type 2 diabetes. *Diabetes Care* 27:2518–2539, 2004

Stevens RJ, Kothari V, Adler AI, Stratton IM: The UKPDS risk engine: a model for the risk of coronary heart disease in Type II diabetes (UKPDS 56). *Clin Sci* (Lond) 101:671–679, 2001

U.S. Preventive Services Task Force: Screening for coronary heart disease: recommendation statement. *Ann Intern Med* 140:569–572, 2004

Wenger NK, Froelicher ES, Smith LK, Ades PA, Berra K, Blumenthal JA, Certo CM, Dattilo AM, Davis D, DeBusk RF, et al.: Cardiac rehabilitation as secondary prevention. Agency for Health Care Policy and Research and National Heart, Lung, and Blood Institute. *Clin Pract Guidel Quick Ref Guide Clin* (17):1–23, 1995

Young LH, Wackers FJ, Chyun DA, Davey JA, Barrett EJ, Taillefer R, Heller GV, Iskandrian AE, Wittlin SD, Filipchuk N, Ratner RE, Inzucchi SE: Cardiac outcomes after screening for asymptomatic coronary artery disease in patients with type 2 diabetes: the DIAD study: a randomized controlled trial. *JAMA* 301:1547–1555, 2009

Chapter 3
Daily Lifestyle Activity

Individuals with all types of diabetes frequently are deconditioned and live a sedentary lifestyle. Therefore, the first major step in assisting them to exercise more regularly is to focus on incorporating more activities of daily living and other less structured physical activity into their lifestyles (Levine 2005, Johannsen 2008). The U.S. Physical Activity Guidelines (2008) refer to such activities as "baseline activity," defined as the light-intensity activities of daily life like standing, walking slowly, and lifting lightweight objects. Although individuals vary in how much baseline activity they do, those engaging only in baseline activity are considered to be inactive. For the purposes of this book, daily lifestyle activity includes any unstructured movement done during each day.

Significant health benefits, such as a reduction in coronary risk factors, can be obtained by incorporating frequent bouts of moderate-intensity activity on most, if not all, days of the week, even if this activity is not a traditional, planned (or structured) one (McBride 2008, Loimaala 2009). A single bout of low-intensity, as opposed to high-intensity, exercise has been shown to substantially reduce the prevalence of hyperglycemia throughout the subsequent 24 h postexercise period in individuals with type 2 diabetes (T2D), demonstrating that activities of daily living also can have a positive effect on blood glucose management (Manders 2010). Although lifestyle physical activity does not entirely take the place of a traditional structured exercise program, in most cases it can be highly effective in helping individuals increase their daily activity level and build a fitness base that will allow them to participate in other, more intense or structured physical activities and exercise programs (Garber 2011).

Case in Point: Finding Time for Daily Movement

DC, a 62-year-old woman who has had T2D for 15 years, wants to do more exercise, but cannot find the time or the motivation to do so. Her medications include a daily evening injection of 70 units of long-acting basal insulin (insulin glargine), as well as a daily antidepressant. DC does not test her blood glucose regularly because of the high cost associated with buying strips for her meter (although she does have one). She has never been regularly physically active, and she has been significantly overweight or obese all of her adult life. Although she knows she needs to exercise, she says she has no time or energy left at the end of the day to do any exercise.

Resting Measurements

Height: 63 inches
Weight: 252 lb
BMI: 44.6 (morbidly obese)
Heart rate: 95 beats per minute (bpm)
Blood pressure: 125/80 mmHg

Fasting Labs

Plasma glucose: 116 mg/dl
A1C: 6.7%
Total cholesterol: 210 mg/dl
Triglycerides: 85 mg/dl
High-density lipoprotein cholesterol: 44 mg/dl
Low-density lipoprotein cholesterol: 149 mg/dl

Questions to Consider

1. Are DC's actual reasons for not being more physically active the same as her stated ones?
2. What would be the most effective way for DC to increase her physical activity level?
3. What precautions (if any) would you recommend that DC take?
4. What strategies will help motivate DC to be more regularly active?

(Continued on page 38.)

HEALTH BENEFITS OF DAILY MOVEMENT (UNSTRUCTURED ACTIVITY)

The health benefits of daily movement are numerous. For example, in sedentary men and women (without diabetes) undertaking either 6 months of fitness training or isocaloric pedometer-measured walking, their BMI, waist circumference, waist-to-hip ratio, and resting heart rate were reduced in both groups, and fasting glucose, glucose tolerance, and total cholesterol were similarly improved (Bell 2010). Thus, although supervised fitness training in previously sedentary adults produces greater improvements in their peak oxygen consumption and other fitness variables, many health-related variables improve similarly from a pedometer-based walking program matched for total energy cost.

Daily movement apparently has a large impact on how well the body handles carbohydrate intake. In a recent study, healthy normally active adults cut their physical activity levels (as monitored with daily steps) from >10,000 a day to <5,000, which is considered a sedentary level (Mikus 2012), over a 3-day period. Despite the fact that they could still release extra insulin in response to a glucose load, their postprandial glucose spikes increased significantly and progressively over the 3 days, which reinforces the importance of daily physical activity as a mediator of glycemic control.

For anyone with diabetes, inclusion of more daily, unstructured physical activity is likely to bestow similar, if not greater, health and glycemic benefits. Nonexercise activity thermogenesis (i.e., energy expended for activities of daily living) can create a large daily caloric deficit to prevent excessive weight gain, which can facilitate body weight and blood glucose management (Levine 2005, 2008). Simply standing counts as unstructured activity: in an observational study, obese individuals sat for ~2.5 h more and walked an average of 3.5 miles less per day than their lean counterparts. Moreover, most of the greater activity done by lean participants resulted from walks of short duration (<15 min) and low velocity (~1 mile/h) (Levine 2005). Health benefits result from concurrently reducing total time engaged in sedentary pursuits and interspersing frequent, short bouts of standing and physical activity between periods of sedentary activity, even in adults who are already physically active (Garber 2011, Dunstan 2012). Thus, how long individuals spend sitting each day and whether they move at all during periods of prolonged inactivity is critical to metabolic health and diabetes management.

PROMOTING LIFESTYLE PHYSICAL ACTIVITY

Engaging in frequent and daily physical activity is an essential part of self-care for all individuals with T2D. For anyone with type 1 diabetes (T1D), however, appropriate medication and dietary regimen changes likely will be needed to maintain control over blood glucose levels. All insulin users (regardless of type of diabetes) need to follow hypoglycemia prevention strategies. In many cases, the success of a physical activity should not simply be gauged by how much blood glucose levels decrease during participation. For insulin users, large drops in blood glucose are more likely to lead to rapid-onset hypoglycemia and worsened control. The focus instead should be on keeping the blood glucose level from interfering with the ability to continue the physical activity.

Although physical activity of any type—including activities of daily living—is not guaranteed to improve acute blood glucose control in insulin users, it is still equally important for them. For instance, one study recently investigated the influence of computer use on glycemic control in 115 patients with T1D. Their A1C levels were not related to age, diabetes duration, television watching, or computer use, but rather were independently and negatively associated with the weekly hours that individuals spent doing any physical exercise (Benevento 2010). Table 3.1 gives some suggestions on how to get individuals started doing more daily physical movement.

BREAKING UP SEDENTARY TIME

Use of physical activity accelerometers has brought a better estimation of total daily movement, along with the time spent doing activities of varying intensities or nothing at all (like sitting or sleeping). In overweight and obese adults, interrupting sitting time with 2-min bouts of light- or moderate-intensity walking lowered their postprandial glucose and insulin levels (Dunstan 2012). Along the same lines, an individual would theoretically expend an additional 24, 59, or 132 kilo-

Table 3.1 Recommendations for Getting Started with More Daily Movement

Following are some suggestions on how to get individuals with any type of diabetes more physically active on a daily basis:

■ Have them begin by focusing on more daily activities that are normal activities of daily living and involve physical movement of any sort, such as taking additional steps or standing longer each day.

■ Once individuals have established a solid base of greater daily movement, encourage participation in other physical activities like brisk walking, but make sure that they start at a low level and progress slowly to enhance compliance and reduce injury risk.

■ Have them include a variety of fitness activities to enhance differing aspects of their health. For example, yoga can reduce stress while improving overall health, well-being, and flexibility; aerobic activities like walking can help boost fitness levels; resistance and core exercises can lead to greater muscle strength; and ballroom or other dancing can improve balance, fitness, sense of enjoyment, and quality of life.

■ Help individuals find ways to decrease the total time that they spend doing sedentary activities, even simply by standing up while talking on the phone or by taking frequent breaks from sitting.

■ Encouraging individuals to move more and sit less will likely lead to their eventually incorporating activity with all types of goals.

calories per day, on average, if he or she chose to stand up and walk around at a normal, self-selected pace for 1, 2, or 5 min every hour, respectively, compared with sitting continuously during an 8 h period (Swartz 2011). Making small changes like taking a 5-min walking break every hour could yield beneficial weight-control or weight-loss results.

In adults with newly diagnosed T2D (ages 30–80 years), each hour of sedentary time during waking hours was associated with a larger waist circumference and lower levels of HDL-C, suggesting that a higher sedentary time is associated with a worse metabolic profile (Cooper 2012). Using similar techniques with accelerometer measurements, others have confirmed that the proportion of time spent in sedentary pursuits on a daily basis is strongly related to metabolic risk, independent of how much physical activity an individual otherwise does (Bankoski 2011). Thus, people with diabetes in particular may benefit from reducing their total sedentary time and avoiding prolonged periods of sedentary behavior, which they can do simply by increasing the number of breaks from sitting that they take during the day.

Case in Point: Continued

A health-care or fitness professional working with DC needs to discuss her personal beliefs, past experiences, preferences, and concerns about increasing her activity levels to figure out how to best assist her in becoming more active on a daily basis. Upon further discussion with DC, it becomes clear that her actual reasons for not exercising differed slightly from what she stated. She agrees that she lacks the motivation to exercise and that she feels too tired after work to do it then. She is also afraid of getting low blood glucose, however, because she takes insulin daily. Moreover, she does not feel safe walking in her neighborhood, especially in the dark during the winter, and she cannot afford to join a fitness center or buy expensive equipment to use at home.

(Continued on page 39.)

KEEPING TRACK OF DAILY MOVEMENT

One way individuals can keep track of how much daily movement they are doing is through the use of pedometers, which are small monitors that record the number of steps taken during the day. They have proven to be useful tools for increasing lifestyle physical activity because they provide immediate feedback, build confidence (in being active), and enhance enjoyment of daily movement. Use of objective measures of daily activity like step counters may enhance reaching goals. A meta-analysis of 26 studies with a total of 2,767 participants (eight random-controlled trials and 18 observational studies) found that pedometer users increased their physical activity by 26.9% over baseline during an average intervention of 18 weeks (Bravata 2007). What best predicted increased levels of physical activity was the establishment of a goal like taking 10,000 steps a day. Tips for the effective use of pedometers are given in Table 3.2.

Although pedometers are most suitable for tracking walking-based activities, they cannot detect changes in type, intensity, or pattern of activity. Some step equivalents for various activities are alternately given in Table 3.3 (based on metabolic equivalents, or MET levels) (Ainsworth 2011). Accelerometers and global positioning system (GPS) devices alternately may be used to detect such movements and are gaining popularity for use in determining total daily movement (Webber 2009).

Case in Point: Wrap-Up

To overcome DC's barriers to and any possible concerns associated with being physically active, a professional makes the following suggestions to her:

1. **Start with more daily movement.** The best way to start is by simply doing more daily movement and by being as active as you can all day long. Every step you take during the day counts. If you are just starting out, start with 10 min a day and add extra minutes a little bit at a time. Work up to 10 min at a time, three times a day, during the day—on breaks, during lunch, or whenever you can fit it in.

2. **Do not wait until you are tired to exercise.** Another trick is to try to fit in more steps and movement at the time of day when you have more energy. Just try walking for as long as possible during your lunch break a few days each week. You'll find that the more you do, the more energy you actually will have.

Table 3.2 Effective Use of Pedometers (Step Counters)

Following are some points to consider when advising diabetic individuals on how to most effectively use pedometers to promote and record daily physical activity:

■ Pedometers are capable of recording ambulatory activity, such as walking, jogging, or running. They will not count steps during cycling, rowing, upper body exercise, swimming, and other activities. However, steps can be estimated using metabolic equivalent (MET) levels for activities (see some equivalent values in Table 3.3).

■ For most adults, 2,000 steps is the equivalent of about 1 mile of walking, but the recorded steps can be affected by stride length, pedometer accuracy, and other factors.

■ The most essential feature of any pedometer is the step count. Pedometers are most accurate in counting steps, less accurate in calculating distance walked, and even less accurate at estimating caloric expenditure.

■ A variety of factors can affect step=counting accuracy, such as walking speed, waistband type, and abdominal size. In general, most pedometers are fairly accurate step counters at speeds of 2.5 mph and above.

■ Pedometers are more accurate at counting steps when attached to a firm waistband in an upright position and placed to the side (directly up from the knee cap on either side); attachment of pedometer to loose waistbands typically leads to an underestimation of steps taken.

■ Having a large waist size can negatively impact step-counting accuracy. For anyone with a large abdomen (or for pregnant women with any type of diabetes), place the pedometer at the small of the back, or use one that can be placed in a pocket or other location (like around the knee).

■ Go for simplicity, but accuracy, in a pedometer: extensive bells and whistles are not required. Recommended brands include most Accusplit, Yamax, and Omron models.

■ To test a pedometer's accuracy, an individual should position the device on his or her belt or waistband in line with one knee on either side of the body and reset the pedometer's count to zero. When taking 20 steps at a typical walking pace, if the pedometer records between 18 and 22 steps, it is reasonably accurate. If not, reposition it and try again. If it repeatedly fails this test, look into buying another type.

■ A "physically active" adult is expected to accumulate at least 10,000 steps per day (or the step equivalent if engaging in activities that a pedometer cannot easily record).

■ Establish a baseline by tracking steps for a few days without intentionally increasing physical activity level.

■ Set appropriate step goals by progressively increasing steps from baseline using small increases to start, such as taking an extra 500–1,000 daily steps.

3. **Stand up more.** Also, instead of sitting down, try standing up for an extra 10 min a day—while you are talking on the phone, stuck in a meeting (stand next to the wall), or just waiting somewhere. Standing is a physical activity that most of us could afford to do more of, so start thinking about ways to stand more every day. It also helps break up your sitting time, which helps use up blood glucose and keep you healthier.

4. **Be active in your home.** Even at home, make physical activity part of your daily routine. For example, exercise while you watch television (even if it just consists of walking in place), do some cleaning around the house, or do something active with your family and friends.

Table 3.3 Step Equivalents for Various Physical Activities

Activity	Minute Step Count	15 Min Step Count	30 Min Step Count
Aerobic dance	197	2,955	5,910
Ballroom dancing, slow to fast	91–167	1,365–2,505	2,730–5,010
Bowling	91	1,365	2,730
Canoeing	106	1,590	3,180
Circuit training	242	3,630	7,260
Climbing, rock or mountain	273	4,095	8,190
Gardening	121	1,815	3,630
Golf	136	2,040	4,080
Gymnastics	121	1,815	3,630
Health club exercise, general	167	2,505	5,010
Hiking	182	2,730	5,460
Jogging	212	3,180	6,360
Jogging on minitrampoline	136	2,040	4,080
Martial arts	303	4,545	9,090
Running, 5–8 mph	242–409	3,630–6,135	7,260–12,270
Shopping	70	1,050	2,100
Stationary cycling, moderate to vigorous	212–318	3,180–4,770	6,360–9,540
Step aerobics	273	4,095	8,190
Swimming laps, moderate to vigorous	212–303	3,180–4,545	6,360–9,090
Swimming leisurely	182	2,730	5,460
Water aerobics	121	1,815	3,630
Water jogging	242	3,630	7,260
Weight lifting, moderate to vigorous	121–182	1,815–2,730	3,630–5,460
Yoga and stretching	76	1,140	2,280

Based on metabolic equivalents (METs) of various physical activities.

5. **Learn how to adjust your insulin dose, and be prepared to treat a low.** Because you use insulin, ask your doctor or health-care provider about how much you might need to lower your insulin dose as you start to be more regularly active. Any physical activity can make insulin work better, so just make sure that you are prepared to treat a low blood glucose level if you have one. Keep some easily absorbed carbohydrates with you during your activity, such as glucose tablets, hard candy, sports drink, or even crackers.

6. **Focus on activities that you can safely do indoors.** Because you cannot walk outside in your neighborhood (at least part of the time), try to find an inexpensive indoor activity that you can do, such as an exercise class at a community center. Also, think of activities you can do in the safety of your home, including

all types of home-based exercise programs and videos. Some programs are also shown on television channels at various times of day. You do not need expensive equipment to work out in your home either. Try walking in place, doing stretching, or using food cans or water bottles for weights. You may want to buy some inexpensive resistance bands to use at home.

7. **Get support from friends and family by involving them.** Finally, if you are still lacking the motivation to exercise, invite a family member or friend to exercise with you on a regular basis (like having a friend walk with you during lunch). Plan when you are going to do each type of activity.

Doing more daily movement is not as effective as most structured exercise programs in increasing fitness levels, but it is important for many other reasons, including expending extra calories, breaking up sitting time, and building a fitness base in individuals who are overweight or sedentary. Use of pedometers may motivate individuals to engage in more unstructured physical activities. In addition, once individuals have successfully implemented more physical activity into their daily lifestyle, they likely will feel more confident, ready, and able to initiate and keep participating in more structured forms of activity.

PROFESSIONAL PRACTICE PEARLS

- All adults should avoid inactivity. Some physical activity is better than none, and participation in any amount of physical activity bestows health and glycemic benefits.
- The best way for deconditioned or overweight individuals with diabetes to start being more physically active is to focus on increasing their daily movement first.
- Daily movement (or unstructured physical activity) includes taking more daily steps, standing more, and doing more activities of daily living like housework.
- Individuals with diabetes will benefit from simply reducing their total sedentary time and avoiding prolonged periods of being sedentary by taking frequent breaks.
- Pedometers are step counters that can be used to track unstructured physical movement throughout the day; go for simplicity, but accuracy, in a pedometer.
- Walking-based activities are the best use for pedometers as they cannot detect changes in type, intensity, or pattern of activity; however, accelerometers and GPS devices can.
- For most adults, 2,000 steps is the equivalent of ~1 mile of walking, but step equivalents of other activities (like swimming) can be estimated based on MET levels.

REFERENCES

Ainsworth BE, Haskell WL, Herrmann SD, Meckes N, Bassett DR Jr, Tudor-Locke C, Greer JL, Vezina J, Whitt-Glover MC, Leon AS: 2011 Compendium of Physical Activities: a second update of codes and MET values. *Med Sci Sports Exerc* 43:1575–1581, 2011

Bankoski A, Harris TB, McClain JJ, Brychta RJ, Caserotti P, Chen KY, Berrigan D, Troiano RP, Koster A: Sedentary activity associated with metabolic syndrome independent of physical activity. *Diabetes Care* 34:497–503, 2011

Bell GJ, Harber V, Murray T, Courneya KS, Rodgers W: A comparison of fitness training to a pedometer-based walking program matched for total energy cost. *J Phys Act Health* 7:203–213, 2010

Benevento D, Bizzarri C, Pitocco D, Crino A, Moretti C, Spera S, Tubili C, Costanza F, Maurizi A, Cipolloni L, Cappa M, Pozzilli P, Imdiab Group: Computer use, free time activities and metabolic control in patients with type 1 diabetes. *Diabetes Res Clin Pract* 88:e32–e34, 2010

Bravata DM, Smith-Spangler C, Sundaram V, Gienger AL, Lin N, Lewis R, Stave CD, Olkin I, Sirard JR: Using pedometers to increase physical activity and improve health: a systematic review. *JAMA* 298:2296–2304, 2007

Cooper AR, Sebire S, Montgomery AA, Peters TJ, Sharp DJ, Jackson N, Fitzsimons K, Dayan CM, Andrews RC: Sedentary time, breaks in sedentary time and metabolic variables in people with newly diagnosed type 2 diabetes. *Diabetologia* 55:589–599, 2012

Dunstan DW, Kingwell BA, Larsen R, Healy GN, Cerin E, Hamilton MT, Shaw JE, Bertovic DA, Zimmet PZ, Salmon J, Owen N: Breaking up prolonged sitting reduces postprandial glucose and insulin responses. *Diabetes Care* 35:976–983, 2012

Garber CE, Blissmer B, Deschenes MR, Franklin BA, Lamonte MJ, Lee IM, Nieman DC, Swain DP, American College of Sports Medicine: American College of Sports Medicine position stand. Quantity and quality of exercise for developing and maintaining cardiorespiratory, musculoskeletal, and neuromotor fitness in apparently healthy adults: guidance for prescribing exercise. *Med Sci Sports Exerc* 43:1334–1359, 2011

Johannsen DL, Welk GJ, Sharp RL, Flakoll PJ: Differences in daily energy expenditure in lean and obese women: the role of posture allocation. *Obesity (Silver Spring)* 16:34–39, 2008

Levine JA, McCrady SK, Lanningham-Foster LM, Kane PH, Foster RC, Manohar CU: The role of free-living daily walking in human weight gain and obesity. *Diabetes* 57:548–554, 2008

Levine JA, Lanningham-Foster LM, McCrady SK, Krizan AC, Olson LR, Kane PH, Jensen MD, Clark MM: Interindividual variation in posture allocation: possible role in human obesity. *Science* 307:584–586, 2005

Loimaala A, Groundstroem K, Rinne M, Nenonen A, Huhtala H, Parkkari J, Vuori I: Effect of long-term endurance and strength training on metabolic control and arterial elasticity in patients with type 2 diabetes mellitus. *Am J Cardiol* 103:972–977, 2009

Manders RJ, Van Dijk JW, van Loon LJ: Low-intensity exercise reduces the prevalence of hyperglycemia in type 2 diabetes. *Med Sci Sports Exerc* 42:219–225, 2010

McBride PE, Einerson JA, Grant H, Sargent C, Underbakke G, Vitcenda M, Zeller L, Stein JH: Putting the Diabetes Prevention Program into practice: a program for weight loss and cardiovascular risk reduction for patients with metabolic syndrome or type 2 diabetes mellitus. *J Nutr Health Aging* 12:745s–749s, 2008

Mikus CR, Oberlin DJ, Libla JL, Taylor AM, Booth FW, Thyfault JP: Lowering physical activity impairs glycemic control in healthy volunteers. *Med Sci Sports Exerc* 44:225–231, 2012

Physical Activity Guidelines Advisory Committee: *Physical Activity Guidelines Advisory Committee Report, 2008*. Washington, DC, U.S. Department of Health and Human Services, p. 1–683, 2008

Swartz AM, Squires L, Strath SJ: Energy expenditure of interruptions to sedentary behavior. *Int J Behav Nutr Phys Act* 8:69, 2011

Webber SC, Porter MM: Monitoring mobility in older adults using global positioning system (GPS) watches and accelerometers: a feasibility study. *J Aging Phys Act* 17:455–467, 2009

Chapter 4

General Principles of Aerobic Exercise Prescription

Aerobic activities involve rhythmic, repeated, and continuous movements of the same large muscle groups for at least 5 min. Anaerobic or resistance activities use muscular strength to move a weight or work against a resistant load and are fully discussed in chapter 8. A program of regular exercise that includes cardiorespiratory, resistance, flexibility, and neuromotor training beyond activities of daily living to improve and maintain physical fitness and health is essential for most adults (Physical Activity Guidelines Advisory Committee 2008, Garber 2011)

All exercise programs need to be designed to address mode (type of activity), intensity (how difficult), frequency (how often), duration (how long), and appropriate progression. Rates of progression depend on an individual's functional capacity, medical and health status, age, individual activity preferences and goals, and tolerance to the current level of activity (Colberg 2011). Empowering individuals to set their own specific goals is the ultimate aim of such programming.

Case in Point: Aerobic Exercise Rx for Uncomplicated T2D

KK is a 50-year-old woman who was recently diagnosed with type 2 diabetes (T2D) during a routine annual checkup with her primary care physician. She has already met with a dietitian to improve her dietary plan, but she wants to get started doing more exercise to manage her blood glucose levels without the need for medications. In the past decade or two, she has gone through phases of being more active—walking daily—and periods of more inactivity, and she was in one of the latter when diagnosed; she does do a lot of standing and walking, though, in her full-time job. Since being diagnosed a month ago, she has lost ~10 lb thanks to dietary improvements, but she has another ~40 lb that she still desires to lose. Her goal with her physical activity is to lose more weight, get more fit, and keep her diabetes in check (without medications).

Resting Measurements

Height: 64 inches
Weight: 170 lb (180 lb at diagnosis)
BMI: 29.2 (high end of "overweight" category)
Heart rate: 80 beats per minute (bpm)
Blood pressure: 135/75 mmHg

Fasting Labs (1 Month after Diagnosis)

Plasma glucose: 105 mg/dl (controlled with lifestyle intervention only)
A1C: 6.2%
Total cholesterol: 180 mg/dl
Triglycerides: 125 mg/dl
High-density lipoprotein cholesterol: 50 mg/dl
Low-density lipoprotein cholesterol: 105 mg/dl

Questions to Consider

1. What type of aerobic exercise should KK start doing?
2. What would be the best exercise Rx for her in terms of exercise frequency, intensity, and duration?
3. How should her exercise training progress over time?
4. Are any precautions needed for KK when she exercises?

(Continued on page 57.)

GENERAL AEROBIC EXERCISE RECOMMENDATIONS

Aerobic (or cardiorespiratory) exercise is defined as continuous, dynamic exercise that uses large muscle groups and requires aerobic metabolic pathways to sustain the activity (Haskell 2007, Physical Activity Guidelines Advisory Committee 2008). Examples include walking, jogging, running, cycling, swimming, water aerobics, rollerblading, and cross-country skiing. Aerobic exercise has been the mode of physical activity traditionally prescribed for diabetes management and prevention. Most of its benefits in terms of management of blood glucose levels are related to acute and chronic improvements in insulin action. The acute effects of a recent bout of exercise account for most of these improvements, but admittedly are short-lived, whereas regular exercise training generally results in a more lasting effect through different mechanisms (Hawley 2008, Winnick 2008).

AEROBIC EXERCISE RECOMMENDATIONS FOR ADULTS

The American College of Sports Medicine (ACSM) recommends that most adults engage in moderate-intensity aerobic training for at least 30 min/day on ≥5 days/week (a total of at least 150 min weekly), vigorous-intensity training for at least 20 min/day on ≥3 days/week (at least 60–75 min/week), or a combination of moderate- and vigorous-intensity exercise to achieve a similar amount of training (Haskell 2007, Nelson 2007, Garber 2011). The latest federal guidelines (2008) are similar, but allow for 150 min of moderate or 75 min of vigorous activity weekly (Physical Activity Guidelines Advisory Committee 2008). For additional and more extensive health benefits, adults should increase their aerobic physical activity to 300 min (5 h) a week of moderate-intensity, or 150 min a week of vigorous-intensity aerobic physical activity, or an equivalent combination of moderate- and vigorous-intensity activity (Physical Activity Guidelines Advisory

Committee 2008). Additional health benefits are gained by engaging in physical activity beyond this amount. The recommended physical activity guidelines and prescription for adults and older adults are available online through the ACSM (www.acsm.org) or U.S. federal guidelines (www.health.gov/paguidelines).

AEROBIC EXERCISE RECOMMENDATIONS FOR ADULTS WITH DIABETES

For individuals with type 1 diabetes (T1D), exercise recommendations are closely aligned with those for apparently healthy people (Haskell 2007, D'Hooge 2011), whereas recommendations for T2D are more reflective of guidelines for obesity, hypertension, and sedentary lifestyles (Sigal 2007; Colberg 2010, 2011) given that ~80% of adults with diabetes are overweight or obese. Most individuals with T2D also have a low aerobic capacity (Boulé 2003), leading to the recommendation that they engage in 150 min of moderate (or higher-intensity) aerobic activity weekly (Colberg 2010, American Diabetes Association 2013). Such individuals should focus on appropriate exercise durations to achieve adequate levels of calorie expenditure (Levine 2005, 2008). Recommendations for women with uncomplicated gestational diabetes (GDM) include engaging in 30 min of moderate intensity activity like brisk walking on most days of the week (150 min weekly) (Committee on Obstetric Practice 2002).

INDIVIDUAL AEROBIC EXERCISE SESSIONS

Each aerobic exercise session generally has three distinct parts or phases:

- Warm-up
- Conditioning phase
- Cooldown

WARM-UP

Doing a warm-up includes 5–10 min of a physical activity done at a slower speed or lower intensity, such as cycling slowly before picking up the pace. Warming up before moderate- or vigorous-intensity aerobic activity allows a gradual increase in heart rate (HR) and breathing at the start of activity (Physical Activity Guidelines Advisory Committee 2008). It may help reduce muscle injury and facilitates a safe transition from rest to exercise by stretching postural muscles, increasing blood flow, elevating body temperature, and increasing oxygen availability and metabolic rate. Alternately, warming up for a muscle-strengthening activity involves doing exercises with lighter weights or resistance to start.

CONDITIONING PHASE

This phase is the most important for achieving fitness and other goals as it includes the actual activities to enhance cardiorespiratory fitness, muscle strength and endurance, or flexibility (depending on the training protocol). Time spent doing the warm-up and cooldown counts toward meeting aerobic activity guidelines only if the activity is of at least moderate intensity (e.g., walking briskly as a warm-up before jogging) (Physical Activity Guidelines Advisory Committee 2008).

COOLDOWN

A cooldown includes at least 3–5 min of doing a lower-intensity activity to help the body gradually recover from the conditioning phase and safely transition back to a resting state. Perhaps most important, cooling down helps prevent blood from pooling in the arms and legs (and thereby lessens the chance of fainting at the end of exercise), as well as aids in the removal of metabolic by-products like lactic acid immediately after exercise. HR monitoring can be effective in monitoring recovery from an exercise bout. If an individual takes medications for hypertension that act as vasodilators, he or she may require a longer period of active cooldown to prevent hypotensive episodes postexercise (Balady 2007).

EXERCISE PRESCRIPTION FOR AEROBIC TRAINING

The exercise prescription is an actual plan for an individual to follow to reach his or her physical fitness or diabetes management goals. The five components of typical aerobic exercise prescription should at a minimum include the following:

- Mode
- Intensity
- Frequency
- Duration
- Progression

MODE

The types, or modes, of aerobic activity that are recommended for individuals with diabetes are highly dependent on their preferences and skill level. Although health-related benefits of improved physical fitness do not depend on the type of aerobic exercise done, the actual fitness gains are somewhat activity specific. Walking is the most common type of physical activity done by individuals with diabetes and often is the most convenient. Other low-impact or non–weight-bearing types of activity, such as cycling, swimming, and aquatic or chair exercises, may be more appropriate for those with complications or coexisting conditions like peripheral or autonomic neuropathy (Browning 2005, Duncan 2005, Colberg 2009). For individuals without lower body joint limitations, jogging and running are acceptable higher-intensity activities.

Although the mode of physical activity (e.g., walking, running, swimming, chair exercises, rowing, etc.) is important to consider, any type of increased movement appears to initially improve an individual's fitness level. Sedentary adults or youth who begin to participate in any physical activity experience measurable results in their fitness levels. Individuals should choose activities that can safely and effectively improve cardiovascular endurance and maximize caloric expenditure (Haskell 2007, Nelson 2007, Colberg 2010). A wide range of physical activities can be included in the exercise prescription, and all possible activities that the individual is interested in doing should be considered, if they are safe to perform. As he or she becomes more successful and confident, options can be expanded and other types of physical activities can be added or substituted.

INTENSITY

Determining appropriate aerobic exercise intensity is important for anyone with diabetes. The prescribed intensity must match the individual's current fitness capabilities. For example, if an activity is too easy, it may not raise fitness levels effectively, but if it is too hard initially, the individual may not be able to complete the workout, may become injured, or may be discouraged from exercising altogether. Physical activity guidelines for adults focus on both moderate-intensity activity and vigorous-intensity activity (Haskell 2007, Physical Activity Guidelines Advisory Committee 2008, Garber 2011). Examples of activities in each of these categories are given in Table 4.1 (Physical Activity Guidelines Advisory Committee 2008). As a rule of thumb, a person doing moderate-intensity aerobic activity can talk, but not sing, during the activity. A person doing vigorous-intensity activity cannot say more than a few words without pausing for a breath.

Individuals can do either moderate-intensity or vigorous-intensity aerobic activities, or a combination of both. It takes less time to get the same benefit from vigorous-intensity activities as from moderate-intensity activities. In general, 2 min of moderate-intensity activity is the equivalent of 1 min of vigorous-intensity activity (Physical Activity Guidelines Advisory Committee 2008). It is also possible to benefit from interspersing faster intervals into any low- or moderate-intensity workouts to make greater gains in fitness levels (Johnson 2006, 2008).

Engaging in moderate- to vigorous-intensity physical activity is generally recommended to achieve aerobic and metabolic improvements in people with diabe-

Table 4.1 Intensity of Various Aerobic Physical Activities (Based on Absolute Intensity)

Moderate	Vigorous
• Walking briskly: 3 mph or faster (but not race-walking) • Water aerobics and pool exercise • Bicycling: slower than 10 mph • Tennis (doubles) • Ballroom dancing • General gardening • Rollerblading • Hiking • Skateboarding • Canoeing • Softball and baseball • Housework (like sweeping)	• Race-walking, jogging, or running • Swimming laps • Tennis (singles) • Aerobic dancing • Bicycling: 10 mph or faster • Jumping rope • Heavy gardening (continuous digging or hoeing, with heart rate increases) • Hiking uphill or with a heavy backpack • Jumping rope • Martial arts (e.g., karate) • Kickboxing or boxing • Sports like basketball, soccer, and tennis • Active games that involve running and chasing

tes (Sigal 2004, 2006; Colberg 2010). Lower-intensity activities will expend calories and help with weight maintenance, but they may or may not have much of an acute impact on blood glucose levels or enhance cardiovascular fitness as much (Duncan 2005, Hansen 2009). Appropriate measures of intensity include the "talk test," perceived exertion, and target HR.

"Talk test." When starting out with an exercise program, the easiest measure of intensity for anyone to use is the "talk test." An individual should be able to carry on a conversation during aerobic activity without struggling to breathe. If he or she is breathing too heavily to talk, the intensity has exceeded the ventilatory threshold and is harder than a moderate workload. The only drawback to the use of this test is that it cannot discern when exercise intensity is too low, but upon starting an exercise program, it is safer for the individual to err on the low side than on the high side.

Perceived exertion. Use of perceived exertion is another easy way for individuals to estimate their exercise intensity. This is a subjective rating based on general fatigue and can be used along with target HR estimations or as a substitute to guide the intensity of activity. Several scales, including the Borg scales, can be used to assign numbers to intensity levels, or individuals can simply state how they feel. When subjective perceived exertion is used, a person should focus on full-body feelings of exertion and general fatigue. Generally, a moderate- to vigorous-intensity exercise corresponds to a subjective rating of "somewhat hard" (for moderate) to "hard" (for vigorous) (Garber 2011). Less fit people generally require a higher level of effort than fitter people require to do the same activity. Relative exertional intensity can be estimated using a scale of 0 to 10, where sitting is 0 and the highest level of effort possible is 10. Moderate-intensity activity is a 5 or 6 out of 10. Vigorous-intensity activity is a 7 or 8 (Physical Activity Guidelines Advisory Committee 2008).

Target HR. Exercise intensity can be prescribed and monitored using HR. The ACSM recommends the following HR measurement: exercise intensity of 40–89% of HR reserve (HRR). (This range roughly corresponds to 64–93% of maximum HR, or HR_{max}.) The recommended intensity range of 40% to 89% is broad because deconditioned individuals can gain improvements in cardiorespiratory fitness at lower intensities, whereas individuals with greater fitness typically require a higher minimal threshold to achieve similar gains (Garber 2011). Therefore, the prescribed intensity range should be based on an individual's fitness level, duration of diabetes, presence and degree of complications, and personal goals. Using this method, moderate-intensity exercise is in the range of 40% to 59% HRR, whereas vigorous-intensity exercise is defined as 60–89% HRR (Garber 2011, Physical Activity Guidelines Advisory Committee 2008). A severely deconditioned person can start even lower than 40% HRR (e.g., light intensity is considered 30–39% and very light is <30%) and progress from there to more moderate levels over time.

Exercise intensity can be calculated most accurately if an individual's maximal HR (MHR) has been determined with an exercise stress test. A true resting HR (RHR) is best measured upon awakening; measuring at other times of day, even at rest, may not yield the same results. The difference between the MHR and RHR is defined as the HRR.

The Karvonen formula, which relies on the calculation of HRR, commonly is used to calculate a single target HR or HR range in bpm (Garber 2011):

$$HRR = MHR - RHR$$

$$\text{Percent HRR (\% HRR)} = HRR \times \text{Desired Intensity (\% as decimal)}$$

$$\text{Karvonen Formula: Target HR} = [(MHR - RHR) \times \text{Desired Intensity}] + RHR$$

If someone's actual MHR has not been measured, target HR ranges can be approximated using the following equation to estimate maximal values:

$$MHR = 220 - \text{Age}$$

This equation should be used with caution because of the large standard deviation, which can cause the HR estimation to be off by 12–15 bpm (Garber 2011). This procedure may overestimate the maximal HR of some individuals with diabetes, particularly those with autonomic neuropathy (Colberg 2010, 2011). If cardiac autonomic neuropathy is present, exercise intensity is better prescribed using the HRR method with MHR directly measured, rather than estimated, for better accuracy (Colberg 2003).

An alternate equation that may be more accurate for estimating maximal HR in an older population utilizes 70% of age rather than full age (Garber 2011):

$$MHR = 208 - (0.7 \times \text{Age})$$

In general, exercise performed at lower levels (<40% HRR) has a lesser glucose-lowering effect than exercise done at higher intensities—unless it is done long enough. Glucose disposal during high-intensity exercise is roughly propor-

---

Table 4.2 Sample Calculation Using Karvonen Formula for Target Heart Rate Range of 40–89% of Heart Rate Reserve

Individual: 50-year-old female (KK from Case in Point) Resting HR (RHR): 80 beats per minute (bpm) Maximal HR (MHR): 170 bpm (estimated with 220 – Age)	
Karvonen Formula: Target HR = [(MHR – RHR) × Desired Intensity)] + RHR	
Lower end of HR range (40%)	= [(170 – 80) × 0.40] + 80 = [90 x 0.40] + 80 = 36 + 80 = 116 bpm
Higher end of HR range (89%)	= [(170 – 80) × 0.89] + 80 = [90 x 0.89] + 80 = 80 + 80 = 160 bpm
Target HR range (40–89% HRR)	= 116 to 160 bpm

tional to the total work performed (time × intensity). On the other hand, vigorous exercise (≥60% HRR) may result in transient hyperglycemia and cause an excessive rise in systolic blood pressure (Colberg 2010).

FREQUENCY

Physical activity sessions can be performed in a variety of combinations of frequency and duration. Most research concludes that physical activity should be performed 3–5 days/week to achieve significant health benefits. The latest guidelines for T2D suggest that individuals should undertake at least 150 min a week of moderate to vigorous aerobic exercise spread over at least 3 days, with no more than 2 consecutive days without aerobic activity, if their goals are to improve glycemic control, enhance fitness, and achieve target caloric expenditure (Colberg 2010, 2011; American Diabetes Association 2013). Exercise that is limited to 2 days/week results in less improvement in cardiovascular fitness.

Moreover, since the duration of glycemic improvement after an exercise session is usually >2 h but <72 h, regular physical activity is needed to lower blood glucose (Boulé 2001, O'Donovan 2005). For individuals taking insulin, being active on a daily basis may help to balance caloric needs with insulin dosages, as well as maintain higher levels of insulin sensitivity to allow for reduced insulin dosing. Obese individuals may need to be active more frequently (5–7 days/week) at lower intensities to optimize weight loss and maintenance (Ross 2000, 2004). In addition, to achieve sustained major weight loss, the optimal level of activity needed is typically greater than that needed to improve glycemic control.

Energy expenditure also can be used to guide exercise programming. The ACSM recommends a target range of 150 to 400 calories/day expended via physical activity (Garber 2011). This represents a minimum threshold of 1,000 calories a week, which is associated with reduction in all-cause mortality risk. For previously sedentary people, this minimal threshold can be an initial goal, but to achieve maximal weight loss, they should work up to expending 300–400 calories/day, or 2,000 calories/week. Energy expenditure in excess of 2,000 calories/week in physical activity has been associated with successful short- and long-term weight loss (Garber 2011).

DURATION

The exercise duration is directly related to caloric expenditure requirements and inversely related to the intensity of exercise required to achieve the same results. In other words, to gain maximum caloric expenditure and glycemic benefits, lower-intensity exercise needs to be performed for longer periods of time compared with higher-intensity exercise.

The recommended weekly exercise duration for adults differs somewhat by guideline. Recent joint guidelines from the ACSM and American Heart Association (2007) recommend 150 min of moderate activity (30 min, 5 days/week) or 60 min of vigorous physical activity (20 min on 3 days) for all adults (Haskell 2007, Nelson 2007). U.S. federal guidelines (2008) recommend 150 min of moderate or 75 min of vigorous activity, or an equivalent combination, spread throughout each week (Physical Activity Guidelines Advisory Committee 2008).

The latter recommends an exercise volume of 500–1,000 metabolic equivalents (METs) min/week, where an MET is the ratio of the rate of energy expended during an activity to the rate of energy expended at rest. For example, 1 MET is the rate of energy expenditure at rest, whereas a 4-MET activity expends four times the energy used by the body at rest. MET minutes are the metabolic equivalent of physical activity times the number of minutes the activity is done. Thus, levels of 500–1,000 METs min/week are achievable with 150 min of weekly walking at 4 mph (6.4 km/h; intensity of 5 METs, or five times resting levels) or 75 min of jogging at 6 mph (9.6 km/h; 10 METs).

Although both of these guidelines apply to most adults with T1D, the majority of people with T2D lack sufficient aerobic capacity to jog for that duration or they have orthopedic or other limitations. The mean maximal aerobic capacity in such individuals is estimated to be only 22.4 ml/kg/min, or the equivalent of 6.4 METs (Boulé 2003), making 4.8 METs (~75% of maximal) the highest, sustainable intensity. Thus, most individuals with T2D have to undertake ≥150 min of moderate to vigorous aerobic exercise per week to achieve optimal cardiovascular risk reduction (Colberg 2010). The ADA's Standards of Medical Care make a similar recommendation that individuals with diabetes perform at least 150 min of weekly moderate-intensity aerobic physical activity (American Diabetes Association 2013).

Although a minimum dose has not been determined, some cardiovascular and glycemic benefits may be gained from lower exercise volumes (Hansen 2009). Additional benefits likely result from engaging in durations beyond recommended amounts, however (Jakicic 2003, Houmard 2004). If someone has a higher aerobic capacity (>10 METs), such as many younger individuals with T1D, T2D, or GDM, he or she may choose to exercise at a higher absolute intensity for less time to achieve the same cardiovascular and glycemic benefits. Bouts of physical activity lasting 60 min or more may be required to achieve weight loss or to prevent weight regain (Physical Activity Guidelines Advisory Committee 2008).

Whether the actual length of each exercise session matters is an interesting question. Although 20 min has been the minimal recommendation for cardiovascular benefits, multiple shorter bouts of 10 min have been shown to result in measurable improvements (Eriksen 2007). Similar gains occur when physical activity is accumulated throughout the day as three bouts of 10 min compared with a single prolonged activity session of similar duration and intensity (i.e., a 30 min bout of continuous activity) (Haskell 2007). Thus, if desired, physical activity may be broken down into sessions of a minimum of 10 min spread throughout the day (Garber 2011). Severely deconditioned individuals may need to exercise in multiple sessions of short duration (5–10 min), begin at low levels with brief rest intervals, and progress slowly to higher-intensity exercise. Initially, sessions can be done for 10–15 min, increasing progressively over time to >30 min (Garber 2011). Closer to 60 min of daily exercise may be necessary to achieve significant weight loss in adults (Ross 2000, 2004).

PROGRESSION

Appropriate progression of aerobic training is required to help individuals effectively and safely achieve aerobic exercise goals. Initially, the focus should be on increasing frequency and duration of the exercise rather than intensity. Individuals should increase physical activity gradually over time whenever more activity is necessary to meet guidelines or health goals, and inactive individuals should "start low and go slow" by gradually increasing how often and how long activities are done (Physical Activity Guidelines Advisory Committee 2008). Progressing in this manner increases the likelihood of creating and sustaining an activity habit and lowers the risk of injury or demotivation (Garber 2011).

A full exercise prescription, to be truly effective, should include both how to start a fitness program and what to reasonably expect in terms of progress, as shown in Table 4.3. The individual must understand the type, quantity, and rate of progress to expect. Over a period of time averaging at least 4–6 months, each individual moves through three distinct stages of a fitness plan: initial, improvement, and maintenance.

Table 4.3 Progressive Stages of Exercise Training

Training Stage	Weeks	Frequency (per week)	Intensity (% HRR)	Duration (minutes)
Initial	1–4	3–4	30–59%	15–30
Improvement	5–24	3–5	40–89%	25–40
Maintenance	24+	3–5	60–89%	20–60

HRR, heart rate reserve.

Initial stage. In this stage, individuals begin to form physical activity habits that can be integrated into their lifestyles. Unfortunately, most people never make it out of this critical stage, either because they attempt activities that are too hard for them given their fitness level or because they develop unrealistic expectations for what they will be able to accomplish and when, which leads to discouragement and a cessation of training. To help ensure success, individuals should be helped to understand that significant changes (like loss of body weight) may not occur during this period. Also, they need to understand that building fitness habits takes 4 weeks or longer, especially when people start out with very poor fitness levels. Setting specific fitness goals can help with motivation during this stage. For individuals who are starting with a higher fitness level, this stage often can be skipped.

Improvement stage. During this second stage, the focus shifts from developing habits to improving fitness levels. The individual now has improved stamina and endurance, is able to spend longer amounts of time doing physical activity, and can begin adding to duration or intensity of workouts. Over the 3 months (or longer for deconditioned and older individuals) of this stage, health benefits begin to become measurable. If individuals see these changes as permanent without further training needed, however, their exercise habit may start to weaken, and they may start missing workouts. Individuals who already have higher levels of fitness will begin their program in this stage when undertaking new types of training or setting new fitness goals. The progression shown is for individuals with an ultimate goal of participating in vigorous aerobic exercise. For many individuals with T2D, however, doing moderate-intensity workouts may be an appropriate endpoint, although frequency and duration may progress.

Maintenance stage. Once someone has successfully met his or her initial fitness or blood glucose management goals, it is important to develop new goals and plans to enhance motivation and continued participation. A new goal may be something like "prevent weight regain" or "train for a competitive event." To ensure continued safety and effectiveness of training in all individuals with diabetes, medications may need to be adjusted or other changes made to training if any existing health comorbidities progress or new ones arise.

SAFETY CONSIDERATIONS

Everyone who engages in physical activity should do so with safety in mind. To do physical activity safely and reduce risk of injuries and other adverse events, people should understand the risks yet should exercise confidently given that physical activity is safe for almost everyone. They should start with and do types of physical activity that are appropriate for their current fitness level and health goals, increase their physical activity gradually over time, start at the lower end of the intensity spectrum and progress slowly to prevent injuries, and use appropriate gear and sports equipment in safe environments.

Although specific safety considerations required for exercise participation by individuals with diabetes will be addressed in many chapters that follow, it is important to mention a few of these guidelines here (also see Table 4.4):

- Individuals should monitor their blood glucose both before and after activity to promote safety and understanding of its glycemic effects.
- All individuals with diabetes who are treated with insulin, sulfonylureas, or meglitinides should carry rapidly absorbed carbohydrates (e.g., glucose tablets or gels) with them while performing physical activity to treat hypoglycemia rapidly.
- They should be aware that certain medications can impair exercise tolerance; for example, β-adrenergic blockers lower the HR response to physical activity, as well as mask hypoglycemic symptoms and lessen the strength of counterregulatory (glucose-raising) hormonal responses.
- All individuals should wear clothing and shoes appropriate for the activity to reduce chance of injury.
- They should wear some form of diabetes and personal identification.
- Individuals need to use caution when exercising—particularly vigorously—in extremely hot, humid, smoggy, or cold environments.
- Because seasonal changes in blood glucose control have been related to environmental temperature, they should find safe and available places to be active indoors when the weather is colder.
- An individual should stop any activity if he or she experiences any symptoms like pain, lightheadedness, or shortness of breath.

Table 4.4 General Guidelines for Safe Exercise Participation with Diabetes

Perform self-monitoring of blood glucose (SMBG)	Check SMBG levels before and after each exercise session to ensure adequate pre-exercise control and to better understand and predict future glycemic responses. If blood glucose is >250–300 mg/dl with moderate or higher levels of urinary or blood ketones, exercise should be postponed; >250–300 mg/dl without ketones, okay to exercise, but use caution; <100 mg/dl, consider eating a snack consisting of easily absorbed carbohydrates (~20–30 g), based on insulin regimen and circulating insulin levels expected during the activity; 100–240 mg/dl, exercise is recommended.
Keep a daily log	Record the time of day the SMBG values are obtained and the dose of any medications taken. Also, approximate the time (min), intensity (heart rate), and distance (miles or meters) of exercise session. Such details aid the individual in understanding the glucose response to an exercise bout.
Plan ahead for exercise sessions	The need for adjustments to medications or food intake can be anticipated based on anticipated exercise (duration and intensity). If needed, carry extra carbohydrate (~10–15 grams for every 30 min) to prevent or treat hypoglycemia.
Ensure hydration	Hydrate before and rehydrate after each exercise session to prevent dehydration.
Modify caloric intake accordingly	Through frequent SMBG, caloric intake can be regulated more carefully on days with and without exercise participation.
Adjust insulin accordingly	If using insulin, reduce rapid- or short-acting insulin dosage to limit hypoglycemic episodes.
Exercise with a partner	Diabetic individuals should exercise with a partner until their glucose response is known and to promote exercise adherence.
Wear a diabetes identification (ID) tag	Diabetes ID with relevant medical information should always be worn. Hypoglycemia and other problems can arise that require immediate attention.
Wear good shoes	Always wear proper-fitting and comfortable footwear with socks to minimize foot irritations and limit orthopedic injury to the feet and lower legs.
Practice good hygiene	Always take extra care to inspect feet for any irritation spots to prevent possible infection. Tend to all sores immediately, and limit any irritations.

Case in Point: Wrap-Up

Because KK has most recently led a sedentary lifestyle, she should start with an initial exercise prescription that allows her to progress slowly toward higher levels of cardiovascular fitness over a period of weeks to months.

Exercise Program Goals

Mode of Activity: KK has stated that she enjoys walking and has done that activity from time to time, so the recommended activity to start will be brisk walking.

Intensity: Because KK already does quite a bit of lifestyle activity, she should be able to start with moderate (brisk) walking at a comfortable pace that feels "somewhat hard" to maintain. To improve her fitness levels faster, she should consider adding short intervals of faster walking interspersed into her normal walking pace. If she wants to monitor her intensity using a target HR, a minimal starting intensity of 40% HRR gives her a target of 117 bpm, or a moderate range (40–59%) of 117 to 135 bpm.

Frequency: KK's goal should be a minimum of 3 nonconsecutive days of walking per week, with a goal of progressing to 5 or more days over the next several months. She should be advised to not go more than 2 consecutive days without doing some aerobic activity (to keep insulin action higher).

Duration: If KK initially cannot walk for 30 min continuously, she should be advised to aim to do 10–15 min at a time spread over the day. Her initial goal should be a minimum of 150 min spread throughout the week, or possibly a lesser total time if she walks more intensely.

Progression: KK's long-term exercise goals should focus on progressively increasing her activity to reach the minimum recommended levels of 150 min of moderate or vigorous exercise spread throughout the week. Her target HR can remain either in the improvement phase (minimum target HR of 117 bpm, equal to 40% HRR) or progress as she is able, as fitness gains will result more quickly with a higher-intensity workout. Once she has reached the maintenance phase, she can substitute some alternative aerobic activities for variety, and she should consider adding in resistance training at least 2 days a week.

Daily Movement: To help with weight loss, KK should engage in as much daily movement as possible, including standing more and taking steps throughout the day. As a possible motivator, she should consider getting a pedometer and setting a daily step goal.

Possible Precautions: KK has minimal risk factors for cardiovascular disease (mainly diabetes), so she should not be required to have an exercise stress test before starting her walking progress. She has had a recent checkup with her doctor with good results (other than the diagnosis of T2D). She should consider, however, investing in a good pair of walking shoes and athletic socks to avoid the development of any orthopedic limitations related to her exercise program.

People with diabetes of any type will benefit from getting specific aerobic exercise prescriptions from their health-care or fitness professional. This prescription should include specifics about what types of activities they should be doing, how hard they should be working out, how often and how long, and when they need to progress and what to expect in terms of reasonable progression through the phases of a training program. Empowering individuals to set their own specific goals is the ultimate aim of such programming.

PROFESSIONAL PRACTICE PEARLS

- Aerobic (or cardiorespiratory) exercise is defined as continuous, dynamic exercise that uses large muscle groups and requires aerobic metabolic pathways to sustain the activity (such as brisk walking, cycling, and swimming).
- Commonly, the warm-up and cooldown involve doing an activity at a slower speed or lower intensity (such as engaging in 5–10 min of brisk walking before and after jogging).
- The aerobic exercise prescription should address mode (type of activity), intensity (how difficult), frequency (how often), duration (how long), and appropriate progression.
- Although doing any physical activity can be beneficial to health, moderate-to vigorous-intensity physical activity is generally recommended to achieve aerobic and metabolic improvements in people with diabetes.
- Lower-intensity activities will expend calories and help with weight maintenance, but may or may not have much of an acute impact on blood glucose levels or enhance cardiovascular fitness as much.
- Appropriate measures of intensity include the "talk test," perceived exertion, and target HR (using the Karvonen formula for HR reserve).
- Physical activity should be performed 3–5 days/week to achieve significant health benefits, with no more than 2 consecutive days without aerobic activity to optimize insulin action; exercise done only 2 days/week results in lesser fitness improvements.
- Both moderate- and vigorous-intensity aerobic activity should be performed in episodes of at least 10 min, with a goal of 30 min or more of continuous activity.
- Progress by increasing physical activity gradually over time whenever more activity is necessary to meet guidelines or health goals; inactive individuals should "start low and go slow" by gradually increasing how often and how long activities are done.
- A full exercise prescription should include both how to start a fitness program and what to expect in terms of progress over a period of 4–6 months, including initial, improvement, and maintenance phases (although fit individuals may skip the initial phase).
- For individuals with T1D without complications, exercise recommendations are similar to those for individuals with no known health problems (i.e., a minimum of 150 min of moderate or 60–75 min of vigorous activity weekly).
- Recommendations for T2D closely align with guidelines for sedentary adults and older adults; most individuals with T2D should at the very least undertake 150 min or more of moderate to vigorous aerobic exercise per week for cardiovascular risk reduction.

■ Women with uncomplicated GDM should engage in 30 min of moderate intensity activity like brisk walking on most days of the week (150 min weekly).

■ Empowering individuals to set their own specific goals is the ultimate aim of providing them with a specific exercise prescription for aerobic training.

REFERENCES

American Diabetes Association: Standards of medical care in diabetes—2013. *Diabetes Care* 36 (Suppl. 1):S11–S66, 2013

Balady GJ, Williams MA, Ades PA, Bittner V, Comoss P, Foody JM, Franklin B, Sanderson B, Southard D, American Heart Association Exercise, Cardiac Rehabilitation, and Prevention Committee, Council on Clinical Cardiology; American Heart Association Council on Cardiovascular Nursing; American Heart Association Council on Epidemiology and Prevention; American Heart Association Council on Nutrition, Physical Activity, and Metabolism; American Association of Cardiovascular and Pulmonary Rehabilitation: Core components of cardiac rehabilitation/secondary prevention programs: 2007 update: a scientific statement from the American Heart Association Exercise, Cardiac Rehabilitation, and Prevention Committee, the Council on Clinical Cardiology; the Councils on Cardiovascular Nursing, Epidemiology and Prevention, and Nutrition, Physical Activity, and Metabolism; and the American Association of Cardiovascular and Pulmonary Rehabilitation. *Circulation* 115:2675–2682, 2007

Boulé NG, Haddad E, Kenny GP, Wells GA, Sigal RJ: Effects of exercise on glycemic control and body mass in type 2 diabetes mellitus: a meta-analysis of ontrolled clinical trials. *JAMA* 286:1218–1227, 2001

Boulé NG, Kenny GP, Haddad E, Wells GA, Sigal RJ: Meta-analysis of the effect of structured exercise training on cardiorespiratory fitness in type 2 diabetes mellitus. *Diabetologia* 46:1071–1081, 2003

Browning RC, Kram R: Energetic cost and preferred speed of walking in obese vs. normal weight women. *Obes Res* 13:891–899, 2005

Colberg SR, Sigal RJ: Prescribing exercise for individuals with type 2 diabetes: recommendations and precautions. *Phys Sportsmed* 39:13–26, 2011

Colberg SR, Sigal RJ, Fernhall B, Regensteiner JG, Blissmer BJ, Rubin RR, Chasan-Taber L, Albright AL, Braun B, American College of Sports Medicine, American Diabetes Association: Exercise and type 2 diabetes: the American College of Sports Medicine and the American Diabetes Association: joint position statement. *Diabetes Care* 33:e147–e167, 2010

Colberg SR, Swain DP, Vinik AI: Use of heart rate reserve and rating of perceived exertion to prescribe exercise intensity in diabetic autonomic neuropathy. *Diabetes Care* 26:986–990, 2003

Colberg SR, Zarrabi L, Bennington L, Nakave A, Thomas Somma C, Swain DP, Sechrist SR: Postprandial walking is better for lowering the glycemic effect of dinner than pre-dinner exercise in type 2 diabetic individuals. *J Am Med Dir Assoc* 10:394–397, 2009

Committee on Obstetric Practice: ACOG committee opinion. Exercise during pregnancy and the postpartum period. Number 267, January 2002. American College of Obstetricians and Gynecologists. *Int J Gynaecol Obstet* 77:79–81, 2002

D'Hooge R, Hellinckx T, Van Laethem C, Stegen S, De Schepper J, Van Aken S, Dewolf D, Calders P: Influence of combined aerobic and resistance training on metabolic control, cardiovascular fitness and quality of life in adolescents with type 1 diabetes: a randomized controlled trial. *Clin Rehabil* 25:349–359, 2011

Duncan GE, Anton SD, Sydeman SJ, Newton RL Jr, Corsica JA, Durning PE, Ketterson TU, Martin AD, Limacher MC, Perri MG: Prescribing exercise at varied levels of intensity and frequency: a randomized trial. *Arch Intern Med* 165:2362–2369, 2005

Eriksen L, Dahl-Petersen I, Haugaard SB, Del F: Comparison of the effect of multiple short-duration with single long-duration exercise sessions on glucose homeostasis in type 2 diabetes mellitus. *Diabetologia* 50:2245–2253, 2007

Garber CE, Blissmer B, Deschenes MR, Franklin BA, Lamonte MJ, Lee IM, Nieman DC, Swain DP, American College of Sports Medicine: American College of Sports Medicine position stand. Quantity and quality of exercise for developing and maintaining cardiorespiratory, musculoskeletal, and neuromotor fitness in apparently healthy adults: guidance for prescribing exercise. *Med Sci Sports Exerc* 43:1334–1359, 2011

Hansen D, Dendale P, Jonkers RA, Beelen M, Manders RJ, Corluy L, Mullens A, Berger J, Meeusen R, van Loon LJ: Continuous low- to moderate-intensity exercise training is as effective as moderate- to high-intensity exercise training at lowering blood HbA(1c) in obese type 2 diabetes patients. *Diabetologia* 52:1789–1797, 2009

Haskell WL, Lee IM, Pate RR, Powell KE, Blair SN, Franklin BA, Macera CA, Heath GW, Thompson PD, Bauman A: Physical activity and public health: updated recommendation for adults from the American College of Sports Medicine and the American Heart Association. *Med Sci Sports Exerc* 39:1423–1434, 2007

Hawley JA, Lessard SJ: Exercise training-induced improvements in insulin action. *Acta Physiol (Oxf)* 192:127–135, 2008

Houmard JA, Tanner CJ, Slentz CA, Duscha BD, McCartney JS, Kraus WE: Effect of the volume and intensity of exercise training on insulin sensitivity. *J Appl Physiol* 96:101–106, 2004

Jakicic JM, Marcus BH, Gallagher KI, Napolitano M, Lang W: Effect of exercise duration and intensity on weight loss in overweight, sedentary women: a randomized trial. *JAMA* 290:1323–1330, 2003

Johnson ST, Boulé NG, Bell GJ, Bell RC: Walking: a matter of quantity and quality physical activity for type 2 diabetes management. *Appl Physiol Nutr Metab* 33:797–801, 2008

Johnson ST, McCargar LJ, Bell GJ, Tudor-Locke C, Harber VJ, Bell RC: Walking faster: distilling a complex prescription for type 2 diabetes management through pedometry. *Diabetes Care* 29:1654–1655, 2006

Levine JA, McCrady SK, Lanningham-Foster LM, Kane PH, Foster RC, Manohar CU: The role of free-living daily walking in human weight gain and obesity. *Diabetes* 57:548–554, 2008

Levine JA, Lanningham-Foster LM, McCrady SK, Krizan AC, Olson LR, Kane PH, Jensen MD, Clark MM: Interindividual variation in posture allocation: possible role in human obesity. *Science* 307:584–586, 2005

Nelson ME, Rejeski WJ, Blair SN, Duncan PW, Judge JO, King AC, Macera CA, Castaneda-Sceppa C: Physical activity and public health in older adults: recommendation from the American College of Sports Medicine and the American Heart Association. *Med Sci Sports Exerc* 39:1435–1445, 2007

O'Donovan G, Kearney EM, Nevill AM, Woolf-May K, Bird SR: The effects of 24 weeks of moderate- or high-intensity exercise on insulin resistance. *Eur J Appl Physiol* 95:522–528, 2005

Physical Activity Guidelines Advisory Committee: Physical Activity Guidelines Advisory Committee Report, 2008. Washington, DC, U.S. Department of Health and Human Services, 2008

Ross R, Dagnone D, Jones PJ, Smith H, Paddags A, Hudson R, Janssen I: Reduction in obesity and related comorbid conditions after diet-induced weight loss or exercise-induced weight loss in men. A randomized, controlled trial. *Ann Intern Med* 133:92–103, 2000

Ross R, Janssen I, Dawson J, Kungl AM, Kuk JL, Wong SL, Nguyen-Duy TB, Lee S, Kilpatrick K, Hudson R: Exercise-induced reduction in obesity and insulin resistance in women: a randomized controlled trial. *Obesity Research* 12:789–798, 2004

Sigal RJ, Kenny GP, Boulé NG, Wells GA, Prud'homme D, Fortier M, Reid RD, Tulloch H, Coyle D, Phillips P, Jennings A, Jaffey J: Effects of aerobic training, resistance training, or both on glycemic control in type 2 diabetes: a randomized trial. *Ann Intern Med* 147:357–369, 2007

Sigal RJ, Kenny GP, Wasserman DH, Castaneda-Sceppa C, White RD: Physical activity/exercise and type 2 diabetes: a consensus statement from the American Diabetes Association. *Diabetes Care* 29:1433–1438, 2006

Sigal RJ, Kenny GP, Wasserman DH, Castaneda-Sceppa C: Physical activity/exercise and type 2 diabetes. *Diabetes Care* 27:2518–2539, 2004

Winnick JJ, Sherman WM, Habash DL, Stout MB, Failla ML, Belury MA, Schuster DP: Short-term aerobic exercise training in obese humans with type 2 diabetes mellitus improves whole-body insulin sensitivity through gains in peripheral, not hepatic insulin sensitivity. *J Clin Endocrinol Metab* 93:771–778, 2008

Chapter 5

Aerobic Exercise Rx for Type 2 Diabetes

Although physical activity is a key element in type 2 diabetes (T2D) management, many people with this chronic disease do not become or remain regularly active (Morrato 2007). Many high-quality studies done to date have established that participation in regular physical activity improves blood glucose control, blood lipids, blood pressure, cardiovascular risk, mortality risk, and quality of life. Acute and chronic improvements in insulin action with aerobic exercise training are primarily responsible for the enhanced glycemic control (King 1995; Boulé 2001, 2005; O'Gorman 2006).

The treatment goal for individuals with T2D is to achieve and maintain optimal blood glucose, lipid, and blood pressure levels to prevent or delay chronic complications of diabetes (American Diabetes Association 2013). Many people with T2D can achieve blood glucose control using the combination of a nutritious meal plan, regular exercise participation, modest weight loss, and medication use (U.S. Department of Health and Human Services 2011). Lifestyle changes that include dietary improvements and regular physical activity are central to diabetes management. When medications are used to control T2D, they should augment lifestyle improvements, not replace them.

Case in Point: Aerobic Exercise Rx for a Typical Older Adult with T2D

DG is a 58-year-old man who has had T2D for at least a decade. Although he golfs for 2–3 h most weekends and does some yard work on occasion, it has been at least 5 years since he has engaged in any structured physical activity, even just regular walking. His motivation to start doing more physical activity comes from the fact that his A1C levels have started creeping up over time, along with his body weight. His doctor put him on exenatide within the past year (in addition to metformin, which he has been on since being diagnosed), but it has only helped him to lose ~10 lb since he started using it. He admits that his job is stressful and that he often puts in long hours that are mostly sedentary in nature (due to lots of meetings and document preparation).

Resting Measurements

Height: 70 inches
Weight: 245 lb
BMI: 35.1 (obese)

Heart rate: 77 beats per minute (bpm)
Blood pressure: 135/85 mmHg (on medication)

Fasting Labs

Plasma glucose: 108 mg/dl (controlled with metformin and exenatide)
A1C: 6.9%
Total cholesterol: 155 mg/dl (on medication)
Triglycerides: 85 mg/dl
High-density lipoprotein cholesterol: 52 mg/dl
Low-density lipoprotein cholesterol: 86 mg/dl

Questions to Consider

1. What type of aerobic exercise should DG consider doing to help lower his blood glucose and his body weight?
2. What exercise frequency, intensity, and duration should DG focus on?
3. How should his exercise training progress over time?
4. Are any precautions needed for DG when he exercises?

(Continued on page 67.)

ACUTE AND CHRONIC METABOLIC AND PSYCHOLOGICAL EFFECTS OF PHYSICAL ACTIVITY

Engaging in physical activity facilitates glucose uptake, improves insulin sensitivity, and aids in glucose homeostasis, with effects that lower blood glucose levels for 2–72 h after the last bout of activity, depending on exercise duration, intensity, and subsequent food intake (King 1995; Boulé 2001, 2005; O'Gorman 2006). Exercised skeletal muscles continue to take up more blood glucose during the ensuing rest period, with the contraction-mediated pathway persisting for several hours (Ivy 1981, Garetto 1984) and insulin-mediated uptake for longer (Richter 1982, Cartee 1989, King 1995, Bajpeyi 2009). Given that these effects are short in duration, remaining physically active is an essential component of diabetes self-management behavior for all individuals with T2D.

ACUTE EFFECTS OF AN EXERCISE SESSION

Low to moderate physical activity. In individuals with T2D exercising moderately, muscular uptake of blood glucose usually rises more than hepatic glucose production, and blood glucose levels decline over the course of the activity (Minuk 1981). At the same time, plasma insulin levels fall, making the risk of exercise-induced hypoglycemia low, as long as someone is not taking insulin or insulin secretagogues (Koivisto 1984). Muscular contractions increase blood glucose uptake to supplement muscular glycogen use (Ploug 1984, Richter 1985). As this uptake pathway is contraction induced and distinct from the one triggered by the binding of insulin to a cell surface receptor (Khayat 2002), glucose uptake into working muscle is normal even when insulin-mediated uptake is impaired (as it usually is in T2D) (Colberg 1996, Zierath 1996, Braun 2004). The glucose-lowering effects of acute moderate aerobic exercise are similar whether the physical activity is performed in a single session or multiple bouts with the same total duration (Baynard 2005).

Glucose production also shifts from hepatic glycogenolysis to enhanced gluconeogenesis as exercise duration increases (Suh 2007, Wahren 2007).

Blood glucose reductions during any physical activity are related to the duration and intensity of the exercise, pre-exercise control, and state of physical training (Colberg 1996, Boulé 2001, Boulé 2005, Sigal 2007). Although prior physical activity of any intensity generally enhances uptake of circulating glucose for glycogen synthesis (Christ-Roberts 2003, Galbo 2007) and stimulates fat oxidation and storage in muscle (Duncan 2003, Goodpaster 2003, Boon 2007), more prolonged or intense activity acutely enhances insulin action for longer periods of time (Braun 1995, Larsen 1999, Houmard 2004, Evans 2005, Sigal 2007, Bajpeyi 2009). Acute improvements in insulin sensitivity in women with T2D have been found for equivalent energy expenditures whether engaging in low-intensity or high-intensity walking (Braun 1995). Moreover, a single 45 min session of either endurance-type exercise (done at 50% of maximum workload capacity) or resistance work (done at 75% of one-repetition maximum) substantially reduces the prevalence of hyperglycemia during the subsequent 24 h period in individuals with insulin-treated and non–insulin-treated T2D (van Dijk 2012b). These benefits are available even when glycemic control is closer to optimal to start with, as demonstrated in adults with well-controlled T2D (A1C level below 7.0%) who still achieved a 28% reduction in the prevalence of hyperglycemia over the 24 h period following a single bout of moderate-intensity aerobic exercise (van Dijk 2012a). While moderate and vigorous aerobic training improve insulin sensitivity more, a lesser intensity still improves insulin action to some degree (Houmard 2004).

Vigorous physical activity. During brief, intense aerobic exercise, plasma catecholamine levels rise markedly, driving a major increase in blood glucose production (Marliss 2002). As a consequence, hyperglycemia can result and persist for up to 1–2 h, likely because plasma catecholamine levels and glucose production do not return to normal immediately with cessation of the intense activity (Marliss 2002). Exercise fuel use is most affected by the intensity of the activity, with harder workouts causing a greater reliance on carbohydrates as a fuel (Sigal 1994, Braun 1995, Colberg 1996, Kang 1996, Larsen 1999, Manetta 2002, Houmard 2004, Galbo 2007, Bajpeyi 2009). Doing any activity, even a lower-intensity one, causes a shift from predominant reliance on free fatty acids at rest to a blend of fat, glucose, and muscle glycogen, with minimal use of amino acids (Bergman 1999, Burke 1999). More carbohydrate is used during intense activity, as long as sufficient amounts are available in muscle or blood (Colberg 1996, Kang 1996, Borghouts 2002, Boon 2007). Early in exercise, muscular glycogen stores provide the bulk of the fuel for working muscles, but during prolonged activities, as glycogen becomes depleted, muscles increase their uptake and use of circulating blood glucose and free fatty acids released from adipose tissue (Bergman 1999, Kang 1999, Watt 2002). Intramuscular lipid stores are more readily used during longer-duration activities and during recovery from intense activities (Borghouts 2002, Pruchnic 2004, Wang 2009).

CHRONIC EFFECTS OF AEROBIC TRAINING

Many long-term studies demonstrate a sustained improvement in glucose control when a regular aerobic training program is maintained (Kirwan 2000, Christ-

Roberts 2004, Holten 2004, O'Gorman 2006, Zoppini 2006, Wang 2009). Such training exerts its beneficial effects primarily through increased insulin sensitivity (Boulé 2001, 2005). Studies have shown that structured exercise training that consists of aerobic exercise, resistance training, or a combination of both is associated with A1C reduction in individuals with T2D (Umpierre 2011). It also may be necessary to combine physical activity advice with dietary advice to most effectively lower glycemic levels (Umpierre 2011). In addition to glycemic benefits, chronic training appears to help with loss and maintenance of body weight and reduction of cardiovascular risk factors (Holten 2004, Zoppini 2006, Wang 2009).

There appears to be a graded dose-response relationship between the aerobic exercise training dose (a product of exercise intensity, duration, and frequency) and improvements in insulin sensitivity (Dubé 2012). In one study, exercise intensity has been shown to be significantly related to improvements in insulin sensitivity, whereas frequency may not be, at least in 55 healthy adults undergoing 16 weeks of supervised endurance training (three to five sessions lasting 45 min/week, with three sessions supervised). Others have shown that engaging in structured exercise training of >150 min/week results in greater glycemic benefits than ≤150 min, so the total exercise dose may be important (Umpierre 2011).

Even 1 week of aerobic training can improve whole-body insulin sensitivity in individuals with T2D, however (Winnick 2008). Training apparently enhances the responsiveness of skeletal muscles to insulin with increased expression or activity of proteins involved in glucose metabolism and insulin signaling (Christ-Roberts 2004, Holten 2004, O'Gorman 2006, Wang 2009). Moderate training may increase glycogen synthase activity and GLUT4 (glucose transporter) protein expression, but not insulin signaling (Christ-Roberts 2004). Fat oxidation is also a key aspect of improved insulin action, and exercise training increases lipid storage in muscle and fat oxidation capacity (Duncan 2003, Goodpaster 2003, Pruchnic 2004, Kelley 2007). Moreover, mitochondrial dysfunction is apparent only in inactive longstanding T2D, which suggests that mitochondrial function and insulin resistance do not depend on each other. Prolonged exercise training can, at least partly, reverse the mitochondrial impairments associated with long-term diabetes (van Tienen 2012).

Recently, low-volume, high-intensity training (HIT) was shown to rapidly improve glucose control and induce adaptations in skeletal muscle that are linked to improved metabolic health in subjects with T2D (Little 2011). In that study, subjects were involved in 2 weeks of thrice-weekly exercise that consisted of a total 10 min of exercise (ten 60 s sessions separated by 1 min of rest) done at 90% of maximal HR. That training reduced their blood glucose levels by 13% over the 24 h period following training, as well as postprandial glucose spikes for several days afterward. Given the intensity of such training, however, each individual's fitness level and cardiovascular risk factors should be carefully considered before HIT is prescribed.

PSYCHOLOGICAL BENEFITS OF PHYSICAL ACTIVITY

Exercise likely has psychological benefits for diabetic individuals, although evidence for acute and chronic psychological benefits is limited. In the Look AHEAD (Action for Health in Diabetes) trial, participants in the intensive lifestyle intervention attempted to lose >7% of their initial weight and increase moderate physical activity participation to >175 min/week. They had improvements in health-related (SF-36 physical component scores) quality-of-life and depression symptoms after 12 months that were mediated by enhanced physical fitness (Williamson 2009). When individuals undertake exercise to prevent a chronic disease, however, they fare better psychologically than those who undertake it to manage an existing health problem. Although psychological well-being is improved among individuals who exercise for disease prevention, it deteriorates when undertaken for management of diagnosed cardiovascular disease, end-stage renal disease, pulmonary disease, neurological disorders, and cancer (Gillison 2009). Thus, the benefits of physical activity participation may vary, with individuals starting these activities with fewer existing health complications benefiting the most.

Both short- and long-term exercise participation result in substantial decreases in depressive symptoms in individuals of all ages (Craft 2004) and in clinical depression and depressive symptoms among the elderly (Sjosten 2006). Potential mechanisms include increased self-efficacy, a sense of mastery, distraction, and changes in self-concept, as well as physiological factors like increased central norepinephrine transmission, changes in the hypothalamic adrenocortical system (Droste 2003), serotonin synthesis and metabolism (Dishman 1997), and endorphin release. In any case, regular physical activity participation may improve psychological well-being, health-related quality of life, and depression in individuals with T2D, among whom depression is more common than in the general population (Egede 2003).

Case in Point: Continued

A more thorough discussion with DG reveals that his biggest barrier to doing structured physical activities is a perceived lack of time during the day and the workweek. He is willing to commit, however, to going 3 days/week to a local gym, either at lunchtime or on his way home from work in the evening. Any more than that, however, he has already decided will not fit into his busy work schedule, and he is not willing to do anything on the weekends except for golfing. Also, one of his knees bothers him from time to time (from an old, college football injury), although he ambulates well most of the time without any problems.

Additional Questions to Consider

1. What type of aerobic exercise should DG consider doing that would fit into his thrice-weekly schedule of structured activities?
2. What exercise intensity, frequency, and duration should DG focus on with only 3 days a week of structured exercise?
3. How should his exercise training progress over time, given his stated time and other constraints?
4. Are any precautions needed for DG when he exercises, particularly with regard to his occasional knee issues?

(Continued on page 71.)

AEROBIC EXERCISE PRESCRIPTION FOR T2D

MODE

Any form of aerobic exercise (including brisk walking) that utilizes large muscle groups and causes sustained increases in heart rate is likely to be beneficial for blood glucose levels and cardiovascular risk management in individuals with T2D (Hu 2001), and undertaking a variety of modes of physical activity is recommended to optimize training effects and lower injury risk (Physical Activity Guidelines Advisory Committee 2008). Examples of acceptable aerobic activities include both weight-bearing and non–weight-bearing ones, including walking, jogging, running, cycling, swimming, water aerobics, aquatic activities, conditioning machines, dancing, chair exercises, rowing, and cross-country skiing, among others. When choosing exercise modes for older and deconditioned individuals in particular, be mindful that walking and moderate-intensity physical activities are associated with a very low risk of musculoskeletal complications, whereas jogging, running, and competitive sports are associated with increased risk of injury (Garber 2011).

INTENSITY

For optimal fitness gains, aerobic exercise should be at least at a moderate intensity, or 40–59% of heart rate reserve (HRR, as discussed in chapter 4), although vigorous-intensity exercise, defined as 60–89% HRR, is likely to confer greater gains in fitness (Garber 2011, Physical Activity Guidelines Advisory Committee 2008). A severely deconditioned person can start as low as 30% HRR and progress from there to higher moderate levels over time. However, doing even 60 min of low-intensity work (30–39%) can improve blood glucose levels over 24 h in individuals with diabetes, maybe even more so than engaging in only 30 min of high-intensity exercise (Manders 2010).

Using subjective ratings, moderate- to vigorous-intensity exercise corresponds to an overall body rating of "somewhat hard" to "hard" (Garber 2011). Less fit people generally require a higher level of effort to complete the same activity, and their initial subjective intensity may need to be lower than "somewhat hard." Subjective intensity can be estimated using a scale of 0 to 10, where resting is 0, maximal effort 10, moderate-intensity activity 5–6, and vigorous-intensity activity 7–8 on that scale (Physical Activity Guidelines Advisory Committee 2008).

For most people with T2D, brisk walking is a moderate-intensity exercise due to their lower cardiorespiratory fitness capacity (Boulé 2003). Including some faster intervals, such as pick-up-the-pace training that involves exercising at even 10% above a person's normal walking or other exercise intensity, can lead to additional fitness gains in individuals with T2D (Johnson 2006, 2008). Greater cardiovascular protection and other benefits may be gained from engaging in vigorous exercise, however, especially if individuals already have a fairly high fitness level or greater physical activity participation. A recent meta-analysis showed that exercise intensity predicts improvements in overall blood glucose control to a greater extent than exercise volume, suggesting that those already fit enough to exercise at a moderate intensity should consider undertaking some vigorous physical activity, at least on occasion, to obtain additional glycemic and cardiovascular benefits (Boulé 2003).

FREQUENCY

Aerobic exercise should be performed at least 3 days/week with no more than 2 consecutive days between bouts of activity due to the short-lived nature of improvements in insulin action (King 1995, Boulé 2005). Most exercise interventions in T2D have used a frequency of three times per week (Boulé 2001, Snowling 2006, Thomas 2006, Sigal 2007), but current guidelines for adults generally recommend five sessions of moderate activity (Haskell 2007, Nelson 2007, Physical Activity Guidelines Advisory Committee 2008). Recently, a study involving adults with diabetes required them to engage in either 30 min of daily, moderate-intensity aerobic activity or 60 min of similar-intensity exercise every other day (van Dijk 2012c). Although both trials substantially reduced the prevalence of hyperglycemia throughout the subsequent day, with total work matched, daily exercise did not lead to further improvements in glycemic control compared with exercise done every other day. The recommended frequency, therefore, is a minimum of 3–5 days/week, with equal caloric expenditure regardless of how many days physical activity is undertaken.

DURATION

Individuals with T2D should engage in a minimum of 150 min/week of exercise undertaken at moderate intensity or greater. Aerobic activity should be performed in bouts of at least 10 min and should be spread throughout the week. Around 150 min/week of moderate-intensity exercise is associated with reduced morbidity and mortality in observational studies in all populations (Physical Activity Guidelines Advisory Committee 2008); however, not all health benefits of physical activity occur at 150 min/week, and engaging in less than this amount still benefits deconditioned individuals. As an individual person moves from 150 min/week toward 300 min (5 h) a week, he or she usually gains additional health benefits. The risk of musculoskeletal injury does rise with increasing exercise durations beyond the recommended amounts, but the type and intensity of the exercise are likely more important factors in the incidence of injury, with the volume of exercise (i.e., total work done or calorie expenditure through activities of varying duration, frequency, or intensity) apparently having less importance (Garber 2011).

Most studies in T2D populations have employed durations of 135–150 min/week of activity (Boulé 2001, Snowling 2006, Thomas 2006), even those that included higher-intensity aerobic exercise (Mourier 1997). Unfortunately, most people with T2D lack a sufficient aerobic capacity to work out vigorously enough to meet federal and other physical activity guidelines that allow for a shorter duration of vigorous work (Haskell 2007, Nelson 2007, Physical Activity Guidelines Advisory Committee 2008, Garber 2011). In a meta-analysis, the mean maximal aerobic capacity in diabetic individuals was only 22.4 ml/kg/min (6.4 metabolic equivalents [METs]), making their highest sustainable intensity only a moderate one in absolute terms (i.e., 4.8 METs, or 75% of maximal) (Boulé 2003). Accordingly, most diabetic individuals will require at least 150 min of moderate to vigorous aerobic exercise per week to achieve optimal cardiovascular disease risk reduction, although some glycemic and other health benefits are likely attained from lower exercise doses. Individuals with higher aerobic capacities may be able to exercise at a higher intensity for less time to gain the same benefits.

PROGRESSION

Deconditioned individuals need to start out on the low end of the intensity scale and work toward gradual progression of both exercise intensity and volume to minimize the risk of injury or noncompliance, particularly if health complications are present (Physical Activity Guidelines Advisory Committee 2008). Initially, their focus should be on increasing frequency and duration of the exercise rather than intensity. Progression over 4–6 months usually has an ultimate goal of inclusion of vigorous aerobic exercise, but for many with T2D, doing moderate-intensity workouts may be an appropriate endpoint (although frequency and duration may progress over time). See Table 5.1 for a summary of these exercise prescription recommendations for individuals with T2D.

If weight loss is a major goal, a greater duration of exercise may be required to maximize caloric expenditure. The most successful weight-control programs involve combinations of exercise, diet, and behavior modification, and people who successfully maintain a large weight loss report exercising ~7 h/week (Pavlou 1989, Schoeller 1997, Weinsier 2002, Saris 2003, Donnelly 2009).

Table 5.1 Recommended Aerobic Exercise Rx for Type 2 Diabetes

Mode	Walking, jogging, cycling, swimming, rowing, aquatic activities, seated exercises, dancing, conditioning machines, and more
Intensity	40–89% HRR (initial intensity may need to be lower, such as 30–39% or light intensity, for sedentary, deconditioned, or overweight individuals)
	Perceived exertion of "somewhat hard" to "hard" (but possibly easier initial intensity only for sedentary, deconditioned, or overweight individuals)
Frequency	3–7 days/week (including structured and lifestyle activity)
	No more than 2 consecutive days without any activity
Duration	30–60 min daily, with minimum of 10 min/session
	At least 150 min/week of moderate- to vigorous-intensity activity
Progression	Start out on the "low" side and progress slowly over weeks to months
	Increase duration and frequency first, intensity last (with the possible exception of adding in faster intervals during exercise sessions)

HRR, heart rate reserve.

Case in Point: Wrap-Up

Because DG has been mostly inactive for a while, he should start with an initial exercise prescription that allows him to start "low" and progress slowly to avoid injury and to prevent his knee irritation from returning. Another important aspect of his program will be to increase his unstructured daily movement throughout the day, particularly on days that he does not plan to work out in the gym doing his structured program.

Exercise Program Goals

Mode of Activity: Given DG's potential for knee issues, his recommended activities to start include stationary cycling, walking on a treadmill, and use of other conditioning machines that are lower impact (such as cross-trainers and elliptical machines).

Intensity: DG should attempt to work up to maintaining a workout pace that feels "somewhat hard" to start, possibly "hard" when he begins to feel more conditioned. On the conditioning machines, he can choose "interval" programs that intersperse harder intervals with easier intervals to gain the most fitness with the least amount of training time. His initial target heart rate should be in the range of 104 to 130 bpm (30–59% HRR), with a later training goal of at least 131 bpm (60% of HRR) due to his limited time in the gym.

Frequency: Because DG has stated that he can only go to the gym 3 days/week, his goal should be to schedule his structured training on 3 nonconsecutive days while increasing his unstructured activities (including golfing) on the other 4 days. In any case, he should avoid letting >2 days lapse without some sustained aerobic activities to optimize his blood glucose management.

Duration: When beginning his exercise program, DG should engage in shorter bouts of exercise training, separated by a rest period, until he can train continuously for 30–60 min. His ultimate training goal is 150 min of physical activity spread throughout the week.

Progression: DG should be advised to focus on increasing the duration of his structured workouts on 3 nonconsecutive days/week to attempt to achieve 150 min/week of moderate or vigorous exercise. Once he has established higher levels of physical fitness, he may choose to do combination training that includes some resistance training on at least 2 of his exercise training days.

Daily Movement: Because of DG's perceived time limitations and to assist with his weight loss, he should attempt to engage in more daily movement, including fidgeting (such as bouncing or swinging one's leg repeatedly while seated), standing, and taking more steps. On days that he has no planned exercise schedule, he should attempt to maximize his unstructured activities throughout the day.

Possible Precautions: Because DG has quite a few risk factors for cardiovascular disease (including elevated lipids, hypertension, diabetes, and obesity), he should consider having a checkup with his doctor and possibly having an exercise stress test before starting regular exercise, to determine his initial fitness level, if nothing else, although neither one is absolutely required before his participation in moderate activities like brisk walking. His medications (metformin and exenatide) should not have any effect on his blood glucose responses to exercise or increase his risk for hypoglycemia, but he should be advised to occasionally monitor his responses to bouts of activity as reductions in glucose levels resulting from exercise can be motivating for many individuals.

People with T2D should embrace lifestyle changes that include regular physical activity to maximize their blood glucose management and lower their cardiovascular disease risk. Engaging in physical activity facilitates glucose uptake, improves insulin sensitivity, and aids in glucose homeostasis, with effects that lower blood glucose levels for 2–72 h after the last bout of activity, depending on exercise duration, intensity, and subsequent food intake. Current recommendations for adults with T2D suggest that such individuals should engage in at least 150 min a week of moderate to vigorous aerobic exercise spread out over at least 3 days during the week, with no more than 2 consecutive days between bouts of aerobic activity.

PROFESSIONAL PRACTICE PEARLS

- Participation in regular physical activity improves blood glucose control, blood lipids, blood pressure, cardiovascular risk, mortality risk, and quality of life in T2D.
- Given that improvements in insulin action that enhance blood glucose control are short lived, aerobic exercise participation should be regular.
- Although moderate and vigorous aerobic training improve insulin sensitivity more, a lower intensity still improves insulin action to some degree.
- Glucose-lowering effects of moderate aerobic exercise are similar whether the physical activity is performed in a single session or in multiple bouts with the same total duration.
- Participation in vigorous exercise may cause a transient increase in blood glucose levels that can last for several hours due to the release of glucose-raising hormones.
- Individuals with T2D should undertake at least 150 min a week of moderate to vigorous aerobic exercise spread out over at least 3 days during the week, with no more than 2 consecutive days between bouts of aerobic activity.
- Most people with T2D lack a sufficient aerobic capacity to work out vigorously enough to meet physical activity guidelines that allow for a lesser duration of vigorous work.
- Each individual's fitness level and cardiovascular risk factors should be carefully considered before prescribing low-volume, high-intensity interval training.
- Progress by increasing physical activity gradually over time whenever more activity is necessary to meet guidelines or health goals; inactive individuals

should "start low and go slow" by gradually increasing how often and how long activities are done.

■ Individuals who successfully maintain a large weight loss report exercising about 7 h/week.

REFERENCES

American Diabetes Association: Standards of medical care in diabetes—2013. *Diabetes Care* 36 (Suppl. 1):S11–S66, 2013

Bajpeyi S, Tanner CJ, Slentz CA, Duscha BD, McCartney JS, Hickner RC, Kraus WE, Houmard JA: Effect of exercise intensity and volume on persistence of insulin sensitivity during training cessation. *J Appl Physiol* 106:1079–1085, 2009

Baynard T, Franklin RM, Goulopoulou S, Carhart R Jr, Kanaley JA: Effect of a single vs multiple bouts of exercise on glucose control in women with type 2 diabetes. *Metabolism* 54:989–994, 2005

Bergman BC, Butterfield GE, Wolfel EE, Casazza GA, Lopaschuk GD, Brooks GA: Evaluation of exercise and training on muscle lipid metabolism. *Am J Physiol* 276:E106–E17, 1999

Boon H, Blaak EE, Saris WH, Keizer HA, Wagenmakers AJ, van Loon LJ: Substrate source utilisation in long-term diagnosed type 2 diabetes patients at rest, and during exercise and subsequent recovery. *Diabetologia* 50:103–112, 2007

Borghouts LB, Wagenmakers AJ, Goyens PL, Keizer HA: Substrate utilization in non-obese Type II diabetic patients at rest and during exercise. *Clin Sci (Lond)* 103:559–566, 2002

Boulé NG, Weisnagel SJ, Lakka TA, Tremblay A, Bergman RN, Rankinen T, Leon AS, Skinner JS, Wilmore JH, Rao DC, Bouchard C: Effects of exercise training on glucose homeostasis: the HERITAGE Family Study. *Diabetes Care* 28:108–114, 2005

Boulé NG, Kenny GP, Haddad E, Wells GA, Sigal RJ: Meta-analysis of the effect of structured exercise training on cardiorespiratory fitness in type 2 diabetes mellitus. *Diabetologia* 46:1071–1081, 2003

Boulé NG, Haddad E, Kenny GP, Wells GA, Sigal RJ: Effects of exercise on glycemic control and body mass in type 2 diabetes mellitus: a meta-analysis of controlled clinical trials. *JAMA* 286:1218–1227, 2001

Braun B, Sharoff C, Chipkin SR, Beaudoin F: Effects of insulin resistance on substrate utilization during exercise in overweight women. *J Appl Physiol* 97:991–997, 2004

Braun B, Zimmermann MB, Kretchmer N: Effects of exercise intensity on insulin sensitivity in women with non-insulin-dependent diabetes mellitus. *J Appl Physiol* 78:300–306, 1995

Burke LM, Hawley JA: Carbohydrate and exercise. *Curr Opin Clin Nutr Metab Care* 2:515–520, 1999

Cartee GD, Young DA, Sleeper MD, Zierath J, Wallberg-Henriksson H, Holloszy JO: Prolonged increase in insulin-stimulated glucose transport in muscle after exercise. *Am J Physiol* 256:E494–E499, 1989

Christ-Roberts CY, Pratipanawatr T, Pratipanawatr W, Berria R, Belfort R, Kashyap S, Mandarino LJ: Exercise training increases glycogen synthase activity and GLUT4 expression but not insulin signaling in overweight non-diabetic and type 2 diabetic subjects. *Metabolism* 53:1233–1242, 2004

Christ-Roberts CY, Pratipanawatr T, Pratipanawatr W, Berria R, Belfort R, Mandarino LJ: Increased insulin receptor signaling and glycogen synthase activity contribute to the synergistic effect of exercise on insulin action. *J Appl Physiol* 95:2519–2529, 2003

Colberg SR, Hagberg JM, McCole SD, Zmuda JM, Thompson PD, Kelley DE: Utilization of glycogen but not plasma glucose is reduced in individuals with NIDDM during mild-intensity exercise. *J Appl Physiol* 81:2027–2033, 1996

Craft LL, Perna FM: The benefits of exercise for the clinically depressed. *Prim Care Companion J Clin Psychiatry* 6:104–111, 2004

Dishman RK, Renner KJ, Youngstedt SD, Reigle TG, Bunnell BN, Burke KA, Yoo HS, Mougey EH, Meyerhoff JL: Activity wheel running reduces escape latency and alters brain monoamine levels after footshock. *Brain Res Bull* 42:399–406, 1997

Donnelly JE, Blair SN, Jakicic JM, Manore MM, Rankin JW, Smith BK: American College of Sports Medicine Position Stand: appropriate physical activity intervention strategies for weight loss and prevention of weight regain for adults. *Med Sci Sports Exerc* 41:459–471, 2009

Droste SK, Gesing A, Ulbricht S, Muller MB, Linthorst AC, Reul JM: Effects of long-term voluntary exercise on the mouse hypothalamic-pituitary-adreno-cortical axis. *Endocrinology* 144:3012–2023, 2003

Dubé JJ, Allison KF, Rousson V, Goodpaster BH, Amati F: Exercise dose and insulin sensitivity: relevance for diabetes prevention. *Med Sci Sports Exerc* 44:793–799, 2012

Duncan GE, Perri MG, Theriaque DW, Hutson AD, Eckel RH, Stacpoole PW: Exercise training, without weight loss, increases insulin sensitivity and pos-theparin plasma lipase activity in previously sedentary adults. *Diabetes Care* 26:557–562, 2003

Egede LE, Zheng D: Independent factors associated with major depressive disorder in a national sample of individuals with diabetes. *Diabetes Care* 26:104–111, 2003

Evans EM, Racette SB, Peterson LR, Villareal DT, Greiwe JS, Holloszy JO: Aerobic power and insulin action improve in response to endurance exercise training in healthy 77-87 yr olds. *J Appl Physiol* 98:40–45, 2005

Galbo H, Tobin L, van Loon LJ: Responses to acute exercise in type 2 diabetes, with an emphasis on metabolism and interaction with oral hypoglycemic agents and food intake. *Appl Physiol Nutr Metab* 32:567–575, 2007

Garber CE, Blissmer B, Deschenes MR, Franklin BA, Lamonte MJ, Lee IM, Nieman DC, Swain DP, American College of Sports Medicine: American College of Sports Medicine position stand. Quantity and quality of exercise for developing and maintaining cardiorespiratory, musculoskeletal, and neuromotor fitness in apparently healthy adults: guidance for prescribing exercise. *Med Sci Sports Exerc* 43:1334–1359, 2011

Garetto LP, Richter EA, Goodman MN, Ruderman NB: Enhanced muscle glucose metabolism after exercise in the rat: the two phases. *Am J Physiol* 246:E471–E475, 1984

Gillison FB, Skevington SM, Sato A, Standage M, Evangelidou S: The effects of exercise interventions on quality of life in clinical and healthy populations; a meta-analysis. *Soc Sci Med* 68:1700–1710, 2009

Goodpaster BH, Katsiaras A, Kelley DE: Enhanced fat oxidation through physical activity is associated with improvements in insulin sensitivity in obesity. *Diabetes* 52:2191–2197, 2003

Haskell WL, Lee IM, Pate RR, Powell KE, Blair SN, Franklin BA, Macera CA, Heath GW, Thompson PD, Bauman A: Physical activity and public health: updated recommendation for adults from the American College of Sports Medicine and the American Heart Association. *Med Sci Sports Exerc* 39:1423–1434, 2007

Holten MK, Zacho M, Gaster M, Juel C, Wojtaszewski JF, Dela F: Strength training increases insulin-mediated glucose uptake, GLUT4 content, and insulin signaling in skeletal muscle in patients with type 2 diabetes. *Diabetes* 53:294–305, 2004

Houmard JA, Tanner CJ, Slentz CA, Duscha BD, McCartney JS, Kraus WE: Effect of the volume and intensity of exercise training on insulin sensitivity. *J Appl Physiol* 96:101–106, 2004

Hu FB, Stampfer MJ, Solomon C, Liu S, Colditz GA, Speizer FE, Willett WC, Manson JE: Physical activity and risk for cardiovascular events in diabetic women. *Ann Intern Med* 134:96–105, 2001

Ivy JL, Holloszy JO: Persistent increase in glucose uptake by rat skeletal muscle following exercise. *Am J Physiol* 241:C200–C203, 1981

Johnson ST, Boulé NG, Bell GJ, Bell RC: Walking: a matter of quantity and quality physical activity for type 2 diabetes management. *Appl Physiol Nutr Metab* 33:797–801, 2008

Johnson ST, McCargar LJ, Bell GJ, Tudor-Locke C, Harber VJ, Bell RC: Walking faster: distilling a complex prescription for type 2 diabetes management through pedometry. *Diabetes Care* 29:1654–1655, 2006

Kang J, Kelley DE, Robertson RJ, Goss FL, Suminski RR, Utter AC, Dasilva SG: Substrate utilization and glucose turnover during exercise of varying intensities in individuals with NIDDM. *Med Sci Sports Exerc* 31:82–89, 1999

Kang J, Robertson RJ, Hagberg JM, Kelley DE, Goss FL, DaSilva SG, Suminski RR, Utter AC: Effect of exercise intensity on glucose and insulin metabolism in obese individuals and obese NIDDM patients. *Diabetes Care* 19:341–349, 1996

Kelley GA, Kelley KS: Effects of aerobic exercise on lipids and lipoproteins in adults with type 2 diabetes: a meta-analysis of randomized-controlled trials. *Public Health* 121:643–655, 2007

Khayat ZA, Patel N, Klip A: Exercise- and insulin-stimulated muscle glucose transport: distinct mechanisms of regulation. *Can J Appl Physiol* 27:129–151, 2002

King DS, Baldus PJ, Sharp RL, Kesl LD, Feltmeyer TL, Riddle MS: Time course for exercise-induced alterations in insulin action and glucose tolerance in middle-aged people. *J Appl Physiol* 78:17–22, 1995

Kirwan JP, del Aguila LF, Hernandez JM, Williamson DL, O'Gorman DJ, Lewis R, Krishnan RK: Regular exercise enhances insulin activation of IRS-1-associated PI3-kinase in human skeletal muscle. *J Appl Physiol* 88:797–803, 2000

Koivisto V, Defronzo R: Exercise in the treatment of type II diabetes. *Acta Endocrinology* 262 (Suppl.):107–116, 1984

Larsen JJ, Dela F, Madsbad S, Galbo H: The effect of intense exercise on postprandial glucose homeostasis in type II diabetic patients. *Diabetologia* 42:1282–1292, 1999

Little JP, Gillen JB, Percival ME, Safdar A, Tarnopolsky MA, Punthakee Z, Jung ME, Gibala MJ: Low-volume high-intensity interval training reduces hyperglycemia and increases muscle mitochondrial capacity in patients with type 2 diabetes. *J Appl Physiol* 111:1554–1560, 2011

Manders RJ, Van Dijk JW, van Loon LJ: Low-intensity exercise reduces the prevalence of hyperglycemia in type 2 diabetes. *Med Sci Sports Exerc* 42:219–225, 2010

Manetta J, Brun JF, Perez-Martin A, Callis A, Prefaut C, Mercier J: Fuel oxidation during exercise in middle-aged men: role of training and glucose disposal. *Med Sci Sports Exerc* 34:423–429, 2002

Marliss EB, Vranic M: Intense exercise has unique effects on both insulin release and its roles in glucoregulation: implications for diabetes. *Diabetes* 51 (Suppl. 1):S271–S283, 2002

Minuk HL, Vranic M, Hanna AK, Albisser AM, Zinman B: Glucoregulatory and metabolic response to exercise in obese noninsulin-dependent diabetes. *Am J Physiol* 240:E458–E464, 1981

Morrato EH, Hill JO, Wyatt HR, Ghushchyan V, Sullivan PW: Physical activity in U.S. adults with diabetes and at risk for developing diabetes, 2003. *Diabetes Care* 30:203–209, 2007

Mourier A, Gautier JF, De Kerviler E, Bigard AX, Villette JM, Garnier JP, Duvallet A, Guezennec CY, Cathelineau G: Mobilization of visceral adipose tissue related to the improvement in insulin sensitivity in response to physical training in NIDDM. Effects of branched-chain amino acid supplements. *Diabetes Care* 20:385–391, 1997

Nelson ME, Rejeski WJ, Blair SN, Duncan PW, Judge JO, King AC, Macera CA, Castaneda-Sceppa C: Physical activity and public health in older adults: recommendation from the American College of Sports Medicine and the American Heart Association. *Med Sci Sports Exerc* 39:1435–1445, 2007

O'Gorman DJ, Karlsson HK, McQuaid S, Yousif O, Rahman Y, Gasparro D, Glund S, Chibalin AV, Zierath JR, Nolan JJ: Exercise training increases insulin-stimulated glucose disposal and GLUT4 (SLC2A4) protein content in patients with type 2 diabetes. *Diabetologia* 49:2983–2992, 2006

Pavlou KN, Krey S, Steffee WP: Exercise as an adjunct to weight loss and maintenance in moderately obese subjects. *Am J Clin Nutr* 49 (5 Suppl.):1115–1123, 1989

Physical Activity Guidelines Advisory Committee: Physical Activity Guidelines Advisory Committee Report, 2008. Washington, DC, U.S. Department of Health and Human Services, 2008

Ploug T, Galbo H, Richter EA: Increased muscle glucose uptake during contractions: no need for insulin. *Am J Physiol* 247:E726–E731, 1984

Pruchnic R, Katsiaras A, He J, Kelley DE, Winters C, Goodpaster BH: Exercise training increases intramyocellular lipid and oxidative capacity in older adults. *Am J Physiol Endocrinol Metab* 287:E857–E862, 2004

Richter EA, Ploug T, Galbo H: Increased muscle glucose uptake after exercise. No need for insulin during exercise. *Diabetes* 34:1041–1048, 1985

Richter EA, Garetto LP, Goodman MN, Ruderman NB: Muscle glucose metabolism following exercise in the rat: increased sensitivity to insulin. *J Clin Invest* 69:785–793, 1982

Saris WH, Blair SN, van Baak MA, Eaton SB, Davies PS, Di Pietro L, Fogelholm M, Rissanen A, Schoeller D, Swinburn B, Tremblay A, Westerterp KR, Wyatt H: How much physical activity is enough to prevent unhealthy weight gain? Outcome of the IASO 1st Stock Conference and consensus statement. *Obes Rev* 4:101–114, 2003

Schoeller DA, Shay K, Kushner RF: How much physical activity is needed to minimize weight gain in previously obese women? *Am J Clin Nutr* 66:551–556, 1997

Sigal RJ, Kenny GP, Boulé NG, Wells GA, Prud'homme D, Fortier M, Reid RD, Tulloch H, Coyle D, Phillips P, Jennings A, Jaffey J: Effects of aerobic training, resistance training, or both on glycemic control in type 2 diabetes: a random-ized trial. *Ann Intern Med* 147:357–369, 2007

Sigal RJ, Purdon C, Bilinski D, Vranic M, Halter JB, Marliss EB: Glucoregulation during and after intense exercise: effects of beta-blockade. *J Clin Endocrinol Metab* 78:359–366, 1994

Sjosten N, Kivela SL: The effects of physical exercise on depressive symptoms among the aged: a systematic review. *Int J Geriatr Psychiatry* 21:410–418, 2006

Snowling NJ, Hopkins WG: Effects of different modes of exercise training on glucose control and risk factors for complications in type 2 diabetic patients: a meta-analysis. *Diabetes Care* 29:2518–2527, 2006

Suh SH, Paik IY, Jacobs K: Regulation of blood glucose homeostasis during pro-longed exercise. *Mol Cells* 23:272–279, 2007

Thomas DE, Elliott EJ, Naughton GA: Exercise for type 2 diabetes mellitus. *Cochrane Database Syst Rev* CD002968, 2006

U.S. Department of Health and Human Services, Centers for Disease Control and Prevention: National Diabetes Fact Sheet: *National Estimates and General Information on Diabetes and Prediabetes in the United States, 2011.* Atlanta, GA, U.S. Department of Health and Human Services, Centers for Disease Control and Prevention, 2011

Umpierre D, Ribeiro PA, Kramer CK, Leitao CB, Zucatti AT, Azevedo MJ, Gross JL, Ribeiro JP, Schaan BD: Physical activity advice only or structured exercise training and association with HbA1c levels in type 2 diabetes: a systematic review and meta-analysis. *JAMA* 305:1790–1799, 2011

van Dijk JW, Manders RJ, Canfora EE, van Mechelen W, Hartgens F, Stehouwer CD, van Loon LJ: Exercise and 24-h glycemic control: Equal effects for all type 2 diabetic patients? *Med Sci Sports Exerc* [Epub ahead of print] 27 Nov 2012a

van Dijk JW, Manders RJ, Tummers K, Bonomi AG, Stehouwer CD, Hartgens F, van Loon LJ: Both resistance- and endurance-type exercise reduce the preva-lence of hyperglycaemia in individuals with impaired glucose tolerance and in insulin-treated and non-insulin-treated type 2 diabetic patients. *Diabetologia* 55:1273–1282, 2012b

van Dijk JW, Tummers K, Stehouwer CD, Hartgens F, van Loon LJ: Exercise therapy in type 2 diabetes: Is daily exercise required to optimize glycemic control? *Diabetes Care* 35:948–954, 2012c

van Tienen FH, Praet SF, de Feyter HM, van den Broek NM, Lindsey PJ, Schoonderwoerd KG, de Coo IF, Nicolay K, Prompers JJ, Smeets HJ, van Loon LJ: Physical activity is the key determinant of skeletal muscle mitochon-drial function in type 2 diabetes. *J Clin Endocrinol Metab* 97:3261–3269, 2012

Wahren J, Ekberg K: Splanchnic regulation of glucose production. *Annu Rev Nutr* 27:329–345, 2007

Wang Y, Simar D, Fiatarone Singh MA: Adaptations to exercise training within skeletal muscle in adults with type 2 diabetes or impaired glucose tolerance: a systematic review. *Diabetes Metab Res Rev* 25:13–40, 2009

Watt MJ, Heigenhauser GJ, Dyck DJ, Spriet LL: Intramuscular triacylglycerol, glycogen and acetyl group metabolism during 4 h of moderate exercise in man. *J Physiol* 541:969–978, 2002

Weinsier RL, Hunter GR, Desmond RA, Byrne NM, Zuckerman PA, Darnell BE: Free-living activity energy expenditure in women successful and unsuccessful at maintaining a normal body weight. *Am J Clin Nutr* 75:499–504, 2002

Williamson DA, Rejeski J, Lang W, Van Dorsten B, Fabricatore AN, Toledo K, Look Ahead Research Group: Impact of a weight management program on health-related quality of life in overweight adults with type 2 diabetes. *Arch Intern Med* 169:163–171, 2009

Winnick JJ, Sherman WM, Habash DL, Stout MB, Failla ML, Belury MA, Schuster DP: Short-term aerobic exercise training in obese humans with type 2 diabetes mellitus improves whole-body insulin sensitivity through gains in peripheral, not hepatic insulin sensitivity. *J Clin Endocrinol Metab* 93:771–778, 2008

Zierath JR, He L, Guma A, Odegoard Wahlstrom E, Klip A, Wallberg-Henriksson H: Insulin action on glucose transport and plasma membrane GLUT4 content in skeletal muscle from patients with NIDDM. *Diabetologia* 39:1180–1189, 1996

Zoppini G, Targher G, Zamboni C, Venturi C, Cacciatori V, Moghetti P, Muggeo M: Effects of moderate-intensity exercise training on plasma biomarkers of inflammation and endothelial dysfunction in older patients with type 2 diabetes. *Nutr Metab Cardiovasc Dis* 16:543–549, 2006

Chapter 6

Aerobic Exercise Rx for Type 1 Diabetes and Latent Autoimmune Diabetes in Adults

Many health benefits of regular physical activity are available to individuals with type 1 diabetes (T1D) or latent autoimmune diabetes in adults (LADA), regardless of their age at onset. For example, regular exercise lowers blood pressure, lipid levels, body weight, cardiovascular and mortality risk, and risk of complications while raising cardiorespiratory fitness levels, muscular strength, quality of life, and sense of well-being (Moy 1993, Laaksonen 2000, Costacou 2007, Herbst 2007, Heyman 2007, Bishop 2009, Conway 2009, Trigona 2010, D'Hooge 2011, Maahs 2011). People with T1D can have lifestyle habits (including sedentary behaviors) that lead to greater insulin resistance and "double diabetes," with symptoms of both T1D and type 2 diabetes (T2D) (Purnell 1998, Orchard 2003, Kilpatrick 2007). Although an acute bout of exercise improves insulin sensitivity in those with T1D as well, little or no improvement in glucose control has been demonstrated after regular exercise training, even though insulin doses generally decrease (Ebeling 1995, Roberts 2002, Ramalho 2006).

Case in Point: Aerobic Exercise Rx for a Young Adult with T1D

MF is a 20-year-old woman currently attending college who has had T1D since the age of 16 years. Although she has achieved reasonable control over her blood glucose levels—even though she is out of the "honeymoon period"—she has gained around 15 lb and is taking higher insulin doses than ever before to keep control over her daily glucose fluctuations. Her college classes are stressful for her this semester, and she has slacked off on doing any regular physical activity (although she rides her bike to classes and walks around a lot). Her goals are to lose the extra 15 lb she gained (her best weight is around 130 lb) and get her A1C value back below 6.5% (ideally no higher than 6.0%, though).

Resting Measurements

Height: 66 inches
Weight: 145 lb
BMI: 23.4 (in a "normal" range, but heavy for her)
Heart rate: 82 beats per minute (bpm)
Blood pressure: 125/70 mmHg

Fasting Labs

Plasma glucose: Variable (65–285 mg/dl, controlled with insulin)
A1C: 6.9%
Cholesterol: Not tested recently but has always been good in the past

Medications

Basal-bolus insulin regimen: 20 units of insulin glargine at bedtime, insulin lispro
for meals, snacks, and corrections (usually 1–6 units per injection, based on carbohydrate intake)

Questions to Consider

1. What type of aerobic exercise should MF start doing to reach her goals?
2. What would be an appropriate exercise Rx for her with regard to exercise
   intensity, frequency, and duration?
3. How should her exercise training progress over time?
4. What precautions should MF take, and does she have any exercise limitations?

(Continued on page 85.)

BENEFICIAL EFFECTS OF AEROBIC EXERCISE

Physical activity in the form of aerobic exercise should be included as part of the
diabetes self-management program for individuals with T1D. Throughout life
such individuals are fully capable of and gain many health benefits from engaging
in a physical fitness plan (Colberg 2009).

HEALTH BENEFITS OF REGULAR ACTIVITY

Appropriate diabetes regimen changes must be made if improved blood glucose management is an expected outcome of regular physical activity by these
individuals. Although regular exercise may not necessarily improve overall glycemic management, it still confers protective effects for individuals with T1D of all
ages. Sedentary behavior has been associated with poor glycemic management in
both adult and pediatric populations of T1D, even though regular exercise training has not been shown to improve glycemic control in most studies, likely due to
the difficulty associated with balancing out appropriate insulin changes and carbohydrate adjustments for exercise (Ebeling 1995, Roberts 2002, Ramalho 2006).
Nonetheless, a recent study showed that children with T1D exercising more than
two times weekly significantly improved their A1C levels and lipid profiles, suggesting that being regularly active for long periods (60 min at a time or more) is
likely beneficial and should be recommended (Aouadi 2011).

In addition to the potential health benefits of regular activity on blood pressure,
lipid levels, body weight, and risk of complications (Moy 1993, Laaksonen 2000,
Costacou 2007, Herbst 2007, Heyman 2007, Bishop 2009, Conway 2009, Trigona

2010, D'Hooge 2011, Maahs 2011), requirements for lower insulin doses that usually result from regular exercise participation are indicative of improved insulin sensitivity and—regardless of changes in glycemic levels—significantly reduce risk of all cardiovascular conditions (Trigona 2010, Seeger 2011). Youth with T1D present early signs of atherosclerosis, as well as low physical activity levels and levels of cardiorespiratory fitness, but endothelial function can be enhanced by engaging >60 min of daily moderate- to vigorous-intensity physical activity (Trigona 2010). Moreover, physical activity can offset some of the potentially negative impact of engaging in more sedentary pursuits: the glycemic impact of greater computer use on metabolic control in individuals with T1D is apparently not related to age, diabetes duration, television watching, or computer use, but rather independently and negatively related to the weekly hours spent on physical exercise (Benevento 2010).

Regular exercise even promotes longevity in people with T1D. One study reported that the 7-year mortality rate in T1D is 50% lower in individuals doing the equivalent of ~7 h a week of brisk walking (i.e., expenditure of ~2,000 kilocalories weekly) compared with <1,000 kilocalories (Moy 1993). The estimated increase in longevity resulting from regular exercise is ~10 years, which exactly counterbalances the number of years that diabetes potentially can shorten a person's life.

CARDIORESPIRATORY FITNESS

Some, but not all, individuals with T1D have the same aerobic capacity as similar-age people without diabetes. For instance, despite having a lower anaerobic threshold and lung capacity, the aerobic capacity in people with T1D doing programmed exercise has been reported to be similar to that of normal athletes (Komatsu 2010). It appears, however, that poor glycemic control impairs pulmonary, cardiac, and vascular responses to exercise (Baldi 2010b). Highly trained individuals with T1D in one study were able to achieve the same cardiopulmonary exercise responses as trained subjects without diabetes, but these responses were reduced by poor glycemic control (i.e., A1C >7.0%) (Baldi 2010a).

Mitochondrial oxidative capacity also depends on glycemic control in untrained women with T1D, although it may not be lower than in untrained healthy women (Item 2011). Others have reported that both sex and diabetes control are significantly associated with cardiorespiratory fitness, with both women and anyone with poorer glycemic control exhibiting a lower level of fitness. At this point, it is not fully clear whether reduced fitness in children and others with T1D is attributable to lower physical activity levels or to physiological changes resulting from diabetes itself (Williams 2011), although exercise training in children improves their overall physical fitness (Seeger 2011).

AEROBIC EXERCISE RESPONSES IN T1D

PHYSIOLOGICAL RESPONSES TO MODERATE PHYSICAL ACTIVITY

Fuel metabolism. Several-fold increments in hormone concentrations contribute to the maintenance of fuel and fluid homeostasis during exercise (Meinders 1988, Koivisto 1992, Galassetti 2001, Kishore 2006, Diabetes Research in Children Network Study Group 2009). When individuals with T1D exercise with normal blood glucose levels, their substrate oxidation is similar to healthy individuals who experience a shift toward lipid oxidation during extended exercise. When exercising in a hyperglycemic state, however, fuel metabolism in T1D is dominated by carbohydrate oxidation, although muscular glycogen is not spared by the greater use of blood glucose (Jenni 2008). Exercise done with higher circulating insulin levels or during insulin peak times also increases blood glucose use (and the potential for hypoglycemia to develop) without sparing muscle glycogen (Chokkalingam 2007a). Some of the additional blood glucose uptake during high-insulin conditions actually may increase glucose flux through nonoxidative pathways (i.e., into glycogen storage). Regimen changes aimed at lowering insulin levels or increasing the availability of exogenous carbohydrates likely will be necessary to counteract the normal decline in blood glucose levels during such activities. During recovery from exercise, fat use dominates, particularly following long-duration exercise and during periods of worse glycemic control (Tuominen 1997b).

Hepatic glycogen. Liver glycogen is affected by glycemic control. In nondiabetic individuals, increases in hepatic glucose production during exercise are almost entirely the result of increased hepatic glycogenolysis; in contrast, in moderately controlled people with T1D, their increased rates of glucose production both at rest and during exercise are primarily accounted for by increased gluconeogenesis (Petersen 2004). In fact, poorly controlled individuals have a marked reduction in both hepatic glycogen synthesis and breakdown, which can be improved, but not normalized, by short-term restoration of normal levels of insulin and blood glucose (Bischof 2001). High levels of insulin and blood glucose during moderate exercise, however, do not suppress hepatic glycogen concentrations (Chokkalingam 2007b).

SPECIFIC RESPONSES TO HIGH-INTENSITY TRAINING

Moderate-intensity exercise has a greater potential to result in blood glucose reductions, but undertaking more vigorous activity actually may cause a deterioration in metabolic control not fully explained by hormonal responses of glucagon or catecholamines (Mitchell 1988). One study compared the blood glucose responses to intermittent high-intensity exercise and moderate-intensity exercise in individuals with T1D (Guelfi 2005a). The high-intensity protocol consisted of 30 min of continuous moderate exercise interspersed with 4-s sprints every 2 min to simulate the activity patterns of team sports, whereas the other involved the same length of moderate activity alone. Although both exercise protocols resulted in a decline in blood glucose, the glycemic decrement was greater with the moderate activity done by itself, despite the performance of a greater amount of total work with intermittent high-intensity protocol. For 1 h, blood glucose levels remained higher following the higher-intensity workout and were associated with elevated levels of lactate, catecholamines, and growth hormone during early recovery from exercise, with no differences in free insulin, glucagon, cortisol, or free fatty acids between the activities.

Thus, intermittent high-intensity exercise does not increase the risk of early postexercise hypoglycemia in individuals with T1D (Guelfi 2005b), which likely is related to a lesser decline in glycemia during exercise (due to greater hepatic glucose output) and attenuated blood glucose uptake during exercise and early recovery (Guelfi 2007). Such training also has been shown to enhanced muscle oxidative metabolism in young adults with T1D, which may have clinically important health benefits (Harmer 2008). It also may protect against nocturnal hypoglycemia in athletes with T1D (Iscoe 2011).

Case in Point: Continued

MF reveals that she used to be on many sports teams in high school: cross-country in fall, swimming in winter, and soccer in spring. She was not talented enough to get recruited to play any sports competitively in college, but she still enjoys many different types of activities. During further discussion, MF admits that she had trouble controlling her blood glucose levels in high school once she developed T1D and that she cut way back on her training because workouts often caused her blood glucose to go too low. In fact, her biggest fear related to starting an exercise training program again is the likelihood of more frequent hypoglycemia. She currently has hypoglycemia 1–2 times/week, and she is able to treat it as soon as symptoms develop, which for her is around a blood glucose level of 55–60 mg/dl. In high school, however, she had a couple of really bad overnight lows that required medical assistance to treat.

Additional Questions to Consider

1. What steps can MF take to prevent hypoglycemia both during and after exercise, given that her concerns about developing it are valid ones?
2. Can treating hypoglycemia have any impact on the possibility of MF reaching her stated body weight goals?

(Continued on page 92.)

MAKING APPROPRIATE EXERCISE-RELATED REGIMEN CHANGES

A better understanding of the physiology of exercise with regard to fuel mobilization and other metabolic changes can suggest which problems may arise in managing diabetes during physical activity and sports participation. Any exercisers with diabetes need to be advised on appropriate diet and insulin management to maximize performance and reduce fatigue (Gallen 2011). With an appropriate adjustment of insulin dose and diet, people with T1D can even participate in competitive events and sports (Koivisto 1992). General management of blood glucose levels during and after exercise, hypoglycemia prevention and treatment, hyperglycemia and dehydration, and balancing insulin use with physical activity are all critical topics associated with exercise prescription for this group, and they are more fully discussed in chapters 11–14 of this book.

SELF-MONITORING OF BLOOD GLUCOSE

Blood glucose responses to physical activity can vary with each exercise session, depending on its duration and intensity, and diabetes regimens (namely, insulin doses and food intake) will require adjustments to keep blood glucose levels balanced. Moderate aerobic exercise usually causes blood glucose levels to drop rapidly, while higher-intensity work may cause them to rise, thereby making glycemic control challenging. Accordingly, people who engage in any physical activity will need to use self-monitoring of blood glucose (SMBG) to better understand their glucose responses to a specific exercise bout and how to make appropriate regimen changes that effectively manage blood glucose levels, keeping in mind that both exercise adaptations and blood glucose responses are specific to the type of training.

Use of continuous monitoring. A more recent technology, continuous glucose monitoring (CGM), provides frequent interstitial glucose readings over a 24 h period and may be particularly helpful for individuals with T1D attempting to establish their usual glycemic responses, trends of hypoglycemia and hyperglycemia, and exercise effects (Riddell 2009, Maran 2010). Short-term use of CGM with alarms, together with appropriate instructions for users, reduces the incidence and duration of hypoglycemia, but only to a limited extent, in part because it tends to overestimate blood glucose levels in the low range and readings lag behind real-time values by 15–20 min (Davey 2010). Having the capacity to know their glucose levels and the direction of change during exercise increases self-efficacy in people who are prone to hypoglycemia and hyperglycemia (Riddell 2009).

CARBOHYDRATE INTAKE

Sports and other carbohydrate drinks. Ingestion of carbohydrate-based drinks (or other sources of carbohydrate) is likely needed to prevent hypoglycemia both during and following physical activity in a T1D population, but the amount varies with the type of activity, exercise duration, and timing of activity relative to insulin dosing and doses. In one study, mean blood glucose levels were reportedly higher during 60 min of moderate treadmill walking in diabetic individuals consuming a glucose polymer sports drink group compared with placebo, and the same drink prevented the onset of postexercise hypoglycemia without causing or contributing to hyperglycemia (Tamis-Jortberg 1996). For 60 min of moderate cycling undertaken 3 h after breakfast (and the last dose of rapid-acting insulin), 40 g of a liquid glucose supplement, ingested 15 min prior exercise, is likely enough to maintain safe blood glucose levels in anyone on a basal-bolus regimen (e.g., Humulin N and lispro) without requiring changes in insulin doses (Dubé 2005). Ingestion of either whole milk or sports drinks designed for quick or long-lasting nutrient replenishment also has been used effectively to avoid late-onset, postexercise hypoglycemia (Hernandez 2000). For anyone using an insulin pump and engaging in moderate or vigorous activity without altering basal rates, ingestion of sugary drinks during exercise, reduction of the overnight basal rate, reduction of the predinner insulin bolus, or a bedtime snack should be considered to prevent hypoglycemia during and following exercise and overnight (Delvecchio 2009).

Daily carbohydrate intake. Endurance-training athletes usually are encouraged to take in a greater proportion of their total daily calories as carbohydrates, in addition to carbohydrate load before events (Burke 1999, American Dietetic Association 2009). This approach, however, may not be the best one for individuals with

T1D. By way of example, an increased carbohydrate intake for 3 weeks in adult athletes with T1D was associated with deterioration in glycemic control, increased insulin requirements, decreased muscle glycogen content, and reduced exercise performance. Thus, consuming a high-carbohydrate diet when doing sport-specific training is not advisable, at least not when compensatory insulin changes are not made and the resulting glycemic control is worse (McKewen 1999). For most individuals, intake of at least 40% of calories from carbohydrates (without overdoing it), along with adequate protein and total daily calories, is more likely to result in optimal glycogen storage (American Dietetic Association 2009).

INSULIN ADJUSTMENTS

Making adjustments to insulin doses and timing of doses can lower the risk of hypoglycemia during and following exercise. For example, consumption of a low–glycemic-index carbohydrate (75 g of isomaltulose) and taking an insulin dose reduced by 75% just 30 min before undertaking 45 min of moderate running improves pre- and postexercise blood glucose responses in T1D (West 2011). Similarly, a 75% reduction of insulin with a meal taken 2 h before 45 min of moderate running results in the greatest preservation of blood glucose during and following exercise (compared with 0%, 25%, and 50% dose reductions) and allows for minimal intake of extra food to maintain euglycemia during the 24 h following the activity (West 2010).

Insulin regimen effects. The types of insulin and insulin regimens used can affect exercise-related adjustments. Insulin detemir is associated with less hypoglycemia than glargine in relatively well-controlled individuals with T1D both during and after exercise (Arutchelvam 2009). People treated with insulin detemir appear to improve their glycemic control with no increases in hypoglycemia, adverse events, or body weight (Marre 2009). Recently, it was reported that athletes with T1D who were treated with rapid-acting insulin analogs and participating in half-marathons required less insulin reductions compared to traditional guidelines, although they needed a significant quantity of carbohydrate supplements to avoid hypoglycemia during and after events (Murillo 2010). For children with T1D using an insulin pump, discontinuing basal insulin during exercise is an effective strategy for reducing hypoglycemia, but the risk of hyperglycemia is increased (Diabetes Research in Children Network Study Group 2006).

Insulin pump use. Other evidence is related to glycemic control in adolescents with T1D on insulin pump therapy doing moderate- or higher-intensity physical activity with their insulin pumps switched on or off (and compared with glargine use) (Delvecchio 2009). Postexercise blood glucose levels were significantly increased with the pump off and were unchanged or lower with the pump on and when compared with glargine. The authors concluded that in that case, it is advisable to leave the basal rate on during activity, but doing so may require consumption of carbohydrate during the exercise, a lower overnight basal rate, less of an insulin bolus for dinner, and a possible bedtime snack to prevent nighttime hypoglycemia.

Exercise timing. Finally, the time of day that exercise is done can also affect insulin requirements. One study compared cycling for 45 min moderately either 1 h after lunch with usual insulin doses or after an overnight fast without morning insulin

(Biankin 2003). Reproducibility of the change in blood glucose levels during exercise after feeding in individuals on nonintensive insulin regimens was poor, but reproducibility was reasonable when fasting. Exercise does decrease the glycemic variability after a meal, meaning that blood glucose levels after exercise seek a reproducible "target." Thus, the absolute glucose level after a typical bout of exercise in the fed state should be a good guide to carbohydrate or insulin adjustment on subsequent occasions.

PREVENTION OF HYPOGLYCEMIA

Fear of hypoglycemia is the strongest barrier to regular physical activity in anyone with T1D, and information about and support for hypoglycemia management is critical (Brazeau 2008). Given the importance of this topic, it is more fully discussed in chapter 12. Various strategies and technologies have been developed to help detect and prevent hypoglycemia, including improved patient education, frequent SMBG, use of rapid-acting and basal insulin analogs, insulin pump therapy, exercise-related insulin modifications, and use of CGM (Realsen 2011).

Later-onset hypoglycemia. A major concern following exercise is the later, delayed onset of hypoglycemia, especially overnight during sleep. Overnight hypoglycemia after afternoon exercise has been shown to be common in children with T1D (Tsalikian 2005). A biphasic increase in glucose requirements to maintain euglycemia after exercise has been reported, suggesting a unique pattern of early and delayed risk for nocturnal hypoglycemia after afternoon exercise (McMahon 2007). Anyone with T1D should be made aware of this possibility to enable them to make adjustments in their management plans before and after any physical activity to minimize or avoid late-onset hypoglycemia (MacDonald 1987, Hernandez 2000, Kalergis 2003, Alemzadeh 2005, Tsalikian 2005, Diabetes Research in Children Network Study Group 2006, McMahon 2007, Tamborlane 2007, Cooperberg 2008, Wilson 2008).

Effects of sprints. A novel approach to hypoglycemia prevention during physical activity is related to the adrenergic effects of sprinting. After moderate-intensity exercise, young individuals with insulin-treated, complication-free T1D have engaged in a 10-s maximal sprint that acutely opposes a further fall in blood glucose compared with rest alone. The addition of the sprint after moderate-intensity exercise is a novel method to reduce the risk of hypoglycemia in active individuals (Bussau 2006). Along the same lines, a 10-s sprint performed immediately before moderate-intensity exercise also prevents blood glucose levels from falling during early recovery from moderate-intensity exercise in individuals with T1D (Bussau 2007). Doing intermittent, high-intensity training may result in a higher incidence of delayed nocturnal hypoglycemia (Maran 2010).

EXERCISE PRESCRIPTION FOR ADULTS AND YOUTH WITH T1D

MODE

Any form of aerobic exercise that utilizes large muscle groups and causes sustained increases in heart rate is likely to be beneficial to cardiovascular risk management (and possibly glycemic control) in children, adolescents, and adults with T1D (Orchard 2003, Costacou 2007, Bishop 2009, Shivu 2010, Maahs 2011). Undertaking a variety of modes of physical activity is recommended for all individuals to optimize training effects and lower injury risk (Physical Activity Guidelines Advisory Committee 2008). Examples of acceptable aerobic activities include both weight-bearing and non–weight-bearing ones, such as walking, jogging, running, cycling, swimming, water aerobics, aquatic activities, conditioning machines, dancing, chair exercises, rowing, and cross-country skiing, among others.

For children and adolescents ages 6 to 17 years, most of their physical activity should be either moderate- or vigorous-intensity aerobic activity, but it can include muscle-strengthening activities (even if unstructured and part of play, such as playing on playground equipment, climbing trees, and playing tug-of-war) and bone-strengthening activities like running, jumping rope, basketball, tennis, and hopscotch. Other more age-specific activities include skateboarding, rollerblading, martial arts, playing tag, wall rock climbing, gymnastics, soccer, and other competitive sports teams. Both adults and youth with T1D can safely and effectively participate in competitive athletic training and sports (Tuominen 1997a, 1997b; Cauza 2005; Graveling 2010; Murillo 2010).

INTENSITY

For adults, aerobic exercise should be moderate or vigorous intensity, corresponding to 40–89% of HRR (heart rate reserve; see chapter 4) (Garber 2011, Haskell 2007, Nelson 2007, Physical Activity Guidelines Advisory Committee 2008). Moderate-intensity exercise equates to 40–59% HRR, whereas vigorous-intensity exercise is 60–89% HRR (Garber 2011). A severely deconditioned person with T1D can start out at 30–39% HRR ("light") and progress to more moderate levels.

For children and adolescents, recommended aerobic activities should be either moderate or vigorous intensity as well (40–89% HRR), but they also should include vigorous-intensity physical activity (60–89% HRR) at least 3 days a week (Physical Activity Guidelines Advisory Committee 2008).

A corresponding overall body rating of "somewhat hard" to "hard" is appropriate for most individuals with T1D (Garber 2011, Haskell 2007, Nelson 2007, Physical Activity Guidelines Advisory Committee 2008). Subjective intensity can be estimated using a scale of 0 to 10, where resting is 0, maximal effort is 10, moderate-intensity activity is 5 to 6, and vigorous-intensity activity is 7 to 8 on that scale (Physical Activity Guidelines Advisory Committee 2008).

FREQUENCY

Adults with T1D should perform aerobic exercise at least 3–5 days/week, depending on exercise intensity and duration, but greater regularity may facilitate diabetes management in these individuals. Increased insulin sensitivity resulting from the last bout of exercise is relatively short lived, and more frequent participation in physical activity confers greater benefits in this regard (King 1995, Kirwan 2000, Clevenger 2002, Houmard 2004, Evans 2005, Hawley 2008, Bajpeyi 2009).

Children and adolescents should engage in daily physical activity, including aerobic, muscle-strengthening, and bone-strengthening activities (Physical Activity Guidelines Advisory Committee 2008). Not all three of these activities necessarily need to be done every day, although some overlap between categories exists.

DURATION

Adults with T1D should engage in a minimum of 60–75 min/week of vigorous activity (>6 metabolic equivalents [METs]) or 150 min/week of moderate-intensity exercise (3–6 METs), performed for at least 20–30 min/session (minimum of 10-min bouts). As with all adults, around 150 min/week of moderate-intensity exercise is associated with reduced morbidity and mortality, but more health benefits may result from longer participation (Physical Activity Guidelines Advisory Committee 2008).

Children and adolescents should engage in 60 min (1 h) or more of physical activity daily, or minimally 420 min a week (Physical Activity Guidelines Advisory Committee 2008). This recommended duration, however, includes aerobic activities, usual play, and muscle- and bone-strengthening activities.

PROGRESSION

If an adult is already normally active or has a reasonable fitness level, he or she can skip the initial training phase and start directly with the improvement phase. Sedentary or deconditioned adults with T1D are advised to begin with low-intensity workouts (<40% HRR), gradually progressing in both exercise intensity and volume to minimize the risk of injury or noncompliance, particularly if he or she has any health complications (Physical Activity Guidelines Advisory Committee 2008). The initial focus should be on increasing frequency and duration of the exercise rather than intensity, although faster training intervals may be used to promote greater fitness and blood glucose management (Guelfi 2005a, 2005b; Guelfi 2007; Iscoe 2011). If weight loss is a major goal, then an exercise duration of ~7 h/week may be necessary (Pavlou 1989, Schoeller 1997, Weinsier 2002, Saris 2003, Donnelly 2009).

Youth should not solely do moderate-intensity activity, but rather they should include vigorous-intensity activities to elicit greater improvements in cardiorespiratory fitness; their activities, therefore, should progress to include ones of a higher intensity. If starting out deconditioned, they should slowly increase their activity in small steps and in ways that they enjoy. Once conditioned or if beginning at that level, they should maintain or increase their activity level beyond 60 min/day and vary the kinds of activities they do to reduce the risk of overtraining or injury. Adolescents and children with T1D may meet recommended levels of physical activity by doing free play, structured programs, or both (Physical Activity Guidelines Advisory Committee 2008). Structured exercise programs can include aerobic activities, such as playing a sport, and muscle-strengthening activities like lifting weights, using resistance bands, or using body weight for resistance (e.g., push-ups, pull-ups, and sit-ups). Muscle-strengthening activities count if they involve a moderate to high level of effort and work the major muscle groups of the body (i.e., legs, hips, back, abdomen, chest, shoulders, and arms). All of these recommendations are summarized for both adults and youth in Table 6.1.

Table 6.1 Recommended Aerobic Exercise Rx for Adults and Youth with Type 1 Diabetes

Mode	Adults: Walking, jogging/running, cycling, swimming, rowing, aquatic activities, team sports, dancing, conditioning machines, seated exercise, and more
	Youth: Running, hopping, skipping, jumping rope, swimming, dancing, bicycling, basketball, tennis, skateboarding, rollerblading, and team sports
Intensity	Adults: 40–89% HRR (initial intensity may need to be lower for sedentary, deconditioned, and overweight individuals)
	Perceived exertion of "somewhat hard" (5–6 on 10-point scale) to "hard" (7–8)
	Youth: moderate or vigorous intensity (40–89% HRR), but vigorous-intensity physical activity (60–89% HRR) at least 3 days a week
	Perceived exertion of "somewhat hard" (5–6) to "hard" (7–8)
Frequency	Adults: 3–7 days/week (including structured and lifestyle activity)
	3 days of vigorous or 5 days of moderate intensity (greater regularity may facilitate diabetes management)
	Youth: 7 days/week of physical activity (including aerobic, muscle-strengthening, and bone-strengthening activities)
Duration	Adults: At least 20–30 min/session (minimum 10-min bouts)
	Minimum of 150 min/week of moderate-intensity (3–6 METs) or 60–75 min/week of vigorous-intensity (>6 METs) physical activity
	Youth: At least 60 min (1 h) of daily physical activity (420 min a week), including aerobic activities, usual play, and muscle- and bone-strengthening activities
Progression	Adults: Start out on the "low" side if deconditioned, and progress slowly over weeks to months; start with the "improvement" phase if fitness levels adequate
	Increase duration and frequency first, intensity last (with the possible exception of adding in faster intervals during exercise sessions)
	Youth: Start out slowly with small increases in activity if deconditioned, but all should progress to engaging in vigorous activity at least three times weekly; once conditioned, maintain or increase activity level and vary activities to reduce the risk of overtraining or injury
	Possible to meet recommended levels of physical activity by doing free play, structured programs, or both

HRR, heart rate reserve; MET, metabolic equivalent.

Case in Point: Wrap-Up

Because MF desires to focus on both weight and diabetes management through her exercise program and her schedule is somewhat flexible in college, she decides to start regularly working out at her university's student recreation center, where she has access to fitness equipment, classes, and other activities.

Exercise Program Goals

Mode of Activity: MF desires to undertake multiple training activities—she likes the idea of cross-training to get more fit and avoid injuries—so she can include conditioning machines (like cross-trainers and elliptical machines), lap swimming, and spinning (cycling) classes as some of her choices.

Intensity: Because MF is starting out somewhat deconditioned (except for walking around campus), she should start with more moderate activities (that feel "somewhat hard" or 5–6 on a 10-point scale) to start and work up to "hard" ones (7–8 using that scale). She should choose interval or hill workouts on the conditioning machines. Her initial target heart rate should start in a moderate-intensity range (130–152 bpm, or 40–59% HRR), with a target goal of 60–89% HRR (153–187 bpm), with a maximal target of 187 bpm (89% HRR). Her intensity during each training session can vary, however, and she may choose to do harder (vigorous) and easier (moderate) workout days to prevent overtraining.

Frequency: Depending on how MF alternates her training intensity, she should do 3–5 days of planned training a week (3 days if vigorous, 5 days if moderate, or a combination of the two intensities and frequencies), keeping in mind that being more regular with her training may make it easier for her to make regimen changes to manage her blood glucose levels. Her insulin action may stay higher following harder workout days, so she should plan to space out her more vigorous training days and intersperse more moderate ones in between them.

Duration: MF's recommended duration is inversely related to her exercise intensity, meaning that working out harder requires a shorter duration. She should aim to do at least 20 min of vigorous physical activity or 30 min/session of moderate training, with a target training goal of 60–75 min of vigorous or 150 min of moderate exercise weekly, or a combination thereof. As a rule of thumb, 1 min of vigorous exercise is equivalent to 2 min of moderate activity.

Progression: Given her initial fitness status and prior sports history, MF can likely begin in the improvement phase of training. Initially, she may choose to only work out 3 nonconsecutive days/week, working up to 5 days/week, depending on her training intensity. Once she has established her aerobic training routine, she should consider adding in some resistance training at least 2 days/week to enhance her muscular strength as well. As she goes into the maintenance phase, she should continue to vary her activities or add in new ones for variety, additional fitness gains, injury prevention, and motivation to continue her training.

Daily Movement: Due to MF's interest in losing weight, she should engage in more daily movement as well, including fidgeting, standing, and taking more steps during the day, to maximize her daily caloric expenditure. Doing so will help keep her blood glucose at a lower level.

Possible Precautions: Because MF has not had T1D for that long and has minimal risk factors for cardiovascular disease, she should not be required to have any testing done before starting an exercise program. MF should be advised to have her health-care provider prescribe a glucagon pen that she can keep in her dorm room as a treatment for severe hypoglycemia. She should instruct both her roommate and her dorm's resident assistant how to give her a glucagon injection, should the need arise.

Regimen Changes: Because weight loss is a stated goal, MF will need to be especially vigilant about preventing hypoglycemia since the extra calories taken in during treatment of lows may sabotage her attempts to lose weight. Her insulin use does require planning ahead with appropriate insulin dosing and food intake changes to prevent hypoglycemia both during and following any physical activity. She will need to use SMBG frequently as she begins her training program—before, possibly during, and several times after exercising—to establish her usual responses to exercise and blood glucose trends. During exercise sessions, she should always have a rapid-acting carbohydrate like glucose tablets or gels readily available to treat low blood glucose with a minimal amount of calories. Once she starts exercising regularly, her basal insulin needs will likely decrease, and she may need to lower her bedtime dose of insulin glargine or eat a bedtime snack (but for weight-loss reasons, it would be better to minimize the need for additional snacking). Furthermore, for exercise sessions done within 1–2 h of a meal, she should consider decreasing her meal insulin (lispro) dose by up to 75% to prevent hypoglycemia during the activity, and she may need less insulin later in the day at subsequent meals.

Individuals of all ages with T1D can and should participate in regular physical activity for better health, although appropriate diabetes regimen changes must be made if improved blood glucose management is an expected outcome. Cardiorespiratory fitness levels may be lower in some individuals with T1D, and their metabolic responses to exercise can be altered by hyperglycemia. Prevention of hypoglycemia related to physical activity will likely require greater carbohydrate intake, reductions in insulin doses (or changes in timing), or both. Fear of hypoglycemia is the biggest barrier to exercise participation, but when diabetes is managed properly, youth and adults with T1D can participate in recommended amounts of physical activity following the same guidelines as their counterparts who do not have diabetes.

PROFESSIONAL PRACTICE PEARLS

- Regular exercise lowers blood pressure, lipid levels, body weight, mortality risk, and risk of complications while raising cardiorespiratory fitness levels, muscular strength, quality of life, and sense of well-being in individuals with T1D.
- Appropriate diabetes regimen changes must be made if improved blood glucose management is an expected outcome of regular physical activity.
- Some, but not all, individuals with T1D have the same aerobic capacity as similar-age people without diabetes.

■ Moderate exercise usually causes a decline in blood glucose levels; conversely, high-intensity training can maintain more stable levels or possibly result in hyperglycemia.

■ When engaging in regular physical activity, individuals with T1D will need to self-monitor their blood glucose levels to establish responses and make regimen changes.

■ Regimen changes to manage glycemic balance with physical activity will likely involve greater food intake, changes in insulin doses and timing, or both.

■ A novel approach to hypoglycemia prevention involves engaging in a 10-s maximal sprint immediately before or at the end of a bout of moderate activity.

■ Adults with T1D should engage in at least 150 min a week of moderate exercise, 60–75 min of vigorous aerobic exercise, or a combination thereof on 3–5 days/week (depending on intensity).

■ Deconditioned adults can start out with lower-intensity activities and progress slowly over weeks to months, or start with the improvement phase if fitness adequate.

■ Youth with T1D should engage in at least 60 min or more of physical activity daily, 7 days/week, including aerobic, muscle-strengthening, and bone-strengthening activities.

■ Children and adolescents should start out slowly if deconditioned, but all should progress to engaging in vigorous activity at least three times weekly.

■ Youth should vary activities, but it is possible for them to meet the recommended levels of physical activity by doing free play, structured programs, or both.

REFERENCES

Alemzadeh R, Berhe T, Wyatt DT: Flexible insulin therapy with glargine insulin improved glycemic control and reduced severe hypoglycemia among preschool-aged children with type 1 diabetes mellitus. *Pediatrics* 115:1320–1324, 2005

American Dietetic Association, Dietitians of Canada, American College of Sports Medicine, Rodriguez NR, Di Marco NM, Langley S: American College of Sports Medicine position stand. Nutrition and athletic performance. *Med Sci Sports Exerc* 41:709–731, 2009

Aouadi R, Khalifa R, Aouidet A, Ben Mansour A, Ben Rayana M, Mdini F, Bahri S, Stratton G: Aerobic training programs and glycemic control in diabetic children in relation to exercise frequency. *J Sports Med Phys Fitness* 51:393–400, 2011

Arutchelvam V, Heise T, Dellweg S, Elbroend B, Minns I, Home PD: Plasma glucose and hypoglycaemia following exercise in people with type 1 diabetes: a comparison of three basal insulins. *Diabet Med* 26:1027–1032, 2009

Bajpeyi S, Tanner CJ, Slentz CA, Duscha BD, McCartney JS, Hickner RC, Kraus WE, Houmard JA: Effect of exercise intensity and volume on persistence of insulin sensitivity during training cessation. *J Appl Physiol* 106:1079–1085, 2009

Baldi JC, Cassuto NA, Foxx-Lupo WT, Wheatley CM, Snyder EM: Glycemic status affects cardiopulmonary exercise response in athletes with type I diabetes. *Med Sci Sports Exerc* 42:1454–1459, 2010a

Baldi JC, Hofman PL: Does careful glycemic control improve aerobic capacity in subjects with type 1 diabetes? *Exerc Sport Sci Rev* 38:161–167, 2010b

Benevento D, Bizzarri C, Pitocco D, Crino A, Moretti C, Spera S, Tubili C, Costanza F, Maurizi A, Cipolloni L, Cappa M, Pozzilli P, IMDIAB Group: Computer use, free time activities and metabolic control in patients with type 1 diabetes. *Diabetes Res Clin Pract* 88:e32–e34, 2010

Biankin SA, Jenkins AB, Campbell LV, Choi KL, Forrest QG, Chisholm DJ: Target-seeking behavior of plasma glucose with exercise in type 1 diabetes. *Diabetes Care* 26:297–301, 2003

Bischof MG, Krssak M, Krebs M, Bernroider E, Stingl H, Waldhausl W, Roden M: Effects of short-term improvement of insulin treatment and glycemia on hepatic glycogen metabolism in type 1 diabetes. *Diabetes* 50:392–398, 2001

Bishop FK, Maahs DM, Snell-Bergeon JK, Ogden LG, Kinney GL, Rewers M: Lifestyle risk factors for atherosclerosis in adults with type 1 diabetes. *Diab Vasc Dis Res* 6:269–275, 2009

Brazeau AS, Rabasa-Lhoret R, Strychar I, Mircescu H: Barriers to physical activity among patients with type 1 diabetes. *Diabetes Care* 31:2108–2109, 2008

Burke LM, Hawley JA: Carbohydrate and exercise. *Curr Opin Clin Nutr Metab Care* 2:515–520, 1999

Bussau VA, Ferreira LD, Jones TW, Fournier PA: A 10-s sprint performed prior to moderate-intensity exercise prevents early post-exercise fall in glycaemia in individuals with type 1 diabetes. *Diabetologia* 50:1815–1818, 2007

Bussau VA, Ferreira LD, Jones TW, Fournier PA: The 10-s maximal sprint: a novel approach to counter an exercise-mediated fall in glycemia in individuals with type 1 diabetes. *Diabetes Care* 29:601–606, 2006

Cauza E, Hanusch-Enserer U, Strasser B, Ludvik B, Kostner K, Dunky A, Haber P: Continuous glucose monitoring in diabetic long distance runners. *Int J Sports Med* 26:774–780, 2005

Chokkalingam K, Tsintzas K, Norton L, Jewell K, Macdonald IA, Mansell PI: Exercise under hyperinsulinaemic conditions increases whole-body glucose disposal without affecting muscle glycogen utilisation in type 1 diabetes. *Diabetologia* 50:414–421, 2007a

Chokkalingam K, Tsintzas K, Snaar JE, Norton L, Solanky B, Leverton E, Morris P, Mansell P, Macdonald IA: Hyperinsulinaemia during exercise does not suppress hepatic glycogen concentrations in patients with type 1 diabetes: a magnetic resonance spectroscopy study. *Diabetologia* 50:1921–1929, 2007b

Clevenger CM, Parker Jones P, Tanaka H, Seals DR, DeSouza CA: Decline in insulin action with age in endurance-trained humans. *J Appl Physiol* 93:2105–2111, 2002

Colberg SR: *Diabetic Athlete's Handbook: Your Guide to Peak Performance.* Champaign, IL, Human Kinetics, 2009

Conway B, Miller RG, Costacou T, Fried L, Kelsey S, Evans RW, Orchard TJ: Adiposity and mortality in type 1 diabetes. *Int J Obes (Lond)* 33:796–805, 2009

Cooperberg BA, Breckenridge SM, Arbelaez AM, Cryer PE: Terbutaline and the prevention of nocturnal hypoglycemia in type 1 diabetes. *Diabetes Care* 31:2271–2272, 2008

Costacou T, Edmundowicz D, Prince C, Conway B, Orchard TJ: Progression of coronary artery calcium in type 1 diabetes mellitus. *Am J Cardiol* 100:1543–1547, 2007

D'Hooge R, Hellinckx T, Van Laethem C, Stegen S, De Schepper J, Van Aken S, Dewolf D, Calders P: Influence of combined aerobic and resistance training on metabolic control, cardiovascular fitness and quality of life in adolescents with type 1 diabetes: a randomized controlled trial. *Clin Rehabil* 25:349–359, 2011

Davey RJ, Jones TW, Fournier PA: Effect of short-term use of a continuous glucose monitoring system with a real-time glucose display and a low glucose alarm on incidence and duration of hypoglycemia in a home setting in type 1 diabetes mellitus. *J Diabetes Sci Technol* 4:1457–1464, 2010

Delvecchio M, Zecchino C, Salzano G, Faienza MF, Cavallo L, De Luca F, Lombardo F: Effects of moderate-severe exercise on blood glucose in type 1 diabetic adolescents treated with insulin pump or glargine insulin. *J Endocrinol Invest* 32:519–524, 2009

Diabetes Research in Children Network Study Group, Tsalikian E, Tamborlane W, Xing D, Becker DM, Mauras N, Fiallo-Scharer R, Buckingham B, Weinzimer S, Steffes M, Singh R, Beck R, Ruedy K, Kollman C: Blunted counterregulatory hormone responses to hypoglycemia in young children and adolescents with well-controlled type 1 diabetes. *Diabetes Care* 32:1954–1959, 2009

Diabetes Research in Children Network Study Group, Tsalikian E, Kollman C, Tamborlane WB, Beck RW, Fiallo-Scharer R, Fox L, Janz KF, Ruedy KJ, Wilson D, Xing D, Weinzimer SA: Prevention of hypoglycemia during exercise in children with type 1 diabetes by suspending basal insulin. *Diabetes Care* 29:2200–2204, 2006

Donnelly JE, Blair SN, Jakicic JM, Manore MM, Rankin JW, Smith BK: American College of Sports Medicine Position Stand. Appropriate physical activity intervention strategies for weight loss and prevention of weight regain for adults. *Med Sci Sports Exerc* 41:459–471, 2009

Dubé MC, Weisnagel SJ, Prud'homme D, Lavoie C: Exercise and newer insulins: how much glucose supplement to avoid hypoglycemia? *Med Sci Sports Exerc* 37:1276–1282, 2005

Ebeling P, Tuominen JA, Bourey R, Koranyi L, Koivisto VA: Athletes with IDDM exhibit impaired metabolic control and increased lipid utilization with no increase in insulin sensitivity. *Diabetes* 44:471–477, 1995

Evans EM, Racette SB, Peterson LR, Villareal DT, Greiwe JS, Holloszy JO: Aerobic power and insulin action improve in response to endurance exercise training in healthy 77-87 yr olds. *J Appl Physiol* 98:40–45, 2005

Galassetti P, Mann S, Tate D, Neill RA, Wasserman DH, Davis SN: Effect of morning exercise on counterregulatory responses to subsequent, afternoon exercise. *J Appl Physiol* 91:91–99, 2001

Gallen IW, Hume C, Lumb A: Fueling the athlete with type 1 diabetes. *Diabetes Obes Metab* 13:130–136, 2011

Garber CE, Blissmer B, Deschenes MR, Franklin BA, Lamonte MJ, Lee IM, Nieman DC, Swain DP, American College of Sports Medicine: American College of Sports Medicine position stand. Quantity and quality of exercise for developing and maintaining cardiorespiratory, musculoskeletal, and neuromotor fitness in apparently healthy adults: guidance for prescribing exercise. *Med Sci Sports Exerc* 43:1334–1359, 2011

Graveling AJ, Frier BM: Risks of marathon running and hypoglycaemia in type 1 diabetes. *Diabet Med* 27:585588, 2010

Guelfi KJ, Ratnam N, Smythe GA, Jones TW, Fournier PA: Effect of intermittent high-intensity compared with continuous moderate exercise on glucose production and utilization in individuals with type 1 diabetes. *Am J Physiol Endocrinol Metab* 292:E865–E870, 2007

Guelfi KJ, Jones TW, Fournier PA: The decline in blood glucose levels is less with intermittent high-intensity compared with moderate exercise in individuals with type 1 diabetes. *Diabetes Care* 28:1289–1294, 2005a

Guelfi KJ, Jones TW, Fournier PA: Intermittent high-intensity exercise does not increase the risk of early postexercise hypoglycemia in individuals with type 1 diabetes. *Diabetes Care* 28:416–418, 2005b

Harmer AR, Chisholm DJ, McKenna MJ, Hunter SK, Ruell PA, Naylor JM, Maxwell LJ, Flack JR: Sprint training increases muscle oxidative metabolism during high-intensity exercise in patients with type 1 diabetes. *Diabetes Care* 31:2097–2102, 2008

Haskell WL, Lee IM, Pate RR, Powell KE, Blair SN, Franklin BA, Macera CA, Heath GW, Thompson PD, Bauman A: Physical activity and public health:

updated recommendation for adults from the American College of Sports Medicine and the American Heart Association. *Med Sci Sports Exerc* 39:1423–1434, 2007

Hawley JA, Lessard SJ: Exercise training-induced improvements in insulin action. *Acta Physiol (Oxf)* 192:127–135, 2008

Herbst A, Kordonouri O, Schwab KO, Schmidt F, Holl RW, D. P. V. Initiative of the German Working Group for Pediatric Diabetology Germany: Impact of physical activity on cardiovascular risk factors in children with type 1 diabetes: a multicenter study of 23,251 patients. *Diabetes Care* 30:2098–2100, 2007

Hernandez JM, Moccia T, Fluckey JD, Ulbrecht JS, Farrell PA: Fluid snacks to help persons with type 1 diabetes avoid late onset postexercise hypoglycemia. *Med Sci Sports Exerc* 32:904–910, 2000

Heyman E, Toutain C, Delamarche P, Berthon P, Briard D, Youssef H, Dekerdanet M, Gratas-Delamarche A: Exercise training and cardiovascular risk factors in type 1 diabetic adolescent girls. *Pediatr Exerc Sci* 19:408–419, 2007

Houmard JA, Tanner CJ, Slentz CA, Duscha BD, McCartney JS, Kraus WE: Effect of the volume and intensity of exercise training on insulin sensitivity. *J Appl Physiol* 96:101–106, 2004

Iscoe KE, Riddell MC: Continuous moderate-intensity exercise with or without intermittent high-intensity work: effects on acute and late glycaemia in athletes with type 1 diabetes mellitus. *Diabet Med* 28:824–832, 2011

Item F, Heinzer-Schweizer S, Wyss M, Fontana P, Lehmann R, Henning A, Weber M, Boesiger P, Boutellier U, Toigo M: Mitochondrial capacity is affected by glycemic status in young untrained women with type 1 diabetes but is not impaired relative to healthy untrained women. *Am J Physiol Regul Integr Comp Physiol* 301:R60–R66, 2011

Jenni S, Oetliker C, Allemann S, Ith M, Tappy L, Wuerth S, Egger A, Boesch C, Schneiter P, Diem P, Christ E, Stettler C: Fuel metabolism during exercise in euglycaemia and hyperglycaemia in patients with type 1 diabetes mellitus—a prospective single-blinded randomised crossover trial. *Diabetologia* 51:1457–1465, 2008

Kalergis M, Schiffrin A, Gougeon R, Jones PJ, Yale JF: Impact of bedtime snack composition on prevention of nocturnal hypoglycemia in adults with type 1 diabetes undergoing intensive insulin management using lispro insulin before meals: a randomized, placebo-controlled, crossover trial. *Diabetes Care* 26:9–15, 2003

Kilpatrick ES, Rigby AS, Atkin SL: Insulin resistance, the metabolic syndrome, and complication risk in type 1 diabetes: "double diabetes" in the Diabetes Control and Complications Trial. *Diabetes Care* 30:707–712, 2007

King DS, Baldus PJ, Sharp RL, Kesl LD, Feltmeyer TL, Riddle MS: Time course for exercise-induced alterations in insulin action and glucose tolerance in middle-aged people. *J Appl Physiol* 78:17–22, 1995

Kirwan JP, del Aguila LF, Hernandez JM, Williamson DL, O'Gorman DJ, Lewis R, Krishnan RK: Regular exercise enhances insulin activation of IRS-1-associated PI3-kinase in human skeletal muscle. *J Appl Physiol* 88:797–803, 2000

Kishore P, Gabriely I, Cui MH, Di Vito J, Gajavelli S, Hwang JH, Shamoon H: Role of hepatic glycogen breakdown in defective counterregulation of hypoglycemia in intensively treated type 1 diabetes. *Diabetes* 55:659–666, 2006

Koivisto VA, Sane T, Fyhrquist F, Pelkonen R: Fuel and fluid homeostasis during long-term exercise in healthy subjects and type 1 diabetic patients. *Diabetes Care* 15:1736–1741, 1992

Komatsu WR, Barros Neto TL, Chacra AR, Dib SA: Aerobic exercise capacity and pulmonary function in athletes with and without type 1 diabetes. *Diabetes Care* 33:2555–2557, 2010

Laaksonen DE, Atalay M, Niskanen LK, Mustonen J, Sen CK, Lakka TA, Uusitupa MI: Aerobic exercise and the lipid profile in type 1 diabetic men: a randomized controlled trial. *Med Sci Sports Exerc* 32:1541–1548, 2000

Maahs DM, Nadeau K, Snell-Bergeon JK, Schauer I, Bergman B, West NA, Rewers M, Daniels SR, Ogden LG, Hamman RF, Dabelea D: Association of insulin sensitivity to lipids across the lifespan in people with type 1 diabetes. *Diabet Med* 28:148–155, 2011

MacDonald MJ: Postexercise late-onset hypoglycemia in insulin-dependent diabetic patients. *Diabetes Care* 10:584–588, 1987

Maran A, Pavan P, Bonsembiante B, Brugin E, Ermolao A, Avogaro A, Zaccaria M: Continuous glucose monitoring reveals delayed nocturnal hypoglycemia after intermittent high-intensity exercise in nontrained patients with type 1 diabetes. *Diabetes Technol Ther* 12:763–768, 2010

Marre M, Pinget M, Gin H, Thivolet C, Hanaire H, Robert JJ, Fontaine P: Insulin detemir improves glycaemic control with less hypoglycaemia and no weight gain: 52-week data from the PREDICTIVE study in a cohort of French patients with type 1 or type 2 diabetes. *Diabetes Metab* 35:469–475, 2009

McKewen MW, Rehrer NJ, Cox C, Mann J: Glycaemic control, muscle glycogen and exercise performance in IDDM athletes on diets of varying carbohydrate content. *Int J Sports Med* 20:349–353, 1999

McMahon SK, Ferreira LD, Ratnam N, Davey RJ, Youngs LM, Davis EA, Fournier PA, Jones TW: Glucose requirements to maintain euglycemia after moderate-intensity afternoon exercise in adolescents with type 1 diabetes are increased in a biphasic manner. *J Clin Endocrinol Metab* 92:963–968, 2007

Meinders AE, Willekens FL, Heere LP: Metabolic and hormonal changes in IDDM during long-distance run. *Diabetes Care* 11:1–7, 1988

Mitchell TH, Abraham G, Schiffrin A, Leiter LA, Marliss EB: Hyperglycemia after intense exercise in IDDM subjects during continuous subcutaneous insulin infusion. *Diabetes Care* 11:311–317, 1988

Moy CS, Songer TJ, LaPorte RE, Dorman JS, Kriska AM, Orchard TJ, Becker DJ, Drash AL: Insulin-dependent diabetes mellitus, physical activity, and death. *Am J Epidemiol* 137:74–81, 1993

Murillo S, Brugnara L, Novials A: One year follow-up in a group of half-marathon runners with type-1 diabetes treated with insulin analogues. *J Sports Med Phys Fitness* 50:506–510, 2010

Nelson ME, Rejeski WJ, Blair SN, Duncan PW, Judge JO, King AC, Macera CA, Castaneda-Sceppa C: Physical activity and public health in older adults: recommendation from the American College of Sports Medicine and the American Heart Association. *Med Sci Sports Exerc* 39:1435–1445, 2007

Orchard TJ, Olson JC, Erbey JR, Williams K, Forrest KY, Smithline Kinder L, Ellis D, Becker DJ: Insulin resistance-related factors, but not glycemia, predict coronary artery disease in type 1 diabetes: 10-year follow-up data from the Pittsburgh Epidemiology of Diabetes Complications Study. *Diabetes Care* 26:1374–1379, 2003

Pavlou KN, Krey S, Steffee WP: Exercise as an adjunct to weight loss and maintenance in moderately obese subjects. *Am J Clin Nutri* 49 (Suppl. 5):1115–1123, 1989

Petersen KF, Price TB, Bergeron R: Regulation of net hepatic glycogenolysis and gluconeogenesis during exercise: impact of type 1 diabetes. *J Clin Endocrinol Metab* 89:4656–4664, 2004

Physical Activity Guidelines Advisory Committee: Physical Activity Guidelines Advisory Committee Report, 2008. Washington, DC, U.S. Department of Health and Human Services, 2008

Purnell JQ, Hokanson JE, Marcovina SM, Steffes MW, Cleary PA, Brunzell JD: Effect of excessive weight gain with intensive therapy of type 1 diabetes on lipid levels and blood pressure: results from the DCCT. Diabetes Control and Complications Trial. *JAMA* 280:140–146, 1998

Ramalho AC, de Lourdes Lima M, Nunes F, Cambui Z, Barbosa C, Andrade A, Viana A, Martins M, Abrantes V, Aragao C, Temistocles M: The effect of resistance versus aerobic training on metabolic control in patients with type-1 diabetes mellitus. *Diabetes Res Clin Pract* 72:271–276, 2006

Realsen JM, Chase HP: Recent advances in the prevention of hypoglycemia in type 1 diabetes. *Diabetes Technol Ther* 13:1177-86, 2011

Riddell M, Perkins BA: Exercise and glucose metabolism in persons with diabetes mellitus: perspectives on the role for continuous glucose monitoring. *J Diabetes Sci Technol* 3:914–923, 2009

Roberts L, Jones TW, Fournier PA: Exercise training and glycemic control in adolescents with poorly controlled type 1 diabetes mellitus. *J Pediatr Endocrinol Metab* 15:621–627, 2002

Saris WH, Blair SN, van Baak MA, Eaton SB, Davies PS, Di Pietro L, Fogelholm M, Rissanen A, Schoeller D, Swinburn B, Tremblay A, Westerterp KR, Wyatt

H: How much physical activity is enough to prevent unhealthy weight gain? Outcome of the IASO 1st Stock Conference and consensus statement. *Obes Rev* 4:101–114, 2003

Schoeller DA, Shay K, Kushner RF: How much physical activity is needed to minimize weight gain in previously obese women? *Am J Clin Nutri* 66:551–556, 1997

Seeger JP, Thijssen DH, Noordam K, Cranen ME, Hopman MT, Nijhuis-van der Sanden MW: Exercise training improves physical fitness and vascular function in children with type 1 diabetes. *Diabetes Obes Metab* 13:382–384, 2011

Shivu GN, Phan TT, Abozguia K, Ahmed I, Wagenmakers A, Henning A, Narendran P, Stevens M, Frenneaux M: Relationship between coronary microvascular dysfunction and cardiac energetics impairment in type 1 diabetes mellitus. *Circulation* 121 :1209–1215, 2010

Tamborlane WV: Triple jeopardy: nocturnal hypoglycemia after exercise in the young with diabetes. *J Clin Endocrinol Metab* 92:815–816, 2007

Tamis-Jortberg B, Downs DA Jr, Colten ME: Effects of a glucose polymer sports drink on blood glucose, insulin, and performance in subjects with diabetes. *Diabetes Educ* 22:471–487, 1996

Trigona B, Aggoun Y, Maggio A, Martin XE, Marchand LM, Beghetti M, Farpour-Lambert NJ: Preclinical noninvasive markers of atherosclerosis in children and adolescents with type 1 diabetes are influenced by physical activity. *J Pediatr* 157:533–539, 2010

Tsalikian E, Mauras N, Beck RW, Tamborlane WV, Janz KF, Chase HP, Wysocki T, Weinzimer SA, Buckingham BA, Kollman C, Xing D, Ruedy KJ, Group Diabetes Research In Children Network Direcnet Study: Impact of exercise on overnight glycemic control in children with type 1 diabetes mellitus. *J Pediatr* 147:528–534, 2005

Tuominen JA, Ebeling P, Koivisto VA: Exercise increases insulin clearance in healthy man and insulin-dependent diabetes mellitus patients. *Clin Physiol* 17:19–30, 1997a

Tuominen JA, Ebeling P, Vuorinen-Markkola H, Koivisto VA: Post-marathon paradox in IDDM: unchanged insulin sensitivity in spite of glycogen depletion. *Diabet Med* 14:301–308, 1997b

Weinsier RL, Hunter GR, Desmond RA, Byrne NM, Zuckerman PA, Darnell BE: Free-living activity energy expenditure in women successful and unsuccessful at maintaining a normal body weight. *Am J Clin Nutri* 75:499–504, 2002

West DJ, Stephens JW, Bain SC, Kilduff LP, Luzio S, Still R, Bracken RM: A combined insulin reduction and carbohydrate feeding strategy 30 min before running best preserves blood glucose concentration after exercise through improved fuel oxidation in type 1 diabetes mellitus. *J Sports Sci* 29:279–289, 2011

West DJ, Morton RD, Bain SC, Stephens JW, Bracken RM: Blood glucose responses to reductions in pre-exercise rapid-acting insulin for 24 h after running in individuals with type 1 diabetes. *J Sports Sci* 28:781–788, 2010

Williams BK, Guelfi KJ, Jones TW, Davis EA: Lower cardiorespiratory fitness in children with type 1 diabetes. *Diabet Med* 28:1005–1007, 2011

Wilson D, Chase HP, Kollman C, Xing D, Caswell K, Tansey M, Fox L, Weinzimer S, Beck R, Ruedy K, Tamborlane W, Group Diabetes Research in Children Network Study: Low-fat vs. high-fat bedtime snacks in children and adolescents with type 1 diabetes. *Pediatr Diabetes* 9:320–325, 2008

Chapter 7
Aerobic Exercise Rx for Gestational Diabetes

Gestational diabetes mellitus (GDM), which is maternal hyperglycemia that arises primarily during the third trimester of pregnancy, is usually diagnosed at 24 to 28 weeks of gestation with an oral glucose challenge (American Diabetes Association 2013a, 2013b). Women who have risk factors for gestational diabetes, however, may have this test earlier in the pregnancy. Using new diagnostic criteria, it is estimated that gestational diabetes affects 18% of pregnancies (American Diabetes Association 2013a).

Physical activity performed during pregnancy benefits a woman's overall health. Instead of detraining, pregnant women undertaking moderate-intensity physical activity can maintain or increase their cardiorespiratory fitness (Ceysens 2006). Furthermore, maternal exercise during pregnancy does not increase the risk of low birth weight, preterm delivery, or early pregnancy loss (Ceysens 2006). On the contrary, regular exercise participation likely reduces the risk of pregnancy complications, such as preeclampsia and GDM, and shortens the duration of active labor (Dyck 2002; Dempsey 2004a, 2004b; Oken 2006; Zhang 2006; Melzer 2010).

Case in Point: Aerobic Exercise Rx for a Woman with GDM

CC is a 32-year-old woman who was recently diagnosed with GDM during week 24 of her pregnancy with a routine oral glucose tolerance test (OGTT). This is her second pregnancy, and although she was not diagnosed with GDM during the first one, her son's birth weight was >9 lb (9 lb, 2 oz) when she gave birth to him at 39 weeks' gestation. She considers herself to be a normally active person, getting plenty of daily movement (i.e., standing and walking) at her job as a retail salesperson in a large department store. She has not been doing any planned activities, however, either before or during this pregnancy, although she claims to be active during her leisure time due to continually chasing after her 18-month-old son.

Resting Measurements

Height: 68 inches
Weight: 160 lb (prepregnancy)
BMI: 24.3 (normal)
Heart rate: 80 beats per minute (bpm)
Blood pressure: 118/78 mmHg

Fasting Labs

Plasma glucose: 90 mg/dl (acceptable)
OGTT (75 g of glucose):
    1 h: 185 mg/dl (positive diagnosis of GDM)
    2 h: 155 mg/dl (positive diagnosis of GDM)

Medications

None currently (although insulin may be initiated if diet and exercise fail to control her blood glucose levels)

Questions to Consider

1. What type of exercise can CC safely start doing at 25 weeks of pregnancy, given her previous sedentary lifestyle?
2. What are an appropriate exercise frequency, intensity, and duration?
3. How should her exercise training progress during the remainder of her pregnancy and after giving birth?
4. What precautions should CC take, and does she have any exercise limitations?

(Continued on page 110.)

ASSESSING AND TREATING GESTATIONAL DIABETES

GDM has been increasing in prevalence and is associated with a significantly elevated risk of developing type 2 diabetes (T2D) in the next 5–10 years (U.S. Department of Health and Human Services 2011, American Diabetes Association 2013a). Uncontrolled hyperglycemia is potentially harmful to both mother and fetus, resulting in a greater need for cesarian-section deliveries, delivery of larger infants with more excess body fat, a greater risk of infant death and stillborn, and an elevated risk of infant hypoglycemia immediately after birth (Hapo Study Cooperative Research Group 2008, Metzger 2010).

CAUSES OF GDM

The pregnant woman's placenta supports the fetus as it grows, releasing its own specific hormones that help the fetus to develop, but at the same time blocking the effect of circulating insulin and making the mother more insulin resistant (and, thereby, sparing maternal blood glucose for the growing fetus). Specifically, placental growth hormone induces maternal insulin resistance and mobilizes maternal nutrients for fetal growth, while human placental lactogen and prolactin increase maternal food intake by induction of central leptin resistance and promote maternal β-cell expansion and insulin production to defend against the development of GDM (Newbern 2011). This state of insulin resistance causes the mother's insulin needs to go up to as much as three or more times normal during the third trimester, resulting in hyperglycemia when the mother's pancreatic β-cells are unable to

Table 7.1 Risk Factors for Development of Gestational Diabetes

Risk for GDM is greatest if a woman:
- Is >25 years old when pregnant
- Has a family history of type 2 diabetes
- Previously gave birth to a baby weighing >9 lb or with a birth defect
- Has high blood pressure
- Has excessive amounts of amniotic fluid
- Has had an unexplained miscarriage or stillbirth
- Was overweight before getting pregnant
- Lives a sedentary lifestyle

keep up with heightened insulin demands. Body fat percentage, physical inactivity, and diet quality are important modifiable risk factors for GDM (Iqbal 2007). These and other important risk factors for GDM are listed in Table 7.1.

SYMPTOMS OF GDM

Given its slow onset during pregnancy, GDM usually has no symptoms, or else the symptoms may be mild and not life threatening to the pregnant woman. In most women, blood glucose levels return to normal shortly after delivery.

If symptoms related to hyperglycemia are present, they may include the following:

- Blurred vision
- Fatigue
- Increased thirst
- Increased urination
- Frequent infections (e.g., bladder, vagina, and skin)
- Weight loss despite increased appetite
- Nausea and vomiting

DIAGNOSIS OF GDM

Maternal hyperglycemia is most common during the third trimester of pregnancy and is commonly diagnosed with a 75-g OGTT given to all women without prior diabetes at 24–28 weeks of gestation. The OGTT should be administered in the morning to women in a fasted state following an overnight fast of at least 8 h (American Diabetes Association 2013b). The diagnostic criteria are listed in Table 7.2. With the increased prevalence of undiagnosed T2D among women of childbearing age, more women with significant risk factors are being screened for preexisting diabetes at their initial prenatal visit and 6–12 weeks postpartum (American Diabetes Association 2013a, 2013b).

Table 7.2 Diagnostic Criteria for Gestational Diabetes

Fasting Plasma Glucose	1 h OGTT Plasma Glucose	2 h OGTT Plasma Glucose
≥92 mg/dl	≥180 mg/dl	≥153 mg/dl
≥5.1 mmol/l	≥10.0 mmol/l	≥8.5 mmol/l

OGTT, oral glucose tolerance test.

TREATMENT OF GDM

Lifestyle changes. The primary goal of treatment of GDM is to keep blood glucose levels within normal limits throughout the pregnancy to ensure appropriate fetal growth. The first recommendation to achieve this goal is to implement lifestyle changes (i.e., diet and exercise) to manage glycemic control (Committee on Obstetric Practice 2002, Davenport 2008, de Barros 2010, Zavorsky 2011a). A recommended diet for women with GDM is moderate in fat and protein and provides controlled levels of carbohydrates (Artal 2007). Foods to avoid include refined carbohydrates, sugary drinks, fruit juices, pastries, and other sweets that require large amount of insulin to remove excess blood glucose after ingestion. Food intake usually is divided into three small- to moderate-size meals and one or more snacks each day. Pregnant women generally will require no more than 300 extra calories daily to cover their increased energy requirements (Committee on Obstetric Practice 2002).

In addition, pregnant women should be under the care of a health-care provider with whom they can discuss how to adjust amounts of physical activity during pregnancy and the postpartum period. Unless a woman has medical reasons to avoid physical activity during pregnancy, she can begin or continue moderate-intensity aerobic physical activity during her pregnancy and after the baby is born, which should help manage her blood glucose levels (Avery 2001, Brankston 2004, Ceysens 2006, Artal 2007, Iqbal 2007, Chasan-Taber 2008, Davenport 2008, de Barros 2010, Tobias 2011).

Diabetes medications. If lifestyle changes are not successful in maintaining target glucose values during a pregnancy complicated by GDM, glucose-lowering medications may be used (Paglia 2009). Insulin has been the traditional treatment, but the use of oral antidiabetic medications in the management of GDM has increased over the past several years. Both glyburide and metformin (discussed further in chapter 15) have similar pregnancy outcomes compared with insulin (Paglia 2009). Although no substantial maternal or neonatal outcome differences have been found with the use of glyburide or metformin compared with the use of insulin in women with GDM (Nicholson 2009, Dhulkotia 2010), given that both of these oral medications cross the placenta and are available to the fetus, they should be used with caution. Physiological changes associated with regular aerobic training may result in a lowering of the daily medication dose (e.g., insulin or oral agents) needed to manage glucose levels during pregnancy in some women with GDM.

Health outcomes related to uncontrolled GDM. If maternal hyperglycemia is not controlled, the elevated blood glucose levels that are the same in the mother and the developing fetus can lead to macrosomia, or an overly fat baby (usually weighing in excess of 9 lb at birth). Depending on the maternal metabolic and proinflammatory derangements, macrosomia is explained by an excessive availability of nutrients and an increase in fetal insulin release (Vambergue 2011). Macrosomic babies can face health problems of their own, including damage to their shoulders during birth, low blood glucose levels following birth, and breathing problems postdelivery. In addition, babies with excess fat and elevated insulin levels are at higher risk for obesity and T2D themselves. Many women with GDM develop T2D within 5–10 years after delivery, and the risk is increased by excess body weight (U.S. Department of Health and Human Services 2011, American Diabetes Association 2013a). Women with a history of GDM should have lifelong screening for T2D or prediabetes at least every 3 years (American Diabetes Association 2013b).

PREVENTION OF GESTATIONAL DIABETES WITH PHYSICAL ACTIVITY

Women diagnosed with GDM have a substantially greater risk of developing T2D at some point later in their lives. In truth, any degree of abnormal glucose homeostasis in pregnancy independently predicts an increased risk of glucose intolerance postpartum (Retnakaran 2008), and women with either GDM or gestational impaired glucose tolerance exhibit declining β-cell function in the first year after giving birth that likely contributes to their future diabetes risk (Retnakaran 2010).

Physical activity during pregnancy may prevent both GDM and possibly later-onset T2D (Dyck 1998). Engaging in regular physical activity before pregnancy frequently has been associated with a reduced risk of developing GDM (Dyck 2002; Dempsey 2004a, 2004b; Oken 2006; Zhang 2006). Studies testing the effects of such activity during pregnancy have had mixed results, with some studies demonstrating protective effects and other not finding them (Dyck 2002, Dempsey 2004b, Oken 2006). In a recent clinical trial, however, a moderate physical activity program performed thrice weekly during pregnancy was found to improve levels of maternal glucose tolerance in healthy, pregnant women (Barakat 2012) and higher levels of physical activity participation before pregnancy or in early pregnancy significantly lower the risk of developing GDM (Tobias 2011).

Similarly a recent meta-analysis reported that pregnant women with GDM who exercised on a cycle or arm ergometer or performed resistance training three times a week for 20–45 min experienced better glycemic control, lower fasting and postprandial glucose levels, and improved cardiorespiratory fitness (Ceysens 2006). The same number of exercising women ended up being prescribed insulin to control their blood sugars compared with sedentary women, however, and pregnancy outcomes were unchanged.

Recent research has also determined that compared with less vigorous activities, exercise intensity that reaches at least 60% of heart rate reserve (HRR) during pregnancy while gradually increasing physical activity energy expenditure reduces the risk of developing GDM (Zavorsky 2011a). The more vigorous the exercise, the less total exercise time is required. Thus, the general consensus is that higher levels of moderate physical activity (aerobic or resistance training) may reduce the risk of developing GDM during pregnancy and lower blood glucose levels in women who do develop it. Prevention of glucose intolerance during pregnancy may be possible, however, if women of reproductive age engage in leisure time physical activity (particularly vigorous) in advance of becoming pregnant (Retnakaran 2009, Baptiste-Roberts 2011).

EXERCISE PRESCRIPTION FOR WOMEN WITH GESTATIONAL DIABETES

MODE

Most moderate and vigorous aerobic exercise is acceptable during pregnancy with GDM, including both weight-bearing and non–weight-bearing activities like walking, jogging or running, cycling, swimming, water aerobics, aquatic activities, conditioning machines, dancing, chair exercises, and rowing (Committee on Obstetric Practice 2002). During pregnancy, however, women should avoid doing exercises involving lying on their back during the second and third trimesters. They should also avoid activities that increase the risk of falling or abdominal trauma, including contact or collision sports, horseback riding, downhill skiing, water skiing, soccer, and basketball. Late in pregnancy, non–weight-bearing activities may be preferable to weight-bearing activities in some women, especially if low back pain is present (Noon 2012).

In addition, resistance training can be safely and effectively undertaken by pregnant women with GDM and may reduce the number of women who need insulin to control hyperglycemia (de Barros 2010). Low- to moderate-intensity muscle-strengthening exercises performed during the second and third trimesters of pregnancy have a minimal effect on newborn body size and overall health (Zavorsky 2011a, 2011b). Thus, women with GDM can experience greater blood glucose uptake through increased insulin sensitivity from both aerobic and resistance training (Avery 2001, Brankston 2004).

INTENSITY

For most healthy women who are not already highly active or doing vigorous-intensity activity, moderate-intensity aerobic activity is recommended during pregnancy and the postpartum period, corresponding to 40–59% HRR, "somewhat hard," or 5–6 on a 10-point rating scale. A more deconditioned woman may start as low as 30% HRR and progress to moderate levels. Women who are already highly active or doing regular vigorous activity (60–89% HRR, "hard," or a rating of 7–8) can continue these activities during pregnancy.

Because the effects of vigorous-intensity aerobic activity during pregnancy have not been studied carefully, there is no basis for recommending that women should begin such activities during pregnancy if they already were not doing so. Women who habitually engage in vigorous or high amounts of activity or strength training should continue to be physically active during pregnancy and after giving birth; they generally do not need to drastically reduce their activity levels, provided that they remain healthy and discuss with their health-care provider how to adjust activity levels during this time.

FREQUENCY

Pregnant women should engage in physical activity on most, if not all, days of the week. Current guidelines for adults generally recommend five sessions of moderate activity, which would also apply to women with GDM (Haskell 2007, Nelson 2007, Physical Activity Guidelines Advisory Committee 2008). Daily exercise may enhance glucose metabolism further, however, and therefore, the recommended frequency for any type of physical activity for women with GDM is 3–7 days, spread throughout the week.

DURATION

Engaging in 30 min of moderate-intensity physical activity on most days of the week, reaching a minimum total of 150 min/week, has been adopted as a recommendation for pregnant women without medical or obstetrical complications (Committee on Obstetric Practice 2002), although studies have shown benefits from daily sessions lasting 20–45 min (Ceysens 2006). Recent research has determined that compared with less vigorous activities, exercise intensity that reaches at least 60% of the HRR during pregnancy while gradually increasing physical-activity energy expenditure reduces the risk of gestational diabetes, and the more vigorous the exercise, the less total exercise time is required. Prolonged-duration physical activity usually is not recommended for pregnant women due to heightened concern over possible hypoglycemia or hyperthermia (Melzer 2010).

PROGRESSION

Sedentary and deconditioned women with GDM should start out on the low end of the intensity scale and gradually progress to moderate-intensity exercise (40–59% HRR or higher). Initially, the focus should be on increasing frequency and duration of the exercise rather than intensity. For previously inactive women, moderate-intensity workouts are likely an appropriate endpoint, but if beginning physical activity during pregnancy, women should increase the amount gradually over time. Women who were active before and during pregnancy and before diagnosis of GDM should continue doing moderate- to vigorous-intensity activities (Zavorsky 2011b).

During a normal postpartum period, regular physical activity continues to benefit a woman's overall health. Moderate-intensity physical activity undertaken after giving birth increases cardiorespiratory fitness and improves mood, with no adverse effects on breast-milk volume, breast-milk composition, or infant growth.

Table 7.3 Recommended Exercise Rx for Women with Gestational Diabetes

Mode	Aerobic: Walk, stationary cycle, swim, aquatic activities, conditioning machines, prenatal exercise classes, prenatal yoga, seated exercises, and possibly jogging or running (if highly active before pregnancy)
	Resistance: Light or moderate resistance exercises
	Exercises to Avoid: Activities lying flat on the back and any that increase the risk of falling or abdominal trauma (e.g., contact or collision sports, horseback riding, downhill skiing, water skiing, soccer, outdoor cycling, basketball, most racquet sports, and scuba diving)
Intensity	If inactive: moderate-intensity aerobic activity (40–59% HRR, or "somewhat hard") during pregnancy and postpartum
	If already active or doing vigorous activity: moderate- to vigorous-intensity activity (40–89% HRR, or "somewhat hard" to "hard")
Frequency	3–7 days, spread throughout the week
	Better done on most, if not all, days of the week
Duration	30 min/session (range of 20–45 min)
	At least 150 min of moderate-intensity physical activity spread throughout the week
Progression	If just starting, increase duration of moderate exercise slowly; if already more active, maintain or lower intensity during pregnancy rather than attempting to progress to higher levels

HRR, heart rate reserve.

An added benefit is that it helps women achieve and maintain a healthy weight postpartum and can promote weight loss when combined with caloric restriction. Pregnant women who habitually engage in vigorous-intensity aerobic activity or are highly active can continue physical activity during pregnancy and the postpartum period, provided that they remain healthy and discuss with their health-care provider how and when activity should be adjusted over time. These recommendations are summarized in Table 7.3.

Case in Point: Wrap-Up

CC plans on working out in the early mornings after dropping her son off at daycare. On her way to work, she can stop at the Y where she is a member and use their exercise equipment and facilities. She enjoys swimming and pool activities, as well as walking on a treadmill and occasionally using some of the aerobic conditioning machines. She thinks that the Y also offers some prenatal exercise classes for pregnant women that she is interested in taking.

Exercise Program Goals

Mode of Activity: Because CC has been mostly sedentary throughout her pregnancy to date (other than daily movement associated with her job), she should start with physical activities that are on the lower end of the intensity scale, such as walking, water aerobics, swimming, stationary cycling, and conditioning machines. She also can consider doing some light resistance training.

Intensity: Given CC's relative inactivity, she should consider working up to an exercise intensity that feels "somewhat hard" (5–6 on a 10-point scale) and not progress beyond that during the remainder of her pregnancy. Her target heart rate should be around 40–59% HRR (123–144 bpm) to receive maximal glycemic benefits from her training. Initially, she can start out as low as 30% HRR (112 bpm) if higher intensities are too difficult for her to do continuously.

Frequency: Because CC wants to avoid having to go on insulin injections, she is willing to engage in daily exercise during the remainder of her pregnancy, if possible. Her recommended frequency, therefore, is at least 5–7 days/week.

Duration: When starting her programmed exercise, CC should try to do at least 20–30 min of activity daily, with a target goal of a minimum of 150 min of physical activity spread throughout the week.

Progression: CC should progress to doing moderate physical activity, but she should not attempt to do vigorous activities during this pregnancy, given her sedentary lifestyle at the start of training. She can, however, continue with her exercise training after delivery and progress to doing a combination of moderate and vigorous training to lower her risk of developing T2D later in her lifetime.

Daily Movement: If possible, CC should continue to engage in as much daily movement as possible to maximize her energy expenditure (to prevent excess weight gain during pregnancy) and to minimize excursions in her blood glucose levels after eating. She should continue standing and taking steps while working and during her leisure time, whenever possible.

Possible Precautions: Because she is young, CC has limited cardiovascular risk factors. Due to that fact and being pregnant, maximal exercise stress testing is neither necessary nor advisable before starting her exercise program. Because she will not initially be taking insulin or oral medications, her risk of developing hypoglycemia related to exercise is low. She should use a blood glucose monitor to determine the effects of physical activity and dietary changes on her glycemic control.

Women at high risk for GDM may be able to prevent it with lifestyle management during pregnancy. In those who develop GDM, dietary improvements and regular physical activity are frequently sufficient to manage hyperglycemia, although insulin and oral medications may be used when these changes are not enough. Management of blood glucose levels ensures better pregnancy outcomes and improves the health of both the mother and the fetus. Engaging in 30 min of moderate-intensity physical activity on most, if not all, days of the week has been adopted as a recommendation for all pregnant women.

PROFESSIONAL PRACTICE PEARLS

- GDM has been increasing in prevalence and is associated with a significantly elevated risk of the woman developing T2D in the next 5–10 years.
- This transient type of diabetes is usually diagnosed in pregnant women at 24 to 28 weeks of gestation using a 75-g oral glucose challenge (OGTT).
- Regular exercise participation during pregnancy likely reduces the risk of pregnancy complications like preeclampsia and shortens the duration of active labor.
- Higher levels of moderate physical activity of any type may reduce the risk of developing GDM during pregnancy and lower blood glucose levels in women who do develop it.
- A state of insulin resistance caused by placental hormone release during the third trimester greatly increases the pregnant woman's insulin, resulting in hyperglycemia when pancreatic β-cells are unable to keep up with heightened insulin demands.
- Diet and exercise are the first line of treatment for GDM, although insulin and oral medications may be considered if lifestyle changes fail to control blood glucose levels.
- Uncontrolled hyperglycemia is potentially harmful to both mother and fetus, possibly resulting in macrosomic babies and other complications.
- Most moderate and vigorous aerobic exercise is acceptable during pregnancy with GDM, although some forms of exercise that increase risk of falls and traumatic injury should be avoided.
- For most healthy women who are not highly active or doing vigorous-intensity activity, moderate-intensity aerobic activity is recommended during pregnancy and postpartum.
- Women who habitually engage in vigorous or high amounts of activity or strength training can continue these activities during pregnancy and after giving birth.
- Pregnant women should engage in physical activity on most, if not all, days of the week for best glycemic results.
- Engaging in 30 min of moderate intensity physical activity on most days of the week, with a target of ≥150 min weekly, is recommended for women with GDM.

REFERENCES

American Diabetes Association: Diagnosis and classification of diabetes mellitus. *Diabetes Care* 36 (Suppl. 1):S67–S74, 2013a

American Diabetes Association: Standards of medical care in diabetes—2013. *Diabetes Care* 36 (Suppl. 1):S11–S66, 2013b

Artal R, Catanzaro RB, Gavard JA, Mostello DJ, Friganza JC: A lifestyle intervention of weight-gain restriction: diet and exercise in obese women with gestational diabetes mellitus. *Appl Physiol Nutr Metab* 32:596–601, 2007

Avery MD, Walker AJ: Acute effect of exercise on blood glucose and insulin levels in women with gestational diabetes. *J Matern Fetal Med* 10:52–58, 2001

Baptiste-Roberts K, Ghosh P, Nicholson WK: Pregravid physical activity, dietary intake, and glucose intolerance during pregnancy. *J Womens Health (Larchmt)* 20:1847–1851, 2011

Barakat R, Cordero Y, Coteron J, Luaces M, Montejo R: Exercise during pregnancy improves maternal glucose screen at 24-28 weeks: a randomised controlled trial. *Br J Sports Med* 46:656–661, 2012

Brankston GN, Mitchell BF, Ryan EA, Okun NB: Resistance exercise decreases the need for insulin in overweight women with gestational diabetes mellitus. *Am J Obstet Gynecol* 190:188–193, 2004

Ceysens G, Rouiller D, Boulvain M: Exercise for diabetic pregnant women. *Cochrane Database Syst Rev* CD004225, 2006

Chasan-Taber L, Schmidt MD, Pekow P, Sternfeld B, Manson JE, Solomon CG, Braun B, and Markenson G: Physical activity and gestational diabetes mellitus among Hispanic women. *J Womens Health (Larchmt)* 17:999–1008, 2008

Committee on Obstetric Practice: ACOG committee opinion. Exercise during pregnancy and the postpartum period. Number 267, January 2002. American College of Obstetricians and Gynecologists. *Int J Gynaecol Obstet* 77:79–81, 2002

Davenport MH, Mottola MF, McManus R, Gratton R: A walking intervention improves capillary glucose control in women with gestational diabetes mellitus: a pilot study. *Appl Physiol Nutr Metab* 33:511–517, 2008

de Barros MC, Lopes MA, Francisco RP, Sapienza AD, Zugaib M: Resistance exercise and glycemic control in women with gestational diabetes mellitus. *Am J Obstet Gynecol* 203:556.e1–6, 2010

Dempsey JC, Butler CL, Sorensen TK, Lee IM, Thompson ML, Miller RS, Frederick IO, Williams MA: A case-control study of maternal recreational physical activity and risk of gestational diabetes mellitus. *Diabetes Res Clin Pract* 66:203–215, 2004a

Dempsey JC, Sorensen TK, Williams MA, Lee IM, Miller RS, Dashow EE, Luthy DA: Prospective study of gestational diabetes mellitus risk in relation to maternal recreational physical activity before and during pregnancy. *Am J Epidemiol* 159:663–670, 2004b

Dhulkotia JS, Ola B, Fraser R, Farrell T: Oral hypoglycemic agents vs insulin in management of gestational diabetes: a systematic review and metaanalysis. *Am J Obstet Gynecol* 203:457.e1–9, 2010

Dyck R, Klomp H, Tan LK, Turnell RW, Boctor MA: A comparison of rates, risk factors, and outcomes of gestational diabetes between aboriginal and non-aboriginal women in the Saskatoon health district. *Diabetes Care* 25:487–493, 2002

Dyck RF, Sheppard MS, Cassidy H, Chad K, Tan L, Van Vliet SH: Preventing NIDDM among aboriginal people: is exercise the answer? Description of a pilot project using exercise to prevent gestational diabetes. *Int J Circumpolar Health* 57 (Suppl. 1):375–378, 1998

Hapo Study Cooperative Research Group, Metzger BE, Lowe LP, Dyer AR, Trimble ER, Chaovarindr U, Coustan DR, Hadden DR, McCance DR, Hod M, McIntyre HD, Oats JJ, Persson B, Rogers MS, Sacks DA: Hyperglycemia and adverse pregnancy outcomes. *N Engl J Med* 358:1991–2002, 2008

Haskell WL, Lee IM, Pate RR, Powell KE, Blair SN, Franklin BA, Macera CA, Heath GW, Thompson PD, Bauman A: Physical activity and public health: updated recommendation for adults from the American College of Sports Medicine and the American Heart Association. *Med Sci Sports Exerc* 39:1423–1434, 2007

Iqbal R, Rafique G, Badruddin S, Qureshi R, Cue R, Gray-Donald K: Increased body fat percentage and physical inactivity are independent predictors of gestational diabetes mellitus in South Asian women. *Eur J Clin Nutr* 61:736–742, 2007

Melzer K, Schutz Y, Boulvain M, Kayser B: Physical activity and pregnancy: cardiovascular adaptations, recommendations and pregnancy outcomes. *Sports Med* 40:493–507, 2010

Metzger BE, Persson B, Lowe LP, Dyer AR, Cruickshank JK, Deerochanawong C, Halliday HL, Hennis AJ, Liley H, Ng PC, Coustan DR, Hadden DR, Hod M, Oats JJ, Trimble ER, Hapo Study Cooperative Research Group: Hyperglycemia and adverse pregnancy outcome study: neonatal glycemia. *Pediatrics* 126:e1545–e1552, 2010

Nelson ME, Rejeski WJ, Blair SN, Duncan PW, Judge JO, King AC, Macera CA, Castaneda-Sceppa C: Physical activity and public health in older adults: recommendation from the American College of Sports Medicine and the American Heart Association. *Med Sci Sports Exerc* 39:1435–1445, 2007

Newbern D, Freemark M: Placental hormones and the control of maternal metabolism and fetal growth. *Curr Opin Endocrinol Diabetes Obes* 18:409–416, 2011

Nicholson W, Bolen S, Witkop CT, Neale D, Wilson L, Bass E: Benefits and risks of oral diabetes agents compared with insulin in women with gestational diabetes: a systematic review. *Obstet Gynecol* 113:193–205, 2009

Noon ML, Hoch AZ: Challenges of the pregnant athlete and low back pain. *Curr Sports Med Rep* 11:43–48, 2012

Oken E, Ning Y, Rifas-Shiman SL, Radesky JS, Rich-Edwards JW, Gillman MW: Associations of physical activity and inactivity before and during pregnancy with glucose tolerance. *Obstet Gynecol* 108:1200–1207, 2006

Paglia MJ, Coustan DR: The use of oral antidiabetic medications in gestational diabetes mellitus. *Curr Diab Rep* 9:287–290, 2009

Physical Activity Guidelines Advisory Committee: Physical Activity Guidelines Advisory Committee Report, 2008. Washington, DC, U.S. Department of Health and Human Services, 2008

Retnakaran R, Qi Y, Sermer M, Connelly PW, Hanley AJ, Zinman B: Beta-cell function declines within the first year postpartum in women with recent glucose intolerance in pregnancy. *Diabetes Care* 33:1798–1804, 2010

Retnakaran R, Qi Y, Sermer M, Connelly PW, Zinman B, Hanley AJ: Pre-gravid physical activity and reduced risk of glucose intolerance in pregnancy: the role of insulin sensitivity. *Clin Endocrinol (Oxf)* 70:615–622, 2009

Retnakaran R, Qi Y, Sermer M, Connelly PW, Hanley AJ, Zinman B: Glucose intolerance in pregnancy and future risk of pre-diabetes or diabetes. *Diabetes Care* 31:2026–2031, 2008

Tobias DK, Zhang C, van Dam RM, Bowers K, Hu FB: Physical activity before and during pregnancy and risk of gestational diabetes mellitus: a meta-analysis. *Diabetes Care* 34:223–229, 2011

U.S. Department of Health and Human Services, Centers for Disease Control and Prevention: National Diabetes Fact Sheet: National Estimates and General Information on Diabetes and Prediabetes in the United States, 2011. Atlanta, GA, U.S. Department of Health and Human Services, Centers for Disease Control and Prevention, 2011

Vambergue A, Fajardy I: Consequences of gestational and pregestational diabetes on placental function and birth weight. *World J Diabetes* 2:196–203, 2011

Zavorsky GS, Longo LD: Adding strength training, exercise intensity, and caloric expenditure to exercise guidelines in pregnancy. *Obstet Gynecol* 117:1399–1402, 2011a

Zavorsky GS, Longo LD: Exercise guidelines in pregnancy: new perspectives. *Sports Med* 41:345–360, 2011b

Zhang C, Solomon CG, Manson JE, Hu FB: A prospective study of pregravid physical activity and sedentary behaviors in relation to the risk for gestational diabetes mellitus. *Arch Intern Med* 166:543–548, 2006

Chapter 8

Resistance Exercise Rx for Type 1 and Type 2 Diabetes

ny type of exercise can acutely improve insulin action in diabetic individuals, but resistance training can be particularly beneficial chronically because of its ability to result in increased muscle mass. The main tissues in the body that are sensitive to insulin are muscles and adipose (fat) cells. By increasing the quantity and insulin sensitivity of skeletal muscles with resistance exercise, most individuals can better manage blood glucose levels and body weight (Ishii 1998, Vincent 2002, Ibanez 2005, Williams 2007).

The goal of resistance training is increased muscular fitness, both muscular strength and endurance. Muscle strength is the ability of the muscle to exert force, whereas muscle endurance is the ability of the muscle to continue to perform without fatigue. Resistance training is recommended for people with diabetes and follows apparently healthy guidelines, with age and experience as prime considerations in program development. Such training has been shown to improve musculoskeletal health, maintain independence in performing daily activities, and reduce the possibility of injury (American College of Sports Medicine 2009, Garber 2011).

Case in Point: Resistance Exercise Rx for T2D

RS is a 60-year-old man who has type 2 diabetes (T2D) that was diagnosed ~8 years ago. His blood sugar control during most of that time has been just marginal since he has not been diligent about including regular physical activity in his routine, and he does not make healthy food choices on a fairly regular basis. His doctor has prescribed daily basal insulin (detemir) to supplement his metformin, which has brought his fasting blood glucose down a bit more. His admitted issue is that he hates doing aerobic exercise, and he is willing only to lift weights if he has to do any physical activity.

Resting Measurements

Height: 70 inches
Weight: 240 lb
BMI: 34.4 (obese)
Heart rate: 74 beats per minute (bpm)
Blood pressure: 130/85 mmHg (on medication); 155/90 mmHg (off medication)

Fasting Labs (1 Month after Diagnosis)

Plasma glucose: 125 mg/dl (controlled with metformin and now also insulin)
A1C: 7.6%
Total cholesterol: 165 mg/dl (on medication)
Triglycerides: 165 mg/dl
High-density lipoprotein cholesterol: 49 mg/dl
Low-density lipoprotein cholesterol: 83 mg/dl

Questions to Consider

1. What type of resistance training program should RS begin?
2. How often should he engage in resistance training each week?
3. How should his resistance training progress over time?
4. Should RS take any precautions related to doing this planned activity?

(Continued on page 119.)

HEALTH AND METABOLIC BENEFITS OF RESISTANCE TRAINING

Resistance (strength) training has been shown to improve musculoskeletal health, enhance the ability to perform activities of daily living, and lower the risk of injury (including from accidental falls) and descent into frailty (Willey 2003, Haskell 2007, Nelson 2007, Physical Activity Guidelines Advisory Committee Report 2009, Garber 2011). In fact, properly designed resistance programs may improve cardiovascular function, glucose tolerance, strength, and body composition, allowing older adults to remain more independent and self-sufficient as they age (Bemben 2000, Castaneda 2002, Dunstan 2002, Cornelissen 2005, Daly 2005, Cohen 2008, American College of Sports Medicine 2009, Church 2010). The prevalence rate for resistance training, however, is estimated at only 10–15% for older adults, despite the leisure time of older adults, access to facilities, and knowledge of its potential benefits (Winett 2009).

GLYCEMIC CONTROL

For people with diabetes, resistance training has additional benefits. It can improve glycemic control, possibly even more so than aerobic training in people with T2D (Ishii 1998, Poehlman 2000, Castaneda 2002, Vincent 2002, Ibanez 2005, Snowling 2006). Despite the fact that intense resistance exercise can acutely raise blood glucose levels due to its high intensity and exaggerated counterregulatory hormonal response (Kreisman 2003), regular resistance work improves overall glycemic control and insulin sensitivity with many training adaptations: It increases levels of GLUT4 (glucose transport protein) in muscle, insulin receptors, protein kinase B, glycogen synthase, and glycogen synthase total activity following acute training (Holten 2004). In another study, 16 weeks of twice-weekly progressive resistance training done by older men with new-onset T2D resulted in a 46% increase in insulin sensitivity, 7% reduction in fasting blood glucose, and loss of visceral fat, all while consuming a 15.5% average higher calorie intake (Ibanez 2005) . Others have found that when combined with moderate weight loss, resistance training was more effective for improving overall glycemic control than moderate weight loss alone, and the training prevented muscle mass loss (Dunstan 2002). An energy-restricted, high-protein diet (33% of daily calories from protein), combined with resistance training, resulted in greater weight loss and more favorable changes in body composition than dieting alone (Wycherley 2010).

EXERCISE INTENSITY

Much of the observed enhancement in insulin action with resistance work may be related to greater muscle mass, which can result from a variety of different training intensities (Bemben 2000, Castaneda 2002, Willey 2003). In fact, engaging in 16 weeks of progressive resistance training not only reduced A1C levels significantly in people with T2D but also increased their muscle glycogen stores and allowed 72% of participants to reduce their prescribed medication doses (Castaneda 2002). Acute resistance exercise sessions at light or moderate intensities are effective for controlling blood glucose levels in individuals with T2D (Moreira 2012). In older, diabetic adults, although improvements in muscle strength and mass can be similar, home-based progressive resistance training following supervised training is less effective for maintaining glycemic control than gymnasium-based work, likely because reductions in adherence and exercise training volume and intensity may somewhat impede the effectiveness of home-based training (Dunstan 2005).

TYPE 1 DIABETES

Fewer studies have investigated the effects of resistance training in type 1 diabetes (T1D). To determine the effect of a single session of resistance training, T1D participants completed five sets of only six repetitions of strenuous (80% 1 RM, or one-repetition maximum) quadriceps and hamstring exercises (Jimenez 2009). Insulin action was assessed before activity and 12 and 36 h postexercise, but no changes were noted. Another study evaluated the effect of 12 weeks of aerobic versus resistance training 3 days/week in people with T1D and found a reduction in insulin requirements in both groups, with no change in A1C levels (Ramalho 2006).

Case in Point: Continued

A second discussion with RS reveals additional points to consider: He has been diagnosed with coronary artery disease for about the past 5 years, and he has had stents placed in two of his coronary arteries; he also has hypertension and high cholesterol levels that are both reasonably under control with medications. Therefore, he has quite a few risk factors for cardiovascular disease, in addition to having diabetes.

Additional Questions to Consider

1. Is his diagnosis of coronary artery disease a contraindication to his participation in resistance training?
2. If RS is able to participate in resistance work, does he need to undergo any specific medical testing first?

(Continued on page 125.)

RESISTANCE TRAINING DEFINITION, DESIGN, AND TESTING

The optimal characteristics of strength-specific programs include the use of concentric, eccentric, and isometric muscle actions, along with bilateral and unilateral single- and multiple-joint exercises. Strength programs should sequence exercises to allow for optimal preservation of exercise intensity: large muscle group exercises should be done before small muscle group ones, multiple-joint exercises should precede single-joint, and higher-intensity exercises should come before lower-intensity choices (American College of Sports Medicine 2009).

DEFINITION OF RESISTANCE TRAINING

Resistance training is the use of resistance to muscular contraction to build the strength, anaerobic endurance, and size of skeletal muscles (American College of Sports Medicine 2009). The most common method of training is the use of gravity or elastic and hydraulic forces to oppose muscle contraction. The terms *resistance training* and *strength training* often are used interchangeably. It is primarily an anaerobic activity, although it can be made somewhat more aerobic when done as circuit training.

This type of training commonly uses the technique of progressively increasing muscular force output through incremental increases of weight, elastic tension, or other resistance and uses a variety of exercises and types of equipment to target specific muscle groups (American College of Sports Medicine 2009). To stimulate further adaptation toward specific training goals, progressive resistance training should be prescribed for all individuals with diabetes (Ghilarducci 1989, Willey 2003, Ibanez 2005, Ramalho 2006, Snowling 2006, Gordon 2009, Kelley 2009). Both strength training and conditioning of the body core are important components of preserving and increasing muscular strength (or 1 RM), muscular endurance (such as the number of push-ups done in a minute), power (e.g., time to run a 50-yard dash), and balance (e.g., time standing on one leg).

Any of the following types of resistance exercises can be used alone or in combination to improve muscular fitness (both muscular strength and endurance):

- Weight lifting with free weights (dumbbells and barbells)
- Weight or resistance machines
- Resistance bands
- Isometric exercises
- Calisthenics using body weight as resistance (e.g., push-ups)

PROGRAM DESIGN

The main factors to consider when designing resistance training programs for anyone with diabetes include the following: *1*) the individual's current activity level; *2*) the primary goals of training; *3*) any medications taken that can interact with physical activity; and *4*) the existence of related health comorbidities. Any or all of these factors can affect the expected outcomes of training.

Current activity level. The current activity level of an individual dictates the overall muscular fitness and strength gains that are attainable. Someone starting out completely sedentary is likely to have greater gains than an already active individual, who may not experience as much of an absolute change in muscle strength from a new resistance training program (Dunstan 2005).

Primary goals of training. The main goals of the resistance training should be determined before program development. Resistance training benefits are specific to the types of exercises and the muscle groups exercised. If the goal of training is either improvements in functional capacity or an increased ability to care for oneself, then the program should be geared more toward such activities (Vincent 2002). If an individual frequently relies on a wheelchair for locomotion, then exercises should be aimed specifically at increasing upper-body strength for movements that assist with rising from the wheelchair. If better glycemic control is the main goal, then activities that utilize large muscle groups and result in increases in muscle mass are appropriate (Ishii 1998, Castaneda 2002, Dunstan 2002, Cuff 2003, Willey 2003, Ibanez 2005, Gordon 2009, Irvine 2009).

Medications. The medications that an individual takes can potentially affect his or her risk for hypoglycemia and alter performance. High-intensity exercises result in significant depletion of muscle glycogen, increasing the risk for later-onset hypoglycemia particularly if certain diabetic medications like supplemental insulin or longer-lasting sulfonylureas are taken (Larsen 1999, Delvecchio 2009). The potential exercise side effects of all of an individual's prescribed medications should be fully discussed with his or her physician or other health-care professional prior to the initiation of any type of exercise training program.

Other health issues. Finally, the presence of other chronic health concerns, such as cardiovascular disease or small vessel damage (e.g., eyes, kidneys, and nerves), is common in individuals with diabetes. Such comorbidities must be addressed when prescribing resistance training. Some exercise precautions with complications are listed in Table 8.1, but all are discussed in more detail in later chapters addressing each comorbidity individually.

ONE-REPETITION MAXIMUM TESTING AND ESTIMATION

Testing an individual to determine his or her maximal strength (1 RM) on each exercise helps determine an appropriate weight or resistance and the number of repetitions. Doing 1 RM testing, however, can cause exaggerated rises in blood pressure, particularly in individuals with preexisting hypertension. If someone has

Table 8.1 Exercise Precautions for Resistance Training with Diabetes

Diabetic individuals should follow these precautions to perform resistance training safely and effectively:

- Consult with a physician before exercising with any of the following conditions:
  - ☐ Proliferative retinopathy or current retinal hemorrhage
  - ☐ Neuropathy (nerve damage), either peripheral or autonomic
  - ☐ Foot injuries (including ulcers)
  - ☐ High blood pressure (especially if not well controlled)
  - ☐ Serious illness or infection
- Have a blood glucose meter accessible to monitor blood glucose levels before, possibly during, or after exercise or any time that symptoms of hypoglycemia occur
- Immediately treat hypoglycemia with glucose tablets or regular soft drinks
- Stay properly hydrated with frequent intake of small amounts of cool water
- Seek immediate medical attention for chest pain or any pain that radiates down the arm, jaw, or neck that may be a sign of a heart attack
- With hypertension or unstable proliferative retinopathy, avoid activities that cause excessive increases in blood pressure, such as heavy resistance work, head-down exercises, jumping or jarring activities, and breath holding
- Never exercise with active retinal hemorrhages, and stop exercise if visual changes occur
- Wear proper footwear, and check feet daily for signs of trauma such as blisters, redness, or other signs of irritation

hypertension or known heart disease, alternately estimating 1 RM from a submaximal lift that takes into account the number of times a certain amount of weight can be lifted is recommended.

An estimated, rather than directly measured, 1 RM can be calculated by determining the weight lifted divided by the percent of 1 RM, where percent of 1 RM = [weight lifted – (# reps × 2)]. For example, if 100 lb can be lifted eight times, then the percent of 1 RM achieved is calculated as [weight lifted – (# reps × 2)] = [100 – (8 × 2)] or 84% (or 0.84). The estimated 1 RM can then be calculated as [weight lifted / % 1 RM], or 100/0.84, which equals 119 lb in this example.

RESISTANCE TRAINING CONSIDERATIONS AND PRECAUTIONS

EXERCISE STRESS TESTING CONSIDERATIONS

For diabetic individuals wishing to begin resistance training workouts, there is no evidence available to determine whether a pre-exercise evaluation involving graded exercise stress testing is necessary or beneficial before participation in anaerobic or resistance training. At present, most testing centers are equipped for maximal stress testing, but not for an alternate form of testing involving resistance exercise. Moreover, coronary ischemia is less likely to occur during resistance compared with aerobic exercise eliciting the same heart rate, and resistance exercise may not induce ischemia (Ghilarducci 1989, Featherstone 1993). For instance, even in men in cardiac rehabilitation programs and with known coronary ischemia and electrocardiogram (ECG) changes inducible by moderate aerobic exercise, no evidence of angina, ST depression, abnormal hemodynamics, ventricular dys-rhythmias, or other complications was documented during high-intensity resistance workouts (Wenger 1995). A study on 12 men with known coronary ischemia and ECG changes inducible by moderate aerobic exercise found that even maximal-intensity resistance exercise did not induce ECG changes (Featherstone 1993).

Resistance training previously was not prescribed to anyone with cardiovascular disease because it was feared that increases in blood pressure would put the individual at increased risk for an adverse cardiac event. Resistance training, however, is now recommended for individuals with known cardiovascular disease and even for those who have suffered a heart attack or stroke as such individuals experience less angina (chest pain due to ischemia) during resistance training compared with aerobic treadmill training (Featherstone 1993). During resistance work, both systolic and diastolic blood pressures rise in parallel, possibly helping to maintain coronary perfusion, whereas in aerobic exercise, systolic pressure rises significantly more than diastolic pressure. There is also a lesser rise in cardiac output with resistance training, and more rest between resistance sets compared with continuous aerobic exercise bouts (Sigal 2004). Thus, for individuals who are diagnosed with coronary artery blockage from plaque buildup, moderate weight training actually may be a safer activity than most high-intensity aerobic ones.

RESISTANCE EXERCISE PRECAUTIONS WITH DIABETES

For safe and effective resistance exercise participation, blood glucose levels should be carefully managed (Sigal 1994, Irvine 2009, Younk 2011). Although resistance training has a similar long-term benefit on glycemic control, the acute effects of a single bout of this type of exercise bestow a lower risk for both postexercise and late-onset hypoglycemia than aerobic training, at least in adults with T2D (Bacchi 2012). In T1D, resistance training consisting of 45 min of exercise (three sets of seven exercises at 8 repetitions maximum) causes less initial decline in blood glucose during the activity compared with a similar length of moderate aerobic work, but resistance exercise is associated with more prolonged reductions in postexercise glycemia (Yardley 2012). Appropriate attention to modifying the intensity of the lifting session may also reduce the risk for elevations in blood pressure, immediate postexercise blood glucose levels, or musculoskeletal injury. Training should progress slowly enough to prevent injury and motivational issues.

Although moderate- to high-intensity resistance training appears not to induce ischemia, resistance exercises should still be dynamic, avoid the Valsalva maneuver, and require breathing out on effort to avoid unduly increasing blood pressure that may contribute to retinal damage (Bernbaum 1989a, 1989b). Individuals with unstable proliferative retinopathy or severe nephropathy should likely refrain from engaging in resistance training because of the increased risk for an excessive systolic blood pressure response that could exacerbate those conditions (Colberg 2010). Finally, any individuals with diabetes-related or other health complications that may be worsened by resistance training need to receive approval from their physician before starting a resistance program. For a list of precautions related to resistance training, refer to Table 8.1.

RESISTANCE EXERCISE PRESCRIPTION FOR T1D AND T2D

MODE

Muscular fitness can be improved by including free weights (dumbbells and barbells), weight or resistance machines, resistance bands, isometric exercises, and calisthenics using body weight as resistance (e.g., push-ups). Resistance machines and free weights result in fairly equivalent gains in strength and mass of targeted muscles (Dunstan 2002, 2005), although no research has specifically evaluated the use of resistance bands or body-weight resistance only. Typically, heavier weights or resistance are needed to optimize insulin action and blood glucose control (Willey 2003, Dunstan 2005).

Individuals should select strengthening exercises that involve the major muscle groups in the upper body, lower body, and core, including the back, legs, hips, chest, shoulders, arms, and abdomen (Haskell 2007, Colberg 2010, Garber 2011). Exercise selection should be based on individual goals, preferences, and skill. Specific muscle groups also may be targeted to enhance other components of the activity program, such as biking, swimming, or golfing.

As far as exercise sequencing goes, individuals should exercise their large muscle groups before small ones, such as doing chest and back exercises before specific arm exercises. In addition, they should do exercises involving multiple joints before those that focus on single joints, for example, leg presses before leg extensions (quadriceps muscle only) or leg curls (hamstrings) (American College of Sports Medicine 2009). Doing them in this sequence helps ensure that adequate energy is available to effectively perform all exercises within a training session and in order to lower injury risk. Abdominal and core muscle exercises should be performed at the end of the training session to avoid premature fatigue.

INTENSITY

The actual resistance used is determined by a person's 1 RM that can be lifted successfully only one time. Training should be either moderate (50% 1 RM) or vigorous (75–80% 1 RM) in intensity to allow for optimal gains in strength and insulin action (Albright 2000; Dunstan 2002, 2005; Vincent 2002; Willey 2003; Sigal 2004, 2006; Gordon 2009). No specific amount of time is recommended for muscle strengthening, but exercises should be performed to the point at which it would be difficult to do another repetition without assistance, at least on the final set. Home-based resistance training is adequate for maintaining muscle mass and strength, but it is less effective than supervised, gym-based training for sustaining blood glucose control as heavier weights or resistance may be needed to optimize insulin action (Willey 2003, Dunstan 2005).

FREQUENCY

Resistance exercise should be undertaken at least twice weekly on nonconsecutive days (with a minimum of 48 h of rest between sessions) (Albright 2000; Sigal 2004, 2006; Haskell 2007; Nelson 2007; Physical Activity Guidelines Advisory Committee Report 2009; Colberg 2010; Garber 2011), but more ideally three times a week (Dunstan 2002, Snowling 2006) as part of a physical activity program for both T1D and T2D, along with regular aerobic activities. Adequate rest periods between sets during a workout session are needed to successfully complete all sets on each exercise. Typically, lower-intensity training requires 15 sec to 1 min of rest, whereas higher-intensity training may necessitate up to 2–3 min of rest between sets.

DURATION

Each training session should minimally include 5–10 exercises involving the major muscle groups in the upper body, lower body, and core, with completion of 10–15 repetitions to near fatigue per set early in training (Albright 2000; Vincent 2002; Sigal 2004, 2006; Gordon 2009), progressing over time to heavier weights or resistance that can be lifted only 8–10 times. A minimum of one set of repetitions to near fatigue, but as many as three to four sets per exercise, is recommended for optimal strength gains. As far as diabetes management is concerned, single-set protocols are generally less effective than multiple-set protocols in lowering fasting blood glucose and raising insulin action, as there is likely a dose-response relationship between volume and intensity on insulin sensitivity and fasting blood glucose (Black 2010).

PROGRESSION

To avoid injury, progression of intensity, frequency, and duration of training sessions should occur slowly. In most progressive resistance training, increases in weight or resistance are undertaken first—but only once the target number of repetitions per set can be exceeded consistently—followed by a greater number of sets and last by increased training frequency (American College of Sports Medicine 2009, Garber 2011). Progression over 6 months to thrice-weekly sessions of three sets of 8–10 repetitions done at 75–80% of 1 RM on 8–10 exercises may be an optimal goal for most individuals with diabetes (Dunstan 2002; Colberg 2010, 2011). Individuals with joint limitations or other health complications, however, should complete one set of exercises for all major muscle groups, starting with 10–15 repetitions and progressing to 15–20 repetitions before additional sets are added (Nelson 2007). Recommended resistance exercise for individuals with T1D and T2D can be found in Table 8.2. A sample program that shows progression of resistance work done twice weekly over 16 weeks is shown in Table 8.3.

Case in Point: Wrap-Up

Given RS's interest in resistance work and his medical history, he should start with a resistance training program to increase muscle mass and whole-body energy

Table 8.2 Recommended Resistance Exercise Rx for Type 1 and Type 2 Diabetes

	Type 1 Diabetes	Type 2 Diabetes
Mode of training	All major muscle groups, using resistance bands, free weights, resistance training machines, isometric exercises, or calisthenics (using body weight) Upper body: 4–5 exercises Lower body/core: 4–5 exercises	All major muscle groups, using resistance bands, free weights, resistance training machines, isometric exercises, and/or calisthenics (using body weight) Upper body: 4–5 exercises Lower body/core: 4–5 exercises
Intensity	60–80% 1 RM 7–8 (10-point scale)	50/60–80% 1 RM (50% 1 RM initially if untrained) 5–8 (10-point scale)
Frequency	2–3 days/week (nonconsecutive) Allow 48 h of rest between training sessions	A minimum of 2 days/week, but preferably 3 days/week (nonconsecutive) Allow 48 h of rest between training sessions
Duration and number of repetitions	8–12 repetitions per exercise 1–3 sets per exercise	8–12 repetitions per exercise as a goal, but 10–15 repetitions initially 1–3 sets per exercise
Progression	Start with 1–2 sets of 8–12 repetitions, progressing to 8–10 harder repetitions, and finally to 2–3 sets of 8–10 repetitions to near fatigue	Start with 1–2 sets of 8–15 repetitions: 1 set of 10–15 repetitions to fatigue initially, progressing to 8–10 harder repetitions, and finally to 2–3 sets of 8–10 repetitions

Note: Certain individuals may need to lower their intensity (more repetitions with less resistance) when diabetic retinopathy, hypertension, or orthopedic limitations are present. 1 RM, one-repetition maximum.

expenditure, along with possibly working with a dietitian to enhance visceral fat loss through dietary changes.

To accommodate his sedentary status, his program will begin with a lower intensity, whole-body resistance training performed two times a week. He also should be advised to use proper lifting techniques to ensure that he does not hold his breath during exercises and cause a greater increase in his blood pressure.

Exercise Program Goals

Mode of Activity: RS currently has access to a local gym that he plans to visit to do his resistance training program. At the onset of training, he will primarily use resistance machines for leg press, leg extension, leg curls, chest press, bench press, lateral pull-down, abdominal curls, and other exercises (a minimum of 5–10 involving all the major muscle groups of his body). As his strength increases, he should incorporate some standing and free weight exercises that complement these.

Intensity: To accommodate his sedentary status at the start of training, RS should aim for working at 50–60% of his 1 RM, which should feel "somewhat hard." His ultimate intensity goal should be closer to 70–80% 1 RM on most exercises. An aerobic cooldown following training also will help lower any elevation in his blood glucose caused by intense resistance training.

Frequency: RS should plan to engage in resistance training a minimum of 2 non-consecutive days/week, with a goal of 3 days/week being optimal for him.

Duration: To make his strength gains progressive, RS should plan on doing one to two sets of 12–15 repetitions to start, with a goal of being able to do two to three sets of 8–10 repetitions to near fatigue after several months of consistent training.

Progression: Given that resistance training is a new activity for RS, he should progress slowly, but steadily, progressively increasing his intensity based on subsequent 1 RM testing after every 4–6 weeks of consistent training. To get optimal strength and blood glucose benefits, he should progress to doing at least two to three sets per exercise, possibly adding in some additional exer-

Table 8.3 Sample Progressive Resistance Training Program for Diabetes

Week	Day 1 (% 1 RM)	Day 2 (% 1 RM)
1	Baseline 1 RM testing	50%, 1 set, 10–15 reps
2	50%, 1–2 sets, 10–15 reps	50%, 1–2 sets, 10–15 reps
3	50%, 1–2 sets, 10–15 reps	50%, 1–2 sets, 10–15 reps
4	50%, 1–2 sets, 10–15 reps	50%, 1–2 sets, 10–15 reps
5	60%, 1–2 sets, 8–10 reps	60%, 1–2 sets, 8–10 reps
6	60%, 1–2 sets, 8–10 reps	60%, 1–2 sets, 8–10 reps
7	60%, 1–2 sets, 8–10 reps	60%, 1–2 sets, 8–10 reps
8	60%, 1–2 sets, 8–10 reps	60%, 1–2 sets, 8–10 reps
9	70%, 1–2 sets, 8–10 reps	70%, 1–2 sets, 8–10 reps
10	70%, 1–2 sets, 8–10 reps	70%, 1–2 sets, 8–10 reps
11	70%, 1–2 sets, 8–10 reps	70%, 1–2 sets, 8–10 reps
12	70–80%, 1–2 sets, 8–10 reps	70–80%, 1–2 sets, 8–10 reps
13	70–80%, 1–2 sets, 8–10 reps	70–80%, 1–2 sets, 8–10 reps
14	70–80%, 1–2 sets, 8–10 reps	70–80%, 1–2 sets, 8–10 reps
15	70–80%, 1–2 sets, 8–10 reps	70–80%, 1–2 sets, 8–10 reps
16	70–80%, 2–3 sets, 8–10 reps	70–80%, 2–3 sets, 8–10 reps

Note: From this point forward, training can progress with the introduction of different resistance exercises, doing additional sets per exercise, or adding in a third training day. 1 RM, one-repetition maximum.

cises (using free weights), and aiming to complete harder sets that allow him to only do 8–10 repetitions before reaching near fatigue on each set.

Possible Precautions: Although RS has known cardiovascular disease, he is not likely to develop symptoms of ischemia while doing resistance training and, therefore, does not necessarily need to undergo any stress testing before beginning his training. Because he does have hypertension (albeit controlled with medications), however, it may advisable to estimate his initial 1 RM for all exercises using a submaximal load on each resistance training machine instead of directly measuring it. He should monitor the effects of training sessions on his blood glucose levels on occasion, particularly when he is starting this activity, to see whether his insulin doses should be lowered to prevent hypoglycemia. Using less insulin (due to heightened sensitivity from regular resistance work) will allow him to lose body fat more easily, assuming he adjusts his diet as well to take in fewer calories than he needs. To be prepared, he also needs to keep rapid-acting carbohydrates readily available to treat hypoglycemia, should it develop during or after exercise sessions.

People with any type of diabetes will benefit from engaging in resistance exercise training a minimum of 2, or more ideally 3, days/week. Resistance training has been shown to be the best exercise not only to maintain muscle mass and to prevent losses of muscle mass and strength but also to potentially increase muscle mass and enhance insulin action. A greater muscle mass generally results in increased resting blood glucose uptake and better glycemic control in individuals with any type of diabetes. Whole-body resistance training actually may be more beneficial than aerobic training in this regard because of the increased utilization of all muscle fibers during resistance exercises.

PROFESSIONAL PRACTICE PEARLS

- Resistance training of all intensities confers many health benefits, and particularly in individuals with T2D, it improves insulin action and lowers blood glucose levels.
- By increasing the quantity and insulin sensitivity of skeletal muscles with resistance exercise, most individuals can better manage blood glucose levels and body weight.
- Resistance training employs progressively increasing muscular force output through incremental increases of weight, elastic tension, or other resistance, and uses a variety of exercises and types of equipment to target specific muscle groups.
- The main factors to consider when designing resistance training programs include the individual's current activity level, the primary goals of training, any medications taken, and the presence of health comorbidities.
- Resistance training is recommended for individuals with known cardiovascular disease (even if they had a prior heart attack or stroke) as they experience less angina during resistance compared with aerobic training.

- Muscular fitness can be improved by including free weights (dumbbells and barbells), weight or resistance machines, resistance bands, isometric exercises, and calisthenics.
- Individuals should select exercises that involve the major muscle groups in the upper body, lower body, and core (i.e., back, legs, hips, chest, shoulders, arms, and abdomen).
- Training should be either moderate (50–60% 1 RM) or vigorous (75–80% 1 RM) in intensity to allow optimal gains in strength and insulin action.
- Resistance exercise should be undertaken at least twice weekly on nonconsecutive days, but more ideally three times a week, by individuals with T1D and T2D.
- Each training session should minimally include 5–10 exercises involving the major muscle groups, with completion of 8–15 repetitions to near fatigue per set.
- A minimum of one set of repetitions to near fatigue, but as many as three to four sets per exercise, is recommended for optimal strength gains.
- To be progressive, increases in weight or resistance should be undertaken once the target number of repetitions per set can be exceeded consistently, followed by a greater number of sets and finally by increased training frequency.

REFERENCES

Albright A, Franz M, Hornsby G, Kriska A, Marrero D, Ullrich I, Verity LS: American College of Sports Medicine position stand. Exercise and type 2 diabetes. *Med Sci Sports Exerc* 32:1345–1360, 2000

American College of Sports Medicine: American College of Sports Medicine position stand. Progression models in resistance training for healthy adults. *Med Sci Sports Exerc* 41:687–708, 2009

Bacchi E, Negri C, Trombetta M, Zanolin ME, Lanza M, Bonora E, Moghetti P: Differences in the acute effects of aerobic and resistance exercise in subjects with type 2 diabetes: Results from the RAED2 randomized trial. *PLoS One* 7:e49937, 2012

Bemben DA, Fetters NL, Bemben MG, Nabavi N, Koh ET: Musculoskeletal responses to high- and low-intensity resistance training in early postmenopausal women. *Med Sci Sports Exerc* 32:1949–1957, 2000

Bernbaum M, Albert SG, Cohen JD: Exercise training in individuals with diabetic retinopathy and blindness. *Arch Phys Med Rehabil* 70:605–611, 1989a

Bernbaum M, Albert SG, Cohen JD, Drimmer A: Cardiovascular conditioning in individuals with diabetic retinopathy. *Diabetes Care* 12:740–742, 1989b

Black LE, Swan PD, Alvar BA: Effects of intensity and volume on insulin sensitivity during acute bouts of resistance training. *J Strength Cond Res* 24:1109–1116, 2010

Castaneda C, Layne JE, Munoz-Orians L, Gordon PL, Walsmith J, Foldvari M, Roubenoff R, Tucker KL, Nelson ME: A randomized controlled trial of resistance exercise training to improve glycemic control in older adults with type 2 diabetes. *Diabetes Care* 25:2335–2341, 2002

Church TS, Blair SN, Cocreham S, Johannsen N, Johnson W, Kramer K, Mikus CR, Myers V, Nauta M, Rodarte RQ, Sparks L, Thompson A, Earnest CP: Effects of aerobic and resistance training on hemoglobin A1c levels in patients with type 2 diabetes: a randomized controlled trial. *JAMA* 304:2253–2262, 2010

Cohen ND, Dunstan DW, Robinson C, Vulikh E, Zimmet PZ, Shaw JE: Improved endothelial function following a 14-month resistance exercise training program in adults with type 2 diabetes. *Diabetes Res Clin Pract* 79:405–411, 2008

Colberg SR, Sigal RJ: Prescribing exercise for individuals with type 2 diabetes: recommendations and precautions. *Phys Sportsmed* 39:13–26, 2011

Colberg SR, Sigal RJ, Fernhall B, Regensteiner JG, Blissmer BJ, Rubin RR, Chasan-Taber L, Albright AL, Braun B, American College of Sports Medicine, American Diabetes Association: Exercise and type 2 diabetes: the American College of Sports Medicine and the American Diabetes Association: joint position statement. *Diabetes Care* 33:e147–e67, 2010

Cornelissen VA, Fagard RH: Effect of resistance training on resting blood pressure: a meta-analysis of randomized controlled trials. *J Hypertens* 23:251–259, 2005

Cuff DJ, Meneilly GS, Martin A, Ignaszewski A, Tildesley HD, Frohlich JJ: Effective exercise modality to reduce insulin resistance in women with type 2 diabetes. *Diabetes Care* 26:2977–2982, 2003

Daly RM, Dunstan DW, Owen N, Jolley D, Shaw JE, Zimmet PZ: Does high-intensity resistance training maintain bone mass during moderate weight loss in older overweight adults with type 2 diabetes? *Osteoporos Int* 16:1703–1712, 2005

Delvecchio M, Zecchino C, Salzano G, Faienza MF, Cavallo L, De Luca F, Lombardo F: Effects of moderate-severe exercise on blood glucose in type 1 diabetic adolescents treated with insulin pump or glargine insulin. *J Endocrinol Invest* 32:519–524, 2009

Dunstan DW, Daly RM, Owen N, Jolley D, Vulikh E, Shaw J, Zimmet P: Home-based resistance training is not sufficient to maintain improved glycemic control following supervised training in older individuals with type 2 diabetes. *Diabetes Care* 28:3–9, 2005

Dunstan DW, Daly RM, Owen N, Jolley D, De Courten M, Shaw J, Zimmet P: High-intensity resistance training improves glycemic control in older patients with type 2 diabetes. *Diabetes Care* 25:1729–1736, 2002

Featherstone JF, Holly RG, Amsterdam EA: Physiologic responses to weight lifting in coronary artery disease. *Am J Cardiol* 71:287–292, 1993

Garber CE, Blissmer B, Deschenes MR, Franklin BA, Lamonte MJ, Lee IM, Nieman DC, Swain DP, American College of Sports Medicine: American College of Sports Medicine position stand. Quantity and quality of exercise for developing and maintaining cardiorespiratory, musculoskeletal, and neuromotor fitness in apparently healthy adults: guidance for prescribing exercise. *Med Sci Sports Exerc* 43:1334–1359, 2011

Ghilarducci LE, Holly RG, Amsterdam EA: Effects of high resistance training in coronary artery disease. *Am J Cardiol* 64:866–870, 1989

Gordon BA, Benson AC, Bird SR, Fraser SF: Resistance training improves metabolic health in type 2 diabetes: a systematic review. *Diabetes Res Clin Pract* 83:157–175, 2009

Haskell WL, Lee IM, Pate RR, Powell KE, Blair SN, Franklin BA, Macera CA, Heath GW, Thompson PD, Bauman A: Physical activity and public health: updated recommendation for adults from the American College of Sports Medicine and the American Heart Association. *Med Sci Sports Exerc* 39:1423–1434, 2007

Holten MK, Zacho M, Gaster M, Juel C, Wojtaszewski JF, Dela F: Strength training increases insulin-mediated glucose uptake, GLUT4 content, and insulin signaling in skeletal muscle in patients with type 2 diabetes. *Diabetes* 53:294–305, 2004

Ibanez J, Izquierdo M, Arguelles I, Forga L, Larrion JL, Garcia-Unciti M, Idoate F, Gorostiaga EM: Twice-weekly progressive resistance training decreases abdominal fat and improves insulin sensitivity in older men with type 2 diabetes. *Diabetes Care* 28:662–667, 2005

Irvine C, Taylor NF: Progressive resistance exercise improves glycaemic control in people with type 2 diabetes mellitus: a systematic review. *Aust J Physiother* 55:237–246, 2009

Ishii T, Yamakita T, Sato T, Tanaka S, Fujii S: Resistance training improves insulin sensitivity in NIDDM subjects without altering maximal oxygen uptake. *Diabetes Care* 21:1353–1355, 1998

Jimenez C, Santiago M, Sitler M, Boden G, Homko C: Insulin-sensitivity response to a single bout of resistive exercise in type 1 diabetes mellitus. *J Sport Rehabil* 18:564–571, 2009

Kelley GA, Kelley KS: Impact of progressive resistance training on lipids and lipoproteins in adults: a meta-analysis of randomized controlled trials. *Prev Med* 48:9–19, 2009

Kreisman SH, Halter JB, Vranic M, Marliss EB: Combined infusion of epinephrine and norepinephrine during moderate exercise reproduces the glucoregulatory response of intense exercise. *Diabetes* 52:1347–1354, 2003

Larsen JJ, Dela F, Madsbad S, Vibe-Petersen J, Galbo H: Interaction of sulfonyl-ureas and exercise on glucose homeostasis in type 2 diabetic patients. *Diabetes Care* 22:1647–1654, 1999

Moreira SR, Simoes GC, Moraes JV, Motta DF, Campbell CS, Simoes HG: Blood glucose control for individuals with type-2 diabetes: acute effects of resistance exercise of lower cardiovascular-metabolic stress. *J Strength Cond Res* 26:2806–2811, 2012

Nelson ME, Rejeski WJ, Blair SN, Duncan PW, Judge JO, King AC, Macera CA, Castaneda-Sceppa C: Physical activity and public health in older adults: recommendation from the American College of Sports Medicine and the American Heart Association. *Med Sci Sports Exerc* 39:1435–1445, 2007

Physical Activity Guidelines Advisory Committee: Physical Activity Guidelines Advisory Committee Report, 2008. Washington, DC, U.S. Department of Health and Human Services, 2008

Physical Activity Guidelines Advisory Committee Report, 2008: To the Secretary of Health and Human Services. Part A: executive summary. *Nutr Rev* 67:114–120, 2009

Poehlman ET, Dvorak RV, DeNino WF, Brochu M, Ades PA: Effects of resistance training and endurance training on insulin sensitivity in nonobese, young women: a controlled randomized trial. *J Clin Endocrinol Metab* 85:2463–2468, 2000

Ramalho AC, de Lourdes Lima M, Nunes F, Cambui Z, Barbosa C, Andrade A, Viana A, Martins M, Abrantes V, Aragao C, Temistocles M: The effect of resistance versus aerobic training on metabolic control in patients with type-1 diabetes mellitus. *Diabetes Res Clin Pract* 72:271–276, 2006

Sigal RJ, Kenny GP, Wasserman DH, Castaneda-Sceppa C, White RD: Physical activity/exercise and type 2 diabetes: a consensus statement from the American Diabetes Association. *Diabetes Care* 29:1433–1438, 2006

Sigal RJ, Kenny GP, Wasserman DH, Castaneda-Sceppa C: Physical activity/exercise and type 2 diabetes. *Diabetes Care* 27:2518–2539, 2004

Sigal RJ, Purdon C, Fisher SJ, Halter JB, Vranic M, Marliss EB: Hyperinsulinemia prevents prolonged hyperglycemia after intense exercise in insulin-dependent diabetic subjects. *J Clin Endocrinol Metab* 79:1049–1057, 1994

Snowling NJ, Hopkins WG: Effects of different modes of exercise training on glucose control and risk factors for complications in type 2 diabetic patients: a meta-analysis. *Diabetes Care* 29:2518–2527, 2006

Vincent KR, Braith RW, Feldman RA, Magyari PM, Cutler RB, Persin SA, Lennon SL, Gabr AH, Lowenthal DT: Resistance exercise and physical performance in adults aged 60 to 83. *J Am Geriatr Soc* 50:1100–1107, 2002

Wenger NK, Froelicher ES, Smith LK, Ades PA, Berra K, Blumenthal JA, Certo CM, Dattilo AM, Davis D, DeBusk RF, et al.: Cardiac rehabilitation as secondary prevention. Agency for Health Care Policy and Research and National

Heart, Lung, and Blood Institute. *Clin Pract Guidel Quick Ref Guide Clin* (17):1–23, 1995

Willey KA, Singh MA: Battling insulin resistance in elderly obese people with type 2 diabetes: bring on the heavy weights. *Diabetes Care* 26:1580–1588, 2003

Williams MA, Haskell WL, Ades PA, Amsterdam EA, Bittner V, Franklin BA, Gulanick M, Laing ST, Stewart KJ: Resistance exercise in individuals with and without cardiovascular disease: 2007 update: a scientific statement from the American Heart Association Council on Clinical Cardiology and Council on Nutrition, Physical Activity, and Metabolism. *Circulation* 116:572–584, 2007

Winett RA, Williams DM, Davy BM: Initiating and maintaining resistance training in older adults: a social cognitive theory-based approach. *Br J Sports Med* 43:114–119, 2009

Wycherley TP, Noakes M, Clifton PM, Cleanthous X, Keogh JB, Brinkworth GD: A high-protein diet with resistance exercise training improves weight loss and body composition in overweight and obese patients with type 2 diabetes. *Diabetes Care* 33:969–976, 2010

Younk LM, Mikeladze M, Tate D, Davis SN: Exercise-related hypoglycemia in diabetes mellitus. *Expert Rev Endocrinol Metab* 6:93–108, 2011

Yardley JE, Kenny GP, Perkins BA, Riddell MC, Balaa N, Malcolm J, Boulay P, Khandwala F, Sigal RJ: Resistance versus aerobic exercise: acute effects on glycemia in type 1 diabetes. *Diabetes Care* [Epub ahead of print] 19 Nov 2012

Chapter 9

Combined Aerobic and Resistance Training for Adults with Diabetes

Exercise guidelines traditionally have addressed aerobic and resistance training separately, likely due to the fact that most studies have examined the two modes of training individually as well. More recently, however, a grouping of studies was designed to examine the glycemic benefits of combined aerobic and resistance training (because both are recommended on a daily or weekly basis), particularly in individuals with type 2 diabetes (T2D) (Maiorana 2002, Tokmakidis 2004, Snowling 2006, Sigal 2007, Marcus 2008, Church 2010, D'Hooge 2011, Touvra 2011, Umpierre 2011).

The results of all these studies have recently been published in a large meta-analysis (Umpierre 2011). In that study focusing on T2D research, structured aerobic, resistance, or combined exercise training was found to be associated with an A1C decrease of 0.67% following ≥12 weeks of training. Structured exercise that exceeded 150 min/week was associated with greater glycemic benefit (0.89% reduction in A1C) than durations of ≤150 min/week (only a 0.36% reduction), and any type of training caused greater declines in glycemic levels than simply giving people physical activity advice.

Case in Point: Combined Training Rx for T2D

JR, a 54-year-old woman with T2D for 3 years, realizes that if she wants to keep up with her grandchildren, she needs to be able to walk faster and be stronger. She has been engaging in daily walking since her diagnosis, but she usually walks only ~1 mile/day. Her diabetes currently is controlled with diet and two medications, daily metformin orally and injections of exenatide once weekly (Bydureon, which recently replaced her shorter-action Byetta). She also uses a cholesterol-lowering medication, but currently she is not taking any others.

Resting Measurements

Height: 65 inches
Weight: 198 lb
BMI: 32.9 (obese)
Heart rate: 84 beats per minute (bpm)
Blood pressure: 135/80 mmHg

Fasting Labs

Plasma glucose: 125 mg/dl (controlled with metformin and Bydureon)
A1C: 7.6%
Total cholesterol: 175 mg/dl (on medication)
Triglycerides: 95 mg/dl
High-density lipoprotein cholesterol: 52 mg/dl
Low-density lipoprotein cholesterol: 104 mg/dl

Questions to Consider

1. What type of combined training program would be appropriate for JR?
2. How often should she engage in structured training each week?
3. How should her training progress over time?
4. Are there any precautions that JR needs to take to engage in combined training safely and effectively?

(Continued on page 143.)

HEALTH BENEFITS OF COMBINED TRAINING

IMPROVEMENTS IN BLOOD GLUCOSE CONTROL IN T2D

It is well established that both resistance- and endurance-type exercise can be integrated in exercise intervention programs designed to improve glycemic control in adults (Umpierre 2011, van Dijk 2012). Moreover, combined aerobic and resistance training done thrice weekly in individuals with T2D may be of greater benefit to blood glucose control than either aerobic or resistance exercise alone (Sigal 2007a, Marcus 2008). The total duration of exercise and caloric expenditure were greatest, however, with combined training in the initial studies done, and both types of training were done on the same days during a single training session.

An early meta-analysis reported that aerobic, resistance, and combined training reduced A1C levels by 0.7%, 0.5%, and 0.8%, respectively (Snowling 2006). Moreover, both aerobic and combined training also reduced systolic and diastolic blood pressures modestly, whereas resistance training alone did not. Others found that both aerobic and resistance exercise training reduce A1C levels (by 0.51% and 0.38%, respectively), and combined aerobic and resistance training reduces them by 0.46% more compared with aerobic training alone and 0.59% more than resistance training alone (Sigal 2007a). In most of these studies, however, a greater total amount of exercise was done in the combined training groups than when either type of training was undertaken alone.

A recent study examined the effects of holding caloric expenditure constant among training groups (Church 2010). In that study, 73 individuals with T2D did resistance training alone 3 days a week, another 72 did aerobic exercise (expending 12 kcal/kg/week), and 76 completed combined aerobic and resistance training (expending 10 kcal/kg/week) and engaged in resistance training twice a week. Surprisingly, only those doing combined training improved their glycemic levels significantly. On a similar note, others have demonstrated that structured exercise training that consists of aerobic exercise, resistance training, or both combined that lasts >150 min/week is associated with greater glycemic declines than training that amounts to ≤150 min/week (Umpierre 2011).

The total duration of exercise and caloric expenditure have been greater with combined training in almost all studies done to date (Cuff 2003, Sigal 2007a, Marcus 2008), and both types of training have been undertaken together on the same days. Unfortunately, no studies have yet investigated whether daily, but alternating, training would be more effective, and the blood glucose impact of various isocaloric combinations of training programs also remains to be fully studied.

EFFECTS ON DAILY INSULIN NEEDS AND HYPOGLYCEMIA RISK IN TYPE 1 DIABETES

Only one study to date has looked at the impact of combination training in type 1 diabetes (T1D), and it was conducted on children who participated twice a week for 20 weeks in combined aerobic and strength training, while age-matched controls continued their normal daily activities. Daily doses of insulin injected were significantly lowered in the training group, but increased in the control group. Thus, combined exercise training lowered daily insulin requirement and improved physical fitness and sense of well-being (D'Hooge 2011). No studies thus far have investigated combination training versus other types of training or no activity in adults with T1D.

A second, recent study investigated the effects of exercise order in active adults with T1D undertaking combined aerobic (45 min of moderate treadmill running) and resistance (three sets of eight repetitions on seven different exercises) training in one session (Yardley 2012). As expected, performing resistance exercise before aerobic exercise rather than the reverse resulted in attenuated declines in blood glucose levels during exercise, less exercise-induced hypoglycemia, and reduced need for carbohydrate supplementation during exercise. The duration and severity of hypoglycemia were reduced for the next 12 h when resistance training was undertaken first during exercise sessions. Thus, individuals who tend to develop exercise-associated hypoglycemia during or following workouts should consider undertaking resistance work first (or another high-intensity exercise) before doing moderate aerobic exercise to lower their need for supplemental carbohydrate during the session and later hypoglycemia risk. Conversely, anyone who usually experiences a hyperglycemic response to exercise should consider engaging in aerobic exercise followed by resistance training when undertaking both in a single exercise session.

OTHER HEALTH AND METABOLIC BENEFITS

In 251 individuals with T2D undertaking aerobic, resistance, or aerobic plus resistance training, a link between changes in fitness and glycemic control has been observed, and improvements in cardiorespiratory fitness with aerobic training may be a better predictor of changes in glycemic control than improvements in strength (Larose 2011). Women with T2D experienced improvements in insulin sensitivity after 6 months of combined, supervised training related to exercise intensity, whereas reductions in A1C in these individuals was related mainly to training volume (calculated as the product of exercise duration and intensity). The authors of the study also observed that metabolic benefits of training may be seen in the absence of improved exercise capacity (Segerstrom 2010).

A combined strength and aerobic exercise program has been shown to have a potential antiatherogenic and anti-inflammatory impact that can reduce the risk of cardiovascular disease and improves the health status in adults with T2D (Touvra 2011). Others have shown that all types of exercise training favorably affect glycemic parameters, lipid profile, blood pressure, and high-sensitivity C-reactive protein (hs-CRP). In addition, resistance and combined training specifically may increase insulin receptor substrate-1 (IRS-1) expression (Jorge 2011).

IMPACT OF TRAINING ON STRENGTH

If strength gains are an individual's primary goal, undertaking combined training may not be as effective. For instance, muscular strength gains were assessed in adults with T2D doing resistance training or resistance plus aerobic training (Larose 2012). Those doing only resistance work experienced greater increases in upper- and lower-body strength. Thus, although both types of training can lead to improved strength over 6 months, gains are greater with resistance training alone, likely because a greater training load is possible when individuals are focused only on that one form of training.

COMBINED AEROBIC AND RESISTANCE EXERCISE PRESCRIPTION FOR ADULTS WITH DIABETES

MODE

Aerobic. Any form of aerobic exercise that utilizes large muscle groups and causes sustained increases in heart rate is likely to be beneficial to cardiovascular risk management (and possibly glycemic control) in adults with diabetes. Undertaking a variety of modes of physical activity is recommended for all individuals to optimize training effects and lower injury risk (Physical Activity Guidelines Advisory Committee 2008). Examples of acceptable aerobic activities include both weight-bearing and non–weight-bearing activities, including walking, jogging, running, cycling, swimming, water aerobics, aquatic activities, conditioning machines, dancing, chair exercises, rowing, and cross-country skiing, among others.

Resistance. Resistance work can include free weights (dumbbells and barbells), weight or resistance machines, resistance bands, isometric exercises, and calisthenics using body weight as resistance (e.g., push-ups). Typically, heavier weights or resistance are needed to optimize insulin action and blood glucose control (Willey 2003, Dunstan 2005). Individuals should select exercises that involve the major muscle groups in the upper body, lower body, and body core (Haskell 2007, Colberg 2010, Garber 2011).

INTENSITY

Aerobic. For adults, aerobic exercise should be moderate or vigorous intensity, corresponding to 50–85% of HRR (heart rate reserve; see chapter 4) (Haskell 2007,

Nelson 2007, Physical Activity Guidelines Advisory Committee 2008, Garber 2011). Moderate-intensity exercise equates to 40–59% HRR, whereas vigorous-intensity exercise is 60–89% HRR (Physical Activity Guidelines Advisory Committee 2008). A severely deconditioned person with any type of diabetes can start out at 30–39% HRR and progress to more moderate levels. For most people with T2D, brisk walking is a moderate-intensity exercise because of their lower cardiorespiratory fitness capacity (Boulé 2003). Including some faster intervals, such as doing pick-up-the-pace training that involves exercising at even 10% above a person's normal walking or other exercise intensity, can lead to additional fitness gains in individuals with T2D (Johnson 2006, 2008).

Using subjective ratings, moderate- to vigorous-intensity exercise corresponds to an overall body rating of "somewhat hard" to "hard" (Garber 2011). Less fit people generally require a higher level of effort to complete the same activity. Subjective intensity also can be estimated using a scale of 0 to 10, where resting is 0, maximal effort 10, moderate-intensity activity 5–6, and vigorous-intensity activity 7–8 on that scale (Physical Activity Guidelines Advisory Committee 2008).

Resistance. Training should be moderate (50% 1 RM) to vigorous (75–80% 1 RM) in intensity to allow for optimal gains in strength and insulin action (Albright 2000; Dunstan 2002, 2005; Vincent 2002; Willey 2003; Sigal 2004, 2006; Gordon 2009). Each exercise should be performed to near fatigue, especially on the final set. Home-based training maintains muscle mass and strength, but it is less effective than supervised, gym-based training for sustaining blood glucose control as heavier weights or resistance may be needed to optimize insulin action (Willey 2003, Dunstan 2005).

FREQUENCY

Aerobic. Aerobic exercise should be performed at least 3 days/week with no more than 2 consecutive days between bouts of activity due to the short-lived nature of improvements in insulin action (King 1995, Boulé 2005). Most exercise interventions in T2D have used a frequency of three times per week (Boulé 2001, Snowling 2006, Thomas 2006, Sigal 2007a), but current guidelines for adults generally recommend five sessions of moderate activity (Haskell 2007, Nelson 2007, Physical Activity Guidelines Advisory Committee 2008). Recommended frequency, therefore, is a minimum of 3–5 days/week. Greater regularity may facilitate diabetes management in individuals with T1D.

Resistance. This should be undertaken at least twice weekly on nonconsecutive days (Albright 2000; Sigal 2004, 2006; Haskell 2007; Nelson 2007; Physical Activity Guidelines Advisory Committee 2008; Colberg 2010; Garber 2011), but more ideally three times a week (Dunstan 2002, Snowling 2006), as part of a physical activity program for both T1D and T2D. Adequate rest periods between sets during a workout session are needed to successfully complete all sets on each exercise.

Combined. If both types of training are done on the same day, adults with diabetes should undertake 2–3 nonconsecutive days/week of combined training, with aerobic activities only on 1–4 other days/week. If both types of training are done on different days, individuals should separate bouts of resistance training by a minimum of 48 h. Individuals with T2D should not go more than 2 consecutive days without any physical activity.

DURATION

Aerobic. Individuals with T2D should engage in a minimum of 150 min/week of exercise undertaken at moderate intensity or greater. Aerobic activity should be performed in bouts of at least 10 min and be spread throughout the week. Engaging in >150 min bestows additional health benefits for most. Adults with T1D should engage in a minimum of 60–75 min/week of vigorous activity or 150 min/week of moderate-intensity exercise, performed for at least 20–30 min in bouts of at least 10 min.

Resistance. Each training session should minimally include 5–10 exercises involving the major muscle groups in the upper body, lower body, and core, with completion of 10–15 repetitions to near fatigue per set early in training (Albright 2000; Vincent 2002; Sigal 2004, 2006; Gordon 2009), progressing over time to heavier weights or resistance that can be lifted only 8–10 times. A minimum of one set of repetitions to near fatigue, but as many as three to four sets per exercise, is recommended for optimal strength gains.

Combined. Structured exercise training that consists of aerobic exercise, resistance training, or both combined is associated with lower A1C levels in T2D, but training of >150 min/week is associated with greater decrements than that of ≤150 min/week (Umpierre 2011). Therefore, individuals with diabetes should attempt to engage in a minimum of 150 min/week, including both types of training in the total duration. Simply adding resistance training time to that minimal aerobic training time to reach a higher total training time, however, may result in greater glycemic and health benefits. For instance, new Australian guidelines for T2D and prediabetes recommend a total combined minimal training time of 210 min of moderate exercise, including two or more resistance training sessions per week (two to four sets of 8–10 repetitions), or ≥125 min of total vigorous activity (Hordern 2012). Prescribed resistance training sessions can usually be completed in 30–60 min (American College of Sports Medicine 2009).

PROGRESSION

Aerobic. Deconditioned individuals with diabetes need to start out on the low end of the intensity scale and work toward gradual progression of both exercise intensity and volume, initially increasing exercise frequency and duration rather than intensity (Physical Activity Guidelines Advisory Committee 2008). Progression over 4–6 months usually has an ultimate goal of including vigorous aerobic exercise, but for many with T2D or others with health complications, doing moderate-intensity workouts may be an appropriate endpoint (although frequency and duration may progress over time). Significant weight loss may require exercising at least 7 h/week (Pavlou 1989, Schoeller 1997, Weinsier 2002, Saris 2003, Donnelly 2009). If an adult is already normally active or has a reasonable fitness level, he or she can skip the "initial" training phase and start directly with the "improvement" one.

Resistance. To avoid injury, progression of intensity, frequency, and duration of training sessions should occur slowly. In most progressive resistance training, increases in weight or resistance are undertaken once the target number of repetitions per set can consistently be exceeded, later followed by a greater number of sets and then increased training frequency (American College of Sports Medicine 2009, Garber 2011). Progression over 6 months to thrice-weekly sessions of three sets of 8–10 repetitions done at 75–80% of 1 RM on 8–10 exercises may be an optimal goal for most individuals with diabetes (Dunstan 2002; Colberg 2010, 2011). Individuals with joint limitations or other health complications, however, should complete one set of exercises for all major muscle groups, starting with 10–15 repetitions and progressing to 15–20 repetitions before additional sets are added (Nelson 2007). Training recommendations for individuals with either T1D or T2D are given in Table 9.1.

Table 9.1 Recommended Combined Training Rx for Type 1 and Type 2 Diabetes

	Type 1 Diabetes	Type 2 Diabetes
Mode of training	Aerobic: Walking, jogging/running, cycling, swimming, rowing, aquatic activities, team sports, dancing, conditioning machines, seated exercises, and more	Aerobic: Walking, jogging, cycling, swimming, rowing, aquatic activities, seated exercises, dancing, conditioning machines, and more
	Resistance: All major muscle groups, using resistance bands, free weights, resistance training machines, isometric exercises, and/or calisthenics (using body weight)	Resistance: All major muscle groups, using resistance bands, free weights, resistance training machines, isometric exercises, and/or calisthenics (using body weight)
	Upper body: 4–5 exercises	Upper body: 4–5 exercises
	Lower body/core: 4–5 exercises	Lower body/core: 4–5 exercises
Intensity	Aerobic: 40–89% HRR (initial intensity may need to be lower for sedentary, deconditioned, and overweight individuals)	Aerobic: 40–89% HRR (initial intensity may need to be lower for sedentary, deconditioned, and overweight individuals)
	Perceived exertion of "somewhat hard" (5 or 6 on 10-point scale) to "hard" (7–8)	Perceived exertion of "somewhat hard" (5 or 6 on 10-point scale) to "hard" (7–8)
	Resistance: 60–80% 1 RM	Resistance: 50/60–80% 1 RM (50% 1 RM initially if untrained)
	7–8 (10-point scale)	5–8 (10-point scale)

Table 9.1 Recommended Combined Training Rx for
Type 1 and Type 2 Diabetes *(Continued)*

	Type 1 Diabetes	Type 2 Diabetes
Frequency	Aerobic: Adults should engage in 3–7 days/week (including structured and lifestyle activity)	Aerobic: 3–7 days/week (including structured and lifestyle activity)
	3 days of vigorous or 5 days of moderate intensity (greater regularity may facilitate diabetes management)	No more than 2 consecutive days without any activity
	Resistance: 2–3 days/week (nonconsecutive)	Resistance: A minimum of 2, but preferably 3, nonconsecutive days/week
	Allow 48 h of rest between training sessions	Allow 48 h of rest between training sessions
	Combined: 2–3 nonconsecutive days/week of combined training, with aerobic activities only on 1–4 other days	Combined: 2–3 nonconsecutive days/week of combined training, with aerobic activities only on 1–4 other days (but no more than 2 consecutive days without activity)
	If both types of training done on different days, allow 48 h of rest between resistance workouts	If both types done on different days, allow 48 h of rest between resistance workouts
Duration and number of repetitions	Aerobic: At least 20–30 min/session (minimum of 10-min bouts)	Aerobic: 30–60 min daily, with minimum of 10 min/session
	Minimum of 150 min/week of moderate-intensity or 60–75 min/week of vigorous-intensity physical activity	At least 150 min/week of moderate- to vigorous-intensity activity
	Resistance: 8–12 repetitions/exercise	Resistance: 8–12 repetitions/exercise as a goal, but 10–15 repetitions initially
	1–3 sets/exercise	1–3 sets/exercise
	Combined: Minimum of 150 min of moderate activity or 60–75 min of vigorous, including aerobic and resistance training	Combined: Minimum of 150 min of moderate- to vigorous-intensity activity, including aerobic and resistance training
	Greater benefits from adding 2–3 resistance training sessions to minimal time, whether moderate or vigorous training	Greater benefits from adding 2–3 resistance training sessions and increasing total exercise time to >210 min/week

Table 9.1 Recommended Combined Training Rx for Type 1 and Type 2 Diabetes *(Continued)*

	Type 1 Diabetes	Type 2 Diabetes
Progression	Aerobic: Start out on the "low" side if deconditioned, and progress slowly over weeks to months; start with the "improvement" phase if fitness levels adequate	Aerobic: Start out on the "low" side and progress slowly over weeks to months
	Increase duration and frequency first, intensity last (with the possible exception of adding in faster intervals during exercise sessions)	Increase duration and frequency first, intensity last (with the possible exception of adding in faster intervals during exercise sessions)
	Resistance: Start with 1–2 sets of 8–12 repetitions, progressing to 8–10 harder repetitions, and finally to 2–3 sets of 8–10 repetitions to near fatigue	Resistance: Start with 1–2 sets of 8–15 repetitions: 1 set of 10–15 repetitions to fatigue initially, progressing to 8–10 harder repetitions, and finally to 2–3 sets of 8–10 repetitions)

HRR, heart rate reserve.

Case in Point: Wrap-Up

JR does not expect to have too many problems increasing her walking to as much as 45 min a day (a little over 2 miles for her), but she is rightfully concerned about doing resistance work. The last time she tried to do any, she got so sore that she could not get out of bed for a day. Accordingly, she should start out on the low side with her resistance training and use the aerobic portion of those combined training days as a warm-up and cooldown for the resistance exercises. She should progress slowly enough that her body has time to fully adapt to each training load before increasing it further.

Exercise Program Goals

Mode of Activity: JR plans to join a local community fitness center to have access to both aerobic and resistance training equipment. Walking is her preferred activity; she usually walks outdoors, weather permitting, but is willing to use a treadmill indoors as well when necessary. Because she has never done much resistance training, she will be starting on the resistance machines and occasionally may use resistance bands at home instead.

Intensity: With regard to her planned walking, JR should aim to be in a moderate training range (40–59%), which for her equates to a HR range of 118–135 bpm. To increase her walking intensity, she will be doing faster intervals interspersed into her walks: her target during the intervals should minimally be in the range of 60–70% HRR, or 136–144 bpm. To prevent injuries or burnout, JR should start with an initial resistance training intensity of 50–60% 1 RM, which should feel "somewhat hard." Her intensity goal should be closer to 70% 1 RM on most exercises after several months of training.

Frequency: Because getting to the community fitness center >2–3 days/week is too difficult for JR, she plans to engage in combined training mainly on those days, meaning that she will be doing resistance training a minimum of 2–3 non-consecutive days/week. Because her walking goal is 5–6 days/week, she will be walking outdoors on 3–4 other days each week.

Duration: JR's walking goal is 15–20 min on combined exercise training days, when she will walk some before or after resistance training, but 20–45 min on the days that she walks outdoors without doing resistance work. JR is a novice to resistance training, so she should start by doing only one to two sets of 12–15 repetitions to start, with a goal of two to three sets of 8–10 repetitions to near fatigue after several months of consistent training. Therefore, her total weekly exercise duration will be 90–220 min of walking, plus resistance training (~30 min/session, or an additional 60–90 min/week).

Progression: Because JR has already been walking and is simply increasing her duration (and to a lesser extent, her intensity), the aerobic portion of her training can progress more rapidly (up to recommended amounts) than her resistance work, which should progress slowly and steadily. To get optimal strength and blood glucose benefits, she should progress to include at least two to three sets per resistance exercise, aiming to complete harder sets that allow her to only do 8–10 repetitions before reaching near fatigue on each set. On days she uses only resistance bands, she should focus on doing more repetitions than normal on similar exercises.

Daily Movement: Another way JR can increase her body's glucose uptake and help control her body weight is to focus on engaging in more daily movement. She should be advised to stand whenever possible and to take more daily steps, especially on the days that she is only doing planned walking as her activity.

Possible Precautions: Because JR will be engaging only in brisk walking and moderate resistance training, she should not be required to undergo a graded exercise stress prior to beginning combination training. If she is intimidated by resistance training, her initial 1 RM values can be estimated using a submaximal load instead of measured directly. Although neither of the diabetes medications that she uses should increase her risk of hypoglycemia, she should occasionally monitor the effects of her differing training sessions on her blood glucose levels. In any case, she should be advised to always carry rapid-acting carbohydrates (like glucose tablets or hard candy) with her on walks and to the fitness center to treat exercise-related hypoglycemia if she develops it.

Combined exercise training likely bestows health and metabolic benefits to people with diabetes, as well as adults with T1D (although the benefits of such training in T1D have not been well studied). Given that structured exercise training of any type that exceeds 150 min/week has a greater glycemic benefit than

≤150 min, all adults with any type of diabetes should consider meeting minimal exercise recommendations with their aerobic training alone and simply add resistance training to that total to achieve a higher total training dose with a combination of aerobic and resistance exercise.

PROFESSIONAL PRACTICE PEARLS

- The total duration of exercise and caloric expenditure have been greater with combined training in almost all studies done to date in individuals with T2D.
- The inclusion of both aerobic and resistance exercise in a weekly exercise program is recommended because combined training (even when isocaloric with other types of training) appears to bestow a greater glycemic benefit.
- Structured exercise training that consists of aerobic exercise, resistance training, or both combined that lasts >150 min/week is associated with greater A1C declines than training that amounts to ≤150 min/week.
- In youth with T1D, combined exercise training lowered daily insulin requirement and improved physical fitness and sense of well-being.
- In active adults with T1D undertaking combined exercise sessions, engaging in resistance training before moderate aerobic work may lead to lower carbohydrate needs during exercise and a lower risk of hypoglycemia later on.
- Although both resistance and combined training can lead to improved strength over 6 months, gains are likely greater with resistance training alone.
- If both aerobic and resistance training are done on the same day, adults with diabetes should undertake 2–3 nonconsecutive days/week of combined training, with aerobic activities only on 1–4 other days/week.
- If both types of training are done on different days, individuals should separate bouts of resistance training by a minimum of 48 h.
- Individuals with diabetes should attempt to engage in a minimum of 150 min/week, including both types of training in the total duration.
- Greater benefits are likely gained from adding two to three resistance training sessions to aerobic training and increasing total exercise time to ≥210 min/week of moderate activity; adults with T1D may do likewise or do more vigorous activity for less time compared with those with T2D.

REFERENCES

Albright A, Franz M, Hornsby G, Kriska A, Marrero D, Ullrich I, Verity LS: American College of Sports Medicine position stand. Exercise and type 2 diabetes. *Med Sci Sports Exerc* 32:1345–1360, 2000

American College of Sports Medicine: American College of Sports Medicine position stand. Progression models in resistance training for healthy adults. *Med Sci Sports Exerc* 41:687–708, 2009

Boulé NG, Weisnagel SJ, Lakka TA, Tremblay A, Bergman RN, Rankinen T, Leon AS, Skinner JS, Wilmore JH, Rao DC, Bouchard C: Effects of exercise training on glucose homeostasis: the HERITAGE Family Study. *Diabetes Care* 28:108–114, 2005

Boulé NG, Kenny GP, Haddad E, Wells GA, Sigal RJ: Meta-analysis of the effect of structured exercise training on cardiorespiratory fitness in type 2 diabetes mellitus. *Diabetologia* 46:1071–1081, 2003

Boulé NG, Haddad E, Kenny GP, Wells GA, Sigal RJ: Effects of exercise on glycemic control and body mass in type 2 diabetes mellitus: a meta-analysis of controlled clinical trials. *JAMA* 286:1218–1227, 2001

Church TS, Blair SN, Cocreham S, Johannsen N, Johnson W, Kramer K, Mikus CR, Myers V, Nauta M, Rodarte RQ, Sparks L, Thompson A, Earnest CP: Effects of aerobic and resistance training on hemoglobin A1c levels in patients with type 2 diabetes: a randomized controlled trial. *JAMA* 304:2253–2262, 2010

Colberg SR, Sigal RJ: Prescribing exercise for individuals with type 2 diabetes: recommendations and precautions. *Phys Sportsmed* 39:13–26, 2011

Colberg SR, Sigal RJ, Fernhall B, Regensteiner JG, Blissmer BJ, Rubin RR, Chasan-Taber L, Albright AL, Braun B, American College of Sports Medicine, American Diabetes Association: Exercise and type 2 diabetes: the American College of Sports Medicine and the American Diabetes Association: joint position statement. *Diabetes Care* 33:e147–e167, 2010

Cuff DJ, Meneilly GS, Martin A, Ignaszewski A, Tildesley HD, Frohlich JJ: Effective exercise modality to reduce insulin resistance in women with type 2 diabetes. *Diabetes Care* 26:2977–2982, 2003

D'Hooge R, Hellinckx T, Van Laethem C, Stegen S, De Schepper J, Van Aken S, Dewolf D, Calders P: Influence of combined aerobic and resistance training on metabolic control, cardiovascular fitness and quality of life in adolescents with type 1 diabetes: a randomized controlled trial. *Clin Rehabil* 25:349–3459, 2011

Donnelly JE, Blair SN, Jakicic JM, Manore MM, Rankin JW, Smith BK: American College of Sports Medicine Position Stand. Appropriate physical activity intervention strategies for weight loss and prevention of weight regain for adults. *Med Sci Sports Exerc* 41:459–471, 2009

Dunstan DW, Daly RM, Owen N, Jolley D, Vulikh E, Shaw J, Zimmet P: Home-based resistance training is not sufficient to maintain improved glycemic control following supervised training in older individuals with type 2 diabetes. *Diabetes Care* 28:3–9, 2005

Dunstan DW, Daly RM, Owen N, Jolley D, De Courten M, Shaw J, Zimmet P: High-intensity resistance training improves glycemic control in older patients with type 2 diabetes. *Diabetes Care* 25:1729–1736, 2002

Garber CE, Blissmer B, Deschenes MR, Franklin BA, Lamonte MJ, Lee IM, Nieman DC, Swain DP, American College of Sports Medicine: American College of Sports Medicine position stand. Quantity and quality of exercise for developing and maintaining cardiorespiratory, musculoskeletal, and neuromotor fitness in apparently healthy adults: guidance for prescribing exercise. *Med Sci Sports Exerc* 43:1334–1359, 2011

Gordon BA, Benson AC, Bird SR, Fraser SF: Resistance training improves metabolic health in type 2 diabetes: a systematic review. *Diabetes Res Clin Pract* 83:157–175, 2009

Haskell WL, Lee IM, Pate RR, Powell KE, Blair SN, Franklin BA, Macera CA, Heath GW, Thompson PD, Bauman A: Physical activity and public health: updated recommendation for adults from the American College of Sports Medicine and the American Heart Association. *Med Sci Sports Exerc* 39:1423–1434, 2007

Hordern MD, Dunstan DW, Prins JB, Baker MK, Singh MA, Coombes JS: Exercise prescription for patients with type 2 diabetes and pre-diabetes: a position statement from Exercise and Sport Science Australia. *J Sci Med Sport* 15:25–31, 2012

Johnson ST, Boulé NG, Bell GJ, Bell RC: Walking: a matter of quantity and quality physical activity for type 2 diabetes management. *Appl Physiol Nutr Metab* 33:797–801, 2008

Johnson ST, McCargar LJ, Bell GJ, Tudor-Locke C, Harber VJ, Bell RC: Walking faster: distilling a complex prescription for type 2 diabetes management through pedometry. *Diabetes Care* 29:1654–1655, 2006

Jorge ML, de Oliveira VN, Resende NM, Paraiso LF, Calixto A, Diniz AL, Resende ES, Ropelle ER, Carvalheira JB, Espindola FS, Jorge PT, Geloneze B: The effects of aerobic, resistance, and combined exercise on metabolic control, inflammatory markers, adipocytokines, and muscle insulin signaling in patients with type 2 diabetes mellitus. *Metabolism* 60:1244–1252, 2011

King DS, Baldus PJ, Sharp RL, Kesl LD, Feltmeyer TL, Riddle MS: Time course for exercise-induced alterations in insulin action and glucose tolerance in middle-aged people. *J Appl Physiol* 78:17–22, 1995

Larose J, Sigal RJ, Khandwala F, Kenny GP: Comparison of strength development with resistance training and combined exercise training in type 2 diabetes. *Scand J Med Sci Sports* 22:e45-e54, 2012

Larose J, Sigal RJ, Khandwala F, Prud'homme D, Boulé NG, Kenny GP, Aerobic Diabetes, Investigators Resistance Exercise trial: Associations between physical fitness and HbA(c) in type 2 diabetes mellitus. *Diabetologia* 54:93–102, 2011

Maiorana A, O'Driscoll G, Goodman C, Taylor R, Green D: Combined aerobic and resistance exercise improves glycemic control and fitness in type 2 diabetes. *Diabetes Res Clin Pract* 56:115–123, 2002

Marcus RL, Smith S, Morrell G, Addison O, Dibble LE, Wahoff-Stice D, Lastayo PC: Comparison of combined aerobic and high-force eccentric resistance exercise with aerobic exercise only for people with type 2 diabetes mellitus. *Phys Ther* 88:1345–1354, 2008

Nelson ME, Rejeski WJ, Blair SN, Duncan PW, Judge JO, King AC, Macera CA, Castaneda-Sceppa C: Physical activity and public health in older adults: recommendation from the American College of Sports Medicine and the American Heart Association. *Med Sci Sports Exerc* 39:1435–1445, 2007

Pavlou KN, Krey S, Steffee WP: Exercise as an adjunct to weight loss and maintenance in moderately obese subjects. *Am J Clin Nutr* 49 (Suppl. 5):1115–1123, 1989

Physical Activity Guidelines Advisory Committee: Physical Activity Guidelines Advisory Committee Report, 2008. Washington, DC, U.S. Department of Health and Human Services, 2008

Saris WH, Blair SN, van Baak MA, Eaton SB, Davies PS, Di Pietro L, Fogelholm M, Rissanen A, Schoeller D, Swinburn B, Tremblay A, Westerterp KR, Wyatt H: How much physical activity is enough to prevent unhealthy weight gain? Outcome of the IASO 1st Stock Conference and consensus statement. *Obes Rev* 4:101–114, 2003

Schoeller DA, Shay K, Kushner RF: How much physical activity is needed to minimize weight gain in previously obese women? *American Journal of Clinical Nutrition* 66:551–556, 1997

Segerstrom AB, Glans F, Eriksson KF, Holmback AM, Groop L, Thorsson O, Wollmer P: Impact of exercise intensity and duration on insulin sensitivity in women with T2D. *Eur J Intern Med* 21:404–408, 2010

Sigal RJ, Kenny GP, Boulé NG, Wells GA, Prud'homme D, Fortier M, Reid RD, Tulloch H, Coyle D, Phillips P, Jennings A, Jaffey J: Effects of aerobic training, resistance training, or both on glycemic control in type 2 diabetes: a randomized trial. *Ann Intern Med* 147:357–369, 2007

Sigal RJ, Kenny GP, Wasserman DH, Castaneda-Sceppa C, White RD: Physical activity/exercise and type 2 diabetes: a consensus statement from the American Diabetes Association. *Diabetes Care* 29:1433–1438, 2006

Sigal RJ, Kenny GP, Wasserman DH, Castaneda-Sceppa C: Physical activity/exercise and type 2 diabetes. *Diabetes Care* 27:2518–2539, 2004

Snowling NJ, Hopkins WG: Effects of different modes of exercise training on glucose control and risk factors for complications in type 2 diabetic patients: a meta-analysis. *Diabetes Care* 29:2518–2527, 2006

Thomas DE, Elliott EJ, Naughton GA: Exercise for type 2 diabetes mellitus. *Cochrane Database Syst Rev* CD002968, 2006

Tokmakidis SP, Zois CE, Volaklis KA, Kotsa K, Touvra AM: The effects of a combined strength and aerobic exercise program on glucose control and insulin action in women with type 2 diabetes. *Eur J Appl Physiol* 92:437–442, 2004

Touvra AM, Volaklis KA, Spassis AT, Zois CE, Douda HD, Kotsa K, Tokmakidis SP: Combined strength and aerobic training increases transforming growth factor-beta1 in patients with type 2 diabetes. *Hormones (Athens)* 10:125–130, 2011

Umpierre D, Ribeiro PA, Kramer CK, Leitao CB, Zucatti AT, Azevedo MJ, Gross JL, Ribeiro JP, Schaan BD: Physical activity advice only or structured exercise training and association with HbA1c levels in type 2 diabetes: a systematic review and meta-analysis. *JAMA* 305:1790–1799, 2011

van Dijk JW, Manders RJ, Tummers K, Bonomi AG, Stehouwer CD, Hartgens F, van Loon LJ: Both resistance- and endurance-type exercise reduce the prevalence of hyperglycaemia in individuals with impaired glucose tolerance and in insulin-treated and non-insulin-treated type 2 diabetic patients. *Diabetologia* 55:1273–1282, 2012

Vincent KR, Braith RW, Feldman RA, Magyari PM, Cutler RB, Persin SA, Lennon SL, Gabr AH, Lowenthal DT: Resistance exercise and physical performance in adults aged 60 to 83. *J Am Geriatr Soc* 50:1100–1107, 2002

Weinsier RL, Hunter GR , Desmond RA, Byrne NM, Zuckerman PA, Darnell BE: Free-living activity energy expenditure in women successful and unsuccessful at maintaining a normal body weight. *Am J Clin Nutr* 75:499–504, 2002

Willey KA, Singh MA: Battling insulin resistance in elderly obese people with type 2 diabetes: bring on the heavy weights. *Diabetes Care* 26:1580–1588, 2003

Yardley JE, Kenny GP, Perkins BA, Riddell MC, Malcolm J, Boulay P, Khandwala F, Sigal RJ: Effects of performing resistance exercise before versus after aerobic exercise on glycemia in type 1 diabetes. *Diabetes Care* 35:669–675, 2012

Chapter 10

Other Physical Activities for All Types of Diabetes

The potential health benefits of other types of physical activities frequently are overlooked. For instance, as individuals age it is important for them to work on maintaining balance, agility, and coordination to lower risk of falling. Individuals with diabetes who have comorbid issues like peripheral neuropathy have an even greater falls risk with aging, which can be lowered with balance and appropriate exercise training (Morrison 2010). On the other end of the athletic spectrum, many individuals with type 1 diabetes (T1D) in particular are training for and participating in extreme athletic events like marathons (Meinders 1988; Tuominen 1996, 1997b; Cauza 2005; Graveling 2010; Murillo 2010).

Current guidelines from the American College of Sports Medicine (ACSM) recommend that adults perform resistance exercises for each of the major muscle groups, and neuromotor exercise involving balance, agility, and coordination 2–3 days/week (Garber 2011). It is critical for all adults, but particularly those with diabetes, to maintain their range of movement around all joints by completing a series of flexibility exercises for each of the major muscle-tendon groups (a total of 60 sec/exercise) on ≥2 days/week (Colberg 2010, Garber 2011). For youth with any type of diabetes, focusing on maintaining greater daily energy expenditure through various physical activities (including active video gaming) is important to prevent weight gain and cardiovascular complications (Maloney 2008, Graf 2009, Murphy 2009, Graves 2010, Bailey 2011).

Case in Point: Other Types of Training Rx for T2D

JR is a 54-year-old woman with type 2 diabetes (T2D) for 3 years who recently started combined aerobic and resistance training at her local community fitness center after getting an exercise prescription during her last appointment with her health-care provider. She currently is doing moderate walking (with some faster intervals interspersed) outdoors 3–4 days/week and another 2 days of combined aerobic and resistance training at the fitness center (see chapter 9 for more details of her actual exercise prescription with combined training). Her diabetes is controlled with physical activity, diet, metformin, and exenatide once weekly (Bydureon), and she takes a statin daily for her cholesterol.

Resting Measurements

Height: 65 inches
Weight: 198 lb
Body mass index: 32.9 (obese)
Heart rate: 84 beats per minute (bpm)
Blood pressure: 135/80 mmHg

Fasting Labs

Plasma glucose: 125 mg/dl (controlled with metformin and Bydureon)
A1C: 7.6%
Total cholesterol: 175 mg/dl (on medication)
Triglycerides: 95 mg/dl
High-density lipoprotein cholesterol: 52 mg/dl
Low-density lipoprotein cholesterol: 104 mg/dl

(Continued on page 155.)

FLEXIBILITY TRAINING

Flexibility is defined as the ability to move a joint though a complete range of motion and is considered an important part of physical fitness (Garber 2011). Some types of physical activity, however, require more flexibility than others. Moreover, limited joint mobility is frequently observed in elderly people and in individuals with all types of diabetes, a contributor likely being formation of advanced glycation end-products (AGEs) that accumulate during the process of normal aging in the plasma and tissues, but to an accelerated degree in individuals with diabetes (Abate 2011). The most extensive accumulation of AGEs occurs in tissues that contain proteins with low turnover, such as the collagen in the extra-cellular matrix of articular capsule, ligaments, and muscle-tendon units. An increase in collagen cross-linking alters the mechanical properties of these tissues, resulting in a decrease in elasticity and tensile strength and an increase in mechanical stiffness. Because of the potential for AGE damage with fluctuations in blood glucose levels, people with diabetes are more prone to developing structural changes to joints that can limit movement. These include shoulder adhesive capsulitis ("frozen shoulder"), carpal tunnel syndrome (wrist pain), metatarsal fractures (of the foot bones), and neuropathy-related joint disorders (e.g., Charcot foot) in people with peripheral neuropathy, among others (Balci 1999, Tighe 2008, Ravindran Rajendran 2011, Rogers 2011). Aging itself also results in a reduction in flexibility and joint movement (Abate 2011).

Finally, flexibility programs are low intensity and easy to perform, thus providing the perfect introduction toward a more physically active lifestyle for deconditioned individuals while bestowing health benefits. By way of example, a recent study reported that flexibility exercises modestly decrease peak plantar pressures in the feet (Goldsmith 2002), although it has not been directly evaluated as to whether such training reduces risk of ulceration or injury in individuals with diabetes.

FLEXIBILITY TRAINING PRESCRIPTION

Exercise recommendations for all adults state that flexibility training is crucial to maintaining joint range of movement. They recommend completing a series of flexibility exercises for each of the major muscle-tendon groups, done for a total of 60 s/exercise, on ≥2 days/week (Garber 2011). The current American Diabetes Association recommendation regarding flexibility training is that it may be included as part of a physical activity program, but not as a substitute for other training (Colberg 2010). Regular stretching should be considered an option to include in the fitness plan for individuals with diabetes. Flexibility exercises, combined with resistance training, have been shown to increase joint range of movement in individuals with T2D (Herriott 2004), thereby allowing them to more easily engage in activities that require greater flexibility.

Both dynamic and static stretching exercises are effective in increasing flexibility and allow individuals with diabetes to more easily do activities that require greater movement around joints. Thus, flexibility exercise is an appropriate part of a physical activity program, even though it is unclear whether it reduces risk of acute, activity-related injury (Shrier 1999, Yeung 2001). Flexibility exercises can be included as part of a warm-up or cooldown, but usually are not counted toward meeting the aerobic or muscle-strengthening guidelines. Recommendations for safe and effective participation in flexibility training are included in Table 10.1.

Table 10.1 Recommendations for Flexibility Exercise

- Flexibility exercises should be done regularly. Better benefits related to joint range of movement are achieved by stretching regularly, at least two to three times a week.

- Warm up before doing flexibility exercises. Stretching "cold" muscles increases the risk of injury, so before stretching, individuals should warm up with light walking, jogging, or biking at low intensity for 5–10 min. An alternative is to stretch after completing an exercise session when muscles already have greater blood flow.

- Stretch the major muscle groups. It is recommended that individuals focus on stretching their calves, thighs, hips, lower back, neck, and shoulders on both side of their bodies.

- Dynamic or static stretches are both effective. While static stretching is more traditionally done, bringing gentle movement into stretches (without bouncing) may improve flexibility in specific movements. (Tai chi exercise is a good example of this principle.)

- Sport-specific stretches are most beneficial. Stretching the muscles and joints that have or will be used during an activity is more effective in preventing injuries to those areas.

- Stretching should not result in pain. Feeling tension during a stretch is normal, but pain is an indicator that the stretch may actually be causing damage instead. Individuals should stretch to the point of tension, but not pain, and hold the stretch.

- Avoid bouncing during stretching. Doing so can cause small tears in the muscle that can ultimately lead to less flexibility. Stretches should ideally last about 15–30 s and be repeated until a total of 60 s exercise is reached.

TAI CHI AND YOGA

Both tai chi and yoga include basic stretching movements as part of the instruction. Gentle movement, such as that undertaken during both of these exercise modalities, can benefit flexibility in doing specific movements, and both activities assist adults in meeting the recommended levels of participation in flexibility exercise (i.e., ≥2 days/week) (Garber 2011).

Glycemic benefits. Mild-intensity exercises like tai chi and yoga have been investigated for their potential to improve blood glucose management in individuals with T2D, with mixed results (Innes 2007, Yeh 2007, Gordon 2008, Lam 2008, Tsang 2008, Wang 2008, Zhang 2008, Chen 2010). Some studies have reported reductions in A1C levels with extended participation in such activities (Innes 2007, Richerson 2007, Yeh 2007, Gordon 2008, Zhang 2008, Hegde 2011, Madanmohan 2012), and others have not (Lam 2008, Tsang 2008, Chen 2010). In addition, the benefits of long-term training (i.e., 16 weeks) on glycemic control may not last >72 h after the last session (Tsang 2008). A meta-analysis of yoga studies stated that the limitations characterizing most studies, such as small sample size and varying forms of yoga, preclude drawing firm conclusions about benefits to diabetes management (Innes 2007), and recent systematic reviews also failed to show any overall glycemic benefit of tai chi participation in individuals with T2D (Lee 2008, 2011). In their position statement, the American Diabetes Association was unable to conclusively support the inclusion of these types of activities due to the variable results with regard to glycemic benefits (Colberg 2010). Accordingly, such exercises can be included based on individual preferences to increase flexibility, muscular strength, and balance and to gain other potential health benefits, but their effects on aerobic fitness are likely minimal and their impact on glycemic control is variable.

Other health benefits. Although the benefits of flexibility training for injury prevention have been questioned (Shrier 1999, Yeung 2001), yoga and tai chi may provide other health and possible fitness benefits not related to glycemic control (Singh 2004, Malhotra 2005, Innes 2007, Gordon 2008, Wang 2008). For instance, participation in either activity has resulted in improvements in BMI (even from yoga in overweight youth) (Benavides 2009), markers of oxidative stress, immune function, blood lipids, blood pressure, balance, reaction time, and cognitive brain function (Taylor-Piliae 2006, Innes 2007, Gordon 2008, Yeh 2009, Chen 2010, Kyizom 2010, Liu 2010, Hegde 2011, Madanmohan 2012). Research performed on tai chi (Yeh 2007, Lam 2008, Tsang 2008, Wang 2008) and yoga (Singh 2004, Malhotra 2005, Innes 2007, Gordon 2008) has additionally reported improvements in cardiovascular fitness levels. Of note, one study demonstrated the effectiveness of 6 months of weekly tai chi training in improving plantar sensation and balance in elderly adults with and without diabetes with a large plantar sensation loss (Richerson 2007), while another showed improvements in auditory reaction time in diabetic adults who underwent thrice-weekly yoga training for only 6 weeks (Madanmohan 2012). Some have argued that yoga's benefits on fasting blood glucose, lipids, oxidative stress markers, and antioxidant status are at least equivalent to more conventional forms of physical activity (Gordon 2008).

Case in Point: Continued

During the course of her combined workouts, JR has been noticing that she has been getting stiffer, and sometimes when she is doing her outdoor walking, she feels like her legs are starting to cramp up a bit. Every once in a while, she feels a bit wobbly on her feet, too, like she is just not as stable as she used to be. She is interested in possibly signing up for some other activities at her local community fitness center, maybe even yoga classes, although she has never tried doing any yoga before. Because her grandkids come to visit her so often, she has a Nintendo Wii system that came with the Wii Sports on it, and she has been interested in trying out the Wii Fit Plus with Balance Board that she has heard others talking about.

Questions to Consider

1. How important is stretching to someone of JR's age, activity level, and diabetes status?
2. What types of other activities would be beneficial to JR?

(Continued on page 159.)

ACTIVE VIDEO GAMING ACTIVITIES

Active video games (exergames) increase energy expenditure and physical activity compared with sedentary video gaming. Exergaming also has the potential to increase overall physical activity and favorably influence energy balance, making it a viable alternative to some types of traditional fitness activities. Dance Dance Revolution (DDR) was among the first exergames available. It can reduce sedentary screen time in children while facilitating slight increases in vigorous physical activity in that population (Maloney 2008) along with improving flow-mediated dilation, aerobic fitness, and mean arterial pressure in overweight children with endothelial dysfunction (Murphy 2009).

Other studies have compared DDR with more recent exergames, like Nintendo's Wii Sports and Wii Fit. In youth (age 11.5 years), energy expenditures associated with participation in DDR, LightSpace (Bug Invasion), Nintendo Wii (Boxing), Cybex Trazer (Goalie Wars), Sportwall, and Xavix (J-Mat) were compared with treadmill walking at 3 mph. All activities increased energy expenditure above rest, with metabolic equivalent (MET) levels of 4.9 for walking, 4.2 for Wii, 5.4 for DDR, 6.4 for LightSpace, 7.0 for Xavix, 5.9 for Cybex Trazer, and 7.1 for Sportwall. Thus, all exergames elevated energy expenditure to a moderate or vigorous intensity in children of varying body weights (Bailey 2011). Energy expenditure in overweight youth ages 10–13 years playing either DDR and Wii Sports also has been found comparable to moderate-intensity walking (Graf 2009).

Simply increasing physical activity with exergaming during leisure time can be beneficial. In one study, cardiorespiratory measurements were compared in adolescents, young adults, and older adults during inactive video gaming, Wii Fit activities (yoga, muscle conditioning, balance, aerobics), and brisk treadmill walking and jogging (Graves 2010). For all groups, energy expenditure and heart rates were higher during Wii Fit activities than inactive gaming, but lower than treadmill exercise.

Wii aerobics provided the equivalent of moderate-intensity activity, but heart rates fell below the recommended intensity for maintaining cardiorespiratory fitness.

Enjoyment was greater for Wii Fit compared with treadmill use, however, suggesting that Wii Fit is a viable exergame for adolescents and adults that replaces sedentary leisure behavior with light- to moderate-intensity activity (Graves 2010). Engaging in Wii Fit games also has been shown to be a feasible alternative to more traditional aerobic exercise in middle-aged and older adults for improving and maintaining cardiorespiratory fitness (Guderian 2010). In older adults doing Wii Fit games, 20-min sessions results in an exercise intensity of 43.4±16.7% heart rate reserve (HRR), or ~3.5 METs, along with net energy expenditure of 116.2±40.9 kilocalories.

Another study compared energy expenditure in adults who performed all five Wii Sports activities (golf, bowling, tennis, baseball, and boxing) and Wii Fit Plus (63 activities classified as yoga, resistance, balance, and aerobic exercises) (Miyachi 2010). Each activity was continued for at least 8 min and resulted in a wide range of energy use ranging from 1.3 METs (Lotus Focus) to 5.6 METs (single-arm stand), with mean MET values of 2.1 (yoga), 2.0 (balance), 3.2 (resistance), 3.4 (Wii Fit Plus aerobic exercise), and 3.0 (Wii Sports). Forty-six activities (67%) were classified as light intensity (<3 METs), and 22 activities (33%) were moderate intensity (3–6 METs), with no vigorous-intensity activities (>6 METs). Thus, time spent playing one-third of the activities supplied by motion- and gesture-controlled Wii video games can count toward the daily amount of exercise based on the latest guidelines for moderate-intensity physical activity (Haskell 2007, Physical Activity Guidelines Advisory Committee 2008, Garber 2011).

BALANCE TRAINING

All older adults are advised to undertake exercises that maintain or improve balance (Nelson 2007, Garber 2011), especially individuals with T2D or peripheral neuropathy with a higher risk of falling (Morrison 2010). Any type of balance training can be beneficial. Older individuals with T2D have been found to have impaired balance, slower reactions, and consequently a higher falls risk than their nondiabetic counterparts; however, all these variables improved after just 6 weeks of thrice-weekly, supervised resistance and balance training, demonstrating that balance training has positive effects on balance, falls risk, postural dynamics, and other physiological function in such individuals (Morrison 2010, 2012). Likewise, in debilitated, ambulatory older adults participating in a home-based exercise and balance training program, their balance confidence, balance performance, and gait improved measurably (Miller 2010). Even engaging in a 10-week traditional Greek dance program improves performance on static and dynamic balance indices in healthy elderly adults (Sofianidis 2009).

Exergaming has been studied with regard to balance improvement. To determine the safety and feasibility of using Wii Fit exergames to improve balance, older adults with impaired balance participated in basic step, soccer heading, ski slalom, and table tilt at home for at least 30 min three times per week for 3 months. Participants rated high enjoyment immediately after exergame play and experienced improved balance during daily activities. Therefore, use of Wii Fit for limited supervised balance training in the home was safe and feasible for a selected sample of older adults (Agmon 2011). Similarly, DDR also provides a low-cost method for older adults to work on balance in the privacy of their own homes (Smith 2011).

Balance training exercises. A balance training program can be effective, even if simple like the following one: Complete a series of stretches of the lower limb muscles followed by lower limb, abdominal, and lower back exercises on 3 nonconsecutive days/week. The lower limb exercises include bilateral calf raises (two sets, 20 repetitions) and bilateral or single-leg calf raises (two sets, 10–15 repetitions). Abdominal crunches (one to three sets), lower back extension exercises, and bilateral single leg extensions (two to three repetitions) are performed while lying prone on a floor mat. Standing balance exercises include standing on a single-leg with eyes closed on a firm surface (two sets, 15 sec), followed by a forward-leaning activity that involves standing on one leg with hands on hips and leaning forward (two sets, 15 sec each exercise, 10 repetitions) (Morrison 2010).

EXTREME ATHLETIC EVENTS

Despite the metabolic and other physical challenges presented by participation in long-duration athletic events, many individuals with diabetes are currently training for and participating in such events. For example, marathon running is growing in popularity, and many diabetic individuals are participating in various marathon races all over the world each year. Research in this area is lacking, but a handful of studies have attempted to investigate the metabolic and hormonal effects of more extreme athletic participation by such individuals.

Long-distance events. An early study examined the metabolic and hormonal effects of a 3-h marathon training run in individuals with T1D (Meinders 1988). Insulin was withheld for 16–26 h before the start of the run, although participants ate a normal breakfast 2.5 h before. Blood glucose levels decreased during the 3-h run, and postexercise ketosis was elevated. Counterregulatory hormone secretion was found to be normal (or even elevated) in response to hypoglycemia during a long-distance run in these reasonably well-controlled, well-trained diabetic subjects without long-term complications. Similarly, nine men with T1D participating in a 75-km cross-country skiing race had insulin dose reductions of 30–40% before the event that resulted in hyperglycemia during the early part of the race, but near normoglycemia during the remainder, likely attributable to several-fold increases in counterregulatory hormone levels (Koivisto 1992). In another study, on the day of a marathon, runners with T1D reduced their prerace insulin doses by an average of 26% and ingested 130 g of carbohydrate before, 91 g during, and 115 g after the race to maintain near euglycemia (Tuominen 1997b).

Impact of insulin analogs. A more recent study involved 14 male amateur athletes with T1D using insulin analogs and examined their responses to participation in two consecutive editions of the same half-marathon (Murillo 2010). On each half-marathon day, athletes reduced total insulin doses by 18.3% the first year, but only by 14.2% the second year; basal insulin was reduced by 23.3% and 20.4% and short-acting insulin at breakfast before the competition by 31.7% and 15.3% in years 1 and 2, respectively. Athletes also consumed more carbohydrates during the event the second year (49.0 vs. 59.1 grams), with fewer glycemic excursions. Thus, T1D athletes treated using insulin analogs may need a lesser insulin reduction compared with traditional guidelines and greater carbohydrate supplementation (amount and timing) to effectively manage blood glucose levels during long-distance competitions.

Effects on insulin action. Others have shown reduced postmarathon insulin needs and increased insulin clearance, resulting in a decreased insulin availability that enhances muscle lipid utilization and spares glucose after long-duration exercise (Tuominen 1997a). After successfully managed marathon running, however, insulin sensitivity was not increased in one study despite low glycogen content and enhanced glycogen synthase activity, likely due to increased lipid oxidation (Tuominen 1997b). Another study examined pre-exercise insulin reductions on consequent metabolic and dietary patterns for 24 h after a bout of running in T1D (West 2010). Participants self-administered 100%, 75%, 50%, or 25% of their full rapid-acting insulin dose immediately before eating a meal and 2 h before completing 45 min of moderate running. Initially, blood glucose levels were unaffected, but were highest 3 h postexercise with the lowest dose (25%) of rapid-acting insulin, which was maintained over the rest of the 24 h period despite less energy and carbohydrate intake.

Use of continuous glucose monitoring devices. The use of continuous glucose monitoring (CGM) devices during and after marathon participation by individuals with T1D and T2D has been studied to determine whether asymptomatic episodes of hypo- and hyperglycemia can be more effectively identified in these exercisers (Cauza 2005). Although such systems are limited in their ability to detect rapid changes in blood glucose levels, use of CGM may help identify asymptomatic hypoglycemia or hyperglycemia during and after a long-distance run, improve understanding about individual changes in glucose during and after a marathon,

Table 10.2 Recommended Other Physical Activities for All Types of Diabetes

Activity	Participation Recommendations
Flexibility training (stretching)	Include a series of flexibility exercises (static or dynamic) for each of the major muscle-tendon groups, done for a total of ~60 s/exercise, on ≥2days/week
Tai chi and yoga	Do as part of or in place of flexibility training on ≥2 days/week (with tai chi being more dynamic, yoga more static in nature)
Active video gaming (exergames)	Use to replace sedentary leisure time with more physical activity; one-third of Wii video game activities can count toward the daily amounts of moderate-intensity physical activity
Balance training	All older adults are advised to undertake exercises that maintain or improve balance at least 3 days/week
Extreme athletic events	Safe participation in longer endurance events like marathons is possible with appropriate training and diabetes regimen changes

and protect against hypoglycemic or hyperglycemic periods in future races. Of note, individuals with T1D are advised not to undertake prolonged intensive exercise after severe hypoglycemia because of increased risk of acute damage to skeletal muscle and to organs such as the liver, severe neuroglycopenia, and the induction of seizures (Graveling 2010).

Case in Point: Wrap-Up

After discussing it with her health-care provider, JR is thrilled with the prospect of adding in some different activities that will help with her stiffness and exercise enjoyment, and she also feels motivated by the social aspect of taking yoga classes with others and doing exergaming activities with her grandchildren on weekends.

Other Physical Activities Goals

Modes of Activity:

Yoga and stretching: At her community fitness center, JR will be signing up for some introductory yoga classes, and once she learns more of the yoga moves, she plans to add some yoga to her home exercise routine. In addition, she should be doing at least some light stretching after structured exercise sessions or whenever she feels stiff during or after physical activities.

Balance training: JR should also add some simple balance training into her weekly routine, even if it simply consists of practicing standing on one leg.

Active video gaming: Finally, she plans on practicing some of the Wii Fit and Wii Sports games on her own so that she can play with her grandkids when they visit on weekends to get them more active, too.

Intensity:

Active video gaming: If JR picks Wii games that elicit a moderate-intensity workload (either from the Wii Sports or Wii Fit activities), she can substitute them for her planned activities on some days. Lower-intensity ones simply increase her daily movement but should not replace other structured activities in that case.

Frequency:

Yoga and stretching: JR can do yoga in place of her usual stretching, and she should aim for doing one or the other at least 2 days/week to meet recommended amounts.

Balance training: JR should undertake some balance training at least 3 days/week.

Active video gaming: This activity is optional but can be done as frequently as desired to replace sedentary leisure time activities.

Duration:

Yoga and stretching: Each flexibility exercise should ideally be done for a total of 60 sec.

Balance training: JR should spend at least 5–10 min doing balance training each time she does it.

Active video gaming: The more time JR can spend being active during leisure time, the better. If she is engaging in moderate-intensity activities that she plans to substitute for her planned activity on a given day, the gaming activity should last for an equivalent amount of time (i.e., 15–45 min for her, depending on the day).

Possible Precautions: All of these activities are relatively low-level ones, so JR should not have any cardiovascular concerns related to her participation in them. Because some studies have shown that yoga can lower blood glucose levels, JR should use her blood glucose meter to find out what effects it has on her diabetes management. As with all physical activities, she should have rapid-acting carbohydrates (like glucose tablets or hard candy) available if she should develop hypoglycemia.

Many physical activities are possible and beneficial for individuals with any type of diabetes. Doing both regular stretching and balance training is increasingly important as people age, and tai chi and yoga are acceptable alternative activities for both of those types of training. Active video gaming activities can be used to work on cardiovascular fitness and balance, and they can be used to reduce leisure time sedentary activities in individuals of all ages. Finally, for anyone who is able to do long-distance training, participation in extreme athletic events is possible with appropriate changes in diabetes regimens.

PROFESSIONAL PRACTICE PEARLS

- Both dynamic and static stretching exercises are effective in increasing flexibility and allow individuals to engage in activities that require greater joint range of movement.
- Completing a series of flexibility exercises for each of the major muscle-tendon groups for a total of 60 sec each on ≥2 days/week is recommended to maintain joint range of movement.
- Both tai chi and yoga include basic stretching movements as part of the instruction and bestow a number of health benefits, although blood glucose changes may be variable.
- Active video gaming (exergames) may increase overall physical activity, favorably influence energy balance, and be a viable alternative to some traditional fitness activities.
- All older adults are advised to undertake exercises that maintain or improve balance, especially individuals with T2D or peripheral neuropathy with a higher risk of falling.
- Despite the challenges presented by participation in long-duration athletic events, many individuals with diabetes are currently training for and participating in such events.

REFERENCES

Abate M, Schiavone C, Pelotti P, Salini V: Limited joint mobility in diabetes and ageing: recent advances in pathogenesis and therapy. *Int J Immunopathol Pharmacol* 23:997–1003, 2011

Agmon M, Perry CK, Phelan E, Demiris G, Nguyen HQ: A pilot study of Wii Fit exergames to improve balance in older adults. *J Geriatr Phys Ther* 34:161–167, 2011

Bailey BW, McInnis K: Energy cost of exergaming: a comparison of the energy cost of 6 forms of exergaming. *Arch Pediatr Adolesc Med* 165:597–602, 2011

Balci N, Balci MK, Tuzuner S: Shoulder adhesive capsulitis and shoulder range of motion in type II diabetes mellitus: association with diabetic complications. *J Diabetes Complications* 13:135–140, 1999

Benavides S, Caballero J: Ashtanga yoga for children and adolescents for weight management and psychological well being: an uncontrolled open pilot study. *Complement Ther Clin Pract* 15:110–114, 2009

Cauza E, Hanusch-Enserer U, Strasser B, Ludvik B, Kostner K, Dunky A, Haber P: Continuous glucose monitoring in diabetic long distance runners. *Int J Sports Med* 26:774–780, 2005

Chen SC, Ueng KC, Lee SH, Sun KT, Lee MC: Effect of t'ai chi exercise on biochemical profiles and oxidative stress indicators in obese patients with type 2 diabetes. *J Altern Complement Med* 16:1153–1159, 2010

Colberg SR, Sigal RJ, Fernhall B, Regensteiner JG, Blissmer BJ, Rubin RR, Chasan-Taber L, Albright AL, Braun B, American College of Sports Medicine, American Diabetes Association: Exercise and type 2 diabetes: the American College of Sports Medicine and the American Diabetes Association: joint position statement. *Diabetes Care* 33:e147–e167, 2010

Garber CE, Blissmer B, Deschenes MR, Franklin BA, Lamonte MJ, Lee IM, Nieman DC, Swain DP, American College of Sports Medicine: American College of Sports Medicine position stand. Quantity and quality of exercise for developing and maintaining cardiorespiratory, musculoskeletal, and neuromotor fitness in apparently healthy adults: guidance for prescribing exercise. *Med Sci Sports Exerc* 43:1334–1359, 2011

Goldsmith JR, Lidtke RH, Shott S: The effects of range-of-motion therapy on the plantar pressures of patients with diabetes mellitus. *J Am Podiatr Med Assoc* 92:483–490, 2002

Gordon LA, Morrison EY, McGrowder DA, Young R, Fraser YT, Zamora EM, Alexander-Lindo RL, Irving RR: Effect of exercise therapy on lipid profile and oxidative stress indicators in patients with type 2 diabetes. *BMC Complement Altern Med* 8:21, 2008

Graf DL, Pratt LV, Hester CN, Short KR: Playing active video games increases energy expenditure in children. *Pediatrics* 124:534–540, 2009

Graveling AJ, Frier BM: Risks of marathon running and hypoglycaemia in type 1 diabetes. *Diabet Med* 27:585–588, 2010

Graves LE, Ridgers ND, Williams K, Stratton G, Atkinson G, Cable NT: The physiological cost and enjoyment of Wii Fit in adolescents, young adults, and older adults. *J Phys Act Health* 7:393–401, 2010

Guderian B, Borreson LA, Sletten LE, Cable K, Stecker TP, Probst MA, Dalleck LC: The cardiovascular and metabolic responses to Wii Fit video game playing in middle-aged and older adults. *J Sports Med Phys Fitness* 50:436–442, 2010

Haskell WL, Lee IM, Pate RR, Powell KE, Blair SN, Franklin BA, Macera CA, Heath GW, Thompson PD, Bauman A: Physical activity and public health: updated recommendation for adults from the American College of Sports Medicine and the American Heart Association. *Med Sci Sports Exerc* 39:1423–1434, 2007

Hegde SV, Adhikari P, Kotian S, Pinto VJ, D'Souza S, D'Souza V: Effect of 3-month yoga on oxidative stress in type 2 diabetes with or without complications: a controlled clinical trial. *Diabetes Care* 34:2208–2210, 2011

Herriott MT, Colberg SR, Parson HK, Nunnold T, Vinik AI: Effects of 8 weeks of flexibility and resistance training in older adults with type 2 diabetes. *Diabetes Care* 27:2988–2989, 2004

Innes KE, Vincent HK: The influence of yoga-based programs on risk profiles in adults with type 2 diabetes mellitus: a systematic review. *Evid Based Complement Alternat Med* 4:469–486, 2007

Koivisto VA, Sane T, Fyhrquist F, Pelkonen R: Fuel and fluid homeostasis during long-term exercise in healthy subjects and type I diabetic patients. *Diabetes Care* 15:1736–1741, 1992

Kyizom T, Singh S, Singh KP, Tandon OP, Kumar R: Effect of pranayama & yoga-asana on cognitive brain functions in type 2 diabetes-P3 event related evoked potential (ERP). *Indian J Med Res* 131:636–640, 2010

Lam P, Dennis SM, Diamond TH, Zwar N: Improving glycaemic and BP control in type 2 diabetes. The effectiveness of tai chi. *Aust Fam Physician* 37:884–887, 2008

Lee MS, Choi TY, Lim HJ, Ernst E: Tai chi for management of type 2 diabetes mellitus: A systematic review. *Chin J Integr Med* [Epub ahead of print] 30 Jul 2011

Lee MS, Pittler MH, Kim MS, Ernst E: Tai chi for type 2 diabetes: a systematic review. *Diabet Med* 25:240–241, 2008

Liu X, Miller YD, Burton NW, Brown WJ: A preliminary study of the effects of Tai Chi and Qigong medical exercise on indicators of metabolic syndrome, glycaemic control, health-related quality of life, and psychological health in adults with elevated blood glucose. *Br J Sports Med* 44:704–709, 2010

Madanmohan, Bhavanani AB, Dayanidy G, Sanjay Z, Basavaraddi IV: Effect of yoga therapy on reaction time, biochemical parameters and wellness score of peri and post-menopausal diabetic patients. *Int J Yoga* 5:10–15, 2012

Malhotra V, Singh S, Tandon OP, Sharma SB: The beneficial effect of yoga in diabetes. *Nepal Med Coll J* 7:145–147, 2005

Maloney AE, Bethea TC, Kelsey KS, Marks JT, Paez S, Rosenberg AM, Catellier DJ, Hamer RM, Sikich L: A pilot of a video game (DDR) to promote physical activity and decrease sedentary screen time. *Obesity (Silver Spring)* 16:2074–2080, 2008

Meinders AE, Willekens FL, Heere LP: Metabolic and hormonal changes in IDDM during long-distance run. *Diabetes Care* 11:1–7, 1988

Miller KL, Magel JR, Hayes JG: The effects of a home-based exercise program on balance confidence, balance performance, and gait in debilitated, ambulatory community-dwelling older adults: a pilot study. *J Geriatr Phys Ther* 33:85–91, 2010

Miyachi M, Yamamoto K, Ohkawara K, Tanaka S: METs in adults while playing active video games: a metabolic chamber study. *Med Sci Sports Exerc* 42:1149–1153, 2010

Morrison S, Colberg SR, Mariano M, Parson HK, Vinik AI: Balance training reduces falls risk in older individuals with type 2 diabetes. *Diabetes Care* 33:748–750, 2010

Morrison S, Colberg SR, Parson HK, Vinik AI: Relation between risk of falling and postural sway complexity in diabetes. *Gait Posture* 35:662–668, 2012

Murillo S, Brugnara L, Novials A: One year follow-up in a group of half-marathon runners with type-1 diabetes treated with insulin analogues. *J Sports Med Phys Fitness* 50:506–510, 2010

Murphy EC, Carson L, Neal W, Baylis C, Donley D, Yeater R: Effects of an exercise intervention using Dance Dance Revolution on endothelial function and other risk factors in overweight children. *Int J Pediatr Obes* 4:205–214, 2009

Nelson ME, Rejeski WJ, Blair SN, Duncan PW, Judge JO, King AC, Macera CA, Castaneda-Sceppa C: Physical activity and public health in older adults: recommendation from the American College of Sports Medicine and the American Heart Association. *Med Sci Sports Exerc* 39:1435–1445, 2007

Physical Activity Guidelines Advisory Committee: Physical Activity Guidelines Advisory Committee Report, 2008. Washington, DC, U.S. Department of Health and Human Services, 2008

Ravindran Rajendran S, Bhansali A, Walia R, Dutta P, Bansal V, Shanmugasundar G: Prevalence and pattern of hand soft-tissue changes in type 2 diabetes mellitus. *Diabetes Metab* 37:312–317, 2011

Richerson S, Rosendale K: Does tai chi improve plantar sensory ability? A pilot study. *Diabetes Technol Ther* 9:276–286, 2007

Rogers LC, Frykberg RG, Armstrong DG, Boulton AJ, Edmonds M, Van GH, Hartemann A, Game F, Jeffcoate W, Jirkovska A, Jude E, Morbach S, Morrison WB, Pinzur M, Pitocco D, Sanders L, Wukich DK, Uccioli L: The Charcot foot in diabetes. *Diabetes Care* 34:2123–2129, 2011

Shrier I: Stretching before exercise does not reduce the risk of local muscle injury: a critical review of the clinical and basic science literature. *Clin J Sport Med* 9:221–227, 1999

Singh S, Malhotra V, Singh KP, Madhu SV, Tandon OP: Role of yoga in modifying certain cardiovascular functions in type 2 diabetic patients. *J Assoc Physicians India* 52:203–206, 2004

Smith ST, Sherrington C, Studenski S, Schoene D, Lord SR: A novel Dance Dance Revolution (DDR) system for in-home training of stepping ability: basic parameters of system use by older adults. *Br J Sports Med* 45:441–445, 2011

Sofianidis G, Hatzitaki V, Douka S, Grouios G: Effect of a 10-week traditional dance program on static and dynamic balance control in elderly adults. *J Aging Phys Act* 17:167–180, 2009

Taylor-Piliae RE, Haskell WL, Stotts NA, Froelicher ES: Improvement in balance, strength, and flexibility after 12 weeks of tai chi exercise in ethnic Chinese adults with cardiovascular disease risk factors. *Altern Ther Health Med* 12:50–58, 2006

Tighe CB, Oakley WS Jr: The prevalence of a diabetic condition and adhesive capsulitis of the shoulder. *South Med J* 101:591–595, 2008

Tsang T, Orr R, Lam P, Comino E, Singh MF: Effects of tai chi on glucose homeostasis and insulin sensitivity in older adults with type 2 diabetes: a randomised double-blind sham-exercise-controlled trial. *Age Ageing* 37:64–71, 2008

Tuominen JA, Ebeling P, Koivisto VA: Exercise increases insulin clearance in healthy man and insulin-dependent diabetes mellitus patients. *Clin Physiol* 17:19–30, 1997a

Tuominen JA, Ebeling P, Vuorinen-Markkola H, Koivisto VA: Post-marathon paradox in IDDM: unchanged insulin sensitivity in spite of glycogen depletion. *Diabet Med* 14:301–308, 1997b

Tuominen JA, Ebeling P, Bourey R, Koranyi L, Lamminen A, Rapola J, Sane T, Vuorinen-Markkola H, Koivisto VA: Postmarathon paradox: insulin resistance in the face of glycogen depletion. *Am J Physiol* 270:E336–E343, 1996

Wang JH: Effects of tai chi exercise on patients with type 2 diabetes. *Med Sport Sci* 52:230–238, 2008

West DJ, Morton RD, Bain SC, Stephens JW, Bracken RM: Blood glucose responses to reductions in pre-exercise rapid-acting insulin for 24 h after running in individuals with type 1 diabetes. *J Sports Sci* 28:781–788, 2010

Yeh SH, Chuang H, Lin LW, Hsiao CY, Wang PW, Liu RT, Yang KD: Regular Tai Chi Chuan exercise improves T cell helper function of patients with type 2 diabetes mellitus with an increase in T-bet transcription factor and IL-12 production. *Br J Sports Med* 43:845–850, 2009

Yeh SH, Chuang H, Lin LW, Hsiao CY, Wang PW, Yang KD: Tai chi chuan exercise decreases A1C levels along with increase of regulatory T-cells and decrease of cytotoxic T-cell population in type 2 diabetic patients. *Diabetes Care* 30: 716–718, 2007

Yeung EW, Yeung SS: Interventions for preventing lower limb soft-tissue injuries in runners. *Cochrane Database Syst Rev* CD001256, 2001

Zhang Y, Fu FH: Effects of 14-week Tai Ji Quan exercise on metabolic control in women with type 2 diabetes. *Am J Chin Med* 36:647–654, 2008

Chapter 11

General Diabetes Management with Physical Activity

L ifestyle improvements (i.e., dietary changes and physical activity) assist in the control of blood glucose levels and reduce the risk of acute and longer-term diabetes-related health complications (American Diabetes Association 2013). Acutely uncontrolled diabetes is a relative contraindication to exercise participation, however. Moreover, precise hormonal and metabolic events that normally regulate glucose homeostasis at rest and during exercise frequently are disrupted in diabetes because of defects in insulin release, action, or both.

Glucose control requires near-normal balance between hepatic glucose production and peripheral glucose uptake, combined with effective insulin responses (Wahren 2007). Although low-level physical activity certainly will expend calories and assist with weight maintenance, it usually results in a lesser or no effect on blood glucose levels compared with moderate-intensity activity. Vigorous exercise, though, may result in transient hyperglycemia as hepatic glucose production tends to exceed muscular glucose uptake under such conditions, particularly immediately following exercise (Sigal 1994).

In a diabetic state, a reduced ability to precisely match glucose production and utilization results in daily glucose fluctuations and may require adjustments in dosages of exogenous insulin and other medications. Consequently, two common perturbations associated with exercise in diabetic individuals are hypoglycemia (low blood glucose) and hyperglycemia (high blood glucose); however, regimen adjustments can be made to reduce the risk of both. These adjustments should be combined with appropriate changes in dietary intake for physical activity (Ploug 1984, Richter 1985). Use of self-monitoring of blood glucose (SMBG) before and after exercise sessions is essential, especially in insulin users, to allow them to make appropriate adjustments in food intake and insulin or other medications (Farmer 2008, St John 2010, Juvenile Diabetes Research Foundation Continuous Glucose Monitoring Study Group 2011, Kapitza 2011).

Case in Point: Aerobic Exercise Rx for an Adult with T1D

LK is a 61-year-old man who has had type 1 diabetes (T1D) for 25 years. He has been normally active most of his life, but now he wants to train to run a 5 K (3.1 mile) race with his son and granddaughter that is coming up in 3 months. He does daily walking now, but not much jogging or running, so he is not sure what effect doing a more intense exercise is likely to have on his blood glucose management.

He currently uses daily basal insulin at bedtime (glargine, or Lantus®), along with sliding-scale doses of insulin aspart (Novolog®) for meals and snacks during the day. He thinks he has a pretty healthy diet, but he does have celiac disease and tries to avoid foods that contain gluten.

Resting Measurements

Height: 73 inches
Weight: 185 lb
BMI: 24.4 (normal)
Heart rate: 75 beats per minute (bpm)
Blood pressure: 118/78 mmHg

Fasting Labs

Plasma glucose: Variable (60–165 mg/dl) (controlled with a basal-bolus insulin regimen)
A1C: 6.8%
Total cholesterol: 165 mg/dl
Triglycerides: 95 mg/dl
High-density lipoprotein cholesterol: 54 mg/dl
Low-density lipoprotein cholesterol: 92 mg/dl

Questions to Consider

1. What type of aerobic training should LK do to get ready to run a 5 K race?
2. What exercise frequency, intensity, and duration should LK focus on?
3. How should his training progress over time?
4. What type of diabetes regimen changes will LK need to make to avoid hypoglycemia or hyperglycemia related to his exercise participation?
5. Are any precautions needed for LK when he trains?

(Continued on page 178.)

ENERGY SYSTEMS AND FUEL METABOLISM DURING PHYSICAL ACTIVITY

Physical activity causes a dramatic increase in energy requirements because of the metabolic needs of working muscles, and exercise-dependent factors regulate fuel use (Mittendorfer 2003). Blood glucose levels can change during and after physical activity based on the physiological responses, which vary with exercise duration and intensity. Some of these pathways for energy production can be affected by diabetes, depending on whether hypoglycemia or hyperglycemia occurs during exercise and on pre-exercise storage of muscle glycogen.

THE FIRST 5 MIN OF PHYSICAL ACTIVITY

At the start of any physical activity, regardless of its duration or intensity, adenosine triphosphate (ATP) in the skeletal muscle provides the direct energy for muscle contraction. Some stored ATP and ATP more immediately replenished from creatine phosphate (CP) is available in the muscles for the first 10 sec of activity, but for any duration beyond that time, muscles are reliant on alternative energy systems to fuel physical activity, which is primarily accomplished via enzymatic pathways that initially break down carbohydrate and later fat and protein. During the first few minutes of physical activity, the majority of energy is derived from intramuscular glycogen through the process of anaerobic (or rapid) glycolysis. This anaerobic pathway provides only a limited amount of energy, peaks at ~30 sec into an activity, and lasts a maximum of 2 min. When an activity is intense, this pathway may result in acid by-products that can cause muscular discomfort (a burning sensation) and a reduced exercise capacity. This energy pathway provides the means to produce additional ATP whenever aerobic conversion of fuels is too slow or unable to compensate or at any time during a workout when the exercise intensity is increased. As physical activity continues, an adequate supply of energy becomes available through the aerobic breakdown of carbohydrate, fat, and protein, although carbohydrate remains as the body's preferred source of energy for almost all activities (Bergman 1999, Watt 2002, Arkinstall 2004).

AFTER 5–10 MIN OF PHYSICAL ACTIVITY

During longer, continuous physical activity, all of the macronutrients (i.e., carbohydrate, fat, and protein) are broken down to provide a steady source of ATP production for the working muscles (Bogardus 1984). During moderate and intense activity, the primary fuel used remains carbohydrate, primarily stored muscle glycogen with a smaller contribution from blood glucose (Burke 1999). After the first 5–10 minutes, circulating blood glucose arising from glycogen breakdown in the liver (hepatic glycogenolysis) and glucose being synthesized there (via hepatic gluconeogenesis) provide additional energy sources for working muscles (Petersen 2004).

BEYOND 20 MIN OF PHYSICAL ACTIVITY

As a physical activity continues beyond 20–30 min, the muscle glycogen stores may start to become depleted. The rate of glycogen utilization is highly dependent on exercise intensity and duration, with more being used at higher workout intensities or during longer-duration activities. Whenever muscle glycogen content decreases significantly, a shift in the fuel mix is required. During low to moderate exercise intensities, free fatty acids (FFA) are always a more significant source of energy (compared with during intense activities), in addition to blood glucose from hepatic sources. As physical exercise continues, hepatic gluconeogenesis becomes increasingly important for providing required amounts of blood glucose. The main substrates for gluconeogenesis are three carbon intermediates in metabolism: lactate, alanine, and glycerol (Petersen 2004).

Figure 11.1—Energy Systems in Use during Physical Activity

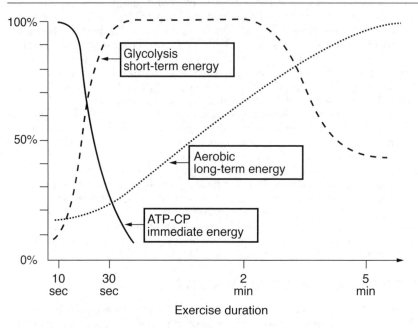

Reprinted, by permission, from Colberg S: *Diabetic Athlete's Handbook: Your Guide to Peak Performance*. Champaign, IL, Human Kinetics, 2009, p. 27.

LONGER DURATION PHYSICAL ACTIVITY

As exercise duration increases further, the contribution of FFA for fuel increases relative to glucose (Manetta 2002). Although carbohydrate remains an important fuel, low- to moderate-intensity exercise relies more on circulating FFA from adipose tissue as the oxidative fuel for muscle, although protein sources may provide up to 5–15% of the total energy during longer-duration activity. The oxidation of fat-derived substrates cannot completely replace carbohydrate use, however, given that a minimum amount of carbohydrate is required for fat to be efficiently used as a fuel (Mittendorfer 2001, 2003). When carbohydrate sources are too limited, fat is not completely oxidized and ketone bodies are formed as a by-product of the incomplete combustion of fat (Devries 2008). Ketones are not an efficient source of energy during exercise. Without an adequate supply of carbohydrate available, the exercise intensity cannot be maintained (e.g., as evidenced by exercisers "bonking" or "hitting the wall" during long-duration activities like marathons).

TRAINING EFFECTS ON EXERCISE FUEL USE

An individual's training status will affect the use of carbohydrate during an aerobic activity. Aerobic training increases fat utilization during a similar-duration bout of low- or moderate-intensity activity done after training, thereby sparing muscle glycogen and blood glucose and resulting in less-acute decreases in glycemia (Braun 2004, Pruchnic 2004, Galbo 2007). Type 2 diabetes (T2D) may be associated with a decrease in lipid oxidation and a shift toward greater carbohydrate oxidation at all exercise intensities compared with their nondiabetic counterparts (Ghanassia 2006). These changes in fuel use also explain why more carbohydrate may be needed to maintain blood glucose levels when beginning training compared with doing the same activity at the same training intensity after several weeks.

Absolute exercise intensity determines the exercise-induced increase in energy demands, whereas exercise intensity relative to an individual's maximal aerobic capacity determines the proportional contribution of different fuel sources (i.e., blood glucose, plasma FFAs, muscle glycogen, and intramuscular fat stores). Although endurance training increases the aerobic capacity in muscle and the oxidation of fat during exercise, when exercise is done at the same relative intensity (i.e., a higher absolute workload after training increases fitness level), carbohydrate use during the activity remains the same (Mittendorfer 2003). Furthermore, training effects are sport or activity specific, with little carryover of the training effect from one activity to the next.

GLYCOGEN STORAGE AND USE IN DIABETES

MUSCLE GLYCOGEN USE AND AVAILABILITY

Glycogen is the storage form of carbohydrates, which primarily is stored in skeletal muscles (about 500g) and the liver (about 100g). Given that blood glucose levels have to be kept within narrow limits for proper brain and nervous system functioning, the human body is adapted to cope with periods of excess carbohydrates (following meals) and periods without any (such as overnight) (Jensen 2011).

Glycogen use during exercise. Muscle glycogen functions mainly as an energy substrate during higher exercise intensities (usually >70% of maximal oxygen uptake), and early fatigue develops when the glycogen stores are depleted in the active muscles. An insulin-resistant state should not affect blood glucose uptake during exercise, given the use of a contraction-induced mechanism for glucose uptake into muscle during exercise (Ploug 1984), but it does appear to affect total carbohydrate use during low-intensity exercise. In obese, insulin-resistant women, total carbohydrate oxidation and estimated muscle glycogen use were significantly lower, even though blood glucose uptake was not impaired (Braun 2004). These results suggest that insulin resistance, independent of body fat, spares muscle glycogen and shifts substrate oxidation toward less carbohydrate use during exercise.

In a study examining the effects of sprint training in young adults with T1D, their pretraining, maximal activities of enzymes involved in carbohydrate use via the second and third energy systems (e.g., hexokinase, citrate synthase, and pyruvate dehydrogenase) were not necessarily different between people with and without T1D when resting (Harmer 2008). Muscle lactate accumulation during sprint exercise, however, was higher at the start of training in T1D and corresponded to pretraining A1C values and fasting plasma glucose. After training, rates of muscular glycogenolysis (muscle glycogen breakdown) and muscular glycolysis rates were similar between groups, suggesting that high-intensity sprint training in young adults with T1D decreases their lactate accumulation during intense activities to more normal levels, while enhancing their muscle oxidative metabolism.

Finally, in a study on active men with T1D, substrate oxidation during 120 min of moderate aerobic cycling during euglycemic metabolic conditions was similar to nondiabetic controls, with a shift toward lipid oxidation during long-duration exercise (Jenni 2008). In a hyperglycemic state, however, fuel metabolism was dominated by carbohydrate oxidation, although muscular glycogen was again not spared by greater availability of blood glucose in T1D. In individuals with T2D, however, low-intensity cycling appeared to increase blood glucose uptake during hyperglycemic conditions without altering total carbohydrate oxidation, suggesting that a decreased oxidation of muscle glycogen occurred (Colberg 1996).

Effects of muscle glycogen content. The effects of altering pre-exercise muscle glycogen content and exercise intensity on endogenous carbohydrate oxidation during exercise of varying intensities are equivocal. In moderately trained individuals, however, muscle glycogen availability (low vs. high) does not appear to greatly influence rates of blood glucose uptake during either low- or moderate-intensity exercise (Arkinstall 2004). In exercisers with T1D, exercise done under peak therapeutic insulin concentrations requires greater carbohydrate supplementation to prevent hypoglycemia, but its intake does not spare muscle glycogen (Chokkalingam 2007a). Moreover, a disproportionate increase in blood glucose uptake relative to increases in carbohydrate oxidation during exercise suggests an increase in glucose flux through nonoxidative pathways (such as storage of glycogen in inactive muscle fibers).

Glycogen storage and replacement. After exercise, synthesis rates are increased to replenish glycogen stores using blood glucose as the substrate (Cartee 1989). Reduced glycogen stores in skeletal muscles after exercise allow carbohydrate to be stored as muscle glycogen and prevent blood glucose from being converted into and stored as fat. In fact, regular participation in physical activity that is moderate or higher allows for the reduction of skeletal muscle glycogen and subsequent storage of ingested carbohydrates after meals postactivity. Individuals without diabetes remove excess amounts of blood glucose rapidly, but insulin-stimulated glucose disposal is reduced in T1D when insulin is deficient and in T2D when insulin resistance prevents normal insulin action. Following meals, normally 70–90% of glucose disposal will be stored as muscle glycogen in nondiabetic individuals; however, muscular glycogen stores are limited because an efficient feedback-mediated inhibition of glycogen synthase prevents accumulation. De novo lipid synthesis can contribute to glucose disposal when glycogen stores are filled (Jensen 2011).

HEPATIC GLYCOGEN AND GLUCOSE PRODUCTION

The liver is responsible for maintaining blood glucose levels in a normal range during resting and exercise conditions, which it accomplishes by balancing storage of glucose as glycogen with release of glucose via hepatic glycogenolysis or de novo production (gluconeogenesis). Hepatic glycogenolysis accounts for the majority of blood glucose production during the first 90 min of exercise or hypoglycemia in nondiabetic subjects. Individuals with T1D, however, frequently exhibit diminished hepatic glycogen stores, augmented gluconeogenesis, and increased basal hepatic glucose production in proportion to the severity of blood glucose elevations (Wahren 2007). In T2D, hyperglycemia associated with a fasting state is in part caused by an overproduction of glucose from the liver that is secondary to inappropriately accelerated gluconeogenesis (Wahren 2007).

Insufficiently insulin-treated T1D individuals may exhibit exaggerated postprandial hyperglycemia and reduction in liver glycogen stores. In fact, marked reduction in both hepatic glycogen synthesis and breakdown has been noted in individuals with poorly controlled diabetes (Bischof 2001). Both defects in hepatic glycogen metabolism are improved, but not normalized, by short-term restoration of more normal insulin and blood glucose levels. In intensively treated individuals with T1D, despite some activation of counterregulatory hormones, hypoglycemia may fail to stimulate hepatic glycogen breakdown or activation of endogenous glucose production (Mevorach 2000, Kishore 2006). Hyperinsulinemic and hyperglycemic conditions during moderate exercise, however, do not appear to suppress hepatic glycogen mobilization during exercise-induced hypoglycemia (Chokkalingam 2007a, 2007b).

Increases in hepatic glucose production in healthy adults with increasing exercise intensity can be entirely attributed to increases in net hepatic glycogenolysis. In contrast, moderately controlled individuals with T1D are likely to exhibit increased rates of glucose production, both at rest and during exercise, entirely accounted for by greater gluconeogenesis (Petersen 2004). Poorly controlled individuals with T1D exhibit a marked reduction in both hepatic glycogen synthesis and breakdown. Both defects in glycogen metabolism are improved but not normalized by short-term restoration of insulinemia and glycemia (Bischof 2001).

CHANGES IN INSULIN ACTION WITH PHYSICAL ACTIVITY

ACUTE CHANGES IN MUSCULAR INSULIN ACTION

Aerobic exercise. Most improvements in diabetes management in T2D are related to acute and chronic improvements in insulin action (Braun 1995, Ishii 1998, Ibanez 2005, Cohen 2008, Winnick 2008). The acute effects of a recent bout of aerobic exercise account for most of the immediate improvements in insulin action, with most individuals experiencing a decrease in their blood glucose levels during mild- and moderate-intensity exercise and for 2–72 h afterward (Boulé 2001, O'Gorman 2006, Galbo 2007). Such glycemic improvements are linked directly to the duration and intensity of the exercise, pre-exercise diabetes control, and an individual's training state (Colberg 1996; Boulé 2001, 2005; Sigal 2007). Although engaging in physical activity of any intensity generally enhances uptake of blood glucose for muscular and hepatic glycogen synthesis (Christ-Roberts 2003, Galbo 2007), by stimulating fat oxidation and storage in muscle (Duncan 2003, Goodpaster 2003, Boon 2007), engaging in longer or more intense activity (and using up greater amounts of stored muscle glycogen) acutely enhances insulin action for longer periods of time (Braun 1995, Larsen 1999, Houmard 2004, Evans 2005, Sigal 2007, Bajpeyi 2009). Acute improvements in insulin sensitivity in women with T2D have been found for equivalent energy expenditures whether engaging in low-intensity or high-intensity walking (Braun 1995), but may be affected by age and training status (Boulé 2001; Rimbert 2004; Evans 2005; Goulet 2005a, 2005b). Although plasma FFA oxidation is not impaired during exercise in nonobese individuals with T2D (Borghouts 2002), increased storage of liver fat common in obesity and T2D is strongly associated with reduced hepatic and peripheral insulin action. Thus, enhanced whole-body insulin action following aerobic training appears to be related to gains in peripheral, not hepatic, insulin action (Winnick 2008, Kirwan 2009).

Resistance exercise. Resistance exercise is an effective treatment for acutely enhancing insulin sensitivity and regulating blood glucose. For example, in adults with insulin resistance, resistance training has been shown to have a dose-response relationship: a high-intensity, multiple-set bout of resistance work had the greatest acute impact on both fasting glucose and insulin sensitivity, whereas single-set protocols were less effective in lowering fasting blood glucose (Black 2010). In another study, however, a single bout of strenuous resistance exercise was not found to necessarily improve insulin sensitivity in people with T1D (Jimenez 2009).

CHRONIC CHANGES IN INSULIN ACTION WITH TRAINING

Aerobic training. Even 1 week of aerobic training can improve whole-body insulin sensitivity in individuals with T2D (Winnick 2008). Moderate and vigorous aerobic training improve insulin sensitivity (Houmard 2004, Evans 2005, Galbo 2007, Bajpeyi 2009), but a lesser intensity also may improve insulin action to some degree (Houmard 2004). Aerobic training can enhance the responsiveness of skeletal muscles to insulin with increased expression or activity of proteins involved in glucose metabolism and insulin signaling (Christ-Roberts 2004, Holten 2004, O'Gorman 2006, Wang 2009), greater glycogen synthase activity, and GLUT4 protein expression (Christ-Roberts 2004). Fat oxidation is a key aspect of improved insulin action, and training increases lipid storage in muscle and fat oxidation capacity (Duncan 2003, Goodpaster 2003, Pruchnic 2004, Kelley 2007).

Resistance training. Resistance training also benefits blood glucose management and insulin action in adults with T2D (Ishii 1998, Dunstan 2002, Ibanez 2005, Snowling 2006, Cohen 2008, Ibanez 2008). Twice-weekly progressive resistance training for 16 weeks by older men with newly diagnosed T2D can result in a 46.3% increase in insulin action, a 7.1% reduction in fasting glycemia, and significant loss of visceral fat (Ibanez 2005). An increase in muscle mass from resistance training may contribute to enhanced blood glucose uptake from a mass effect, and heavy weight training in particular may reverse or prevent further loss of skeletal muscle due to disuse and aging (Castaneda 2002, Willey 2003). Diabetic women undergoing 12 weeks of low-intensity training with resistance bands had gains in strength and muscle mass and loss of fat mass but no change in insulin sensitivity (Kwon 2010).

Combined training. Combined strength and aerobic exercise training also has been shown to result in positive adaptations in glucose control, insulin action, muscular strength, and exercise tolerance in women with T2D (Tokmakidis 2004), and such training results in lower daily insulin requirements in adolescents with T1D (D'Hooge 2011). Benefits to insulin action from adding resistance training to aerobic training in women with T2D are likely related to loss of visceral fat and increases in muscle density (Cuff 2003).

SELF-MANAGEMENT STRATEGIES FOR PHYSICAL ACTIVITY

Frequent self-monitoring of blood glucose (SMBG) benefits glycemic control, regardless of the type of diabetes (St John 2010). It usually involves at least three to six glucose checks per day by individuals with T1D, but less frequent blood glucose monitoring by non–insulin users with T2D (Farmer 2008). More recently, continuous glucose monitoring (CGM) has been used to detect patterns in blood glucose across multiple days and evaluate both acute and delayed effects of exercise (Allen 2008, Fritschi 2010). Adjustments in insulin dose, oral medications, or carbohydrate intake can be fine-tuned using the detailed information provided by SMBG and CGM. Overall glycemic control assessed with A1C (or estimated average glucose, eAG) should ideally be assessed every 3–4 months (American Diabetes Association 2013).

SELF-MONITORING BLOOD GLUCOSE FOR PHYSICAL ACTIVITY

SMBG is useful to determine if and when a snack or other regimen changes are required to keep the blood glucose within the established goals and to anticipate and prevent hypoglycemic events. Blood glucose readings taken at the start and end of an exercise session allow the individual to gauge the amount of change happening during physical activity and to determine whether additional carbohydrates are needed at that time (Biankin 2003). For example, if an individual's blood glucose usually drops 30–40 mg/dl during a physical activity and the goal is to stay >90 mg/dl, a pre-exercise snack should be eaten for readings <130 mg/dl. For pre-exercise glucose levels between the target starting value and the goal, some—albeit a lesser amount of—carbohydrate may still be needed.

FACTORS AFFECTING EXERCISE BLOOD GLUCOSE RESPONSES

Anticipating blood glucose responses to every exercise session is problematic given that many factors can affect the outcome on a given day. For example, each person's blood glucose responses will be affected by the type of diabetes that he or

Table 11.1 Factors Affecting Blood Glucose Responses

Exercise intensity and duration	Time of day exercise is undertaken
Blood glucose level at start of activity	Prior hypoglycemia
Training status (i.e., new versus usual activity)	Timing of last insulin dose (i.e., circulating insulin levels)
Prior exercise (same day or day before)	Use of other glucose-lowering medications
Types of insulin used	Type of food last eaten
Timing of last meal or snack	Level of hydration
Temperature and other environmental conditions	Seasonal variations
Recent or current illness	Presence of diabetic complications
Mental stress	Sleep patterns
Recent weight loss or gain	Pregnancy (women only)
Type of exercise	Phase of menstrual cycle (women only)

she has; type and delivery method of insulin (if taken); use of other diabetes medications; type, intensity, and duration of exercise; fitness level of the individual; and his or her starting blood glucose (Sigal 1994, Braun 1995, Larsen 1999, Arkinstall 2004, Houmard 2004, O'Donovan 2005, Ghanassia 2006, Bajpeyi 2009). Even the time of day that exercise is done can result in a differing effect (Poirier 2001, Dubé 2006, Colberg 2009b, Taplin 2010). Other factors can change over time, such as weight gain or loss, seasonal variations, and changes in medication doses, as well as physical issues like sleep patterns, illness or injury, orthopedic limitations, and the development of diabetes-related complications (Table 11.1) (Ferriss 2006, Costacou 2007, Richerson 2007, Lemaster 2008, Lee 2009, Salem 2010, Hegde 2011).

FOOD INTAKE TO PREVENT HYPOGLYCEMIA

Snacking is the easiest strategy that individuals with any type of diabetes can learn to implement on their own. By adequately replacing carbohydrates during exercise, almost all hypoglycemia can be prevented, even if insulin doses are not adjusted for activity (Kilbride 2011). Furthermore, the amount of extra carbohydrates required to maintain glycemia is easier to anticipate than the correct reduction in insulin dosing (Grimm 2004, Riddell 2011). Adequate carbohydrate replacement during and after exercise is likely the most important measure to prevent hypoglycemia, with insulin dosage adjustments playing a less important role, although an insulin decrease of 20–30% may be needed during long-duration exercise (>60 min) (Grimm 2004). (Insulin adjustments for physical activity are fully discussed in chapter 14.)

Table 11.2 Estimated Carbohydrate Requirements during Aerobic Physical Activity

Intensity	Carbohydrate Replacement	Frequency
Mild	0–10 g	Every 30 min
Moderate	5–10 g	Every 15 min
High	0–15 g	Every 15 min

Adapted from Colberg S: *Diabetic Athlete's Handbook: Your Guide to Peak Performance*. Champaign, IL, Human Kinetics, p. 29, 2009.

Correctly estimating the amount of food needed also can be difficult, however. When the snack is not sufficient, hypoglycemia can still occur, whereas if too much is eaten, some degree of hyperglycemia may result. When weight loss is a goal of the fitness plan, both of these circumstances can result in the intake of more total calories, and if enough calories are consumed, weight gain can result instead of weight loss. If a lesser carbohydrate intake is desired, individuals should consider carefully choosing an exercise time that corresponds to lower circulating levels of insulin to lower their risk of developing hypoglycemia that has to be treated either during or following a bout of physical activity (Larsen 1999; Poirier 2001; Dubé 2005, 2006; Colberg 2009b). Table 11.2 gives some general guidelines for carbohydrate requirements during aerobic exercise; a longer version of this table can be found in chapter 12 (Colberg 2009a).

CHOOSING THE RIGHT SNACK

The type of snack eaten should reflect both immediate and future glycemic needs. People with diabetes frequently choose to consume glucose tablets, juice, or regular soda at the start of the physical activity, knowing that these options are used to treat hypoglycemic events and assuming they are useful as a preventative as well. While they work in the short term, simple sugars alone are likely not the best snacking options for longer-term prevention of hypoglycemia during extended exercise and afterward.

Before and during exercise snacking. To prevent hypoglycemia during exercise, a pre-exercise snack with carbohydrates that are more slowly absorbed or containing a small amount of protein may be a better match for exercise fuel requirements than a rapidly absorbed carbohydrate source used to treat hypoglycemia (Nathan 1985). During exercise, a general guideline is that a snack containing 10–30 g of carbohydrate should be consumed for every 30–45 min of moderate physical activity (Grimm 2004, Colberg 2009a, Kilbride 2011, Riddell 2011). The actual carbohydrate requirement will vary from person to person and even among activities done by one individual or on differing days, making SMBG critical for predicting snack requirements to optimize exercise performance and blood glucose control. A number of factors can influence actual carbohydrate needs, including intensity and duration of exercise, starting blood glucose level, circulating insulin levels, medication regimens, recent food and fluid consumption, and timing of exercise, to name a few. For example, even in individuals with T2D, blood glucose levels are likely to decrease more during physical activity undertaken in the fed state (postmeal) compared with the fasted or premeal state at varying times of day (Poirier 2001, Colberg 2009b).

Diabetic exercisers consume a variety of carbohydrate-based snacks during exercise, including sports bars, gels, and drinks, some of which contain some protein and fat along with carbohydrate (Colberg 2009a). Some carbohydrates that are more slowly absorbed can be found in whole grains, many whole fruits, yogurt, and many snack bars. The choice of the best option should be based on the desired blood glucose level throughout the activity, duration and intensity of the activity, an individual's unique glucose response to exercise and tolerance to foods, and personal preferences.

Postexercise snacking. After a bout of physical activity, additional snacks may be needed to prevent late-onset hypoglycemia. The first 30–60 min after exercise is generally when muscles are taking up blood glucose to replace glycogen at the fastest rate and with the least insulin needed (Cartee 1989). Eating a small carbohydrate snack within 30–120 min postexercise may prevent hypoglycemia during that time. The actual number of carbohydrates required will vary with the type of activity that was done, any regimen changes implemented for the activity (lower insulin or higher carbohydrate intake), and an individual's postexercise blood glucose level. Hypoglycemia is more common again 7–11 h after exercise, and precautions may be needed to prevent its later occurrence (McMahon 2007). Postexercise and bedtime snacks for insulin users to prevent late-onset and nighttime lows should likely contain higher relative amounts of protein and fat (such as found in whole milk, chocolate milk, or yogurt), which are metabolized more slowly and keep blood glucose levels more stable over time than carbohydrate alone (Hernandez 2000).

Exercise timing effects. Generally speaking, if an activity is being performed after a meal or usual snack, no extra food may be needed unless insulin levels are higher than normal during that time or exercise is prolonged. If more food is required, the amount of carbohydrate can be adjusted upward to achieve the desired blood glucose level. If an activity is being undertaken >2 h after a meal, then a snack should be eaten within 15 min of beginning the physical activity to avoid pre-exercise hyperglycemia (Nathan 1985). Doing so also gives the glucose sufficient time to be absorbed and to enter the bloodstream to be available to active muscles.

Case in Point: Wrap-Up

LK's new exercise goals revolve around a specific training goal: in 3 months, he wants to be able to finish a 5 K run. He does not have any orthopedic limitations to running that he knows of; he just has not been running in the past couple of decades. He should progress slowly enough to avoid developing any overuse injuries, while increasing his exercise program sufficiently to allow him to develop the endurance to run that distance at a reasonable race pace without needing to walk.

Exercise Program Goals

Mode of Activity: To be able to run a 5 K race without stopping, LK will need to work up to running continuously for ≥30 min. He can do this with a combination of fast walking, jogging, and running during his workouts on various days.

Intensity: LK should work up to maintaining a jogging or running pace that feels "somewhat hard" to start to "hard." His initial target heart rate should be in the range of 111–128 bpm, equivalent to 40–59% heart rate reserve (HRR), with a later training goal of at least 129 bpm (60% HRR, the low end of the vigorous range). He should consider alternating "hard" and "easy" days, focusing on interval training and longer distances at a slower pace, respectively.

Frequency: LK's training for running will progress more effectively with adequate recovery time between harder workouts. He should likely do some walking or jogging on 3–5 days/week from now until his race day, with at least 1 day a week as a rest day.

Duration: When beginning his exercise program, DG should engage in shorter bouts of exercise training (15–20 min), until he can train continuously for ≥30 min on his longer-duration days. He should ideally engage in a combination of brisk walking and jogging for that duration (with alternating bouts of each, with jogging or running segments getting longer over time), with a training goal of doing 75–150 min of physical activity (depending on intensity) each week.

Progression: To avoid developing an overuse injury during run training, LK should increase the duration of his structured workouts first, then the intensity, and lastly the frequency. He can start jogging for as long as possible and alternate it with walking until he is able to cover a 5 K distance at a constant running pace over a period of 6–8 weeks. On nonrunning days, he should consider doing some resistance work or an alternate aerobic activity.

Possible Precautions: Since LK has no risk factors for cardiovascular disease other than diabetes and he is only planning to work up to doing moderate-intensity jogging at this point, he does not necessarily need to have a checkup or an exercise stress test before starting his training. He has been regularly active for many years (although not doing much running), and he has already been doing moderate exercise. He will need to use SMBG, however, to establish his body's usual response to varying types and durations of training, and he will need to make appropriate food and insulin adjustments to maintain normal blood glucose levels. On all training runs, he should carry a rapid-acting carbohydrate and either exercise with a partner or carry a cellular phone and diabetes identification with him.

Almost all physical activity participation by individuals who use exogenous insulin requires diabetes regimen changes to manage blood glucose levels. Muscular fuel use during physical activity is dictated by a number of factors, including the duration of exercise, its intensity, and circulating insulin levels, among other things. With appropriate regimen management, people with diabetes can safely and effectively participate in regular physical activity without experiencing major metabolic perturbations.

PROFESSIONAL PRACTICE PEARLS

- Precise hormonal and metabolic events that normally regulate glucose homeostasis are frequently disrupted in diabetes due to defects in insulin release, action, or both.
- Glucose control requires near-normal balance between hepatic glucose production and peripheral glucose uptake, combined with effective insulin responses.
- Use of SMBG before and after exercise sessions allows individuals to make appropriate adjustments in food intake and insulin or other medications.
- Physical activity causes a dramatic increase in energy requirements because of the metabolic needs of working muscles, and exercise-dependent factors regulate fuel use.
- Blood glucose levels can change during and after physical activity based on the physiological responses, which vary with exercise type, duration, and intensity.
- At the start of any physical activity, ATP in skeletal muscle provides the direct energy for muscle contraction.
- During moderate and intense activity, the primary fuel used remains carbohydrate, primarily stored muscle glycogen with a smaller contribution from blood glucose.
- Muscle glycogen stores may become depleted during physical activity, but its rate of use is highly dependent on exercise intensity and duration.
- Although carbohydrate remains an important fuel, exercise of low to moderate intensity relies more on circulating FFAs from adipose tissue as the oxidative fuel for muscle.
- An individual's training status will affect the use of carbohydrate during an activity, given that aerobic training increases fat utilization during a similar-duration bout of moderate or easier activity, thereby sparing muscle glycogen and blood glucose.
- Greater carbohydrate supplementation may prevent hypoglycemia in individuals with diabetes, but its intake does not appear to spare muscle glycogen.
- Diabetes can alter the normal hepatic balance of storage of glucose as glycogen in the liver with release of glucose via glycogenolysis or gluconeogenesis.
- Most improvements in blood glucose management in T2D are related to acute and chronic improvements in insulin action.
- Adjustments to insulin dose, oral medications, or carbohydrate intake can be fine-tuned using the detailed glycemic information provided by SMBG and CGM.
- Anticipating blood glucose responses to every exercise session is problematic given that a large number of factors can affect the outcome on a given day.
- Adequate carbohydrate replacement during and after exercise is likely the most important measure to prevent hypoglycemia, with insulin dosage adjustments playing a lesser role.

- The type of snack eaten should reflect both immediate and future glycemic needs, with those used to treat hypoglycemia likely differing from ones more effective to prevent it.
- To prevent hypoglycemia in insulin users, a snack containing 10–30 g of carbohydrate should likely be consumed for every 30–45 min of moderate physical activity.

REFERENCES

Allen NA, Fain JA, Braun B, Chipkin SR: Continuous glucose monitoring counseling improves physical activity behaviors of individuals with type 2 diabetes: a randomized clinical trial. *Diabetes Res Clin Pract* 80:371–379, 2008

American Diabetes Association: Standards of medical care in diabetes—2013. *Diabetes Care* 36 (Suppl. 1):S11–S66, 2013

Arkinstall MJ, Bruce CR, Clark SA, Rickards CA, Burke LM, Hawley JA: Regulation of fuel metabolism by preexercise muscle glycogen content and exercise intensity. *J Appl Physiol* 97:2275–2283, 2004

Bajpeyi S, Tanner CJ, Slentz CA, Duscha BD, McCartney JS, Hickner RC, Kraus WE, Houmard JA: Effect of exercise intensity and volume on persistence of insulin sensitivity during training cessation. *J Appl Physiol* 106:1079–1085, 2009

Bergman BC, Butterfield GE, Wolfel EE, Casazza GA, Lopaschuk GD, Brooks GA: Evaluation of exercise and training on muscle lipid metabolism. *Am J Physiol* 276:E106–E117, 1999

Biankin SA, Jenkins AB, Campbell LV, Choi KL, Forrest QG, Chisholm Dj: Target-seeking behavior of plasma glucose with exercise in type 1 diabetes. *Diabetes Care* 26:297–301, 2003

Bischof MG, Krssak M, Krebs M, Bernroider E, Stingl H, Waldhausl W, Roden M: Effects of short-term improvement of insulin treatment and glycemia on hepatic glycogen metabolism in type 1 diabetes. *Diabetes* 50:392–388, 2001

Black LE, Swan PD, Alvar BA: Effects of intensity and volume on insulin sensitivity during acute bouts of resistance training. *J Strength Cond Res* 24:1109–1116, 2010

Bogardus C, Ravussin E, Robbins DC, Wolfe RR, Horton ES, Sims EA: Effects of physical training and diet therapy on carbohydrate metabolism in patients with glucose intolerance and non-insulin-dependent diabetes mellitus. *Diabetes* 33:311–318, 1984

Boon H, Blaak EE, Saris WH, Keizer HA, Wagenmakers AJ, van Loon LJ: Substrate source utilisation in long-term diagnosed type 2 diabetes patients at rest, and during exercise and subsequent recovery. *Diabetologia* 50:103–112, 2007

Borghouts LB, Wagenmakers AJ, Goyens PL, Keizer HA: Substrate utilization in non-obese Type II diabetic patients at rest and during exercise. *Clin Sci (Lond)* 103:559–566, 2002

Boulé NG, Weisnagel SJ, Lakka TA, Tremblay A, Bergman RN, Rankinen T, Leon AS, Skinner JS, Wilmore JH, Rao DC, Bouchard C: Effects of exercise training on glucose homeostasis: the HERITAGE family study. *Diabetes Care* 28:108–114, 2005

Boulé NG, Haddad E, Kenny GP, Wells GA, Sigal RJ: Effects of exercise on glycemic control and body mass in type 2 diabetes mellitus: a meta-analysis of controlled clinical trials. *JAMA* 286:1218–1227, 2001

Braun B, Sharoff C, Chipkin SR, Beaudoin F: Effects of insulin resistance on substrate utilization during exercise in overweight women. *J Appl Physiol* 97:991–997, 2004

Braun B, Zimmermann MB, Kretchmer N: Effects of exercise intensity on insulin sensitivity in women with non-insulin-dependent diabetes mellitus. *J Appl Physiol* 78:300–306, 1995

Burke LM, Hawley JA: Carbohydrate and exercise. *Curr Opin Clin Nutr Metab Care* 2:515–520, 1999

Cartee GD, Young DA, Sleeper MA, Zierath J, Wallberg-Henriksson H, Holloszy JO: Prolonged increase in insulin-stimulated glucose transport in muscle after exercise. *Am J Physiol* 256:E494–E499, 1989

Castaneda C, Layne JE, Munoz-Orians L, Gordon PL, Walsmith J, Foldvari M, Roubenoff R, Tucker KL, Nelson ME: A randomized controlled trial of resistance exercise training to improve glycemic control in older adults with type 2 diabetes. *Diabetes Care* 25:2335–2341, 2002

Chokkalingam K, Tsintzas K, Norton L, Jewell K, Macdonald IA, Mansell PI: Exercise under hyperinsulinaemic conditions increases whole-body glucose disposal without affecting muscle glycogen utilisation in type 1 diabetes. *Diabetologia* 50:414–421, 2007a

Chokkalingam K, Tsintzas K, Snaar JE, Norton L, Solanky B, Leverton E, Morris P, Mansell P, Macdonald IA: Hyperinsulinaemia during exercise does not suppress hepatic glycogen concentrations in patients with type 1 diabetes: a magnetic resonance spectroscopy study. *Diabetologia* 50:1921–1929, 2007b

Christ-Roberts CY, Pratipanawatr T, Pratipanawatr W, Berria R, Belfort R, Kashyap S, Mandarino LJ: Exercise training increases glycogen synthase activity and GLUT4 expression but not insulin signaling in overweight non-diabetic and type 2 diabetic subjects. *Metabolism* 53:1233–1242, 2004

Christ-Roberts, CY, Pratipanawatr T, Pratipanawatr W, Berria R, Belfort R, Mandarino LJ: Increased insulin receptor signaling and glycogen synthase activity contribute to the synergistic effect of exercise on insulin action. *J Appl Physiol* 95:2519–2529, 2003

Cohen ND, Dunstan DW, Robinson C, Vulikh E, Zimmet PZ, Shaw JE: Improved endothelial function following a 14-month resistance exercise training program in adults with type 2 diabetes. *Diabetes Res Clin Pract* 79:405–411, 2008

Colberg SR: *Diabetic Athlete's Handbook*. Champaign, IL, Human Kinetics, p. 28–32, 2009a

Colberg SR, Zarrabi L, Bennington L, Nakave A, Thomas Somma C, Swain DP, Sechrist SR: Postprandial walking is better for lowering the glycemic effect of dinner than pre-dinner exercise in type 2 diabetic individuals. *J Am Med Dir Assoc* 10:394–397, 2009b

Colberg SR, Hagberg JM, McCole SD, Zmuda JM, Thompson PD, Kelley DE: Utilization of glycogen but not plasma glucose is reduced in individuals with NIDDM during mild-intensity exercise. *J Appl Physiol* 81:2027–2033, 1996

Costacou T, Edmundowicz D, Prince C, Conway B, Orchard TJ: Progression of coronary artery calcium in type 1 diabetes mellitus. *Am J Cardiol* 100:1543–1547, 2007

Cuff DJ, Meneilly GS, Martin A, Ignaszewski A, Tildesley HD, Frohlich JJ: Effective exercise modality to reduce insulin resistance in women with type 2 diabetes. *Diabetes Care* 26:2977–2982, 2003

D'Hooge R, Hellinckx T, Van Laethem C, Stegen S, De Schepper J, Van Aken S, Dewolf D, Calders P: Influence of combined aerobic and resistance training on metabolic control, cardiovascular fitness and quality of life in adolescents with type 1 diabetes: a randomized controlled trial. *Clin Rehabil* 25:349–359, 2011

Devries MC, Samjoo IA, Hamadeh MJ, Tarnopolsky MA: Effect of endurance exercise on hepatic lipid content, enzymes, and adiposity in men and women. *Obesity (Silver Spring)* 16:2281–2288, 2008

Dubé MC, Weisnagel SJ, Prud'homme D, Lavoie C: Is early and late post-meal exercise so different in type 1 diabetic lispro users? *Diabetes Res Clin Pract* 72:128–134, 2006

Dubé MC, Weisnagel SJ, Prud'homme D, Lavoie C: Exercise and newer insulins: how much glucose supplement to avoid hypoglycemia? *Med Sci Sports Exerc* 37:1276–1282, 2005

Duncan GE, Perri MG, Theriaque DW, Hutson AD, Eckel RH, Stacpoole PW: Exercise training, without weight loss, increases insulin sensitivity and postheparin plasma lipase activity in previously sedentary adults. *Diabetes Care* 26:557–562, 2003

Dunstan DW, Daly RM, Owen N, Jolley D, De Courten M, Shaw J, Zimmet P: High-intensity resistance training improves glycemic control in older patients with type 2 diabetes. *Diabetes Care* 25:1729–1736, 2002

Evans EM, Racette SB, Peterson LR, Villareal DT, Greiwe JS, Holloszy JO: Aerobic power and insulin action improve in response to endurance exercise training in healthy 77-87 yr olds. *J Appl Physiol* 98:40–45, 2005

Farmer A, Balman E, Gadsby R, Moffatt J, Cradock S, McEwen L, Jameson K: Frequency of self-monitoring of blood glucose in patients with type 2 diabetes: association with hypoglycaemic events. *Curr Med Res Opin* 24:3097–3104, 2008

Ferriss JB, Webb D, Chaturvedi N, Fuller JH, Idzior-Walus B, Eurodiab Prospective Complications Group: Weight gain is associated with improved glycaemic control but with adverse changes in plasma lipids and blood pressure in type 1 diabetes. *Diabet Med* 23:557–564, 2006

Fritschi C, Quinn L, Penckofer S, Surdyk PM: Continuous glucose monitoring: the experience of women with type 2 diabetes. *Diabetes Educ* 36:250–257, 2010

Galbo H, Tobin L, van Loon LJ: Responses to acute exercise in type 2 diabetes, with an emphasis on metabolism and interaction with oral hypoglycemic agents and food intake. *Appl Physiol Nutr Metab* 32:567–575, 2007

Ghanassia E, Brun JF, Fedou C, Raynaud E, Mercier J: Substrate oxidation during exercise: type 2 diabetes is associated with a decrease in lipid oxidation and an earlier shift towards carbohydrate utilization. *Diabetes Metab* 32:604–610, 2006

Goodpaster BH, Katsiaras A, Kelley DE: Enhanced fat oxidation through physical activity is associated with improvements in insulin sensitivity in obesity. *Diabetes* 52:2191–2197, 2003

Goulet ED, Melancon MO, Aubertin-Leheudre M, Dionne IJ: Aerobic training improves insulin sensitivity 72-120 h after the last exercise session in younger but not in older women. *Eur J Appl Physiol* 95:146–152, 2005a

Goulet ED, Melancon MO, Dionne IJ, Aubertin-Leheudre M: No sustained effect of aerobic or resistance training on insulin sensitivity in nonobese, healthy older women. *J Aging Phys Act* 13:314–326, 2005b

Grimm JJ, Ybarra J, Berne C, Muchnick S, Golay A: A new table for prevention of hypoglycaemia during physical activity in type 1 diabetic patients. *Diabetes Metab* 30:465–470, 2004

Harmer AR, Chisholm DJ, McKenna MJ, Hunter SK, Ruell PA, Naylor JM, Maxwell LJ, Flack JR: Sprint training increases muscle oxidative metabolism during high-intensity exercise in patients with type 1 diabetes. *Diabetes Care* 31:2097–2102, 2008

Hegde SV, Adhikari P, Kotian S, Pinto VJ, D'Souza S, D'Souza V: Effect of 3-month yoga on oxidative stress in type 2 diabetes with or without complications: a controlled clinical trial. *Diabetes Care* 34:2208–2210, 2011

Hernandez JM, Moccia T, Fluckey JD, Ulbrecht JS, Farrell PA: Fluid snacks to help persons with type 1 diabetes avoid late onset postexercise hypoglycemia. *Med Sci Sports Exerc* 32:904–910, 2000

Holten MK, Zacho M, Gaster M, Juel C, Wojtaszewski JF, Dela F: Strength training increases insulin-mediated glucose uptake, GLUT4 content, and insulin signaling in skeletal muscle in patients with type 2 diabetes. *Diabetes* 53:294–305, 2004

Houmard JA, Tanner CJ, Slentz CA, Duscha BD, McCartney JS, Kraus WE: Effect of the volume and intensity of exercise training on insulin sensitivity. *J Appl Physiol* 96:101–106, 2004

Ibanez J, Gorostiaga EM, Alonso AM, Forga L, Arguelles I, Larrion JL, Izquierdo M: Lower muscle strength gains in older men with type 2 diabetes after resistance training. *J Diabetes Complications* 22:112–118, 2008

Ibanez J, Izquierdo M, Arguelles I, Forga L, Larrion JL, Garcia-Unciti M, Idoate F, Gorostiaga EM: Twice-weekly progressive resistance training decreases abdominal fat and improves insulin sensitivity in older men with type 2 diabetes. *Diabetes Care* 28:662–667, 2005

Ishii T, Yamakita T, Sato T, Tanaka S, Fujii S: Resistance training improves insulin sensitivity in NIDDM subjects without altering maximal oxygen uptake. *Diabetes Care* 21:1353–1355, 1998

Jenni S, Oetliker C, Allemann S, Ith M, Tappy L, Wuerth S, Egger A, Boesch C, Schneiter P, Diem P, Christ E, Stettler C: Fuel metabolism during exercise in euglycaemia and hyperglycaemia in patients with type 1 diabetes mellitus—a prospective single-blinded randomised crossover trial. *Diabetologia* 51:1457–1465, 2008

Jensen J, Rustad PI, Kolnes AJ, Lai YC: The role of skeletal muscle glycogen breakdown for regulation of insulin sensitivity by exercise. *Front Physiol* 2:112, 2011

Jimenez C, Santiago M, Sitler M, Boden G, Homko C: Insulin-sensitivity response to a single bout of resistive exercise in type 1 diabetes mellitus. *J Sport Rehabil* 18:564–571, 2009

Juvenile Diabetes Research Foundation Continuous Glucose Monitoring Study Group, Fiallo-Scharer R, Cheng J, Beck RW, Buckingham BA, Chase HP, Kollman C, Laffel L, Lawrence JM, Mauras N, Tamborlane WV, Wilson DM, Wolpert H: Factors predictive of severe hypoglycemia in type 1 diabetes: analysis from the Juvenile Diabetes Research Foundation continuous glucose monitoring randomized dontrol trial dataset. *Diabetes Care* 34:586–590, 2011

Kapitza C, Hovelmann U, Nosek L, Kurth HJ, Essenpreis M, Heinemann L: Continuous glucose monitoring during exercise in patients with type 1 diabetes on continuous subcutaneous insulin infusion. *J Diabetes Sci Technol* 4:123–131, 2011

Kelley GA, Kelley KS: Effects of aerobic exercise on lipids and lipoproteins in adults with type 2 diabetes: a meta-analysis of randomized-controlled trials. *Public Health* 121:643–655, 2007

Kilbride L, Charlton J, Aitken G, Hill GW, Davison RC, McKnight JA: Managing blood glucose during and after exercise in type 1 diabetes: reproducibility of glucose response and a trial of a structured algorithm adjusting insulin and carbohydrate intake. *J Clin Nurs* 20:3423–3429, 2011

Kirwan JP, Solomon TP, Wojta DM, Staten MA, Holloszy JO: Effects of 7 days of exercise training on insulin sensitivity and responsiveness in type 2 diabetes mellitus. *Am J Physiol Endocrinol Metab* 297:E151–E156, 2009

Kishore P, Gabriely I, Cui MH, Di Vito J, Gajavelli S, Hwang JH, Shamoon H: Role of hepatic glycogen breakdown in defective counterregulation of hypoglycemia in intensively treated type 1 diabetes. *Diabetes* 55:659–666, 2006

Kwon HR, Han KA, Ku YH, Ahn HJ, Koo BK, Kim HC, Min KW: The effects of resistance training on muscle and body fat mass and muscle strength in type 2 diabetic women. *Korean Diabetes J* 34:101–110, 2010

Larsen JJ, Dela F, Madsbad S, Galbo H: The effect of intense exercise on postprandial glucose homeostasis in type II diabetic patients. *Diabetologia* 42:1282–1292, 1999

Lee DC, Sui X, Church TS, Lee IM, Blair SN: Associations of cardiorespiratory fitness and obesity with risks of impaired fasting glucose and type 2 diabetes in men. *Diabetes Care* 32:257–262, 2009

Lemaster JW, Mueller MJ, Reiber GE, Mehr DR, Madsen RW, Conn VS: Effect of weight-bearing activity on foot ulcer incidence in people with diabetic peripheral neuropathy: feet first randomized controlled trial. *Phys Ther* 88:1385–1398, 2008

Manetta J, Brun JF, Perez-Martin A, Callis A, Prefaut C, Mercier J: Fuel oxidation during exercise in middle-aged men: role of training and glucose disposal. *Med Sci Sports Exerc* 34:423–429, 2002

McMahon SK, Ferreira LD, Ratnam N, Davey RJ, Youngs LM, Davis EA, Fournier PA, Jones TW: Glucose requirements to maintain euglycemia after moderate-intensity afternoon exercise in adolescents with type 1 diabetes are increased in a biphasic manner. *J Clin Endocrinol Metab* 92:963–968, 2007

Mevorach M, Kaplan J, Chang CJ, Rossetti L, Shamoon H: Hormone-independent activation of EGP during hypoglycemia is absent in type 1 diabetes mellitus. *Am J Physiol Endocrinol Metab* 278:E421–E429, 2000

Mittendorfer B, Klein S: Physiological factors that regulate the use of endogenous fat and carbohydrate fuels during endurance exercise. *Nutr Res Rev* 16:97–108, 2003

Mittendorfer B, Klein S: Effect of aging on glucose and lipid metabolism during endurance exercise. *Int J Sport Nutr Exerc Metab* 11 (Suppl.):S86–S91, 2001

Nathan DM, Madnek SF, Delahanty L: Programming pre-exercise snacks to prevent post-exercise hypoglycemia in intensively treated insulin-dependent diabetics. *Ann Intern Med* 102:483–486, 1985

O'Donovan G, Kearney EM, Nevill AM, Woolf-May K, Bird SR: The effects of 24 weeks of moderate- or high-intensity exercise on insulin resistance. *Eur J Appl Physiol* 95:522–528, 2005

O'Gorman DJ, Karlsson HK, McQuaid S, Yousif O, Rahman Y, Gasparro D, Glund S, Chibalin AV, Zierath JR, Nolan JJ: Exercise training increases insulin-stimulated glucose disposal and GLUT4 (SLC2A4) protein content in patients with type 2 diabetes. *Diabetologia* 49:2983–2992, 2006

Petersen KF, Price TB, Bergeron R: Regulation of net hepatic glycogenolysis and gluconeogenesis during exercise: impact of type 1 diabetes. *J Clin Endocrinol Metab* 89:4656–4664, 2004

Ploug T, Galbo H, Richter EA: Increased muscle glucose uptake during contractions: no need for insulin. *Am J Physiol* 247:E726–E731, 1984

Poirier P, Mawhinney S, Grondin L, Tremblay A, Broderick T, Cleroux J, Catellier C, Tancrede G, Nadeau A: Prior meal enhances the plasma glucose lowering effect of exercise in type 2 diabetes. *Med Sci Sports Exerc* 33:1259–1264, 2001

Pruchnic R, Katsiaras A, He J, Kelley DE, Winters C, Goodpaster BH: Exercise training increases intramyocellular lipid and oxidative capacity in older adults. *Am J Physiol Endocrinol Metab* 287:E857–E862, 2004

Richerson S, Rosendale K: Does Tai Chi improve plantar sensory ability? A pilot study. *Diabetes Technol Ther* 9:276–286, 2007

Richter EA, Ploug T, Galbo H: Increased muscle glucose uptake after exercise. No need for insulin during exercise. *Diabetes* 34:1041–1048, 1985

Riddell MC, Milliken J: Preventing exercise-induced hypoglycemia in type 1 diabetes using real-time continuous glucose monitoring and a new carbohydrate intake algorithm: an observational field study. *Diabetes Technol Ther* 13:819–825, 2011

Rimbert V, Boirie Y, Bedu M, Hocquette JF, Ritz P, Morio B: Muscle fat oxidative capacity is not impaired by age but by physical inactivity: association with insulin sensitivity. *FASEB J* 18:737–739, 2004

Salem MA, Aboelasrar MA, Elbarbary NS, Elhilaly RA, Refaat YM: Is exercise a therapeutic tool for improvement of cardiovascular risk factors in adolescents with type 1 diabetes mellitus? A randomised controlled trial. *Diabetol Metab Syndr* 2:47, 2010

Sigal RJ, Kenny GP, Boulé NG, Wells GA, Prud'homme D, Fortier M, Reid RD, Tulloch H, Coyle D, Phillips P, Jennings A, Jaffey J: Effects of aerobic training, resistance training, or both on glycemic control in type 2 diabetes: a randomized trial. *Ann Intern Med* 147:357–369, 2007

Sigal RJ, Purdon C, Bilinski D, Vranic M, Halter JB, Marliss EB: Glucoregulation during and after intense exercise: effects of beta-blockade. *J Clin Endocrinol Metab* 78:359–366, 1994

Snowling NJ, Hopkins WG: Effects of different modes of exercise training on glucose control and risk factors for complications in type 2 diabetic patients: a meta-analysis. *Diabetes Care* 29:2518–2527, 2006

St John A, Davis WA, Price CP, Davis TM: The value of self-monitoring of blood glucose: a review of recent evidence. *J Diabetes Complications* 24:129–141, 2010

Taplin CE, Cobry E, Messer L, McFann K, Chase HP, Fiallo-Scharer R: Preventing post-exercise nocturnal hypoglycemia in children with type 1 diabetes. *J Pediatr* 157:784–788 e1, 2010

Tokmakidis SP, Zois CE, Volaklis KA, Kotsa K, Touvra AM: The effects of a combined strength and aerobic exercise program on glucose control and insulin action in women with type 2 diabetes. *Eur J Appl Physiol* 92:437–442, 2004

Wahren J, Ekberg K: Splanchnic regulation of glucose production. *Annu Rev Nutr* 27:329–345, 2007

Wang Y, Simar D, Fiatarone Singh MA: Adaptations to exercise training within skeletal muscle in adults with type 2 diabetes or impaired glucose tolerance: a systematic review. *Diabetes Metab Res Rev* 25:13–40, 2009

Watt MJ, Heigenhauser GJ, Dyck DJ, Spriet LL: Intramuscular triacylglycerol, glycogen and acetyl group metabolism during 4 h of moderate exercise in man. *J Physiol* 541:969–978, 2002

Willey KA, Singh MA: Battling insulin resistance in elderly obese people with type 2 diabetes: bring on the heavy weights. *Diabetes Care* 26:1580–1588, 2003

Winnick JJ, Sherman WM, Habash DL, Stout MB, Failla ML, Belury MA, Schuster DP: Short-term aerobic exercise training in obese humans with type 2 diabetes mellitus improves whole-body insulin sensitivity through gains in peripheral, not hepatic insulin sensitivity. *J Clin Endocrinol Metab* 93:771–778, 2008

Chapter 12
Hypoglycemia Treatment and Prevention

Iatrogenic hypoglycemia (i.e., blood glucose levels of <70 mg/dl or <3.9 mmol/L caused by diabetes treatment) is one of the chief barriers to optimal glycemic control in people with type 1 diabetes (T1D) (Realsen 2011). Severe hypoglycemia is a common contributor to morbidity and mortality and is a major source of fear for people with diabetes and their families. Fear of hypoglycemia and avoiding hypoglycemia are predominant limiting factors in achieving normal or near-normal blood glucose levels (ter Braak 2000, Brazeau 2008, Ross 2011).

In prediabetic individuals or those who have type 2 diabetes (T2D) controlled with diet and exercise alone, the risk of developing hypoglycemia related to physical activity is minimal, even though undertaking longer-duration and lower-intensity exercise generally reduces glycemic levels (Larsen 1999b, Houmard 2004, Evans 2005). In anyone who uses insulin or select insulin secretagogues (that stimulate the secretion of insulin)—whether someone with T1D, T2D, or gestational diabetes (GDM)—engaging in physical activity has the potential to significantly lower blood glucose levels both during and after exercise (MacDonald 1987, Ertl 2004, Admon 2005, Tsalikian 2005, Diabetes Research in Children Network Study Group 2006, Arutchelvam 2009, Delvecchio 2009, Chu 2011, West 2011). Since the absorption and release of injected insulin cannot always be effectively controlled or anticipated, the additive uptake of blood glucose by muscle contractions and excess insulin in anyone taking insulin may result in hypoglycemia.

Physical activity can cause hypoglycemia both during and following sessions, and its risk is affected by a number of factors, including exercise type, duration, and intensity; insulin and other medication doses; and food intake. Diabetic individuals at higher risk of developing hypoglycemia will benefit from gaining a better understanding of its causes, symptoms, treatments and learning preventative measures. Both severe hypoglycemia and hypoglycemia unawareness are prevalent obstacles in its detection, treatment, and prevention. Various strategies and technologies currently are used to help detect and prevent it, including improved patient education, frequent self-monitoring of blood glucose (SMBG), use of rapid-acting and basal insulin analogs, insulin pump therapy, exercise-related insulin adjustments, and continuous glucose monitors (Realsen 2011).

Case in Point: Diabetes Regimen Concerns for an Active Adolescent with T1D

SB is a 16-year-old girl who has had T1D since the age of 12 years. She is physically active in high school as a member of the cheerleading squad in the fall, swim and dive team during the winter season, and gymnastics in the spring. She has had a few problems of late controlling her blood glucose levels effectively, however, especially when she transitions from one season into the next, but she does not want to stop doing any of her sports at this point. For insulin delivery, she uses an insulin pump (filled with insulin aspart), and she also has a continuous glucose monitoring (CGM) device (DexCom) that she wears on occasion, only not much during the swim season because the sensors do not last long when she puts in many hours of training in the pool.

Resting Measurements

Height: 67 inches
Weight: 125 lb
Body mass index: 19.6 (normal)
Heart rate: 72 beats per minute (bpm)
Blood pressure: 115/65 mmHg

Fasting Labs

Plasma glucose: Variable (45–325 mg/dl, using an insulin pump)
A1C: 7.5%

Questions to Consider

1. What type of activities should SB focus on doing?
2. Does she need to make any diabetes regimen changes to maintain blood glucose control?
3. Are any precautions needed for SB when she exercises?

(Continued on page 197.)

SYMPTOMS OF HYPOGLYCEMIA

The blood glucose level at which symptomatic hypoglycemia occurs is relative (Diabetes Research in Children Network Study Group 2006, Graveling 2010). For example, rapid drops in blood glucose may occur with exercise and cause symptoms even when blood glucose is well above 70 mg/dl or may occur without generating noticeable symptoms. Sulfonylurea-treated individuals with T2D are more symptomatic at a higher glucose level than insulin-treated individuals, thereby protecting them from developing severe hypoglycemia, but hindering their attainment of glycemic goals (Choudhary 2009).

Common adrenergic symptoms (mostly related to the release of epinephrine and norepinephrine) associated with hypoglycemia include shakiness, heart palpitations, weakness, nervousness, anxiety, tingling sensations, and hunger. Neuroglycopenic symptoms (resulting from insufficient glucose for brain and nervous system function) may include headache, visual disturbances, mental dullness, confusion, amnesia, seizures, and coma. Typical symptoms of both types are grouped together in Table 12.1. Counterregulatory hormones released during exercise result in some of the same symptoms as hypoglycemia, which can make it hard to distinguish between the onset of hypoglycemia and normal physical sensations associated with physical activity like fatigue (Meinders 1988, Koivisto 1992, Galassetti 2003, Kishore 2006, Galbo 2007). Symptoms may also vary among people and are affected by type of physical activity, fitness levels, rate of blood glucose decline, and environmental conditions.

Table 12.1 Common Symptoms of Hypoglycemia

Buzzing in ears	Nausea
Cold or clammy skin	Nervousness
Dizziness or lightheadedness	Nightmares
Double or blurred vision	Poor physical coordination
Elevated pulse rate	Restlessness
Fatigue	Shakiness
Hand tremors	Slurred speech
Headache	Sweating
Inability to do basic math	Tingling of hands or tongue
Insomnia	Tiredness
Irritability	Visual spots
Mental confusion	Weakness

TREATMENT OF HYPOGLYCEMIA

All incidences of hypoglycemia should be treated with ingestion of rapidly absorbed carbohydrate sources, such as glucose tablets or gels, hard candy, regular soda, skim milk, cake icing, or juice (Taplin 2010, Chu 2011, Realsen 2011). Ingestion of 15–20 g of glucose is the preferred treatment for hypoglycemia when an individual is conscious, although any form of carbohydrate that contains glucose may be used (American Diabetes Association 2013). If blood glucose levels measured with SMBG 15 min after treatment are still too low, the treatment can be repeated, and a later meal or snack may be needed to prevent recurrence.

If an individual is unable to self-treat with glucose ingestion or is unconscious, treatment with glucagon injection by a family member, friend, or caregiver instructed on its administration is advised. Individuals at risk for severe hypoglycemia are advised to keep glucagon on hand at all times (American Diabetes Association 2013). If no glucagon is available, medical treatment should be initiated with a phone call to emergency services.

CAUSES OF HYPOGLYCEMIA

Hypoglycemia can result from a number of factors, including defective counter-regulatory mechanisms, acutely increased insulin mobilization and sensitivity, increased glucose utilization, and replenishment of glycogen stores. Any of these factors, or a combination of them, can result in hypoglycemia, with or without symptoms.

IMPAIRED COUNTERREGULATORY RESPONSES

When blood glucose levels fall below threshold glycemic levels, neuroendo-crine, autonomic nervous system, and metabolic glucose counterregulatory mechanisms are activated in nondiabetic individuals. These hypoglycemia prevention mechanisms can be blunted irreversibly by disease duration or by acute episodes of prior stress in individuals with T1D, and reduced or absent counterregulation results in a threefold increase in severe hypoglycemia when intensive glycemic control is implemented (Ertl 2004). Even in T2D, intensive insulin or oral combination therapy and antecedent hypoglycemia both blunt physiological defenses against subsequent hypoglycemia, resulting in counterregulatory failure and impaired hypoglycemia prevention in intensively treated individuals with subop-timal control (Davis 2009).

ACUTE AND DELAYED EFFECTS OF PHYSICAL ACTIVITY

In individuals whose diabetes is being controlled with lifestyle management alone, the risk of developing hypoglycemia during exercise is minimal, making stringent measures unnecessary to maintain blood glucose levels (Sigal 2004). Activities of longer duration and lower intensity generally cause a decline toward euglycemia, but not to the level of hypoglycemia (Braun 1995, Larsen 1999a, Houmard 2004, Evans 2005, Bajpeyi 2009). While very intense activities can cause transient elevations in blood glucose levels (Kreisman 2003; Szewieczek 2007, 2009), intermittent high-intensity exercise done immediately after breakfast in individuals with T2D treated with diet only reduces blood glucose levels and insulin secretion (Larsen 1999a).

In insulin or insulin secretagogue users, however, who frequently have to contend with the additive effects of insulin-independent glucose uptake stimulated by muscular contractions during exercise and insulin-dependent uptake, the inclusion of physical activity as part of the diabetes regimen can complicate its management and result in hypoglycemia, both during and following a bout of exercise (Zierath 1996, Kennedy 1999, Musi 2001, Rosenstock 2004). Although moderate- and high-intensity exercise have differing effects on acute blood glucose levels, participation in any physical activity can increase the risk of experiencing mild or severe hypoglycemia, with the latter being a potentially life-threatening condition, both during exercise and for up to 31 h during recovery (Guelfi 2007a). High-intensity exercises like repeated interval or resistance training result in significant depletion of muscle glycogen and heightened insulin sensitivity, and the accelerated uptake of blood glucose after exercise to restore muscle glycogen levels increases the risk for late-onset hypoglycemia (Larsen 1999b).

EFFECTS OF PRIOR EXERCISE AND HYPOGLYCEMIA

Much recent research has focused on determining the in vivo mechanisms responsible for causing the increased incidence of severe hypoglycemia in T1D. Even in adults without diabetes, prior episodes of short-duration moderate hypoglycemia can produce significant blunting of key neuroendocrine and metabolic counterregulatory responses to subsequent hypoglycemia, whereas longer-duration events have an even great impact (Davis 2000).

Both episodes of antecedent exercise and prior hypoglycemia are now known to blunt counterregulatory responses during subsequent exposures of hypoglycemia or exercise (Davis 2000; Galassetti 2001c; Sandoval 2004, 2006b; Bao 2009). Vicious cycles can be created in T1D when an episode of hypoglycemia or exercise can feed forward to downregulate neuroendocrine and autonomic nervous system responses to a subsequent episode of either stressor, thereby creating further hypoglycemia (Ertl 2004).

In individuals with T1D, antecedent hypoglycemia produces acute counterregulatory failure during a subsequent episode of prolonged moderate-intensity exercise, resulting in blunted neuroendocrine and autonomic nervous system responses and the inability of endogenous glucose production to match increased glucose requirements during exercise (Galassetti 2003). Antecedent physiologic increases in cortisol (equivalent to levels occurring during hypoglycemia) also appear to blunt neuroendocrine, autonomic nervous system, and metabolic counterregulatory responses during subsequent exercise and may play a role in the development of exercise-related counterregulatory failure in T1D (Bao 2009).

The severity of antecedent hypoglycemia also affects subsequent responses to moderate physical activity. After a day of euglycemia, normal counterregulatory responses to next-day exercise are evident in T1D. Conversely, when identical exercise was performed the day after 2-h episodes of hypoglycemia of increasing depth (70 mg/dl, 60 mg/dl, or 50 mg/dl, or 3.9 mmol/l, 3.3 mmol/l, or 2.8 mmol/l), a progressively greater blunting of glucagon, catecholamine, cortisol, glucose production, and lipolytic responses to exercise occurs. Acute counterregulatory failure during prolonged, moderate-intensity exercise may be induced in a dose-dependent fashion by differing depths of antecedent hypoglycemia starting at 70 mg/dl (3.9 mmol/l) in adults with T1D (Galassetti 2006).

Male–female differences. Sex differences in responses to hypoglycemia have also been noted. Heart rate and blood pressure responses to induced hypoglycemia on the day following a 90-min bout of moderate exercise are higher in men than in women, although men have a lesser glucagon, catecholamines, and muscle sympathetic nerve activity and metabolic response to next-day hypoglycemia (Galassetti 2001c). Along similar lines, engaging in morning exercise significantly impairs a T1D individual's ability to maintain euglycemia during later exercise of similar intensity and duration by modifying metabolic and neuroendocrine responses to subsequent exercise, but more so in men who exercise (Galassetti 2001b).

NOCTURNAL HYPOGLYCEMIA
FOLLOWING PHYSICAL ACTIVITY

A state of sleep has been demonstrated to impair counterregulatory hormone responses to hypoglycemia in individuals with and without diabetes (Jones 1998), thereby increasing the risk of undetected hypoglycemic episodes overnight following bouts of physical activity. For example, DirecNet (Diabetes Research in Children Network) studied the effects of 60 min of moderate aerobic exercise done in the late afternoon by 50 youth with T1D with unchanged basal and bolus insulin doses. Even on sedentary days, 28% of these youth experienced at least one nighttime glucose of ≤60 mg/dl, but the frequency of nocturnal hypoglycemia nearly doubled on nights following moderate afternoon exercise (Tsalikian 2005). In another study, youth undertaking 45 min of vigorous activity exhibited increased blood glucose uptake during and shortly following exercise, as well as again 7–11 h postexercise, suggesting a biphasic increase in glucose requirements and a pattern of early risk for hypoglycemia and a delayed risk for nocturnal hypoglycemia after afternoon exercise (McMahon 2007). Others have shown that 16% of individuals with T1D have a symptomatic hypoglycemic event, usually during sleep, 6–16 h after strenuous exercise (MacDonald 1987).

HYPOGLYCEMIA UNAWARENESS

Hypoglycemia unawareness is largely the result of reduced sympathetic neural responses to falling glucose levels. As discussed, either prior hypoglycemia or exercise can result in defective glucose counterregulation that reduces epinephrine and norepinephrine responses to subsequent hypoglycemia and increases the risk of hypoglycemia unawareness (Davis 2000; Sandoval 2004, 2006a, 2006b, 2007). Even young children and adolescents with T1D are prone to develop hypoglycemia-associated autonomic failure regardless of diabetes duration (Diabetes Research in Children Network Study Group 2009). Hypoglycemia unawareness is less common in individuals with T2D (Levy 1998), but it is frequently more severe when it does occur (Davis 2009). In people with T2D aged ≥65 years, unawareness of hypoglycemia that does not depend on altered neuroendocrine counterregulation may contribute to the increased probability of severe hypoglycemia frequently reported in such individuals (Bremer 2009). In their case, it is likely the result of some level of hypoglycemia unawareness combined with deteriorated cognitive function.

Thankfully, hypoglycemia unawareness is now known to be largely reversible by as little as 2–3 weeks of scrupulous avoidance of hypoglycemia even in individuals with autonomic neuropathy at higher risk and without full recovery of epinephrine responses (Fanelli 1997). Although people often experience diminished glucagon release in response to hypoglycemia after 2–10 years of diabetes, the most common reason that unawareness develops is frequent low blood glucose levels. Some diabetes educators also provide hypoglycemia unawareness training, which can teach individuals to become more cognizant of changes in blood glucose levels.

ASSESSMENT OF HYPOGLYCEMIA RISK

Fear of hypoglycemia is the strongest barrier to regular physical activity in adults and youth with T1D diabetes (Brazeau 2008), and they need to be informed and supported in hypoglycemia risk management (Galassetti 2001a, 2001b). Even though individuals with T2D not taking any diabetes medications have a low risk of exercise-induced hypoglycemia, this risk varies from person to person, based on medication regimen, food intake, and physical activity choices, and also is important to assess (Neumiller 2009). For example, individuals with a low carbohydrate intake are more likely to deplete muscle glycogen stores rapidly during exercise and increase their risk of exercise-associated hypoglycemia. Other variables that may contribute to or protect the individual from hypoglycemia include the usual timing of activity, type or duration of diabetes, and food preferences. The best risk indicator for hypoglycemia may be the individual's own personal experience. For example, the strongest predictor of severe hypoglycemia in one study on children and adults with T1D was having an episode of severe hypoglycemia during the 6 months before the study (Juvenile Diabetes Research Foundation Continuous Glucose Monitoring Study Group 2011). In another study, the presence of long-term complications of diabetes, a threshold for hypoglycemic symptoms that was <54 mg/dl (3 mmol/l), alcohol intake, and use of (nonselective) β-blockers were associated with severe hypoglycemia during the previous year (ter Braak 2000).

Physical activity is extremely beneficial and an essential health-management behavior for everyone with diabetes, but pathophysiology and treatment options may affect blood glucose differently in T1D, T2D, and GDM. As discussed, individuals with T1D for >10 years frequently experience a blunted release of counterregulatory hormones (e.g., glucagon and adrenaline) in response to hypoglycemia (Ertl 2004), and intensive diabetes management in individuals with T2D can have similar negative effects (Davis 2009). Furthermore, antecedent hypoglycemia and exercise can both inhibit the ability to maintain more stable blood glucose levels during subsequent same-day or next-day hypoglycemia or exercise (Davis 2000, 2009; Galassetti 2001a, 2001b, 2003, 2006; Ertl 2004). The severity of prior hypoglycemia also has an effect (Galassetti 2006) as does the sex of the individual with T1D (Galassetti 2001b, 2001c). Understanding these differences aids identification and avoidance of associated blood glucose concerns.

EFFECTS OF VARIOUS MEDICATIONS

A major factor affecting hypoglycemia risk is medication use. Pharmacological regimens for people with diabetes vary greatly, and although treatment of T1D always includes insulin in varying regimens, T2D treatment more frequently includes combinations of different classes of antihyperglycemic agents or insulin. Since hypoglycemia is one of the most common concerns associated with physical activity, individuals must understand whether this risk is present with or increased by the medication regimen in use (Table 12.2). The best indicator of risk is likely the individual's past experiences with physical activity while using a particular medication.

Insulin. The use of exogenous insulin poses the greatest risk for hypoglycemia because of its ability to lower blood glucose levels both at rest and during exercise. Although normally reduced naturally by the body during exercise, exogenous insulin—whether injected or pumped—cannot be regulated in parallel without pre-exercise planning. Administration of short- or rapid-acting human insulin or insulin analogs within 2–3 h before onset of physical activity increases hypoglycemia risk, particularly if doses are not reduced in anticipation. Hypoglycemia risk is higher with the use of certain basal insulins (Arutchelvam 2009). Basal insulin generally has a less acute impact on glycemic balance during most activities, but it may need to be adjusted before participation in long-duration events. Both insulin detemir and neutral protamine hagedorn (NPH, an intermediate-acting insulin) are associated with less hypoglycemia than insulin glargine in relatively well-controlled people with T1D during and after 30 min of moderate exercise undertaken 5 h after the last mealtime and basal insulin injection (Arutchelvam 2009). In individuals with T2D, use of once-weekly exenatide results in a lower hypoglycemia risk than insulin glargine (Diamant 2012).

Newer medication use. Whereas use of some of the older oral medications that act as insulin secretagogues (sulfonlyureas) increases risk of hypoglycemia during exer-

Table 12.2 Risk of Hypoglycemia with Use of Diabetes Medications

No Risk or Minimal Risk (Generic name: Brand name)	Higher Risk (Generic name: Brand name)
Acarbose: Precose	Glimepiride: Amaryl
Metformin and Combinations: Glucophage Janumet (metformin/sitagliptin)	Glipizide and Combinations: Glucotrol, Glucotrol XL MetaGlip (glipizide/metformin)
Miglitol: Glyset	Glyburide and Combinations: DiaBeta, Glynase, Micronase, Pres Tab Glucovance (glyburide/metformin)
Pioglitazone: Actos	
Rosiglitizone: Avandia	Nateglinide: Starlix
Exenatide: Byetta (daily), Bydureon (weekly)	Repaglinide: Prandin
Liraglutide: Victoza	Insulin: All types and delivery methods
Linagliptin: Tradjenta	
Sitagliptin: Januvia	
Saxagliptin: Onglyza	
Pramlintide: Symlin	

cise (Larsen 1999b), most of the newer prescribed medications (i.e., exenatide, sitagliptin, saxagliptin, liraglutide, and pramlintide) likely confer little or no such risk (Neumiller 2009, 2010). Exenatide has been shown to cause an exaggerated release of catecholamines and a rise in blood glucose during aerobic exercise in nondiabetic men (Khoo 2010). Pramlintide also has been found to have no effect on the counterregulatory hormonal, metabolic, and symptomatic responses to hypoglycemia, suggesting that its use may not affect responses to hypoglycemia (Amiel 2005). Anecdotal reports of hard-to-treat episodes of hypoglycemia related to physical activity when exenatide and pramlintide doses were taken close to initiation of activity have been noted (Colberg 2009).

DELAYED EFFECTS OF PHYSICAL ACTIVITY

Not all hypoglycemic episodes associated with physical activity occur during it or even immediately afterward. Low blood glucose levels may be biphasic for up to ≥24 h after the exercise is stopped (McMahon 2007). Delayed-onset hypoglycemia becomes a greater concern when carbohydrate stores (i.e., muscle and liver glycogen) are more fully depleted during an acute exercise session that is higher intensity or longer duration. In particular, repeated interval workouts or intense resistance training can result in substantial depletion of muscle glycogen, thereby increasing risk for hypoglycemia particularly if supplemental insulin or longer-lasting secretagogues are used (Larsen 1999b, Galbo 2007). Consuming moderate amounts of carbohydrates (5–30 g, depending on postexercise blood glucose levels) during and within 30–120 min after exhaustive, glycogen-depleting exercise will lower hypoglycemia risk and allow for more efficient and timely restoration of muscle glycogen (Cartee 1989, Garcia-Roves 2003, Jensen 2012).

EXERCISE FOLLOWING SEVERE HYPOGLYCEMIA

People with T1D are advised to avoid undertaking prolonged intensive exercise after a bout of severe hypoglycemia as metabolic events occurring in the 48 h period before the exercise can influence the risk of and responses to exercise-induced hypoglycemia. In a recent case report, a 27-year-old man with T1D suffered an episode of nocturnal hypoglycemia that provoked a seizure (Graveling 2010). Nevertheless, he ran a marathon race the following day during which he collapsed with severe hypoglycemia and another seizure. Subsequently, he developed severe myalgia, elevated plasma creatine kinase (rhabdomyolysis), and deranged liver function (hypoxic hepatitis), all of which persisted for several weeks. Thus, undertaking intense and prolonged physical exercise following severe hypoglycemia may increase the risk of severe hypoglycemia resulting from neuroglycopenia, seizures, and acute damage to skeletal muscle and organs.

Case in Point: Continued

SB has been experiencing hypoglycemia frequently both during and after workouts, particularly during the swim and dive training season, and she is getting discouraged about ever being able to prevent it. Recently, she experienced a bout of severe hypoglycemia overnight while she was sleeping that required her parents to give her an injection of glucagon, and she really wants to avoid ever having to go through that again.

Additional Questions to Consider

1. What type of insulin or dietary regimen changes does SB need to make to avoid hypoglycemia related to physical activity?
2. Does she need to change anything related to her workouts or training seasons to specifically prevent overnight low blood glucose levels?

(Continued on page 207.)

PREVENTION OF HYPOGLYCEMIA ASSOCIATED WITH PHYSICAL ACTIVITY

Participation in exercise can increase the risk of experiencing hypoglycemia, which if severe can be a potentially life-threatening condition, both during exercise and for up to 31 h of recovery (Guelfi 2007a). Fortunately, with the use of SMBG and CGM, hypoglycemia frequently can be prevented with adjustments to doses of exogenous insulin and food intake to maintain more normal blood glucose levels during and following physical activity. Some general rules for prevention of hypoglycemia are given in Table 12.3.

Table 12.3 General Rules for Prevention of Hypoglycemia

- Learn unique reactions to specific foods, activities, and stress by using frequent self-monitoring of blood glucose to establish individual patterns and trends.
- Test blood glucose levels more frequently when engaging in new activities, traveling, or doing anything outside the usual routines.
- If an individual takes rapid-acting analogs to cover food intake, he or she needs to learn how much is needed for a certain intake of carbohydrate to avoid taking excess insulin.
- Use the insulin-on-board rules: it takes at least 2 h for most rapid-acting insulin analogs to clear the bloodstream; if chasing a high with insulin, an individual should wait a while for it to exert its full effects before taking additional units.
- An individual should never skip meals or food for which he or she has already taken insulin or medications.
- If someone is not certain when food will arrive (such as in a restaurant), he or she should wait to take a full dose of insulin until the food has been delivered.
- Following blood glucose levels for several hours after exercise can help detect and prevent delayed-onset hypoglycemia.
- Consumption of a carbohydrate snack of at least 15 g within 1 h after completing strenuous or prolonged exercise can help restore muscle glycogen more rapidly, and adding some protein and fat may help prevent hypoglycemia.

SELF-MONITORING OF BLOOD GLUCOSE

Use of blood glucose monitors. Use of SMBG is critical to the prevention of hypoglycemia associated with participation in physical activity. Monitoring related to physical activity participation can provide important feedback that can be used to adjust insulin or carbohydrate to avoid hypoglycemia. Readings obtained at the start and end of activity are the most common to gather, but checking within 15–45 min before exercise, in the midst of exercise, or periodically for a few hours after its completion can better establish patterns and trends (Temple 1995). More frequent SMBG should be used to monitor for possible declines in blood glucose when hypoglycemia unawareness is present in T1D or T2D.

In adults with T2D, individuals treated with insulin used SMBG more frequency than those not treated with insulin, but increased frequency of testing was associated with a greater number of self-reported episodes of low blood glucose, even among patients not taking insulin or sulfonylureas (Farmer 2008). The exercise effects of lowering blood glucose after exercise may be compounded due to medication use (e.g., supplemental insulin or longer-lasting sulfonylureas) (Larsen 1999b). Thus, it is important even for individuals with T2D to regularly check their blood glucose levels after exercise to protect against hypoglycemic situations.

Continuous glucose monitors. Nowadays, many active individuals with T1D also have the option of using CGM systems to track glucose trends, although rapid changes in blood glucose (e.g., during exercise or after meals) are still better detected with fingerstick readings (Cauza 2005). Individuals with T1D exhibit wide variability in glucose profiles before, during, and after physical exercise (both moderate and intense), and use of CGM helps reduce the risk of acute, undetected metabolic deteriorations (Kapitza 2010). Its use in individuals with hypoglycemia unawareness is also advisable for quicker detection of decreases in blood glucose levels and better tracking of trends (Riddell 2009), although short-term use of the device with alarm reduces the incidence and duration of hypoglycemia to a limited extent because it tends to overestimate blood glucose levels in the low range (Davey 2010). Hypoglycemia measured with CGM over a 24-h span was found to be highly associated with severe hypoglycemia the following day, but the predictive value was very low (<5%). CGM also has demonstrated that participation in intermittent, high-intensity exercise is associated with delayed nocturnal hypoglycemia (Maran 2010). CGM use combined with a carbohydrate-intake algorithm has been shown to be effective in preventing hypoglycemia and maintaining euglycemia during exercise in adolescents with T1D participating in a 2-week-long sports camp, particularly if they ingested carbohydrate when trend arrows alerted them of a decrease in blood glucose levels (Riddell 2011).

ESTABLISHMENT OF BLOOD GLUCOSE GOALS

Once an individual understands if he or she is at greater risk for hypoglycemia, the next step is to establish reasonable blood glucose goals for physical activity, taking into account any complications or circumstances that may affect responses. For example, steroids and β-adrenergic blocking agents are two classes of prescription medications that need to be considered when predicting or interpreting an individual's blood glucose response to physical activity, given that steroids are likely to result in hyperglycemia, whereas β-blockers can cause hypoglycemia. Moreover, β-blockers also lower the heart rate response to submaximal and maximal exercise and may result in early fatigue. Complications like gastroparesis can make blood glucose levels erratic at times.

If individuals are unable to detect their hypoglycemic episodes or experience one or more episodes of severe hypoglycemia, they should raise their glycemic targets to strictly avoid further hypoglycemia for several weeks, in an attempt to at least partially reverse hypoglycemia unawareness and prevent future episodes (American Diabetes Association 2013). If more blood glucose readings cannot be performed because of finances or the individual's unwillingness to do so, other options should be explored to ensure that any risks, including those associated with hypoglycemia, are minimized during and after participation in physical activity. Modifications may include exercising after meals when blood glucose levels may be higher (in T2D, or in T1D with insulin modifications); engaging in more intense, shorter exercise sessions; exercising at times of day when glucose levels are highest; or exercising in the presence of trained helpers or peers who can help detect symptoms of hypoglycemia.

To keep blood glucose levels above the target goal before, during, and after physical activity (Table 12.4), most people will need to consider making adjustments to other aspects of the diabetes regimen as well. These adjustments are intended to either raise the amount of glucose available (with ingestion of carbohydrates) or normalize the amount of insulin circulating during physical activity using medication or exogenous insulin timing adjustments. Both strategies may result in the blood glucose level drifting higher for a short period of time, but this glucose will be used as a fuel for active muscles once the physical activity begins. While working out at higher exercise intensities, adjustments that lower blood glucose levels rather than raise them may be needed.

CARBOHYDRATE (AND OTHER FOOD) INTAKE

Recommended carbohydrate intake during physical activity. Rapidly absorbed carbohydrates remain the best treatment for acute hypoglycemia, and a greater intake is frequently used to prevent declines in blood glucose levels during exercise as

---

Table 12.4 General Blood Glucose Goals during Physical Activity

Individuals with any type of diabetes are advised to follow these guidelines to avoid hypoglycemia during physical activity:

- If using oral diabetes medications with possible hypoglycemia side effects, aim to keep blood glucose level >90 mg/dl (5 mmol/l) during all physical activities.
- If using insulin, a reasonable target is blood glucose levels >110 mg/dl (6.1 mmol/l).
- With other complications or circumstances that increase hypoglycemia risk, keep levels >120 mg/dl (6.7 mmol/l).
- If using oral agents that do not cause hypoglycemia or if not taking any medications for diabetes, no minimal blood glucose threshold is necessary.

well. Hypoglycemia treatment during exercise depends on its severity and whether the individual plans to continue exercising. Mild-to-moderate hypoglycemia generally can be treated with 15–20 g of simple carbohydrate (or ~0.3 grams of carbohydrate/kg body mass) using glucose tablets, soft drinks, dextrose gels, or juice (American Diabetes Association 2013). It is recommended that the carbohydrate source be low in fat to increase the rate of absorption. Individuals should check glucose levels again after 15 min and treat again if glucose levels have not elevated to a normal range. In situations in which exercise is to be continued, higher amounts of fast-acting carbohydrate should be consumed, along with a lower–glycemic index snack once euglycemia is attained. In the postexercise period, a meal containing complex carbohydrate should be consumed, with an appropriate (albeit

Table 12.5 General Carbohydrate Increases for Endurance Sports (Grams from Rapidly Absorbed Sources)

		Starting Blood Glucose Level in mg/dl (mmol/l)			
Duration	Intensity	<100 (<5.6)	100–150 (5.6–8.3)	150–200 (8.3–11.1)	>200 (>11.1)*
15 min	Low	0–5	None	None	None
	Moderate	5–10	0–10	0–5	None
	High	0–15	0–15	0–10	0–5
30 min	Low	5–10	0–10	None	None
	Moderate	10–25	10–20	5–15	0–10
	High	15–35	15–30	10–25	5–20
45 min	Low	5–15	5–10	0–5	None
	Moderate	15–35	10–30	5–20	0–10
	High	20–40	20–35	15–30	10–25
60 min	Low	10–15	10–15	5–10	0–5
	Moderate	20–50	15–40	10–30	5–15
	High	30–45	25–40	20–35	15–30
90 min	Low	15–20	10–20	5–15	0–10
	Moderate	30–60	25–50	20–35	10–20
	High	45–70	40–60	30–50	25–40
120 min	Low	15–30	15–25	10–20	5–15
	Moderate	40–80	35–70	30–50	15–30
	High	60–90	50–80	40–70	30–60
180 min	Low	30–45	25–40	20–30	10–20
	Moderate	60–120	50–100	40–80	25–45
	High	90–135	75–120	60–105	45–90

*For blood glucose levels well over 200 mg/dl or when ketones are present, an additional dose of rapid-acting insulin may be required to reduce these levels during an activity, and the recommended carbohydrate intake may be higher than actually needed.

Adapted from Colberg S: *Diabetic Athlete's Handbook.* Champaign, IL, Human Kinetics, p. 29, 2009.

likely reduced) amount of bolus insulin so that muscle and liver glycogen stores may be replenished.

General guidelines for carbohydrate intake during aerobic activities are included in Table 12.5, based on exercise duration, exercise intensity, and starting blood glucose levels. These guidelines assume that little or no reduction in insulin dosing is being done concurrently.

An older American Diabetes Association guideline (Sigal 2004) suggests that carbohydrate ingestion of at least 15 g is needed for pre-exercise blood glucose levels of <100 mg/dl (5.5 mmol/l), but only in people with T1D or those with T2D also using supplemental short- or rapid-acting insulin or select insulin secretagogues (Larsen 1999b, Rosenstock 2004). The exact quantity required to be ingested, however, depends on other variables such as when insulin peaks, exercise duration, and training status (Murillo 2010, Chu 2011). Recent research estimated that 40 g of a liquid glucose supplement may be necessary to prevent hypoglycemia during and after 1 h of late postprandial exercise in people using rapid-acting analog (lispro) in basal-bolus therapy (Dubé 2005). Even higher amounts of glucose may be needed if peak insulin levels are in circulation and hepatic glucose production is at a minimum. For example, one study in youth with T1D showed that matching glucose intake with endogenous carbohydrate utilization (~1 g carbohydrate/kg body mass/h) prevented blood glucose levels from dropping during 60 min of exercise (Kilbride 2011). Most exercise undertaken >2–3 h after the last administration of rapid-acting insulin likely will require only a small carbohydrate intake to prevent hypoglycemia, if any (Murillo 2010).

In individuals controlled with diet, exercise, or oral diabetic medications alone, hypoglycemia is uncommon, and extra carbohydrates are not generally required during exercise lasting <1 h. Intense, short-duration exercise also requires no or little carbohydrate intake due to a greater release of counterregulatory hormones that raise blood glucose (Kreisman 2003; Guelfi 2005a, 2005b, 2007b). As an alternative to ingesting extra carbohydrate, insulin pump users may reduce or eliminate their basal infusion of insulin during exercise (Mitchell 1988, Admon 2005, Delvecchio 2009).

Composition of snacks. Carbohydrates may not be the only food source that can be used to prevent exercise-induced hypoglycemia, however. In adolescents with T1D doing exercise 2 h after breakfast, drinking a pre-exercise carbohydrate beverage was the best method of preventing a large decrease in blood glucose levels during the activity. Although these results suggest that carbohydrate supplements before unplanned exercise are still most effective in preventing hypoglycemia, using a protein supplement was shown to have some benefit in limiting hypoglycemic events during and immediately after exercise (Dubé 2012).

As discussed in chapter 11, a pre-exercise snack containing carbohydrates that are more slowly absorbed and a small amount of protein may be a better match for exercise fuel requirements than a rapidly absorbed carbohydrate source used to treat hypoglycemia (Nathan 1985). During exercise, preventative snacks may include sports bars, gels, sports drinks, and snack bars (like Power bars), many of which contain some protein and fat with the carbohydrate (Colberg 2009). Postexercise snacks may contain a balance of carbohydrate, protein, and fat (such as found in whole milk, chocolate milk, ice cream, and yogurt), which are metabolized more slowly and keep blood glucose levels more stable over time than carbohydrate alone (Hernandez 2000).

Carbohydrate storage as glycogen. Participation in muscle glycogen–depleting activities increases risk of delayed-onset hypoglycemia. In such cases, the consumption of 5–30 g of carbohydrate during and within 30 min after exhaustive, glycogen-depleting exercise will lower hypoglycemia risk and allow for more efficient restoration of muscle glycogen (Burke 1999, Halse 2001, Stellingwerff 2007). To maximize muscle and liver glycogen stores before an event or training session, all that individuals with diabetes likely need is a single day in which they combine adequate rest, a carbohydrate-rich diet, and excellent blood glucose control throughout the day (Burke 1999, McKewen 1999, Bischof 2001). By way of example, T1D athletes who consumed a diet with 59% of calories from carbohydrates compared with only 50% over a 3-week period actually experienced a deterioration in glycemic control, increased insulin requirements, decreased muscle glycogen, and reduced performance, suggesting that consuming more carbohydrates is not effective when glycemic control worsens upon following more typical carbohydrate loading advice. Maintenance of more normal blood glucose levels has been shown to be the most effective strategy to optimize liver glycogen stores in T1D as well (Bischof 2001).

INSULIN DOSAGE ADJUSTMENTS

Although a typical response in individuals without diabetes, a decrease in circulating insulin levels during exercise does not naturally occur in everyone treated with exogenous insulin. If the level of circulating insulin from exogenous sources is elevated during activities, hypoglycemia is likely to occur (Yamakita 2002).

Bolus insulin adjustments. Doses of rapid-acting insulin analogs and regular (short-acting) human insulin taken within 2–3 h before prolonged, moderate-intensity exercise may need to be reduced by a minimum of 25%, particularly if individuals do not eat any additional food to compensate (West 2010, Bracken 2011). Newer synthetic insulin analogs (e.g., lispro, aspart, and glulisine) may result in reduced hypoglycemia overall and decreased frequency of both severe and nocturnal hypoglycemia because of their more rapid onset and shorter duration of action compared with regular human insulin (Yamakita 2002, Kitabchi 2012). All of the insulin reductions in Table 12.6 apply to the specific insulin peaking during exercise (usually the rapid-acting ones), although adjustments should be tailored to each individual's specific response to physical activity and goals and may require a combination of both additional carbohydrates and insulin adjustments.

For intense, near-maximal exercise, an actual increase in rapid-acting insulin (rather than a decrease) may be necessary to counter the glucose-raising effects of hormones released during exercise. Moreover, a lesser insulin reduction may be needed if exercise occurs >3 h following the last injection of rapid-acting insulin. Doses administered within 1 h after the activity may need to be decreased to prevent postexercise hypoglycemia.

Table 12.6 General Rapid- and Short-Acting Insulin Reductions for Aerobic Activities Done within 2 h of a Meal

Duration	Low-Intensity	Moderate-Intensity	High-Intensity
15 min	None	5–10%	0–15%
30 min	None	10–20%	10–30%
60 min	10–20%	20–40%	30–60%
120 min	20–40%	40–70%	60–90%

Adapted from Colberg S: *Diabetic Athlete's Handbook.* Champaign, IL, Human Kinetics, p. 32, 2009 (for a longer version, see chapter 14).

Insulin pump use. For insulin pump users, basal rate reductions during an activity can be done alone or along with reduced bolus amounts (Table 12.6) (Admon 2005, Diabetes Research in Children Network Study Group 2006, Maahs 2010). When using insulin pump therapy, individuals can adjust their basal rates and boluses based on the timing, duration, intensity, and type of activity performed. The degree of insulin reduction or carbohydrate supplementation depends on an individual's fitness level and the duration and intensity of the activity. Pump users have the following options to prevent hypoglycemia during periods of physical activity: reduce the basal infusion rates at various times (before, during, or after physical activity), temporarily suspend the pump, or consume extra carbohydrates (Admon 2005, Diabetes Research in Children Network Study Group 2006, Maahs 2010). One option may be preferred, but use of another strategy or a combination of these strategies may better serve to achieve the desired blood glucose results in different circumstances. The strategies included in Table 12.7 are applicable to both insulin injections and insulin pump use.

Basal insulin adjustments. If only longer-acting insulin (e.g., glargine or detemir) is injected, immediate glycemic declines during physical activity are not as likely. Reductions in basal insulins (not given via an insulin pump) may be needed only following especially prolonged activities or once a regular plan of physical activity is established that results in overall lower insulin requirements.

Table 12.7 Diabetes Regimen Changes to Prevent Hypoglycemia with Physical Activity

Consume additional carbohydrate if—
- Pre-exercise blood glucose is not sufficient to prevent hypoglycemia during activity
- Long-duration physical activity is undertaken
- Physical activity is unplanned or erratic
- Insulin adjustments are not possible or desired
- Oral hypoglycemic medications are used (but only for elevated hypoglycemia risk)
- Prevention of delayed-onset hypoglycemia is a goal

Injection sites. Insulin should always be injected into the subcutaneous fat layer, taking care to avoid intramuscular injections because contractions accelerate the absorption of insulin injected in muscle into the circulation (Saltiel-Berzin 2012). Changing a subcutaneous injection site to a part of the body not involved in the activity is not likely to be helpful in preventing hypoglycemia, however.

USE OF HIGH-INTENSITY EXERCISE

Short sprints. After moderate-intensity exercise, young individuals with T1D who engage in a 10-s maximal sprint prevent further declines in their blood glucose levels and reduce their risk of hypoglycemia (Bussau 2006). Accordingly, it may be advisable for them to sprint as hard as they can for ≥10 s to induce a greater release of glucose-raising hormones following activities, and possibly during them as well, to prevent hypoglycemia. Moreover, doing a 10-s sprint immediately before moderate-intensity exercise also prevents blood glucose levels from falling during early recovery (Bussau 2007). Blood glucose levels still fall similarly during 20 min of moderate exercise done following a pre-exercise sprint, but the larger increase in hormones elicited may keep them from limiting their postexercise declines.

Intermittent high-intensity exercise. Blood glucose responses to a combination of moderate- and high-intensity exercise, a pattern of physical activity referred to as intermittent high-intensity exercise (IHE), recently have been studied, given that this type of activity characterizes most team and field sports and spontaneous play in children. Fundamental differences have been noted in the metabolic responses to IHE compared with other types of exercise, requiring alternative recommendations for managing blood glucose levels during IHE (Guelfi 2007a).

For example, blood glucose levels decline less during IHE (simulated with interspersed 4-s sprints every 2 min during moderate activity) compared with moderate exercise during both exercise and recovery in individuals with T1D (Guelfi 2005a, Dubé 2013). This stabilization of blood glucose levels with IHE is related to elevated levels of lactate, catecholamines, and growth hormone during early recovery from exercise. In fact, the decline in blood glucose levels is lower with IHE compared with sustained moderate activity during both exercise and recovery (Guelfi 2005a), which likely is attributable to a greater hepatic glucose production during exercise and attenuated glucose uptake by muscles during exercise and early recovery (Guelfi 2007b). The latest study using intermittent sprints every 2 min during 60 min of moderate exercise reported that although ingesting 30 g of glucose pre-exercise was the most effective way to prevent hypoglycemia during the activity, using intermittent high-intensity sprints also may be a safe strategy in individuals with T1D on a combination of insulin glargine and insulin glulisine (Dubé 2013). IHE does not increase the risk of early postexercise hypoglycemia (Guelfi 2005b). It is, however, associated with delayed nocturnal hypoglycemia (likely the result of greater depletion of muscle glycogen during the activity) (Maran 2010).

In individuals with T2D, only one study has examined the glycemic effects of high-intensity training, with participants undertaking one session of training consisting of 10 bouts of cycling lasting 60 sec each done at ~90% of their maximal heart rate, interspersed with 1 min of rest (Gillen 2012). In that case, a total of 10 min of intense activity reduced time spent in hyperglycemia over the following 24-h period, as well as postprandial glucose peaks, compared with a sedentary control day, suggesting that harder exercise may be a more time-efficient means by which individuals with T2D can at least temporarily lower their blood glucose levels and improve their glycemic responses to food intake without necessarily resulting in hypoglycemia.

Resistance training. In active adults with T1D undertaking combined aerobic (45 min of moderate treadmill running) and resistance (three sets of eight repetitions on seven different exercises) training in one session, exercise order has been shown to affect glycemic responses (Yardley 2012). Engaging in resistance training before aerobic exercise rather than the reverse resulted in attenuated declines in blood glucose levels during exercise, less exercise-induced hypoglycemia, and reduced need for carbohydrate supplementation during exercise, and even the duration and severity of hypoglycemia monitored using CGM were reduced for the next 12 h when resistance training was undertaken first. To lower the risk of exercise-associated hypoglycemia, then, individuals who are willing and able to do combination training should undertake resistance work (or another high-intensity exercise) first before doing moderate aerobic exercise to lower their hypoglycemia risk. Conversely, anyone who usually experiences a hyperglycemic response to resistance exercise should consider engaging in aerobic exercise first when doing both during an exercise session.

STRATEGIES FOR DELAYED-ONSET HYPOGLYCEMIA

Many strategies can be used to prevent hypoglycemia during and following physical activity. Hypoglycemia may be delayed and can occur up to 12 h (or more) postexercise, even with reductions in insulin doses (Admon 2005), although inclusion of intermittent high-intensity work may lower the risk (Iscoe 2011). Blood glucose use is elevated during and shortly following 45 min of moderate aerobic exercise and again from 7–11 h afterward, suggesting a biphasic glycemic response to physical activity (McMahon 2007). The best strategy for hypoglycemia prevention is to use SMBG before, during, and after exercise and compensate with appropriate dietary or medication regimen changes. For instance, consumption of either whole milk or sports drinks before, during, and after 1 h of moderate exercise may lower the risk of late-onset hypoglycemia in T1D (Hernandez 2000). Similarly, the risk of nocturnal hypoglycemia following physical activity may be lowered with ingestion of a bedtime snack or reduced basal rates of insulin overnight (Kalergis 2003, Delvecchio 2009, Taplin 2010).

As far as bedtime snack composition is concerned, fat intake usually has no immediate impact on preventing hypoglycemia during an activity, and at least one study reported no difference between high- and low-fat bedtime snacks on the frequency of overnight hyperglycemia or hypoglycemia when carbohydrate content was held constant at 30 g (Wilson 2008). In T1D adults using lispro insulin before meals and NPH insulin at bedtime, the need for and composition of a bedtime snack depends on the blood glucose level, with no snack needed at levels

>180 mg/dl (10 mmol/l), any snack effective for 126–180 mg/dl (7–10 mmol/l), and a standard or protein snack recommended for <126 mg/dl (7 mmol/l) (Kalergis 2003). With that insulin regimen, only higher blood glucose levels at bedtime were protective against hypoglycemia but also were associated with a greater incidence of morning hyperglycemia.

Some studies have investigated the use of terbutaline, a β-2-adrenergic agonist, at bedtime, which appears to prevent most nocturnal hypoglycemia, but may cause morning hyperglycemia in individuals with T1D (Cooperberg 2008, Taplin 2010). For example, when T1D youth using insulin pumps were treated with oral terbutaline (2.5 mg) or a 20% reduction in basal insulin rates for 6 h overnight, terbutaline eliminated nocturnal hypoglycemia but resulted in significantly more hyperglycemia (Taplin 2010). The basal insulin rate reduction was also safe and effective in raising postexercise nocturnal blood glucose nadirs and preventing hypoglycemia.

Case in Point: Wrap-Up

To manage her blood glucose levels effectively, SB should use frequent SMBG (and CGM) to monitor her daily fluctuations—her monitoring tools will truly be her best defense against hypoglycemia and hyperglycemia. Using an insulin pump also allows her to make frequent temporary changes to basal insulin rates to compensate for varying amounts and intensities of physical training on a day-to-day basis.

Insulin Regimen Changes: To adjust to different types of training by season, SB needs to use SMBG and CGM to establish trends and patterns from differing types of training. For instance, she is likely to discover that longer-duration practices (regardless of which sport she is doing) will cause greater reductions in her blood glucose levels, both during the activity and for several hours afterward, necessitating pre-exercise reductions in bolus doses for meals and lower basal settings on her pump during and following workouts, along with overall reduced basal rates during the season. Cheerleading, diving, and gymnastics all incorporate elements of IHE training that can keep her blood glucose levels more stable during practices, but that raise her risk for delayed-onset and overnight hypoglycemia. Following harder training days, she should use her CGM to alert her to such decreases in glycemia and to keep basal insulin rates lower overnight. On easier workout days, she will likely need smaller insulin adjustments.

Dietary Changes: Frequent snacking will serve a twofold purpose for SB during her training season: first, it will help her take in enough carbohydrates to restore glycogen between workouts, along with protein and fat to keep her blood glucose levels more balanced for longer periods of time; and, second, snacking will allow her to replace the extra calories that she is expending while she is physically active. On all high-activity days, SB should plan on consuming a larger bedtime snack (with a balance of carbohydrate, protein, and fat), along with frequent, similarly balanced snacks during extended practices.

Sport-Specific Changes: Seasonal variations in sports and training make preventing hypoglycemia more of a challenge for SB, but she certainly has the tools that she needs to make it happen. For more aerobic sports and workouts (like swimming), SB needs to understand that her blood glucose levels are more likely to decrease during and immediately following practices, and she will likely need to make both food and insulin adjustments to compensate. For more intense training during cheerleading, diving, and gymnastics practices, she may need lesser adjustments to both, but she should be prepared to counter the effects of greater muscle glycogen use during IHE training that can cause late-onset hypoglycemia, particularly overnight.

Additional Concerns: Given that SB has already experienced at least one severe hypoglycemic episode related to prior physical activity participation, she should be advised to keep a glucagon pen with her at all times. In addition, her coaches, family members, and close friends should likely be educated on the symptoms of severe hypoglycemia and be trained on how to give SB a glucagon injection, if she is ever unable to self-treat her hypoglycemia.

Detection, treatment, and prevention of hypoglycemia related to physical activity participation are critical and frequently require SMBG and diabetic regimen changes. Given that fear of hypoglycemia is a significant barrier to exercise participation, diabetic exercisers need to better understand its causes and how to prevent it effectively. Individuals may choose to reduce doses of certain insulins before, during, and after activities to accomplish this, or they may increase their intake of carbohydrates and other foods. Making appropriate regimen changes to compensate for prior physical activity may also be effective in preventing delayed-onset and overnight hypoglycemia.

PROFESSIONAL PRACTICE PEARLS

- Hypoglycemia (blood glucose levels of <70 mg/dl) is one of the chief barriers to optimal glycemic control in people with T1D and some with T2D.
- The blood glucose level at which symptomatic hypoglycemia occurs is relative, and symptoms can vary by occurrence.
- All incidences of hypoglycemia should be treated with ingestion of rapidly absorbed carbohydrate sources, such as glucose tablets or gels, hard candy, or regular soda.
- If an individual is unable to self-treat with glucose ingestion or is unconscious, treatment with glucagon injection by a family member, friend, or caregiver is advised; individuals at risk for severe hypoglycemia should have glucagon available at all times.
- Hypoglycemia can result from a number of factors, including defective counterregulatory mechanisms, acutely increased insulin mobilization and sensitivity, increased glucose utilization, and replenishment of glycogen stores.
- Physical activity can cause hypoglycemia both during and following sessions, and its risk is affected by a number of factors, including exercise type,

duration, and intensity; insulin and other medication doses; and food intake.

- Not all hypoglycemic episodes associated with physical activity occur during it or even immediately afterward, with many occurring up to ≥24 h afterward.
- Episodes of both antecedent exercise and prior hypoglycemia can blunt counterregulatory responses and increase risk during subsequent exposures of hypoglycemia or exercise.
- SMBG allows for adjustments to doses of exogenous insulin and food intake to prevent hypoglycemia during and following physical activity.
- Intake of additional carbohydrates both during and following more prolonged physical activities may be used to prevent hypoglycemia in individuals with T1D and T2D.
- In insulin users, doses of short-duration insulin analogs taken before prolonged, moderate-intensity exercise may need to be reduced by a minimum of 20–30%.
- As an alternative or in addition to carbohydrate ingestion, insulin pump users may reduce or eliminate their basal infusion of insulin during exercise or adjust bolus doses.
- Reductions in basal insulin may be needed only following prolonged activities or after establishment of a regular plan of physical activity that lowers overall insulin needs.
- Both intermittent high-intensity training and sprinting may be effective means to maintain blood glucose levels during exercise, but delayed hypoglycemia is a greater risk.

REFERENCES

Admon G, Weinstein Y, Falk B, Weintrob N, Benzaquen H, Ofan R, Fayman G, Zigel L, Constantini N, Phillip M: Exercise with and without an insulin pump among children and adolescents with type 1 diabetes mellitus. *Pediatrics* 116:e348–e355, 2005

American Diabetes Association: Standards of medical care in diabetes—2013. *Diabetes Care* 36 (Suppl. 1):S11–S66, 2013

Amiel SA, Heller SR, Macdonald IA, Schwartz SL, Klaff LJ, Ruggles JA, Weyer C, Kolterman OG, Maggs DG: The effect of pramlintide on hormonal, metabolic or symptomatic responses to insulin-induced hypoglycaemia in patients with type 1 diabetes. *Diabetes Obes Metab* 7:504–516, 2005

Arutchelvam V, Heise T, Dellweg S, Elbroend B, Minns I, Home PD: Plasma glucose and hypoglycaemia following exercise in people with type 1 diabetes: a comparison of three basal insulins. *Diabet Med* 26:1027–1032, 2009

Bajpeyi S, Tanner CJ, Slentz CA, Duscha BD, McCartney JS, Hickner RC, Kraus WE, Houmard JA: Effect of exercise intensity and volume on persistence of insulin sensitivity during training cessation. *J Appl Physiol* 106:1079–1085, 2009

Bao S, Briscoe VJ, Tate DB, Davis SN: Effects of differing antecedent increases of plasma cortisol on counterregulatory responses during subsequent exercise in type 1 diabetes. *Diabetes* 58:2100–2108, 2009

Bischof MG, Krssak M, Krebs M, Bernroider E, Stingl H, Waldhausl W, Roden M: Effects of short-term improvement of insulin treatment and glycemia on hepatic glycogen metabolism in type 1 diabetes. *Diabetes* 50:392–398, 2001

Bracken RM, West DJ, Stephens JW, Kilduff LP, Luzio S, Bain SC: Impact of pre-exercise rapid-acting insulin reductions on ketogenesis following running in type 1 diabetes. *Diabet Med* 28:218–222, 2011

Braun B, Zimmermann MB, Kretchmer N: Effects of exercise intensity on insulin sensitivity in women with non-insulin-dependent diabetes mellitus. *J Appl Physiol* 78:300–306, 1995

Brazeau AS, Rabasa-Lhoret R, Strychar I, Mircescu H: Barriers to physical activity among patients with type 1 diabetes. *Diabetes Care* 31:2108–2109, 2008

Bremer JP, Jauch-Chara K, Hallschmid M, Schmid S, Schultes B: Hypoglycemia unawareness in older compared with middle-aged patients with type 2 diabetes. *Diabetes Care* 32:1513–1517, 2009

Burke LM, Hawley JA: Carbohydrate and exercise. *Curr Opin Clin Nutr Metab Care* 2:515–520, 1999

Bussau VA, Ferreira LD, Jones TW, Fournier PA: The 10-s maximal sprint: a novel approach to counter an exercise-mediated fall in glycemia in individuals with type 1 diabetes. *Diabetes Care* 29:601–606, 2006

Bussau VA, Ferreira LD, Jones TW, Fournier PA: A 10-s sprint performed prior to moderate-intensity exercise prevents early post-exercise fall in glycaemia in individuals with type 1 diabetes. *Diabetologia* 50:1815–1818, 2007

Cartee GD, Young DA, Sleeper MD, Zierath J, Wallberg-Henriksson H, Holloszy JO: Prolonged increase in insulin-stimulated glucose transport in muscle after exercise. *Am J Physiol* 256:E494–E499, 1989

Cauza E, Hanusch-Enserer U, Strasser B, Kostner K, Dunky A, Haber P: Strength and endurance training lead to different post exercise glucose profiles in diabetic participants using a continuous subcutaneous glucose monitoring system. *Eur J Clin Invest* 35:745–751, 2005

Choudhary P, Lonnen K, Emery CJ, MacDonald IA, MacLeod KM, Amiel SA, Heller SR: Comparing hormonal and symptomatic responses to experimental hypoglycaemia in insulin- and sulphonylurea-treated type 2 diabetes. *Diabet Med* 26:665–672, 2009

Chu L, Hamilton J, Riddell MC: Clinical management of the physically active patient with type 1 diabetes. *Phys Sportsmed* 39:64–77, 2011

Colberg SR: *Diabetic Athlete's Handbook.* Champaign, IL, Human Kinetics, 2009

Cooperberg BA, Breckenridge SM, Arbelaez AM, Cryer PE: Terbutaline and the prevention of nocturnal hypoglycemia in type 1 diabetes. *Diabetes Care* 31:2271–2272, 2008

Davey RJ, Jones TW, Fournier PA: Effect of short-term use of a continuous glucose monitoring system with a real-time glucose display and a low glucose alarm on incidence and duration of hypoglycemia in a home setting in type 1 diabetes mellitus. *J Diabetes Sci Technol* 4:1457–1464, 2010

Davis SN, Mann S, Briscoe VJ, Ertl AC, Tate DB: Effects of intensive therapy and antecedent hypoglycemia on counterregulatory responses to hypoglycemia in type 2 diabetes. *Diabetes* 58:701–709, 2009

Davis SN, Mann S, Galassetti P, Neill RA, Tate D, Ertl AC, Costa F: Effects of differing durations of antecedent hypoglycemia on counterregulatory responses to subsequent hypoglycemia in normal humans. *Diabetes* 49:1897–1903, 2000

Delvecchio M, Zecchino C, Salzano G, Faienza MF, Cavallo L, De Luca F, Lombardo F: Effects of moderate-severe exercise on blood glucose in type 1 diabetic adolescents treated with insulin pump or glargine insulin. *J Endocrinol Invest* 32:519–524, 2009

Diabetes Research in Children Network Study Group, Tsalikian E, Kollman C, Tamborlane WB, Beck RW, Fiallo-Scharer R, Fox L, Janz KF, Ruedy KJ, Wilson D, Xing D, Weinzimer SA: Prevention of hypoglycemia during exercise in children with type 1 diabetes by suspending basal insulin. *Diabetes Care* 29:2200–2204, 2006

Diabetes Research in Children Network Study Group, Tsalikian E, Tamborlane W, Xing D, Becker DM, Mauras N, Fiallo-Scharer R, Buckingham B, Weinzimer S, Steffes M, Singh R, Beck R, Ruedy K, Kollman C: Blunted counterregulatory hormone responses to hypoglycemia in young children and adolescents with well-controlled type 1 diabetes. *Diabetes Care* 32:1954–1959, 2009

Diamant M, Van Gaal L, Stranks S, Guerci B, MacConell L, Haber H, Scism-Bacon J, Trautmann M: Safety and efficacy of once-weekly exenatide compared with insulin glargine titrated to target in patients with type 2 diabetes over 84 weeks. *Diabetes Care* 35:683–689, 2012

Dubé MC, Lavoie C, Weisnagel SJ: Glucose or intermittent high-intensity exercise in glargine/glulisine users with T1DM. *Med Sci Sports Exerc* 45:3–7, 2013

Dubé MC, Lavoie C, Galibois I, Weisnagel SJ: Nutritional strategies to prevent hypoglycemia at exercise in diabetic adolescents. *Med Sci Sports Exerc* 44:1427–1432, 2012

Dubé MC, Weisnagel SJ, Prud'homme D, Lavoie C: Exercise and newer insulins: how much glucose supplement to avoid hypoglycemia? *Med Sci Sports Exerc* 37:1276–1282, 2005

Ertl AC, Davis SN: Evidence for a vicious cycle of exercise and hypoglycemia in type 1 diabetes mellitus. *Diabetes Metab Res Rev* 20:124–130, 2004

Evans EM, Racette SB, Peterson LR, Villareal DT, Greiwe JS, Holloszy JO: Aerobic power and insulin action improve in response to endurance exercise training in healthy 77-87 yr olds. *J Appl Physiol* 98:40–45, 2005

Fanelli C, Pampanelli S, Lalli C, Del Sindaco P, Ciofetta M, Lepore M, Porcellati F, Bottini P, Di Vincenzo A, Brunetti P, Bolli GB: Long-term intensive therapy of IDDM patients with clinically overt autonomic neuropathy: effects on hypoglycemia awareness and counterregulation. *Diabetes* 46:1172–1181, 1997

Farmer A, Balman E, Gadsby R, Moffatt J, Cradock S, McEwen L, Jameson K: Frequency of self-monitoring of blood glucose in patients with type 2 diabetes: association with hypoglycaemic events. *Curr Med Res Opin* 24:3097–3104, 2008

Galassetti P, Tate D, Neill RA, Richardson A, Leu SY, Davis SN: Effect of differing antecedent hypoglycemia on counterregulatory responses to exercise in type 1 diabetes. *Am J Physiol Endocrinol Metab* 290:E1109–E1117, 2006

Galassetti P, Tate D, Neill RA, Morrey S, Wasserman DH, Davis SN: Effect of antecedent hypoglycemia on counterregulatory responses to subsequent euglycemic exercise in type 1 diabetes. *Diabetes* 52:1761–1769, 2003

Galassetti P, Mann S, Tate D, Neill RA, Costa F, Wasserman DH, Davis SN: Effects of antecedent prolonged exercise on subsequent counterregulatory responses to hypoglycemia. *Am J Physiol Endocrinol Metab* 280:E908–E917, 2001a

Galassetti P, Mann S, Tate D, Neill RA, Wasserman DH, Davis SN: Effect of morning exercise on counterregulatory responses to subsequent, afternoon exercise. *J Appl Physiol* 91:91–99, 2001b

Galassetti P, Neill AR, Tate D, Ertl AC, Wasserman DH, Davis SN: Sexual dimorphism in counterregulatory responses to hypoglycemia after antecedent exercise. *J Clin Endocrinol Metab* 86:3516–3524, 2001c

Galbo H, Tobin L, van Loon LJ: Responses to acute exercise in type 2 diabetes, with an emphasis on metabolism and interaction with oral hypoglycemic agents and food intake. *Appl Physiol Nutr Metab* 32:567–575, 2007

Garcia-Roves PM, Han DH, Song Z, Jones TE, Hucker KA, Holloszy JO: Prevention of glycogen supercompensation prolongs the increase in muscle GLUT4 after exercise. *Am J Physiol Endocrinol Metab* 285:E729–E736, 2003

Gillen JB, Little JP, Punthakee Z, Tarnopolsky MA, Riddell MC, Gibala MJ: Acute high-intensity interval exercise reduces the postprandial glucose response and prevalence of hyperglycaemia in patients with type 2 diabetes. *Diabetes Obes Metab* 14: 575–577, 2012

Graveling AJ, Frier BM: Risks of marathon running and hypoglycaemia in type 1 diabetes. *Diabet Med* 27:585–588, 2010

Guelfi KJ, Jones TW, Fournier PA: New insights into managing the risk of hypo-glycaemia associated with intermittent high-intensity exercise in individuals with type 1 diabetes mellitus: implications for existing guidelines. *Sports Med* 37:937–946, 2007a

Guelfi KJ, Ratnam N, Smythe GA, Jones TW, Fournier PA: Effect of intermittent high-intensity compared with continuous moderate exercise on glucose pro-duction and utilization in individuals with type 1 diabetes. *Am J Physiol Endo-crinol Metab* 292 (3):E865–E870, 2007b

Guelfi KJ, Jones TW, Fournier PA: The decline in blood glucose levels is less with intermittent high-intensity compared with moderate exercise in individuals with type 1 diabetes. *Diabetes Care* 28:1289–1294, 2005a

Guelfi KJ, Jones TW, Fournier PA: Intermittent high-intensity exercise does not increase the risk of early postexercise hypoglycemia in individuals with type 1 diabetes. *Diabetes Care* 28:416–418, 2005b

Halse R, Bonavaud SM, Armstrong JL, McCormack JG, Yeaman SJ: Control of glycogen synthesis by glucose, glycogen, and insulin in cultured human mus-cle cells. *Diabetes* 50:720–726, 2001

Hernandez JM, Moccia T, Fluckey JD, Ulbrecht JS, Farrell PA: Fluid snacks to help persons with type 1 diabetes avoid late onset postexercise hypoglycemia. *Med Sci Sports Exerc* 32:904–910, 2000

Houmard JA, Tanner CJ, Slentz CA, Duscha BD, McCartney JS, Kraus WE: Effect of the volume and intensity of exercise training on insulin sensitivity. *J Appl Physiol* 96:101–106, 2004

Iscoe KE, Riddell MC: Continuous moderate-intensity exercise with or without intermittent high-intensity work: effects on acute and late glycaemia in ath-letes with type 1 diabetes mellitus. *Diabet Med* 28:824–832, 2011

Jensen J, Rustad PI, Kolnes AJ, Lai YC: The role of skeletal muscle glycogen breakdown for regulation of insulin sensitivity by exercise. *Front Physiol* 2:112, 2012

Jones TW, Porter P, Sherwin RS, Davis EA, O'Leary P, Frazer F, Byrne G, Stick S, Tamborlane WV: Decreased epinephrine responses to hypoglycemia during sleep. *N Engl J Med* 338:1657–1662, 1998

Juvenile Diabetes Research Foundation Continuous Glucose Monitoring Study Group, Fiallo-Scharer R, Cheng J, Beck RW, Buckingham BA, Chase HP, Kollman C, Laffel L, Lawrence JM, Mauras N, Tamborlane WV, Wilson DM, Wolpert H: Factors predictive of severe hypoglycemia in type 1 diabetes: anal-ysis from the Juvenile Diabetes Research Foundation continuous glucose monitoring randomized control trial dataset. *Diabetes Care* 34:586–590, 2011

Kalergis M, Schiffrin A, Gougeon R, Jones PJ, Yale JF: Impact of bedtime snack composition on prevention of nocturnal hypoglycemia in adults with type 1 diabetes undergoing intensive insulin management using lispro insulin before meals: a randomized, placebo-controlled, crossover trial. *Diabetes Care* 26:9–15, 2003

Kapitza C, Hovelmann U, Nosek L, Kurth HJ, Essenpreis M, Heinemann L: Continuous glucose monitoring during exercise in patients with type 1 diabetes on continuous subcutaneous insulin infusion. *J Diabetes Sci Technol* 4:123–131, 2010

Kennedy JW, Hirshman MF, Gervino EV, Ocel JV, Forse RA, Hoenig SJ, Aronson D, Goodyear LJ, Horton ES: Acute exercise induces GLUT4 translocation in skeletal muscle of normal human subjects and subjects with type 2 diabetes. *Diabetes* 48:1192–1197, 1999

Khoo EY, Wallis J, Tsintzas K, Macdonald IA, Mansell P: Effects of exenatide on circulating glucose, insulin, glucagon, cortisol and catecholamines in healthy volunteers during exercise. *Diabetologia* 53:139–143, 2010

Kilbride L, Charlton J, Aitken G, Hill GW, Davison RC, McKnight JA: Managing blood glucose during and after exercise in type 1 diabetes: reproducibility of glucose response and a trial of a structured algorithm adjusting insulin and carbohydrate intake. *J Clin Nurs* 20:3423–3429, 2011

Kishore P, Gabriely I, Cui MH, Di Vito J, Gajavelli S, Hwang JH, Shamoon H: Role of hepatic glycogen breakdown in defective counterregulation of hypoglycemia in intensively treated type 1 diabetes. *Diabetes* 55:659–666, 2006

Kitabchi AE, Gosmanov AR: Safety of rapid-acting insulin analogs versus regular human insulin. *Am J Med Sci* 344:136–141, 2012

Koivisto VA, Sane T, Fyhrquist F, Pelkonen R: Fuel and fluid homeostasis during long-term exercise in healthy subjects and type I diabetic patients. *Diabetes Care* 15:1736–1741, 1992

Kreisman SH, Halter JB, Vranic M, Marliss EB: Combined infusion of epinephrine and norepinephrine during moderate exercise reproduces the glucoregulatory response of intense exercise. *Diabetes* 52:1347–1354, 2003

Larsen JJ, Dela F, Madsbad S, Galbo H: The effect of intense exercise on postprandial glucose homeostasis in type II diabetic patients. *Diabetologia* 42:1282–1292, 1999a

Larsen JJ, Dela F, Madsbad S, Vibe-Petersen J, Galbo H: Interaction of sulfonylureas and exercise on glucose homeostasis in type 2 diabetic patients. *Diabetes Care* 22:1647–1654, 1999b

Levy CJ, Kinsley BT, Bajaj M, Simonson DC: Effect of glycemic control on glucose counterregulation during hypoglycemia in NIDDM. *Diabetes Care* 21:1330–1338, 1998

Maahs DM, Horton LA, Chase HP: The use of insulin pumps in youth with type 1 diabetes. *Diabetes Technol Ther* 12 (Suppl. 1):S59–S65, 2010

MacDonald MJ: Postexercise late-onset hypoglycemia in insulin-dependent diabetic patients. *Diabetes Care* 10:584–588, 1987

Maran A, Pavan P, Bonsembiante B, Brugin E, Ermolao A, Avogaro A, Zaccaria M: Continuous glucose monitoring reveals delayed nocturnal hypoglycemia after intermittent high-intensity exercise in nontrained patients with type 1 diabetes. *Diabetes Technol Ther* 12:763–768, 2010

McKewen MW, Rehrer NJ, Cox C, Mann J: Glycaemic control, muscle glycogen and exercise performance in IDDM athletes on diets of varying carbohydrate content. *Int J Sports Med* 20:349–353, 1999

McMahon SK, Ferreira LD, Ratnam N, Davey RJ, Youngs LM, Davis EA, Fournier PA, Jones TW: Glucose requirements to maintain euglycemia after moderate-intensity afternoon exercise in adolescents with type 1 diabetes are increased in a biphasic manner. *J Clin Endocrinol Metab* 92:963–968, 2007

Meinders AE, Willekens FL, Heere LP: Metabolic and hormonal changes in IDDM during long-distance run. *Diabetes Care* 11:1–7, 1988

Mitchell TH, Abraham G, Schiffrin A, Leiter LA, Marliss EB: Hyperglycemia after intense exercise in IDDM subjects during continuous subcutaneous insulin infusion. *Diabetes Care* 11:311–317, 1988

Murillo S, Brugnara L, Novials A: One year follow-up in a group of half-marathon runners with type-1 diabetes treated with insulin analogues. *J Sports Med Phys Fitness* 50:506–510, 2010

Musi N, Fujii N, Hirshman MF, Ekberg I, Froberg S, Ljungqvist O, Thorell A, Goodyear LJ: AMP-activated protein kinase (AMPK) is activated in muscle of subjects with type 2 diabetes during exercise. *Diabetes* 50:921–927, 2001

Nathan DM, Madnek SF, Delahanty L: Programming pre-exercise snacks to prevent post-exercise hypoglycemia in intensively treated insulin-dependent diabetics. *Ann Intern Med* 102:483–486, 1985

Neumiller JJ, Setter SM: Pharmacologic management of the older patient with type 2 diabetes mellitus. *Am J Geriatr Pharmacother* 7:324–342, 2009

Neumiller JJ, Wood L, Campbell RK: Dipeptidyl peptidase-4 inhibitors for the treatment of type 2 diabetes mellitus. *Pharmacotherapy* 30:463–484, 2010

Realsen JM, Chase HP: Recent advances in the prevention of hypoglycemia in type 1 diabetes. *Diabetes Technol Ther* 13:1177–1186, 2011

Riddell MC, Milliken J: Preventing exercise-induced hypoglycemia in type 1 diabetes using real-time continuous glucose monitoring and a new carbohydrate intake algorithm: an observational field study. *Diabetes Technol Ther* 13:819–825, 2011

Riddell M, Perkins BA: Exercise and glucose metabolism in persons with diabetes mellitus: perspectives on the role for continuous glucose monitoring. *J Diabetes Sci Technol* 3:914–923, 2009

Rosenstock J, Hassman DR, Madder RD, Brazinsky SA, Farrell J, Khutoryansky N, Hale PM, Repaglinide Versus Nateglinide Comparison Study Group: Repaglinide versus nateglinide monotherapy: a randomized, multicenter study. *Diabetes Care* 27:1265–1270, 2004

Ross SA, Tildesley HD, Ashkenas J: Barriers to effective insulin treatment: the persistence of poor glycemic control in type 2 diabetes. *Curr Med Res Opin* 27 (Suppl. 3):13–20, 2011

Sandoval DA, Gong B, Davis SN: Antecedent short-term central nervous system administration of estrogen and progesterone alters counterregulatory responses to hypoglycemia in conscious male rats. *Am J Physiol Endocrinol Metab* 293:E1511–E1516, 2007

Sandoval DA, Davis SN: Metabolic consequences of exercise-associated autonomic failure. *Exercise & Sport Sciences Reviews* 34:72–76, 2006a

Sandoval DA, Guy DL, Richardson MA, Ertl AC, Davis SN: Acute, same-day effects of antecedent exercise on counterregulatory responses to subsequent hypoglycemia in type 1 diabetes mellitus. *Am J Physiol Endocrinol Metab* 290:E1331–E1318, 2006b

Sandoval DA, Guy DL, Richardson MA, Ertl AC, Davis SN: Effects of low and moderate antecedent exercise on counterregulatory responses to subsequent hypoglycemia in type 1 diabetes. *Diabetes* 53:1798–1806, 2004

Saltiel-Berzin R, Cypress M, Gibney M: Translating the research in insulin injection technique: implications for practice. *Diabetes Educ* 38:635–643, 2012

Sigal RJ, Kenny GP, Wasserman DH, Castaneda-Sceppa C: Physical activity/exercise and type 2 diabetes. *Diabetes Care* 27:2518–2539, 2004

Stellingwerff T, Boon H, Gijsen AP, Stegen JH, Kuipers H, van Loon LJ: Carbohydrate supplementation during prolonged cycling exercise spares muscle glycogen but does not affect intramyocellular lipid use. *Pflugers Arch* 454:635–647, 2007

Szewieczek J, Dulawa J, Strzalkowska D, Batko-Szwaczka A, Hornik B: Normal insulin response to short-term intense exercise is abolished in type 2 diabetic patients treated with gliclazide. *J Diabetes Complications* 23:380–386, 2009

Szewieczek J, Dulawa J, Strzalkowska D, Hornik B, Kawecki G: Impact of the short-term, intense exercise on postprandial glycemia in type 2 diabetic patients treated with gliclazide. *J Diabetes Complications* 21:101–107, 2007

Taplin CE, Cobry E, Messer L, McFann K, Chase HP, Fiallo-Scharer R: Preventing post-exercise nocturnal hypoglycemia in children with type 1 diabetes. *J Pediatr* 157:784–788 e1, 2010

Temple MY, Bar-Or O, Riddell MC: The reliability and repeatability of the blood glucose response to prolonged exercise in adolescent boys with IDDM. *Diabetes Care* 18:326–332, 1995

ter Braak EW, Appelman AM, van de Laak M, Stolk RP, van Haeften TW, Erkelens DW: Clinical characteristics of type 1 diabetic patients with and without severe hypoglycemia. *Diabetes Care* 23:1467–1471, 2000

Tsalikian E, Mauras N, Beck RW, Tamborlane WV, Janz KF, Chase HP, Wysocki T, Weinzimer SA, Buckingham BA, Kollman C, Xing D, Ruedy KJ, Diabetes Research In Children Network Group DirecNet Study: Impact of exercise on overnight glycemic control in children with type 1 diabetes mellitus. *J Pediatr* 147:528–534, 2005

West DJ, Stephens JW, Bain SC, Kilduff LP, Luzio S, Still R, Bracken RM: A combined insulin reduction and carbohydrate feeding strategy 30 min before running best preserves blood glucose concentration after exercise through improved fuel oxidation in type 1 diabetes mellitus. *J Sports Sci* 29:279–289, 2011

West DJ, Morton RD, Bain SC, Stephens JW, Bracken RM: Blood glucose responses to reductions in pre-exercise rapid-acting insulin for 24 h after running in individuals with type 1 diabetes. *J Sports Sci* 28:781-788, 2010

Wilson D, Chase HP, Kollman C, Xing D, Caswell K, Tansey M, Fox L, Weinzimer S, Beck R, Ruedy K, Tamborlane W, Diabetes Research in Children Network Study Group: Low-fat vs. high-fat bedtime snacks in children and adolescents with type 1 diabetes. *Pediatr Diabetes* 9:320–325, 2008

Yamakita T, Ishii T, Yamagami K, Yamamoto T, Miyamoto M, Hosoi M, Yoshioka K, Sato T, Onishi S, Tanaka S, Fujii S: Glycemic response during exercise after administration of insulin lispro compared with that after administration of regular human insulin. *Diabetes Res Clin Pract* 57:17–22, 2002

Yardley JE, Kenny GP, Perkins BA, Riddell MC, Malcolm J, Boulay P, Khandwala F, Sigal RJ: Effects of performing resistance exercise before versus after aerobic exercise on glycemia in type 1 diabetes. *Diabetes Care* 35:669–675, 2012

Zierath JR, He L, Guma A, Odegoard Wahlstrom E, Klip A, Wallberg-Henriksson H: Insulin action on glucose transport and plasma membrane GLUT4 content in skeletal muscle from patients with NIDDM. *Diabetologia* 39:1180–1189, 1996

Chapter 13

Hyperglycemia and Dehydration Concerns

Hyperglycemia, or elevated blood glucose levels, is associated with unique causes, problems, and treatments (Avogaro 1993). Technically, any blood glucose value in excess of 125 mg/dl (6.9 mmol/l) qualifies as hyperglycemia for the purposes of diabetes diagnosis. Abnormal responses to physical activity, however, are not usually experienced until glucose levels exceed twice that concentration (i.e., 250 mg/dl, or 13.9 mmol/l) (American Diabetes Association 2004), particularly when ketones are present; thus, hyperglycemia is more frequently considered to be a blood glucose level >180 mg/dl (10 mmol/l). Intense exercise has the potential to cause a rise in blood glucose levels instead of the usual decline experienced with most aerobic activities (Mitchell 1988; Sigal 1994a, 1999; Marliss 2002; Kreisman 2003), and any physical work undertaken during hyperglycemic conditions has the potential to cause a worsening of metabolic control (Avogaro 1993). Moreover, highly trained individuals with type 1 diabetes (T1D) can achieve the same cardiorespiratory exercise responses, but these responses are reduced by poor glycemic control (A1C >7.0%) (Baldi 2010a).

A related issue is that frequent or sustained hyperglycemia increases the likelihood of dehydration (Ugale 2012), which is a concern when undertaking any physical activity. Although it is important to ensure proper hydration during physical activity done in any environmental conditions (American College of Sports Medicine 2007), exercising in a thermally challenging environment (e.g., hot or humid) can pose additional difficulties for those with diabetes because of hydration issues and heightened glucose metabolism. Thus, strategies to avoid dehydration are needed for physically active individuals with any type of diabetes (Hernandez 2000, Diabetes Research in Children Network Study Group 2006, American College of Sports Medicine 2007).

Case in Point: Exercise Concerns for an Athlete with T1D

JH is a 45-year-old man who trains for and participates in triathlons. When he was diagnosed with T1D at the age of 28 years, he was a semiprofessional athlete, but now his training is more for his own benefit and less competitive. He typically trains for 2–3 h on weekdays doing a combination of running, cycling, and swimming workouts, and on weekends he does at least one long training day that takes 6–8 h. At the present time, he manages his diabetes with an insulin pump, in which he uses a rapid-acting insulin analog (lispro).

Resting Measurements

Height: 69.5 inches
Weight: 155 lb
BMI: 22.6 (normal)
Heart rate: 58 beats per minute (bpm)
Blood pressure: 110/70 mmHg

Fasting Labs

Plasma glucose: variable (45–185 mg/dl) (using an insulin pump)
A1C: 6.1%

Questions to Consider

1. Does JH need to make any routine regimen changes to prevention hyperglycemia or hydration related to his training?
2. Are any other precautions needed for JH when he engages in long-duration training?

(Continued on page 223.)

HYPERGLYCEMIA AND PHYSICAL ACTIVITY

CAUSES AND INTERPRETATION OF HYPERGLYCEMIA

Hyperglycemia can be an acute condition that follows consumption of a meal, or it can be indicative of a more chronic, relative state of insulin deficiency. People with type 2 diabetes (T2D) can have high blood glucose readings resulting from a combination of insulin resistance and inadequate insulin secretion, either acutely or chronically. In T2D, extremely elevated blood glucose levels accompanied by severe dehydration can result in a condition known as hyperosmolar hyperglycemia, which may be precipitated by severe illness, and infections. Individuals with T2D typically do not produce ketones; if ketones do develop, it is frequently the result of inadequate calories and starvation ketosis rather than due to insulin deficiency and acidosis.

Individuals with T1D, however, are more susceptible to insulin deficiency because they lack the ability to produce their own; therefore, they need to receive instruction on why and when to check for the production of ketones, particularly if using an insulin pump. If urinary or blood ketones are present, then hyperglycemia is the result of insulin deficiency and corrective action should be taken immediately to prevent diabetic ketoacidosis (DKA).

In the presence of low insulin levels, insulin-stimulated glucose uptake in skeletal muscle is reduced, and exercise-induced hepatic glucose output is increased, frequently resulting in hyperglycemia (Sigal 1994b). In T1D and other insulin-deficient states, after glucose levels exceed 250–300 mg/dl (13.9–16.7 mmol/l), ketones can begin to form as a result of ineffective fat metabolism and can contribute to DKA if hyperglycemia persists (Kitabchi 2006, Ugale 2012). This scenario requires exogenous insulin to be administered to lower the glucose level and reestablish euglycemia before the initiation of physical activity. When blood glucose levels are elevated (e.g., >250–300 mg/dl) before exercise, an acute bout may exacerbate hyperglycemia if moderate or higher levels of ketones are evident. Poor glycemic control in athletes with T1D may negatively impact their cardiopulmonary exercise training responses, such as maximal oxygen consumption, heart rate, stroke volume, and cardiac output (Baldi 2010a, 2010b).

EFFECTS ON EXERCISE METABOLISM

The metabolic adjustments that preserve euglycemia during physical activity are in large part hormonally mediated. A decrease in plasma insulin and the presence of glucagon appear to be necessary for the early increase in hepatic glucose production during physical activity, and during prolonged exercise, increases in plasma glucagon and catecholamines appear to play a key role (Kjaer 1991, Manetta 2002). These hormonal adaptations, however, are essentially lost in insulin-deficient individuals (Meinders 1988, Koivisto 1992, Admon 2005). Consequently, when such individuals have too little insulin in their circulation due to inadequate therapy, an excessive release of counterregulatory hormones during physical activity may increase already high levels of glucose and ketone bodies and can even precipitate the onset of DKA (Burge 2001).

Oxidation of fuels. Substrate oxidation in people with T1D performing aerobic exercise during euglycemic conditions is similar to that in healthy individuals, revealing a shift toward lipid oxidation during prolonged, moderate exercise. Under hyperglycemic conditions, however, fuel metabolism is dominated by carbohydrate oxidation, assumed to be increased blood glucose use given that muscular glycogen is not spared (Jenni 2008). Likewise, in nondiabetic individuals undertaking prolonged cycling exercise, glycogen is not spared under hyperglycemic conditions, although blood glucose uptake is increased (Coyle 1991). Moreover, individuals with T1D have been shown to experience a greater increase in muscular levels of acetylcarnitine (involved in transportation of free fatty acids into the mitochondria for oxidation) during moderate exercise undertaken with normal blood glucose levels compared with hyperglycemia (blood glucose clamped at ~200 mg/dl, or 11 mmol/l), suggesting that hyperglycemic conditions may alter fuel use and specifically depress fat oxidation (Boss 2011). Growth hormone levels are also reduced in T1D during exercise undertaken with hyperglycemia (Jenni 2010).

Intense exercise effects. Intense physical activity can result in hyperglycemia in individuals with T1D (Marliss 2002). The catecholamine hormone response to intense activity results in an exaggerated hepatic production of glucose for fuel. After the activity is stopped, the insulin need can double during the postactivity period. If insulin needs are not met with correct dosing, this state of hyperglycemia may last for several hours before returning to the desired level or may never return without additional insulin (Sigal 1994a, 1994b; Marliss 2002).

Individuals using insulin pump therapy sometimes find it useful to bolus a small amount of insulin to address this physiological need, or if insulin is injected, additional short- or rapid-acting insulin also can be administered. In a recent study, among individuals performing regular moderate- to heavy-intensity aerobic exercise, use of an insulin pump actually helped to limit postexercise hyperglycemia compared with other basal-bolus insulin regimens and was not associated with increased risk for postexercise late-onset hypoglycemia (Yardley 2012). In any case, the timing and amount of insulin given need careful consideration and monitoring to accomplish the desired blood glucose result, taking into account any insulin remaining from the last injection or bolus and residual effects of the last bout of activity on blood glucose use (i.e., postexercise enhancements in insulin action). Regardless of the delivery method, this additional insulin dose can still result in hypoglycemia and may not be advisable in all cases.

In intense exercise, glucose is the exclusive muscle fuel and is mobilized from muscle and liver glycogen in both the fed and fasted states. Therefore, regulation of glucose production and glucose utilization are different than during lower-intensity exercise. At lower intensities, blood glucose is constant during postabsorptive exercise and declines during postprandial exercise even though insulin secretion is reduced. In contrast, in intense exercise, glucose production rises seven- to eightfold and glucose uptake rises three- to fourfold; therefore, glycemia increases and plasma insulin decreases minimally, if at all. At exhaustion, glucose uptake initially decreases more than glucose production, which leads to greater hyperglycemia postexercise and requiring a substantial rise in insulin for 40–60 min after such exercise to restore pre-exercise levels. Absence of this response in T1D leads to sustained hyperglycemia without insulin administration (Marliss 2002).

HYPERGLYCEMIC EXERCISE RECOMMENDATIONS

T1D. To prevent a worsening of metabolic control with physical activity, the American Diabetes Association put forth the following recommendation: "Avoid physical activity if blood glucose levels are >250 mg/dl and ketosis is present, and use caution if glucose levels are >300 mg/dl and no ketosis is present" (American Diabetes Association 2004). In other words, exercise should be avoided with hyperglycemia accompanied by a relative state of insulin deficiency given that any physical activity performed under such conditions would likely result in an exaggerated counterregulatory hormone response, causing blood glucose levels and ketones to rise excessively (Avogaro 1993). Hyperglycemia during intense exercise in individuals with T1D results in deteriorations in diabetic control and may require different regimen changes compared with moderate exercise (Mitchell 1988). After intense exercise, the postexercise increase in insulin levels normally observed is essential to return blood glucose to resting levels in individuals with diabetes (Sigal 1994b).

On the basis of this medical concern, most individuals with T1D may need to check for ketones when their blood glucose levels exceed 250 mg/dl (Avogaro 1993). In the absence of ketones (such as with acute hyperglycemia following a meal), these higher readings are transient and should not pose a medical threat (Avogaro 1993). Some people, however, report headaches, blurry vision, or lack of energy while exercising with elevated blood glucose levels, which may provide reason enough to avoid physical activity until the glucose level is lower. Modern insulin regimens paired with frequent self-monitoring of blood glucose (SMBG) greatly diminish the chance of insulin deficiency developing, and ketones are rarely found when performing blood or urine checks. In most circumstances, slightly elevated blood glucose levels should not interfere with exercise performance.

Some people with T1D capitalize on the faster absorption of rapid-acting insulin to lower hyperglycemia rapidly with moderate exercise. For instance, if they start out with elevated blood glucose levels (>300 mg/dl) without significant ketones, they may take 0.5–2.5 units of rapid-acting insulin before starting physical activity to cause a speedy decrease in glycemia down to a more normal range (Ploug 1984, Richter 1985, Colberg 2009a). Such practices should be undertaken with extreme caution, however, given that the additive effects of contraction- and insulin-induced blood glucose uptake can rapidly result in hypoglycemia.

T2D. Although hyperglycemia can be worsened by exercise in individuals with T1D who are insulin deficient and ketotic (due to missed or insufficient insulin), few people with T2D develop such a profound degree of insulin deficiency because they still produce much of their own insulin. Therefore, individuals with T2D or gestational diabetes mellitus (GDM) generally do not need to postpone exercise because of hyperglycemia, provided that they are feeling well (Avery 2001, Colberg 2010, Manders 2010). If they undertake strenuous physical activities with elevated glucose levels (>300 mg/dl), it is prudent to ensure that they are adequately hydrated (American Diabetes Association 2004).

Moderate aerobic exercise has been shown to be beneficial, however, in dampening the acute hyperglycemia that occurs following a meal in individuals with T2D by increasing muscle glucose uptake (Larsen 1999, Poirier 2001). More intense activities can cause transient blood glucose elevations in all individuals with diabetes (Sigal 1994a; Kreisman 2003; Szewieczek 2007, 2009), but intermittent high-intensity exercise done immediately after breakfast in individuals with T2D treated with diet alone reduces blood glucose levels and insulin secretion (Larsen 1999). Even if hyperglycemic after eating, they will still likely experience a reduction in glycemia during aerobic work as endogenous insulin levels will likely be higher at that time (Poirier 2001, Colberg 2009b). As a precaution, however, glucose monitoring can be performed before and after physical activity to assess its individualized effect.

Furthermore, a single bout of low-intensity exercise done for 60 min compared to high-intensity work for 30 min has been shown to substantially reduce the prevalence of hyperglycemia throughout the subsequent 24 h postexercise period (Manders 2010). Likewise, a single session of resistance- or endurance-type exercise substantially reduces the prevalence of hyperglycemia during the subsequent 24 h period in both insulin-treated and non–insulin-treated individuals with T2D (van Dijk 2012). Thus, both resistance- and endurance-type exercise can be integrated in exercise intervention programs designed to improve their glycemic control.

Case in Point: Continued

JH participated in a full Ironman triathlon that took place in 85°F weather with 90% humidity and mostly sunny skies. The day before, he experienced some unexplained hyperglycemia, but his starting blood glucose levels on the day of the race were fairly normal for him (135 mg/dl). Although he thought he was drinking plenty of water, halfway through the event he experienced severe fatigue, muscle cramps in his calf muscles, and an inability to finish the race. Discouraged, he dropped out, but vowed to train better for the next race to avoid experiencing a repeat of that disastrous event.

Additional Questions to Consider

1. What type of regimen changes should JH make to maintain glycemic control during physical activity done under those extreme environmental conditions?
2. Did JH's hydration or electrolyte status have anything to do with his experiences during that event?

(Continued on page 228.)

HYDRATION, ELECTROLYTES, AND PHYSICAL ACTIVITY

EFFECTS OF DIABETES ON HYDRATION STATUS

Ensuring proper hydration in any environmental condition is important for sports and athletic performance (American College of Sports Medicine 2007), but poorly controlled diabetes increases the likelihood of dehydration (Ugale 2012). Healthcare and fitness professionals, therefore, should offer precautionary measures and prevention strategies to avoid exercise-associated dehydration or hyperglycemia in those with diabetes (Hernandez 2000, Diabetes Research in Children Network Study Group 2006, American College of Sports Medicine 2007). Exercising in a hot or humid environment in particular can pose difficulties for individuals with diabetes because of hydration issues and alterations in glucose metabolism. For instance, if individuals with T2D undertake strenuous physical activity with glucose levels >300 mg/dl, they need to be adequately hydrated, given that dehydration resulting from polyuria (excessive urination associated with hyperglycemia) may contribute to a compromised thermoregulatory response (Vinik 2007). In some cases, outdoor exercise should be postponed to ensure a safe environment in which to participate.

If individuals have autonomic neuropathy, they may be more likely to become dehydrated during exercise without realizing it, making fluid intake during activities particularly critical. Normally, thirst centers in the brain are not activated until a person has already lost 1–2% of body weight, but autonomic neuropathy can make it harder for the body to activate thirst receptors to drive fluid intake in a timely manner and can lead to a greater risk of postural hypotension (Purewal 1995).

MAINTENANCE OF HYDRATION

Because of potentially greater water losses with hyperglycemia (Burge 2001), all exercisers with diabetes must focus on staying adequately hydrated before, during, and after any physical activity. Starting several hours before exercise, individuals should take in normal amounts of fluids and meals to attain a state of euhydration before exercising, particularly if they have recently experienced hyperglycemia, either acutely or chronically (Burge 2001). Hydration state at the start of exercise, sweating rates, and environmental conditions all affect fluid requirements during physical activity (American College of Sports Medicine 2007). Individual sweat rates can be estimated by measuring body weight before and after exercise. Excessive weight loss is indicative of a state of dehydration and should be prevented (Noakes 2007), whereas weight gain from excess fluid intake during activities may lead to hyponatremia (water intoxication) and also should be avoided (Noakes 2007, Hubing 2011).

WATER INTAKE DURING EXERCISE

The goal of drinking fluids during exercise is to prevent excessive dehydration (>2% body weight loss from water deficit) and electrolyte imbalances but not necessarily to replace all water losses during exercise as long as plasma osmolality is maintained (American College of Sports Medicine 2007, Noakes 2007). Drinking cool, plain water is generally adequate for hydration during moderate exercise lasting up to 1 h. In most cases, taking in too much fluid is worse than dehydrating, as the former greatly increases the risk of developing hyponatremia (Noakes 2007, Hubing 2011). Body weight should never increase during a physical activity, or else excessive amounts of fluid are being consumed by an individual. Drinking ~1 oz (30 ml) of fluid every 10–15 min to replace up to 80% of sweat losses should be adequate for most exercise participation, using thirst as the guide for its intake (Coyle 1992, Noakes 2007, Hubing 2011). If water is being consumed during the activity, additional carbohydrates can be consumed in a sports or other drink or in solid form (Table 13.1) (American College of Sports Medicine 2007).

CARBOHYDRATE AND ELECTROLYTE INTAKE

Generally, it is unnecessary to replace electrolytes (i.e., sodium, potassium, chloride, and magnesium) during shorter athletic endeavors because sweating does not immediately unbalance their levels given that sweat is more dilute than blood and contains less sodium and other electrolytes (American College of Sports Medicine 2007, Noakes 2007), Inclusion of electrolytes in beverages, however, can enhance their palatability and voluntary intake during activity (Maughan 1997). Any drinks taken in during exercise ideally should contain <10% carbohydrate, be cold, have a volume of <500 ml, and contain some replacement electrolytes for exercise lasting >1 h (American College of Sports Medicine 2007).

Carbohydrate and electrolyte replacement. Beverages containing electrolytes and carbohydrates can provide benefits over water alone under certain circumstances (Hubing 2011, Peacock 2011), including when carbohydrate is needed to prevent hypoglycemia (Tamis-Jortberg 1996) and during more prolonged activities when glucose ingestion provides an alternate fuel that can delay fatigue when muscle glycogen stores are declining (Yaspelkis 1993, American College of Sports Medicine 2007, Peacock 2011). By way of example, adolescents with T1D undertaking

Table 13.1 Products Available for Carbohydrate, Electrolyte, and Fluid Replacement

Product	Carbohydrate Content	Electrolytes and Other Ingredients
Gatorade	14 g/8 oz (240 ml) (6% carbohydrate solution)	Sodium, 110 mg; potassium, 25 mg
PowerAde	21 g/8 oz (240 ml) (8% carbohydrate solution)	Sodium, 55 mg; potassium, 30 mg
All-Sport	21 g/8 oz (240 ml) (9% carbohydrate solution)	Sodium, 55 mg; potassium, 55 mg
Cytomax	19 g/8 oz (240 ml) (8% carbohydrate solution)	Sodium, 10 mg; potassium, 150 mg
Ultra Fuel	50 g/8 oz (240 ml) (21% carbohydrate solution)	None
Accel Gel	20 g carbohydrate/41 g pouch	Protein, 5 g (whey protein from milk); fat, 0 g; sodium, 100 mg; potassium, 50 mg; vitamins E and C (100%); various flavors
Gu Energy Gel	25 g (85% maltodextrin, 15% fructose) in 1.1 oz (31 g) pouch	Sodium, 50 mg; potassium, 35 mg; vitamins C and E, 100% of daily value
Hammer Gel	23 g/36 g serving (about 2 Tbsp, or 30 ml)	Amino acids (L-leucine, L-alanine, L-valine, L-isoleucine); sodium chloride; potassium
PowerBar	43 g/65 g bar	Protein, 9 g; fat, 2.5 g; fiber, 2 g; sodium, 200 mg; potassium, 115 mg; vitamins; minerals; essential amino acids; various flavors
PowerBar Gel	27 g/41 g packet	Sodium, 200 mg; potassium, 20 mg; chloride, 90 mg; many flavors with 25 or 50 mg of caffeine added
Clif Bar	45 g/68 g bar	Protein, 10–11 g; fat, 3–6 g; fiber, 5 g; sodium, 125 mg; potassium, 310 mg; vitamins; minerals; various flavors
Clif Shot Bloks Chews	24 g per three pieces (30 g)	Sodium, 70 mg; potassium, 20 mg; various flavors, some with more sodium or caffeine
Jelly Belly Sport Beans	24 g in 1 oz (30 g)	Sodium, 80 mg; potassium, 40 mg; some thiamin, riboflavin, niacin, and vitamin C; various flavors; Extreme Sport Beans only: caffeine, 50 mg
GlucoBurst	15 g glucose in 1.3 oz (37 g) pouch	Sodium, 30 mg; potassium, 10 mg
Dex4 Glucose Gel	15 g glucose/tube	None
Dex4 Glucose Tablets	4 g glucose/tablet	None

60 min of moderate cycling maintained hydration status when consuming either an 8% or a 10% carbohydrate drink, but the latter containing extra carbohydrate preserved euglycemia more effectively (Perrone 2005).

Since the carbohydrates in sports drinks are absorbed quickly, every 5–10 min a few ounces must be consumed to provide a consistent supply of fuel to prevent peaks and valleys in blood glucose levels (Tamis-Jortberg 1996). A 24-oz bottle of a typical sports drink contains ~42 g of carbohydrate, which satisfies the recommended hourly intake for most endurance workouts, along with supplying important electrolytes crucial for fluid and pH balance, electrical impulses of neurons and muscles, and prevention of muscle cramps. Ingestion of ~30–60 g of carbohydrate during each hour of exercise generally will be sufficient to maintain blood glucose oxidation late in prolonged bouts of exercise and to delay fatigue (Coyle 1992).

Optimal carbohydrate concentration. A carbohydrate-based fluid consumed during exercise should ideally be a 5–10% solution (i.e., containing 5–10 g of carbohydrate per 100 ml of fluid); such fluids empty from the stomach as rapidly as plain water, hydrate effectively, and provide adequate replacement carbohydrates (Perrone 2005). More concentrated carbohydrate solutions (above 10%) should be consumed only before or after exercise because their gastric emptying is somewhat delayed and may cause fluid shifts into the gut (reverse osmosis) (American College of Sports Medicine 2007). Fruit juices and most regular soft drinks contain ~12% carbohydrate and can lead to gastrointestinal upset, such as cramps, nausea, vomiting, diarrhea, or bloating during exercise, if not diluted with water (American College of Sports Medicine 2007). A list of some of the more common products used to replace fluids, carbohydrates, and electrolytes during physical activity are given in Table 13.1.

HYPONATREMIA AND SODIUM INTAKE

During prolonged physical activity, some replacement of electrolytes may be necessary while the event is ongoing especially when fluid intake is greater to prevent exercise-associated hyponatremia, a rare but serious condition that is more likely to occur during physical activity done in a hot environment (Hubing 2011). Hyponatremia is diagnosed as a serum sodium concentration below 135 mmol/l. Symptoms of hyponatremia can include light-headedness, headaches, nausea, repeated vomiting, and malaise. Possible causes include sodium loss, sweat loss and its replacement with dilute solutions, elevations in antidiuretic hormone, increases in interleukin-6, and depletion of muscle glycogen stores, all of which can occur during prolonged exercise (Hubing 2011). Fluid intake that exceeds the thirst drive is also an important causal mechanism, even with the ingestion of beverages containing low levels of sodium (Noakes 2004). In the presence of dehydration, postexercise hyponatremia is actually more common than its onset during activity because sweat is dilute. Intake of excessive amounts of any fluid during exercise, even if it contains sodium and other electrolytes, can result in this condition, although a higher carbohydrate status (i.e., greater muscle glycogen stores) and electrolyte intake may be somewhat protective (American Dietetic Association 2009, Hubing 2011).

MAGNESIUM IN DIABETES AND MUSCLE CRAMPS

Although aging itself has been associated with lower serum magnesium levels (Barbagallo 2009), individuals with T2D in particular frequently have a low magnesium status, indicative of deficiency (Simmons 2010, Sales 2011, Lecube 2012). Magnesium has been shown to play an important role in blood glucose control and may contribute to the onset of T2D (Sales 2011). In individuals with T1D, a low magnesium status has been found to be associated with greater oxidation of low-density lipoprotein (LDL) cholesterol (Djurhuus 2001, Wegner 2010). In that population, it is unclear whether a lesser dietary intake or diabetes itself reduces serum magnesium levels, but replenishment with supplements may decrease both atherogenic lipid fractions and insulin-stimulated glucose uptake (Djurhuus 2001). Oral-magnesium oxide supplementation also increases muscle potassium content in individuals with T1D (Djurhuus 2003).

Depletion of certain electrolytes, such as magnesium, also has been suggested as causative in the onset of exercise-associated muscle cramps. Neither clinically significant alterations in serum electrolytes nor dehydration, however, has been observed in runners with exercise-associated muscle cramps participating in an ultradistance race (Schwellnus 2004), and muscle cramping in Ironman triathletes was not found to be associated with greater body mass loss or changes in serum electrolyte concentrations (Sulzer 2005). Recently, others have alternatively suggested that a past history of cramps, faster running pace at the early stage of a race, and possibly pre-race muscle damage are more likely associated with and predictive of muscle cramps in distance runners than dehydration or changes in serum sodium levels (Schwellnus 2011a, 2011b).

HYDRATION FOLLOWING EXERCISE

After exercise, the focus should be on replacing any fluid and electrolyte deficits, which usually can be accomplished with water intake (that restores pre-exercise body weight) and a healthy, balanced diet containing foods that are naturally rich in electrolytes (such as nuts, legumes, many vegetables and fruits, whole grains, and salted foods) (Maughan 1996). Plasma volume and fluid status may recover faster when food is ingested before consuming any water in the 2 h after exercise (Sharp 2007). Whole milk and sports drinks that are designed for both quick and long-lasting nutrient replenishment (including carbohydrates) can be used by anyone with T1D to lower the risk of late-onset hypoglycemia associated with prior exercise (Tamis-Jortberg 1996, Hernandez 2000).

Case in Point: Wrap-Up

To his credit, JH manages his blood glucose levels effectively most of the time, and he uses frequent SMBG to prevent both hyperglycemia and hypoglycemia during and after his extensive exercise training. Using an insulin pump helps him to maintain control most of the time as well. His starting blood glucose levels likely had little to do with his outcome in the race that he failed to finish during hot weather, although experiencing some hyperglycemia the day before may have left him more dehydrated than usual as he did not compensate for excessive water losses via urine. What he likely experienced during the race was some dehydration, possible electrolyte imbalances, and lower muscle glycogen levels exacerbated by the extreme heat and humidity.

Insulin Regimen Changes: Exercising in the heat can actually increase blood glucose use, so JH will have to perform SMBG more frequently in such environments to prevent hyperglycemia. He should be aware of the possibility for elevations in blood glucose levels resulting from dehydration, which fluid intake may assist in lowering without the need for additional insulin. On exercise days when JH will be subject to more extreme environmental conditions, he should plan on modifying his basal rates on his insulin pump to compensate for any resulting changes in his blood glucose levels based on testing results.

Dietary Changes: JH will need to focus on adequate intake of foods rich in electrolytes in the days leading up to events or training where hydration and electrolyte balance may be a concern. Such foods include leafy green and other vegetables, nuts, legumes (dried beans), whole grains, many fruits, and salty foods. He also needs to maintain nearly normal blood glucose levels while consuming adequate carbohydrates on the day before races to maximize his muscle glycogen storage before starting; doing so may require greater insulin doses and more frequent SMBG.

Hydration Concerns: JH should focus on taking in enough fluid before, during, and after all physical activity, particularly when he exercises in more extreme environments (i.e., hot, humid, and sunny). He also needs to ensure that he takes in adequate amounts of electrolytes (i.e., sodium, potassium, and magnesium) before and during long-duration exercise and recovery from workouts. Most of the time he can do this effectively by taking in a balanced diet, maintaining his blood glucose levels as close to normal as possible, and consuming some drinks containing some electrolytes during training and competitive events. On days when he experiences some hyperglycemia, he should increase his intake of fluids to compensate for any potential losses from polyuria.

Environment-Specific Changes: When JH knows that he will be exercising in hot and humid conditions, he should try to hyperhydrate before starting his workout or event by taking in extra fluid and electrolytes. He will need to concentrate on drinking more frequently during exercise when his sweating rate is accelerated.

Both hyperglycemia and dehydration are valid concerns for individuals with diabetes involved in physical activity. Physical activities undertaken during hyperglycemic conditions have the potential to worsen metabolic control, particularly if they are intense and cause a greater release of counterregulatory hormones. Paying attention to maintaining hydration and electrolyte balance will lower any risks associated with imbalances in either during participation in physical activity, especially when undertaken in more extreme environmental conditions.

PROFESSIONAL PRACTICE PEARLS

■ Exercise undertaken with hyperglycemia (blood glucose levels of >180 mg/dl) can potentially worsen metabolic control, particularly when ketones are present.

■ Intense exercise has the potential to cause a rise in blood glucose levels instead of the usual decline experienced with most activities.

■ In T2D, extremely elevated blood glucose levels accompanied by severe dehydration can result in a condition known as hyperosmolar hyperglycemia.

■ In T1D, sustained hyperglycemia accompanied by increased ketone production and dehydration can result in DKA, which is potentially life threatening.

■ When insulin levels are too low, insulin-stimulated glucose uptake in muscle is reduced, and exercise-induced hepatic glucose output is increased, resulting in hyperglycemia.

■ Under hyperglycemic conditions, exercise fuel metabolism is dominated by carbohydrate oxidation, likely increasing blood glucose use given that muscular glycogen is not spared.

■ Individuals should avoid physical activity if glucose levels are >250 mg/dl and ketosis is present and should use caution if glucose levels are >300 mg/dl and no ketosis is present.

■ Because they make some insulin on their own, people with T2D or GDM generally do not need to postpone exercise because of hyperglycemia, provided that they are feeling well.

■ Hyperglycemia increases the likelihood of dehydration; thus, all exercisers with diabetes must focus on staying adequately hydrated before, during, and after any physical activity.

■ Hydration state at the start of exercise, sweating rates, and environmental conditions all affect fluid requirements during physical activity.

■ Drinking cool, plain water is generally adequate for hydration during moderate exercise lasting up to 1 h.

■ It is unnecessary to replace electrolytes during shorter bouts of exercise because sweating does not immediately unbalance their levels given that it is more dilute than blood.

■ Beverages like sports drinks can be used when 30–60 g/h of carbohydrate is needed to prevent hypoglycemia and to delay the onset of fatigue during longer activities.

■ Drinks should ideally contain <10% carbohydrate, be cold, have a volume of <500 ml, and contain some electrolytes for exercise >1 h.

■ Intake of excessive amounts of any fluid during exercise can cause hyponatremia, although greater muscle glycogen stores and electrolyte intake may be protective.

■ Many individuals with diabetes have a low magnesium status that can exacerbate blood glucose control, but low levels are unlikely to be the cause of exercise muscle cramps.

■ After exercise, individuals should focus on replacing any fluid and electrolyte deficits, which usually can be accomplished with water intake and a healthy, balanced diet.

REFERENCES

Admon G, Weinstein Y, Falk B, Weintrob N, Benzaquen H, Ofan R, Fayman G, Zigel L, Constantini N, Phillip M: Exercise with and without an insulin pump among children and adolescents with type 1 diabetes mellitus. *Pediatrics* 116:e348–e355, 2005

American College of Sports Medicine, Sawka MN, Burke LM, Eichner ER, Maughan RJ, Montain SJ, Stachenfeld NS: American College of Sports Medicine position stand. Exercise and fluid replacement. *Med Sci Sports Exerc* 39:377–390, 2007

American Diabetes Association: Physical activity/exercise and diabetes. *Diabetes Care* 27 (Suppl. 1):S58–S62, 2004

American Dietetic Association, Canada Dietitians of, American College of Sports Medicine, Rodriguez NR, Di Marco NM, Langley S: American College of Sports Medicine position stand. Nutrition and athletic performance. *Med Sci Sports Exerc* 41:709–731, 2009

Avery MD, Walker AJ: Acute effect of exercise on blood glucose and insulin levels in women with gestational diabetes. *J Matern Fetal Med* 10:52–58, 2001

Avogaro A, Gnudi L, Valerio A, Maran A, Miola M, Opportuno A, Tiengo A, Bier DM: Effects of different plasma glucose concentrations on lipolytic and ketogenic responsiveness to epinephrine in type I (insulin-dependent) diabetic subjects. *J Clin Endocrinol Metab* 76:845–850, 1993

Baldi JC, Cassuto NA, Foxx-Lupo WT, Wheatley CM, Snyder EM: Glycemic status affects cardiopulmonary exercise response in athletes with type I diabetes. *Med Sci Sports Exerc* 42:1454–1459, 2010a

Baldi JC, Hofman PL: Does careful glycemic control improve aerobic capacity in subjects with type 1 diabetes? *Exercise & Sport Sciences Reviews* 38:161–167, 2010b

Barbagallo M, Belvedere M, Dominguez LJ: Magnesium homeostasis and aging. *Magnes Res* 22:235–246, 2009

Boss A, Kreis R, Jenni S, Ith M, Nuoffer JM, Christ E, Boesch C, Stettler C: Non-invasive assessment of exercise-related intramyocellular acetylcarnitine in euglycemia and hyperglycemia in patients with type 1 diabetes using (1)H magnetic resonance spectroscopy: a randomized single-blind crossover study. *Diabetes Care* 34:220–222, 2011

Burge MR, Garcia N, Qualls CR, Schade DS: Differential effects of fasting and dehydration in the pathogenesis of diabetic ketoacidosis. *Metabolism* 50:171–177, 2001

Colberg SR: *Diabetic Athlete's Handbook.* Champaign, IL, Human Kinetics, 2009a

Colberg SR, Sigal RJ, Fernhall B, Regensteiner JG, Blissmer BJ, Rubin RR, Chasan-Taber L, Albright AL, Braun B, American College of Sports Medicine, American Diabetes Association: Exercise and type 2 diabetes: the American College of Sports Medicine and the American Diabetes Association: joint position statement. *Diabetes Care* 33:e147–e167, 2010

Colberg SR, Zarrabi L, Bennington L, Nakave A, Thomas Somma C, Swain DP, Sechrist SR: Postprandial walking is better for lowering the glycemic effect of dinner than pre-dinner exercise in type 2 diabetic individuals. *J Am Med Dir Assoc* 10:394–397, 2009b

Coyle EF, Montain SJ: Benefits of fluid replacement with carbohydrate during exercise. *Med Sci Sports Exerc* 24 (Suppl. 9):S324–S330, 1992

Coyle EF, Hamilton MT, Alonso JG, Montain SJ, Ivy JL: Carbohydrate metabolism during intense exercise when hyperglycemic. *J Appl Physiol* 70:834–840, 1991

Diabetes Research in Children Network Study Group, Tsalikian E, Kollman C, Tamborlane WB, Beck RW, Fiallo-Scharer R, Fox L, Janz KF, Ruedy KJ, Wilson D, Xing D, Weinzimer SA: Prevention of hypoglycemia during exercise in children with type 1 diabetes by suspending basal insulin. *Diabetes Care* 29:2200–2204, 2006

Djurhuus MS, Klitgaard NA, Pedersen KK: Effect of glucose/insulin infusion and magnesium supplementation on serum and muscle sodium and potassium and muscle [3H]ouabain binding capacity in type 1 diabetes mellitus. *Scand J Clin Lab Invest* 63:93–102, 2003

Djurhuus MS, Klitgaard NA, Pedersen KK, Blaabjerg O, Altura BM, Altura BT, Henriksen JE: Magnesium reduces insulin-stimulated glucose uptake and serum lipid concentrations in type 1 diabetes. *Metabolism* 50:1409–1417, 2001

Hernandez JM, Moccia T, Fluckey JD, Ulbrecht JS, Farrell PA: Fluid snacks to help persons with type 1 diabetes avoid late onset postexercise hypoglycemia. *Med Sci Sports Exerc* 32:904–910, 2000

Hubing KA, Bassett JT, Quigg LR, Phillips MD, Barbee JJ, Mitchell JB: Exercise-associated hyponatremia: the influence of pre-exercise carbohydrate status combined with high volume fluid intake on sodium concentrations and fluid balance. *Eur J Appl Physiol* 111:797–807, 2011

Jenni S, Christ ER, Stettler C: Exercise-induced growth hormone response in euglycaemia and hyperglycaemia in patients with type 1 diabetes mellitus. *Diabet Med* 27:230–233, 2010

Jenni S, Oetliker C, Allemann S, Ith M, Tappy L, Wuerth S, Egger A, Boesch C, Schneiter P, Diem P, Christ E, Stettler C: Fuel metabolism during exercise in euglycaemia and hyperglycaemia in patients with type 1 diabetes mellitus—a prospective single-blinded randomised crossover trial. *Diabetologia* 51:1457–1465, 2008

Kitabchi AE, Umpierrez GE, Murphy MB, Kreisberg RA: Hyperglycemic crises in adult patients with diabetes: a consensus statement from the American Diabetes Association. *Diabetes Care* 29:2739–2748, 2006

Kjaer M, Kiens B, Hargreaves M, Richter EA: Influence of active muscle mass on glucose homeostasis during exercise in humans. *J Appl Physiol* 71:552–557, 1991

Koivisto VA, Sane T, Fyhrquist F, Pelkonen R: Fuel and fluid homeostasis during long-term exercise in healthy subjects and type I diabetic patients. *Diabetes Care* 15:1736–1741, 1992

Kreisman SH, Halter JB, Vranic M, Marliss EB: Combined infusion of epinephrine and norepinephrine during moderate exercise reproduces the glucoregulatory response of intense exercise. *Diabetes* 52:1347–1354, 2003

Larsen JJ, Dela F, Madsbad S, Galbo H: The effect of intense exercise on postprandial glucose homeostasis in type II diabetic patients. *Diabetologia* 42:1282–1292, 1999

Lecube A, Baena-Fustegueras JA, Fort JM, Pelegri D, Hernandez C, Simo R: Diabetes is the main factor accounting for hypomagnesemia in obese subjects. *PLoS One* 7:e30599, 2012

Manders RJ, Van Dijk JW, van Loon LJ: Low-intensity exercise reduces the prevalence of hyperglycemia in type 2 diabetes. *Med Sci Sports Exerc* 42:219–225, 2010

Manetta J, Brun JF, Perez-Martin A, Callis A, Prefaut C, Mercier J: Fuel oxidation during exercise in middle-aged men: role of training and glucose disposal. *Med Sci Sports Exerc* 34:423–429, 2002

Marliss EB, Vranic M: Intense exercise has unique effects on both insulin release and its roles in glucoregulation: implications for diabetes. *Diabetes* 51 (Suppl. 1):S271–S283, 2002

Maughan RJ, Leiper JB, Shirreffs SM: Restoration of fluid balance after exercise-induced dehydration: effects of food and fluid intake. *Eur J Appl Physiol Occup Physiol* 73:317–325, 1996

Maughan RJ, Leiper JB, Shirreffs SM: Factors influencing the restoration of fluid and electrolyte balance after exercise in the heat. *Br J Sports Med* 31:175–182, 1997

Meinders AE, Willekens FL, Heere LP: Metabolic and hormonal changes in IDDM during long-distance run. *Diabetes Care* 11:1–7, 1988

Mitchell TH, Abraham G, Schiffrin A, Leiter LA, Marliss EB: Hyperglycemia after intense exercise in IDDM subjects during continuous subcutaneous insulin infusion. *Diabetes Care* 11:311–317, 1988

Noakes T: Sodium ingestion and the prevention of hyponatraemia during exercise. *Br J Sports Med* 38:790–792, 2004

Noakes TD: Hydration in the marathon: using thirst to gauge safe fluid replacement. *Sports Med* 37:463–466, 2007

Peacock OJ, Thompson D, Stokes KA: Voluntary drinking behaviour, fluid balance and psychological affect when ingesting water or a carbohydrate-electrolyte solution during exercise. *Appetite* 58:56–63, 2011

Perrone C, Laitano O, Meyer F: Effect of carbohydrate ingestion on the glycemic response of type 1 diabetic adolescents during exercise. *Diabetes Care* 28:2537–2538, 2005

Ploug T, Galbo H, Richter EA: Increased muscle glucose uptake during contractions: no need for insulin. *Am J Physiol* 247 (6 Pt 1):E726–E731, 1984

Poirier P, Mawhinney S, Grondin L, Tremblay A, Broderick T, Cleroux J, Catellier C, Tancrede G, Nadeau A: Prior meal enhances the plasma glucose lowering effect of exercise in type 2 diabetes. *Med Sci Sports Exerc* 33:1259–1264, 2001

Purewal TS, Watkins PJ: Postural hypotension in diabetic autonomic neuropathy: a review. *Diabet Med* 12:192–200, 1995

Richter EA, Ploug T, Galbo H: Increased muscle glucose uptake after exercise. No need for insulin during exercise. *Diabetes* 34:1041–1048, 1985

Sales CH, Pedrosa LF, Lima JG, Lemos TM, Colli C: Influence of magnesium status and magnesium intake on the blood glucose control in patients with type 2 diabetes. *Clin Nutr* 30:359–364, 2011

Schwellnus MP, Allie S, Derman W, Collins M: Increased running speed and pre-race muscle damage as risk factors for exercise-associated muscle cramps in a 56 km ultra-marathon: a prospective cohort study. *Br J Sports Med* 45:1132–1136, 2011a

Schwellnus MP, Drew N, Collins M: Increased running speed and previous cramps rather than dehydration or serum sodium changes predict exercise-associated muscle cramping: a prospective cohort study in 210 Ironman triathletes. *Br J Sports Med* 45:650–656, 2011b

Schwellnus MP, Nicol J, Laubscher R, Noakes TD: Serum electrolyte concentrations and hydration status are not associated with exercise associated muscle cramping (EAMC) in distance runners. *Br J Sports Med* 38:488–492, 2004

Sharp RL: Role of whole foods in promoting hydration after exercise in humans. *J Am Coll Nutr* 26 (Suppl. 5):592S–596S, 2007

Sigal RJ, Fisher SJ, Halter JB, Vranic M, Marliss EB: Glucoregulation during and after intense exercise: effects of beta-adrenergic blockade in subjects with type 1 diabetes mellitus. *J Clin Endocrinol Metab* 84:3961–3671, 1999

Sigal RJ, Purdon C, Bilinski D, Vranic M, Halter JB, Marliss EB: Glucoregulation during and after intense exercise: effects of beta-blockade. *J Clin Endocrinol Metab* 78:359–366, 1994a

Sigal RJ, Purdon C, Fisher SJ, Halter JB, Vranic M, Marliss EB: Hyperinsulinemia prevents prolonged hyperglycemia after intense exercise in insulin-dependent diabetic subjects. *J Clin Endocrinol Metab* 79:1049–1057, 1994b

Simmons D, Joshi S, Shaw J: Hypomagnesaemia is associated with diabetes: not pre-diabetes, obesity or the metabolic syndrome. *Diabetes Res Clin Pract* 87:261–266, 2010

Sulzer NU, Schwellnus MP, Noakes TD: Serum electrolytes in Ironman triathletes with exercise-associated muscle cramping. *Med Sci Sports Exerc* 37:1081–1085, 2005

Szewieczek J, Dulawa J, Strzalkowska D, Batko-Szwaczka A, Hornik B: Normal insulin response to short-term intense exercise is abolished in Type 2 diabetic patients treated with gliclazide. *J Diabetes Complications* 23:380–386, 2009

Szewieczek J, Dulawa J, Strzalkowska D, Hornik B, Kawecki G: Impact of the short-term, intense exercise on postprandial glycemia in type 2 diabetic patients treated with gliclazide. *J Diabetes Complications* 21:101–107, 2007

Tamis-Jortberg B, Downs DA Jr, Colten ME: Effects of a glucose polymer sports drink on blood glucose, insulin, and performance in subjects with diabetes. *Diabetes Educ* 22:471–487, 1996

Ugale J, Mata A, Meert KL, Sarnaik AP: Measured degree of dehydration in children and adolescents with type 1 diabetic ketoacidosis. *Pediatr Crit Care Med* 13:e103–e107, 2012

van Dijk JW, Manders RJ, Tummers K, Bonomi AG, Stehouwer CD, Hartgens F, van Loon LJ: Both resistance- and endurance-type exercise reduce the prevalence of hyperglycaemia in individuals with impaired glucose tolerance and in insulin-treated and non-insulin-treated type 2 diabetic patients. *Diabetologia* 55:1273–1282, 2012

Vinik AI, Ziegler D: Diabetic cardiovascular autonomic neuropathy. *Circulation* 115:387–397, 2007

Wegner M, Araszkiewicz A, Zozulinska-Ziolkiewicz D, Wierusz-Wysocka B, Piorunska-Mikolajczak A, Piorunska-Stolzmann M: The relationship between concentrations of magnesium and oxidized low density lipoprotein and the activity of platelet activating factor acetylhydrolase in the serum of patients with type 1 diabetes. *Magnes Res* 23:97–104, 2010

Yardley JE, Iscoe KE, Sigal RJ, Kenny GP, Perkins BA, Riddell MC: Insulin pump therapy is associated with less post-exercise hyperglycemia than multiple daily injections: An observational study of physically active type 1 diabetes patients. *Diabetes Technol Ther* 2012

Yaspelkis BB III, Patterson JG, Anderla PA, Ding Z, Ivy JL: Carbohydrate supplementation spares muscle glycogen during variable-intensity exercise. *J Appl Physiol* 75:1477–1485, 1993

Chapter 14
Balancing Insulin Use with Physical Activity

Youth and adults with type 1 diabetes (T1D) or latent autoimmune diabetes of adults (LADA) can be treated using a basal-bolus insulin regimen (that utilizes multiple daily insulin injections) or continuous subcutaneous insulin infusion (i.e., insulin pump) to facilitate resting blood glucose uptake and control blood glucose levels (American Diabetes Association 2013). Regardless of the delivery method, insulin dosages can and frequently should be reduced before, during, or after exercise to avoid hypoglycemia, depending on the intensity, duration, and timing of the activity (Rabasa-Lhoret 2001, Admon 2005, Diabetes Research in Children Network Study Group 2006, Delvecchio 2009). Making appropriate insulin adjustments involves a trial-and-error process and requires a greater understanding of insulin action and the impact of exercise, food intake, and medication on glucose variability, combined with frequent self-monitoring of blood glucose (SMBG) (Boulé 2001; Admon 2005; Diabetes Research in Children Network Study Group 2006; Szewieczek 2007, 2009; Delvecchio 2009). Using SMBG to guide appropriate regimen changes provides the cornerstone for safe and effective blood glucose control during and following physical activity in all insulin users (Farmer 2008, St John 2010).

Many individuals with type 2 diabetes (T2D) are prescribed insulin to assist in blood glucose management (Vinik 2007). Multiple insulin secretory defects are present in T2D, including absence of pulsatility, loss of early phase of insulin secretion after glucose, decreased basal and stimulated insulin release, and progressive decrease in insulin secretory capacity over time (Kahn 2001, Guillausseau 2008). Their exogenous insulin use may only be basal in nature (such as a once-daily injection of long-acting insulin like glargine or detemir) or also may involve premeal injections of faster-acting insulin to correspond to postprandial increases in blood glucose levels (Morello 2011, Shanik 2012). All insulin users, however, regardless of diabetes type, have a higher risk of exercise-induced hypoglycemia and should use SMBG, along with decreased insulin doses or increased carbohydrate intake, to prevent hypoglycemia (Hernandez 2000, Kalergis 2003, Schutt 2006, Taplin 2010).

Case in Point: Exercise Blood Glucose Management in an Adult with LADA

HW is a 48-year-old married man and a father of two active boys. Athletic throughout his life, his family time often has included sports or outdoor pursuits. Everyone was shocked when he was told at age 45 years that he had diabetes, initially diagnosed as T2D. Although the addition of medications helped at first, his blood glucose levels continued to rise over time on oral agents. As exercise became more physically difficult for him in the past few years, he had begun to accept the fact that hiking, camping, hunting, biking, kayaking, and ice hockey refereeing were all a thing of the past until his wife convinced him to see his health-care provider. Autoimmunity tests diagnosed LADA, a form of T1D, which explained why his blood glucose levels had stayed so high despite his best efforts. He is now using a set amount of insulin on a basal-bolus therapy (aspart for meals and detemir twice a day) and is hopeful that he may be able to resume the active lifestyle he and his family enjoy.

Resting Measurements

Height: 70 inches
Weight: 155 lb
BMI: 22.2 (normal)
Heart rate: 65 beats per minute (bpm)
Blood pressure: 115/70 mmHg

Fasting Labs

Plasma glucose: variable (65–215 mg/dl) (following a set basal-bolus insulin regimen)
A1C: 7.8% (right before going on insulin therapy)

Questions to Consider

1. Are there any limitations as to what types of exercise HW can engage in safely with a new diagnosis of LADA?
2. Are any precautions needed for HW when he exercises?

(Continued on page 242.)

INSULINS AND ACTIONS

Different insulins have varying times to peak action and unique durations (as shown in Table 14.1), both of which can make physical activities (especially spontaneous ones) harder to handle. In general, insulin is considered rapid- or short-, intermediate-, long-acting, or ultra–long-acting depending on its onset, peak, and duration (Morello 2011, Kitabchi 2012). Each distinct insulin potentially has a different effect on blood glucose responses to exercise. It is critical for an individual to understand his or her insulin peaks and total duration to be able to anticipate the exercise response and make appropriate regimen changes, particularly when activity is unplanned. See appendix A for a listing of generic and brand names of all insulins.

Table 14.1 Human Insulin Action Times

Insulin	Onset	Peak	Duration
Humalog (insulin lispro)	15 min	1–1.5 h	2–5 h
NovoLog (insulin aspart)	10–20 min	1–3 h	3–5 h
Apidra (insulin glulisine)	10–20 min	55 min	3 h
Humulin R, Novolin R (human insulin regular)	30–60 min	2–5 h	6–8 h
Humulin N, Novolin N (insulin isophane or NPH)	60–90 min	6–12 h	15–24 h
Lantus (insulin glargine)	60 min	None	16–24 h
Levemir (insulin detemir)	30–60 min	None	16–24 h
Tresiba (insulin degludec)	30–90 min	None	>24 h

Note: Individual action times may vary depending on environmental conditions, activity level, injection site, and dosage taken.

SHORT- AND RAPID-ACTING INSULIN

A few human-synthetic, short-acting regular insulins (most common brand names, Humulin R, Novolin R, and Actrapid) are still available, but almost all beef and pork insulins have been discontinued. Insulins of synthetic origin that have the same structure as human insulin generally have faster onset, quicker peak time, and shorter duration than their previous animal counterparts and are less likely to cause allergic reactions. A benefit of the short-action profile of regular human insulin is that it may be used more effectively in individuals with gastroparesis and slowed gastric emptying who have delayed carbohydrate absorption (compared with more rapid-acting insulins) (Rave 2006).

More recently, several rapid-acting insulins have been developed, including Humalog (generic name, insulin lispro), NovoLog or NovoRapid (insulin aspart), and Apidra (insulin glulisine). These are actually insulin analogs, meaning that they have a structure similar to that of human insulin, but the order of the amino acids is slightly modified to result in faster absorption and shorter duration (Hanaire-Broutin 2000; Bode 2002; Rave 2006; Becker 2007, 2008; van Bon 2011). Most insulin pumps are loaded with one of these rapid-acting analogs for both basal and bolus insulin coverage.

The choice of injection or infusion site for such insulin causes only slight variation, with one study reporting a slightly faster absorption of insulin lispro from the abdomen compared with thigh sites, whereas insulin glulisine is less affected by injection site (ter Braak 1996). The benefit of these analogs is that for exercise done before meals and at least 2–3 h after the last injection, most of the effect has peaked and waned and hypoglycemia risk is lowered, although any intensity of postprandial exercise done within 2 h after eating increases this risk unless doses of short-acting insulin are reduced premeal (Rabasa-Lhoret 2001).

In one study, well-controlled adult men with T1D undertook exercise starting 90 min after a mixed breakfast (containing 600 kilocalories and 75 g of carbohydrate). All were on intensive insulin therapy and treated with a basal-bolus insulin regimen (i.e., with ultralente, a basal insulin that is no longer on the market, and lispro) (Rabasa-Lhoret 2001). Their risk of developing hypoglycemia was minimized during postprandial exercise of different intensities and different durations by appropriate reduction of prebreakfast insulin lispro only, as shown in Table 14.2.

INTERMEDIATE-ACTING INSULIN

Some intermediate-acting insulins are available as Humulin N or Novolin N in the U.S. (Protophane elsewhere) and have the generic name of insulin isophane. In individuals with T1D using one of these insulins, a usual regimen is insulin isophane at breakfast along with a short- or rapid-acting insulin to cover breakfast, an optional rapid-acting injection at lunch, a mandatory dose at dinner, and another dose of insulin isophane at bedtime. Overall, however, combination therapy using insulin isophane and regular human insulin does not closely approximate physiologic insulin secretion, may provide limited control over fasting and postprandial blood glucose levels, and may be associated with a higher risk for hypoglycemia than other basal-bolus insulin combinations (Luzio 2003). An alternative regimen is to take rapid-acting insulin doses during the day with a single bedtime dose of insulin isophane to cover basal insulin requirements overnight.

Individuals with T2D may use intermediate-acting insulin alone (usually at bedtime) or a mixture with a shorter-acting insulin (e.g., Humulin or Novolin 70/30 mix with insulin isophane and regular). Other premixed insulins include insulin lispro protamine and insulin aspart protamine, which are suspensions of crystals produced by combining insulin lispro or aspart with protamine sulfate. The addition of protamine converts insulin lispro and insulin aspart, which are rapid-acting insulin, into intermediate-acting insulin. In individuals with T1D, use of intermediate-acting insulin conveys a higher risk of nocturnal and severe hypoglycemia than supplying basal insulin needs with an ultra–long-acting insulin (Monami 2009).

Table 14.2 Reductions in Prebreakfast Insulin Lispro Dosing for Postprandial Exercise of Varying Intensities and Durations

Intensity of Aerobic Exercise	30 min	60 min
Mild (~25% of maximal aerobic capacity)	25%	50%
Moderate (~50% of maximal aerobic capacity)	50%	75%
Heavy (~75% of maximal aerobic capacity)	75%	NA

NA, not available.

LONG-ACTING AND ULTRA–LONG-ACTING BASAL INSULIN AND BASAL-BOLUS REGIMENS

Ultra–long-acting basal insulin analogs, such as Lantus (insulin glargine) and Levemir (insulin detemir), have replaced the use of older, long-lasting insulins like Ultralente (Humulin U). The main difference between these two newer basal insulins is that insulin glargine lasts up to 24 h and usually is taken once daily, and insulin detemir generally requires once-daily dosing in T2D or possibly twice-daily dosing in T1D, depending on the dosage taken (King 2009, Nelson 2011). Both analogs are essentially peakless and provide coverage for basal insulin needs, but meal and snack intake for all individuals with T1D and some with T2D are additionally covered with shorter-acting insulin. In at least one study in T1D, the likelihood of weight gain was reduced with insulin detemir compared with insulin glargine (McAdam-Marx 2010). In preschool-age children with T1D, use of a flexible daily regimen of premeal lispro plus bedtime glargine resulted in improved overall glycemic control and decreased frequency of severe hypoglycemia (Alemzadeh 2005). Use of insulin detemir with insulin aspart as mealtime insulin is well tolerated and also reduces the risks of nocturnal hypoglycemia and weight gain compared with the use of insulin isophane in people with T1D (De Leeuw 2005), possibly because of a lower energy intake when using detemir for basal needs (Zachariah 2011).

Insulin glargine. Use of either insulins glargine or isophane alone in individuals with T2D does not increase the risk of exercise-associated hypoglycemia (Plockinger 2008). Notably, insulin glargine can have a significantly shorter duration when small doses are injected, and for many insulin-sensitive individuals or youth with T1D, twice-daily dosing is required for 24 h basal coverage. In general, with all types of insulin, even basal ones, the smaller the dose, the more rapidly it is absorbed because of the surface area of the insulin depot (the spot where the insulin is injected) under the skin (Lindholm 2001; Becker 2007, 2008; Heise 2007; Danne 2008; Dailey 2010; Wang 2010), and this faster absorption of small doses must be taken into consideration when anticipating blood glucose responses to physical activity. Furthermore, a recent study also demonstrated that blood glucose levels in anyone using insulin glargine usually rise around the time that the next dose is due, whether it is usually given once a day at bedtime, at dinner, or at another time of day. Bedtime injections, in particular, lead to hyperglycemia in the early part of the night, which may be improved by giving a single daily dose at lunch or dinner instead (Danne 2008).

Another issue associated with the use of long-acting insulin is that its absorption can be inconsistent due to the choice of injection site, activity level, massage, hot tub use, or other factors that may increase the rate at which the insulin is absorbed, resulting in basal insulin levels that are first excessive and later deficient (Guerci 2005). One study in individuals with T1D, however, reported that subcutaneous injection of insulin glargine in the thigh region on the evening before engaging in 30 min of intense exercise did not increase its absorption rate (Peter 2005).

Insulin detemir. To achieve the same glycemic control, insulin detemir often must be injected twice daily in a higher dose (though the likelihood of weight gain is lower with insulin detemir), whereas insulin glargine may be injected only once a day (King 2009, McAdam-Marx 2010, Swinnen 2011). Insulin detemir was associated with less hypoglycemia than insulin glargine in relatively well-controlled people with T1D during and after 30 min of moderate exercise performed 5 h after the last injection of rapid-acting insulin (Arutchelvam 2009). The duration of basal insulin, however, makes it harder to implement short-term corrections in basal coverage for unusual or prolonged activities unless the basal dose is lowered in advance or following an activity (Arutchelvam 2009, Delvecchio 2009).

Insulin degludec. The latest submitted for U.S. Food and Drug Administration (FDA) approval, insulin degludec (trade name Tresiba, or Ryzodeg when premixed with insulin glulisine) is basal insulin that has an ultralong action profile (lasting >24 h and possibly up to 40 h), giving it the option of being used once a day or only three times per week in some individuals. When compared with its rival basal insulin analogs (glargine and levemir), a longer duration of action and lower incidence of hypoglycemic events in individuals with both T1D and T2D has been demonstrated (Nasrallah 2012). In adults with T2D, use of insulin degludec provides comparable glycemic control when compared with insulin glargine without additional adverse events and may reduce dosing frequency because of its ultralong action profile (Zinman 2011). In people with T1D, use of daily injection of insulin degludec results in improved mental well-being scores, likely resulting from a decreased incidence of hypoglycemia, compared with use of insulin glargine (Home 2012).

Case in Point: Continued (Part 2)

HW is eager to do what he needs to get his diabetes under better control, and he is especially happy to be able to start back into his fitness routine. He likes to work out in the evenings, the time of day he can most easily get to his fitness club. Assuming that hypoglycemia can be prevented by exercising after a meal because eating food makes blood glucose go higher and exercise usually makes it drop (so the two should balance out), he takes his usual premeal, rapid-acting insulin dose and eats dinner before going to his club. Twenty-five minutes into his moderate aerobic workout, however, he has to stop and treat a blood glucose level of 57 mg/dl with some regular soda. Unsure how to proceed, he goes home early, discouraged.

Additional Question to Consider (Part 2)

1. What type of diabetes regimen changes does HW need to make to avoid hypoglycemia related to physical activity?

(Continued on page 244.)

INSULIN PUMP USE

Pump features. Individuals with any types of diabetes can deliver replacement insulin using continuous subcutaneous insulin infusion, otherwise known as an insulin pump, although its use is most common among individuals with T1D (Admon 2005, Diabetes Research in Children Network Study Group 2006, Vinik 2007, Delvecchio 2009, Maahs 2010, Chu 2011, Jankovec 2011). All pumps use a subcutaneous plastic catheter through which small, basal doses of insulin (usually one of the rapid-acting analogs or insulin regular) are delivered continually to mimic normal insulin release by the pancreas (Hanaire-Broutin 2000, Monami 2009). Pumps must be programmed to give basal doses at a set rate, along with bolus doses to cover food intake at meals and snacks (mainly to cover carbohydrates) or for correction of hyperglycemia. Most require a new infusion set to be placed every 3 days to avoid excessive buildup of scar tissue that can compromise insulin delivery.

Many insulin pumps are now available, and the features vary by manufacturer and model. Most of the manufacturers' respective pumps have features like small basal increments (≤ 0.05 unit/h), temporary basal rates, menu-driven programming, and various bolus patterns (e.g., normal, extended, and combination) (Kordonouri 2011). Normal boluses, for instance, give the insulin dose all at once, but extended boluses allow a programmed dose to be given over a longer period to avoid peaks and valleys in insulin coverage for foods that are more slowly absorbed; combination boluses simply combine these two strategies for optimal coverage of foods like pizza. At least two pumps even have self-contained food databases or blood glucose meters, and most pumps are waterproof at shallow depths.

Although a physiological insulin delivery pattern can be closely mimicked using any of the newer basal or bolus regimens (e.g., insulin levemir for basal, insulin aspart for boluses), insulin pumps make the delivery of that insulin easier and offer more flexibility by allowing the user to change basal rates of insulin delivery at any time during the day (or set up different programmed profiles of delivery). The exercise responses of people who use either basal insulin or pumps are often similar because both regimens attempt to provide basal insulin levels (Admon 2005, Diabetes Research in Children Network Study Group 2006, Maahs 2010). Pump users, however, can suspend the pump and immediately reduce basal rates of insulin, which is not possible with the use of injected doses without planning ahead (Admon 2005, Diabetes Research in Children Network Study Group 2006).

Type of insulin used in pumps. Although any type of rapid- or short-acting insulin can be used in a pump, most individuals now use one of the rapid-acting analogs that is delivered to cover both basal and bolus insulin needs. In external pumps, lispro provides better glycemic control and stability with much lower doses of insulin and does not increase the frequency of hypoglycemic episodes compared with the use of a basal-bolus injection regimen (Hanaire-Broutin 2000). Use of lispro and aspart in pumps is acceptable and essentially equivalent in outcomes in youth and adults with T1D (Bode 2002, Weinzimer 2008). Moreover, use of insulin glulisine in pump therapy was not found to be superior to the use of insulin aspart or lispro, and no significant differences were seen among these insulins with respect to unexplained hyperglycemia or perceived catheter set occlusion (van Bon 2011). Glulisine in one study was associated with a higher frequency of symptomatic hypoglycemia, however, possibly because of slight overdosing as previous trials suggested lower insulin requirements when this analog was initiated for T1D (van Bon 2011).

Case in Point: Continued (Part 3)

HW remembers being told that he may need to reduce his insulin dose before he exercises to prevent low blood glucose levels. The next time he goes to his fitness club, he takes one unit less than his normal 6-unit dinner dose of aspart with his meal, which results in a preworkout blood glucose of 154 mg/dl. He hopes that this is high enough to get him through his aerobic workout, but it again drops: 15 min into his workout he has to stop and treat another low, this time 63 mg/dl.

He decides to reduce his insulin by half for the following night's workout. He is alarmed, however, when his blood glucose reading the next night ends up at 287 mg/dl before his workout. He remembers something about not exercising with his blood glucose >250 mg/dl and ketones. Because he does not have urine ketone strips with him, he skips the workout and goes home, discouraged yet again.

Additional Questions to Consider (Part 3)

1. What additional diabetes regimen changes should HW make to avoid hyperglycemia related to physical activity?
2. Should he consider doing another type of physical activity to avoid these glycemic balance issues?

(Continued on page 246.)

SELF-MONITORING OF BLOOD GLUCOSE WITH INSULIN USE

Two guidelines from the American Diabetes Association (ADA) address blood glucose monitoring practices related to physical activity participation by insulin users (American Diabetes Association 2004). The first ADA guideline recommends that exercisers with diabetes identify when changes in insulin or food intake are necessary. Although most insulin users agree that glucose monitoring is essential to establish a pattern and make changes to maintain better control of blood glucose levels, doing so still involves significant trial and error (Colberg 2000). Many insulin users minimally check their blood glucose before and after exercise, and sometimes during, particularly when participating in new or unusual physical activity compared with established routines (Kilbride 2011). Many insulin users who exercise regularly self-monitor their blood glucose levels more frequently (Schutt 2006). A recent study, however, reported that SMBG was performed daily by only 39% of individuals with T1D and less than weekly by 24%, although 67% did perform routine testing and the other 33% only tested when hypo- or hyperglycemia was suspected; not surprisingly, a lower A1C was associated with more frequent testing (Hansen 2009).

Use of continuous glucose monitoring (CGM) devices alternatively provides blood glucose readings every 5 min 24 h/day, but frequently these readings must be calibrated against fingerstick values. CGM identifies significantly more episodes of hypoglycemia and hyperglycemia during the day and night than frequent blood glucose tests (Cauza 2005). Even during days that include episodic strenuous physical exercise in adolescents with T1D participating in sports camps, CGM can provide useful information on glucose fluctuations during day and night, albeit with significant failure rates (Adolfsson 2011). CGM glucose readings are somewhat time delayed and may not always indicate hypoglycemia during exercise before it actually occurs.

The second ADA guideline recommends that exercisers with diabetes learn the glycemic response to different exercise conditions (American Diabetes Association 2004). Establishing patterns, even with a blood glucose meter or CGM technology, is still an inexact science because of the multitude of variables that can affect responses. Often, information from multiple workout sessions is needed as well as frequent blood glucose readings and patience. General trends are predictable for most activities with use of trial and error, however, allowing for a more predictable pattern to emerge that will allow individuals to anticipate responses to future bouts of similar exercise (Biankin 2003, West 2010). Although these two recommendations are followed more closely than a number of the previous ones, the significant number of reported modifications made by individuals indicates that a substantial need exists to modify and individualize them (Colberg 2000).

INSULIN ADJUSTMENTS WITH PHYSICAL ACTIVITY

When engaging in physical activity, the main focus for individuals using insulin is the blood glucose level, which is affected by circulating levels of insulin and release of glucose-raising, counterregulatory hormones. Individuals must understand that if the circulating level of insulin is greater than physiological needs, hypoglycemia can occur, and if circulating insulin is insufficient, hyperglycemia may result. The interpretation of this information—particularly glycemic trends during an activity—can lead to a better understanding of the insulin and food adjustments required to support exercise energy needs.

Physical activity is one of the main causes of hypoglycemia in people with tightly controlled diabetes (MacDonald 1987, Ertl 2004, Admon 2005, Tsalikian 2005, Diabetes Research in Children Network Study Group 2006, Arutchelvam 2009, Delvecchio 2009, Chu 2011, West 2011). Exercising with low levels of insulin is indeed a much more normal physiological response, which can be replicated with pre-exercise insulin adjustments, primarily made to rapid- or short-acting insulins rather than basal ones. Discontinuing basal insulin normally delivered with an insulin pump during an hour of moderate exercise is an effective strategy for reducing hypoglycemia in youth with T1D, although their risk for hyperglycemia is increased until insulin delivery is restored (Diabetes Research in Children Network Study Group 2006). Fortunately, temporarily lowering or suspending basal insulin doses is not likely to increase risk of diabetic ketoacidosis (DKA). For instance, ketogenesis following 45 min of moderate running in adults with T1D was not found to be influenced by reductions in pre-exercise rapid-acting insulin dose, meaning that this important preparatory strategy aids in the preservation of blood glucose without increasing the risk of exercise-induced ketone body formation (Bracken 2011). General strategies for lowering rapid- or

Table 14.3 General Rapid- or Short-Acting Insulin Reductions for Dosing before Aerobic Activities

Duration	Low Intensity	Moderate Intensity	High Intensity
15 min	None	5–10%	0–15%
30 min	None	10–20%	10–30%
45 min	5–15%	15–30%	20–45%
60 min	10–20%	20–40%	30–60%
90 min	15–30%	30–55%	45–75%
120 min	20–40%	40–70%	60–90%
180 min	30–60%	60–90%	75–100%

Adapted from Colberg SR: *Diabetic Athlete's Handbook.* Champaign, IL, Human Kinetics, p. 32, 2009.

short-acting insulin doses for exercise of varying durations and intensities are given in Table 14.3. These strategies may be used as a starting point to determine an individual's unique responses, based on differences in insulin regimens, usual food intake, body weight, and more.

The insulin reductions in Table 14.3 apply to the specific insulin peaking during exercise (usually rapid-acting ones); however, smaller or no insulin reductions may be needed if exercise occurs >3 h following the last injection of rapid-acting insulin, but postexercise decreases may be necessary to prevent delayed-onset hypoglycemia. Moreover, these recommendations assume that no additional food is eaten before or during the activity to compensate. For insulin pump users, basal rate reductions during an activity may be greater or lesser than these recommendations, and they may be done alone or along with reduced bolus amounts. For intense, near-maximal exercise, an actual increase in rapid-acting insulin (rather than a decrease) may be necessary to counter the glucose-raising effects of hormones released during exercise (Kreisman 2003; Mitchell 1988; Sigal 1994, 1999).

Case in Point: Continued (Part 4)

The next day HW decides to try another type of workout with reductions in his insulin dose: a heavy session of resistance training instead of an aerobic workout. Because his blood glucose had gone too high the last time when he cut his predinner insulin in half, he only reduces it by 25% this time. About 30 min into his resistance workout, he starts to feel funny and checks his blood glucose. He is shocked to find that his reading is even higher than before, reaching 318 mg/dl. He really has no idea why it has gone higher even with taking more insulin than the previous time, but he knows it is not supposed to get that high. He stops his workout immediately and again goes home not knowing what to do again.

In the middle of the night, he wakes up feeling shaky and sweating profusely with a blood glucose of 54 mg/dl, which is puzzling to him as he had not taken any extra insulin to bring down his high postworkout sugar and it was still elevated (188 mg/dl) at bedtime. Now he is really confused about how to handle his blood glucose and still engage in any type of workout, and he hates getting low blood glucose levels all the time (especially at night).

Additional Question to Consider (Part 4)

1. Should he consider working out at another time of day instead of after dinner to avoid these issues?

(Continued on page 248.)

FOOD INTAKE AND EXERCISE TIMING

Another exercise guideline recommends that individuals ingest added carbohydrates if glucose levels are <100 mg/dl (5.6 mmol/l). The need for food intake (or even insulin adjustments), however, is largely dependent on exercise type and duration and circulating plasma insulin levels during the activity (Sigal 1994). Insulin pump users who can easily lower basal insulin infusion or make other adjustments for exercising >3 h after the last injection of rapid-acting insulin may not need to consume any carbohydrates (Mitchell 1988, Admon 2005, Delvecchio 2009). Moreover, although most insulin users consume extra carbohydrates before prolonged, less intense activities, they may not necessarily do the same before undertaking weight training, sprinting, or other intense but shorter workouts.

The time of day that exercise is undertaken also affects diabetes regimen adjustments (Larsen 1999, Poirier 2001). Engaging in early morning activities (before food intake or faster-insulin use) when levels of the hormone cortisol are higher is unlikely to cause as significant or any decrease in blood glucose levels as later-day ones, and prebreakfast, intense workouts are even more likely to raise levels at that time of day (although even moderate exercise can do so then as well) (Poirier 2000, 2001). Depending on all of these factors, an individual's pre-exercise carbohydrate requirements may be based on a different starting blood glucose level, such as 75 mg/dl (4.2 mmol/l) instead of 100 mg/dl. Insulin pump users always have the option of simply maintaining or decreasing basal insulin rates during early morning exercise (Mitchell 1988, Admon 2005, Delvecchio 2009), and in some cases, they actually may need to raise basal infusions instead to prevent hyperglycemia.

Anyone with T2D with the capacity to release some insulin naturally will experience a decrease in blood glucose levels when exercising after breakfast or another meal as opposed to before breakfast because of higher circulating insulin levels stimulated by food consumption. For instance, 1 h of aerobic exercise has a minimal impact on blood glucose when undertaken by fasted, moderately hyperglycemic men with T2D treated with oral agents only, but this same exercise causes a significant decrease in glycemia when performed 2 h after breakfast (Poirier 2001). Similarly, although intense activities usually elevate blood glucose levels at most times of day (Kreisman 2003; Szewieczek 2007, 2009), intermittent high-intensity exercise done immediately after breakfast in individuals with T2D treated with diet only reduces blood glucose levels and insulin secretion (Larsen 1999). Thus, individuals with any type of diabetes are unlikely to develop hypoglycemia when exercising moderately (or harder) early in the morning before breakfast or whenever their circulating insulin levels are lower.

In some cases, modulation of insulin, food intake, and exercise timing may work most effectively. For instance, ingestion of 75 g of a low–glycemic-index carbohydrate (isomaltulose) combined with 75% reduction in rapid-acting insulin doses administered 30 min before undertaking 45 min of moderate running improved pre- and postexercise blood glucose responses in individuals with T1D (West 2011). Waiting 60, 90, or 120 min before starting exercise, however, resulted in a greater incidence of hypoglycemia.

Case in Point: Wrap-Up

HW is totally frustrated by the large fluctuations in his blood glucose levels caused by his physical activity participation, especially since his health-care providers told him he could continue to be physically active while using insulin. He decides that he will just have to stop trying to work out because it is too hard to manage his blood glucose levels. On a follow-up appointment with his diabetes educator the next week, his educator not only explains what happened to his blood glucose numbers but also encourages him to keep trying different things until he finds out what works best for him. Encouraged that it is possible to find the right balance of food, insulin, and workouts, he also decides to join a support group to get more ideas about how to better manage his exercise blood glucose levels.

Glycemic Effects of Mode of Activity: To his surprise, HW learns that although most moderate aerobic activity lowers blood glucose levels, intense resistance workouts release more hormones that raise levels and result in transient hyperglycemia. Aerobic workouts, therefore, likely will need more regimen changes before engaging in them (especially right after a meal and injection of insulin), whereas resistance training instead may need more regimen changes following the activity.

Regimen Changes for Aerobic Activity: On evenings that HW plans to mainly engage in moderate aerobic activity, he reduces his premeal insulin aspart dose by 25–75%, depending on the planned workout duration and what he eats for dinner.

Regimen Changes for Resistance Activity: For after-dinner resistance work, HW finds that he does not need to reduce his premeal insulin at all. He checks his blood glucose at bedtime, however, and consumes a balanced snack (with carbohydrate, protein, and fat) that works to prevent overnight lows.

Balancing insulin use with physical activity presents its own set of challenges. Regular activity participation by all insulin users with any type of diabetes is possible, however, with frequent use of self-monitoring as well as a trial-and-error process in learning how to make appropriate insulin adjustments or make decisions about compensatory food intake to prevent hypoglycemia and hyperglycemia both during and after exercise at different times of day.

PROFESSIONAL PRACTICE PEARLS

- All individuals with T1D and some with T2D use exogenous insulin administered by injection or via an insulin pump to better control their blood glucose levels.
- All insulin users have a higher risk of exercise-induced hypoglycemia and should use SMBG, along with regimen changes, to prevent hypoglycemia.
- Insulin dosages may need to be reduced before, during, or after exercise to avoid hypoglycemia, depending on the intensity, duration, and timing of the activity.
- Different types of insulin are considered rapid- or short-, intermediate-, long-acting, or ultra–long-acting depending on their unique onset, peak, and duration.
- Most individuals with T1D use either a basal-bolus insulin regimen or an insulin pump filled with rapid-acting insulin for basal insulin delivery and boluses for food intake.
- Any intensity of postprandial exercise done within 2 h after eating increases the risk of hypoglycemia unless doses of short-acting insulin are reduced premeal.
- Absorption of insulin can be inconsistent because of the choice of injection site, activity level, massage, hot tub use, or other factors that increase the absorption rate.
- In general, with all types of insulin, the smaller the dose, the more rapidly it is absorbed because of the surface area of the subcutaneous insulin depot.
- During physical activity, if the circulating level of insulin is greater than physiological needs, hypoglycemia can occur, and if it is less, hyperglycemia may result.
- The time of day that exercise is undertaken also affects diabetes regimen adjustments, and morning, prebreakfast activity usually conveys a lower hypoglycemia risk.

REFERENCES

Admon G, Weinstein Y, Falk B, Weintrob N, Benzaquen H, Ofan R, Fayman G, Zigel L, Constantini N, Phillip M: Exercise with and without an insulin pump among children and adolescents with type 1 diabetes mellitus. *Pediatrics* 116:e348–e355, 2005

Adolfsson P, Nilsson S, Lindblad B: Continuous glucose monitoring system during physical exercise in adolescents with type 1 diabetes. *Acta Paediatr* 100:1603–1609, 2011

Alemzadeh R, Berhe T, Wyatt DT: Flexible insulin therapy with glargine insulin improved glycemic control and reduced severe hypoglycemia among pre-school-aged children with type 1 diabetes mellitus. *Pediatrics* 115:1320–1324, 2005

American Diabetes Association: Physical activity/exercise and diabetes. *Diabetes Care* 27 (Suppl. 1):S58–S62, 2004

American Diabetes Association: Standards of medical care in diabetes—2013. *Diabetes Care* 36 (Suppl. 1):S11–S66, 2013

Arutchelvam V, Heise T, Dellweg S, Elbroend B, Minns I, Home PD: Plasma glucose and hypoglycaemia following exercise in people with type 1 diabetes: a comparison of three basal insulins. *Diabet Med* 26:1027–1032, 2009

Becker RH, Frick AD: Clinical pharmacokinetics and pharmacodynamics of insulin glulisine. *Clin Pharmacokinet* 47:7–20, 2008

Becker RH, Frick AD, Nosek L, Heinemann L, Rave K: Dose-response relationship of insulin glulisine in subjects with type 1 diabetes. *Diabetes Care* 30:2506–2507, 2007

Biankin SA, Jenkins AB, Campbell LV, Choi KL, Forrest QG, Chisholm DJ: Target-seeking behavior of plasma glucose with exercise in type 1 diabetes. *Diabetes Care* 26:297–301, 2003

Bode B, Weinstein R, Bell D, McGill J, Nadeau D, Raskin P, Davidson J, Henry R, Huang WC, Reinhardt RR: Comparison of insulin aspart with buffered regular insulin and insulin lispro in continuous subcutaneous insulin infusion: a randomized study in type 1 diabetes. *Diabetes Care* 25:439–444, 2002

Boulé NG, Haddad E, Kenny GP, Wells GA, Sigal RJ: Effects of exercise on glycemic control and body mass in type 2 diabetes mellitus: a meta-analysis of controlled clinical trials. *JAMA* 286:1218–1227, 2001

Bracken RM, West DJ, Stephens JW, Kilduff LP, Luzio S, Bain SC: Impact of pre-exercise rapid-acting insulin reductions on ketogenesis following running in type 1 diabetes. *Diabet Med* 28:218–222, 2011

Cauza E, Hanusch-Enserer U, Strasser B, Ludvik B, Kostner K, Dunky A, Haber P: Continuous glucose monitoring in diabetic long distance runners. *Int J Sports Med* 26:774–780, 2005

Chu L, Hamilton J, Riddell MC: Clinical management of the physically active patient with type 1 diabetes. *Phys Sportsmed* 39:64–77, 2011

Colberg SR: *Diabetic Athlete's Handbook*. Champaign, IL, Human Kinetics, 2009

Colberg SR: Use of clinical practice recommendations for exercise by individuals with type 1 diabetes. *Diabetes Educ* 26:265–271, 2000

Dailey G, Admane K, Mercier F, Owens D: Relationship of insulin dose, A1c lowering, and weight in type 2 diabetes: comparing insulin glargine and insulin detemir. *Diabetes Technol Ther* 12:1019–1027, 2010

Danne T, Datz N, Endahl L, Haahr H, Nestoris C, Westergaard L, Fjording MS, Kordonouri O: Insulin detemir is characterized by a more reproducible pharmacokinetic profile than insulin glargine in children and adolescents with type

1 diabetes: results from a randomized, double-blind, controlled trial. *Pediatr Diabetes* 9:554–560, 2008

De Leeuw I, Vague P, Selam JL, Skeie S, Lang H, Draeger E, Elte JW: Insulin detemir used in basal-bolus therapy in people with type 1 diabetes is associated with a lower risk of nocturnal hypoglycaemia and less weight gain over 12 months in comparison to NPH insulin. *Diabetes Obes Metab* 7:73–82, 2005

Delvecchio M, Zecchino C, Salzano G, Faienza MF, Cavallo L, De Luca F, Lombardo F: Effects of moderate-severe exercise on blood glucose in type 1 diabetic adolescents treated with insulin pump or glargine insulin. *J Endocrinol Invest* 32:519–524, 2009

Diabetes Research in Children Network Study Group, Tsalikian E, Kollman C, Tamborlane WB, Beck RW, Fiallo-Scharer R, Fox L, Janz KF, Ruedy KJ, Wilson D, Xing D, Weinzimer SA: Prevention of hypoglycemia during exercise in children with type 1 diabetes by suspending basal insulin. *Diabetes Care* 29:2200–2204, 2006

Ertl AC, Davis SN: Evidence for a vicious cycle of exercise and hypoglycemia in type 1 diabetes mellitus. *Diabetes Metab Res Rev* 20:124–130, 2004

Farmer A, Balman E, Gadsby R, Moffatt J, Cradock S, McEwen L, Jameson K: Frequency of self-monitoring of blood glucose in patients with type 2 diabetes: association with hypoglycaemic events. *Curr Med Res Opin* 24:3097–3104, 2008

Guerci B, Sauvanet JP: Subcutaneous insulin: pharmacokinetic variability and glycemic variability. *Diabetes Metab* 31 (4 Pt 2):4S7–4S24, 2005

Guillausseau PJ, Meas T, Virally M, Laloi-Michelin M, Medeau V, Kevorkian JP: Abnormalities in insulin secretion in type 2 diabetes mellitus. *Diabetes Metab* 34 (Suppl. 2):S43–S48, 2008

Hanaire-Broutin H, Melki V, Bessieres-Lacombe S, Tauber JP: Comparison of continuous subcutaneous insulin infusion and multiple daily injection regimens using insulin lispro in type 1 diabetic patients on intensified treatment: a randomized study. The Study Group for the Development of Pump Therapy in Diabetes. *Diabetes Care* 23:1232–1235, 2000

Hansen MV, Pedersen-Bjergaard U, Heller SR, Wallace TM, Rasmussen AK, Jorgensen HV, Pramming S, Thorsteinsson B: Frequency and motives of blood glucose self-monitoring in type 1 diabetes. *Diabetes Res Clin Pract* 85:183–188, 2009

Heise T, Nosek L, Spitzer H, Heinemann L, Niemoller E, Frick AD, Becker RH: Insulin glulisine: a faster onset of action compared with insulin lispro. *Diabetes Obes Metab* 9:746–753, 2007

Hernandez JM, Moccia T, Fluckey JD, Ulbrecht JS, Farrell PA: Fluid snacks to help persons with type 1 diabetes avoid late onset postexercise hypoglycemia. *Med Sci Sports Exerc* 32:904–910, 2000

Home PD, Meneghini L, Wendisch U, Ratner RE, Johansen T, Christensen TE, Jendle J, Roberts AP, Birkeland KI: Improved health status with insulin degludec compared with insulin glargine in people with type 1 diabetes. *Diabet Med* 29:716–720, 2012

Jankovec Z, Krcma M, Gruberova J, Komorousova J, Tomesova J, Zourek M, Rusavy Z: Influence of physical activity on metabolic state within a 3-h interruption of continuous subcutaneous insulin infusion in patients with type 1 diabetes. *Diabetes Technol Ther* 13:1234–1239, 2011

Kahn SE, Montgomery B, Howell W, Ligueros-Saylan M, Hsu CH, Devineni D, McLeod JF, Horowitz A, Foley JE: Importance of early phase insulin secretion to intravenous glucose tolerance in subjects with type 2 diabetes mellitus. *J Clin Endocrinol Metab* 86:5824–5829, 2001

Kalergis M, Schiffrin A, Gougeon R, Jones PJ, Yale JF: Impact of bedtime snack composition on prevention of nocturnal hypoglycemia in adults with type 1 diabetes undergoing intensive insulin management using lispro insulin before meals: a randomized, placebo-controlled, crossover trial. *Diabetes Care* 26:9–15, 2003

Kilbride L, Charlton J, Aitken G, Hill GW, Davison RC, McKnight JA: Managing blood glucose during and after exercise in type 1 diabetes: reproducibility of glucose response and a trial of a structured algorithm adjusting insulin and carbohydrate intake. *J Clin Nurs* 20:3423–3429, 2011

King AB: Once-daily insulin detemir is comparable to once-daily insulin glargine in providing glycaemic control over 24 h in patients with type 2 diabetes: a double-blind, randomized, crossover study. *Diabetes Obes Metab* 11:69–71, 2009

Kitabchi AE, Gosmanov AR: Safety of rapid-acting insulin analogs versus regular human insulin. *Am J Med Sci* 344:136–141, 2012

Kordonouri O, Hartmann R, Danne T: Treatment of type 1 diabetes in children and adolescents using modern insulin pumps. *Diabetes Res Clin Pract* 93 (Suppl. 1):S118–S124, 2011

Kreisman SH, Halter JB, Vranic M, Marliss EB: Combined infusion of epinephrine and norepinephrine during moderate exercise reproduces the glucoregulatory response of intense exercise. *Diabetes* 52:1347–1354, 2003

Larsen JJ, Dela F, Madsbad S, Galbo H: The effect of intense exercise on postprandial glucose homeostasis in type II diabetic patients. *Diabetologia* 42:1282–1292, 1999

Lindholm A, Jacobsen: Clinical pharmacokinetics and pharmacodynamics of insulin aspart. *Clin Pharmacokinet* 40:641–659, 2001

Luzio SD, Beck P, Owens DR: Comparison of the subcutaneous absorption of insulin glargine (Lantus) and NPH insulin in patients with type 2 diabetes. *Horm Metab Res* 35:434–438, 2003

Maahs DM, Horton LA, Chase HP: The use of insulin pumps in youth with type 1 diabetes. *Diabetes Technol Ther* 12 (Suppl. 1):S59–S65, 2010

MacDonald MJ: Postexercise late-onset hypoglycemia in insulin-dependent diabetic patients. *Diabetes Care* 10:584–588, 1987

McAdam-Marx C, Bouchard J, Aagren M, Nelson R, Brixner D: Analysis of glycaemic control and weight change in patients initiated with human or analog insulin in an US ambulatory care setting. *Diabetes Obes Metab* 12:54–64, 2010

Mitchell TH, Abraham G, Schiffrin A, Leiter LA, Marliss EB: Hyperglycemia after intense exercise in IDDM subjects during continuous subcutaneous insulin infusion. *Diabetes Care* 11:311–317, 1988

Monami M, Marchionni N, Mannucci E: Long-acting insulin analogues vs. NPH human insulin in type 1 diabetes. A meta-analysis. *Diabetes Obes Metab* 11:372–378, 2009

Morello CM: Pharmacokinetics and pharmacodynamics of insulin analogs in special populations with type 2 diabetes mellitus. *Int J Gen Med* 4:827–835, 2011

Nasrallah SN, Reynolds LR: Insulin degludec, the new generation basal insulin or just another basal insulin? *Clin Med Insights Endocrinol Diabetes* 5:31–37, 2012

Nelson SE: Detemir as a once-daily basal insulin in type 2 diabetes. *Clin Pharmacol* 3:27–37, 2011

Peter R, Luzio SD, Dunseath G, Miles A, Hare B, Backx K, Pauvaday V, Owens DR: Effects of exercise on the absorption of insulin glargine in patients with type 1 diabetes. *Diabetes Care* 28:560–565, 2005

Plockinger U, Topuz M, Riese B, Reuter T: Risk of exercise-induced hypoglycaemia in patients with type 2 diabetes on intensive insulin therapy: comparison of insulin glargine with NPH insulin as basal insulin supplement. *Diabetes Res Clin Pract* 81:290–295, 2008

Poirier P, Mawhinney S, Grondin L, Tremblay A, Broderick T, Cleroux J, Catellier C, Tancrede G, Nadeau A: Prior meal enhances the plasma glucose lowering effect of exercise in type 2 diabetes. *Med Sci Sports Exerc* 33:1259–1264, 2001

Poirier P, Tremblay A, Catellier C, Tancrede G, Garneau C, Nadeau A: Impact of time interval from the last meal on glucose response to exercise in subjects with type 2 diabetes. *J Clin Endocrinol Metab* 85:2860–2864, 2000

Rabasa-Lhoret R, Bourque J, Ducros F, Chiasson JL: Guidelines for premeal insulin dose reduction for postprandial exercise of different intensities and durations in type 1 diabetic subjects treated intensively with a basal-bolus insulin regimen (ultralente-lispro). *Diabetes Care* 24:625–630, 2001

Rave K, Klein O, Frick AD, Becker RH: Advantage of premeal-injected insulin glulisine compared with regular human insulin in subjects with type 1 diabetes. *Diabetes Care* 29:1812–1817, 2006

Schutt M, Kern W, Krause U, Busch P, Dapp A, Grziwotz R, Mayer I, Rosenbauer J, Wagner C, Zimmermann A, Kerner W, Holl RW, DPV Initiative: Is the frequency of self-monitoring of blood glucose related to long-term metabolic control? Multicenter analysis including 24,500 patients from 191 centers in Germany and Austria. *Exp Clin Endocrinol Diabetes* 114:384–388, 2006

Shanik MH: Intensifying insulin therapy with insulin analog premixes: transitioning from basal insulin in type 2 diabetes. *Diabetes Technol Ther* 14:533–539, 2012

Sigal RJ, Fisher SJ, Halter JB, Vranic M, Marliss EB: Glucoregulation during and after intense exercise: effects of beta-adrenergic blockade in subjects with type 1 diabetes mellitus. *J Clin Endocrinol Metab* 84:3961–3971, 1999

Sigal RJ, Purdon C, Fisher SJ, Halter JB, Vranic M, Marliss EB: Hyperinsulinemia prevents prolonged hyperglycemia after intense exercise in insulin-dependent diabetic subjects. *J Clin Endocrinol Metab* 79:1049–1057, 1994

St John A, Davis WA, Price CP, Davis TM: The value of self-monitoring of blood glucose: a review of recent evidence. *J Diabetes Complications* 24:129–141, 2010

Swinnen SG, Simon AC, Holleman F, Hoekstra JB, Devries JH: Insulin detemir versus insulin glargine for type 2 diabetes mellitus. *Cochrane Database Syst Rev* 6):CD006383, 2011

Szewieczek J, Dulawa J, Strzalkowska D, Batko-Szwaczka A, Hornik B: Normal insulin response to short-term intense exercise is abolished in type 2 diabetic patients treated with gliclazide. *J Diabetes Complications* 23:380–386, 2009

Szewieczek J, Dulawa J, Strzalkowska D, Hornik B, Kawecki G: Impact of the short-term, intense exercise on postprandial glycemia in type 2 diabetic patients treated with gliclazide. *J Diabetes Complications* 21:101–107, 2007

Taplin CE, Cobry E, Messer L, McFann K, Chase HP, Fiallo-Scharer R: Preventing post-exercise nocturnal hypoglycemia in children with type 1 diabetes. *J Pediatr* 157:784–788 e1, 2010

ter Braak EW, Woodworth JR, Bianchi R, Cerimele B, Erkelens DW, Thijssen JH, Kurtz D: Injection site effects on the pharmacokinetics and glucodynamics of insulin lispro and regular insulin. *Diabetes Care* 19:1437–1440, 1996

Tsalikian E, Mauras N, Beck RW, Tamborlane WV, Janz KF, Chase HP, Wysocki T, Weinzimer SA, Buckingham BA, Kollman C, Xing D, Ruedy KJ, Group Diabetes Research in Children Network DirecNet Study: Impact of exercise on overnight glycemic control in children with type 1 diabetes mellitus. *J Pediatr* 147:528–534, 2005

van Bon AC, Bode BW, Sert-Langeron C, DeVries JH, Charpentier G: Insulin glulisine compared to insulin aspart and to insulin lispro administered by continuous subcutaneous insulin infusion in patients with type 1 diabetes: a randomized controlled trial. *Diabetes Technol Ther* 13:607–614, 2011

Vinik A: Advancing therapy in type 2 diabetes mellitus with early, comprehensive progression from oral agents to insulin therapy. *Clin Ther* 29 (Spec No.):1236–1253, 2007

Wang Z, Hedrington MS, Gogitidze Joy N, Briscoe VJ, Richardson MA, Younk L, Nicholson W, Tate DB, Davis SN: Dose-response effects of insulin glargine in type 2 diabetes. *Diabetes Care* 33:1555–1560, 2010

Weinzimer SA, Ternand C, Howard C, Chang CT, Becker DJ, Laffel LM, Insulin Aspart Pediatric Pump Study Group: A randomized trial comparing continuous subcutaneous insulin infusion of insulin aspart versus insulin lispro in children and adolescents with type 1 diabetes. *Diabetes Care* 31:210–215, 2008

West DJ, Morton RD, Bain SC, Stephens JW, Bracken RM: Blood glucose responses to reductions in pre-exercise rapid-acting insulin for 24 h after running in individuals with type 1 diabetes. *J Sports Sci* 28:781–788, 2010

West DJ, Stephens JW, Bain SC, Kilduff LP, Luzio S, Still R, Bracken RM: A combined insulin reduction and carbohydrate feeding strategy 30 min before running best preserves blood glucose concentration after exercise through improved fuel oxidation in type 1 diabetes mellitus. *J Sports Sci* 29:279–289, 2011

Zachariah S, Sheldon B, Shojaee-Moradie F, Jackson NC, Backhouse K, Johnsen S, Jones RH, Umpleby AM, Russell-Jones DL: Insulin detemir reduces weight gain as a result of reduced food intake in patients with type 1 diabetes. *Diabetes Care* 34:1487–1491, 2011

Zinman B, Fulcher G, Rao PV, Thomas N, Endahl LA, Johansen T, Lindh R, Lewin A, Rosenstock J, Pinget M, Mathieu C: Insulin degludec, an ultra-long-acting basal insulin, once a day or three times a week versus insulin glargine once a day in patients with type 2 diabetes: a 16-week, randomised, open-label, phase 2 trial. *Lancet* 377:924–931, 2011

Chapter 15

Other Medication Effects on Physical Activity

The majority of people with type 2 diabetes (T2D) rely on a combination of diet, exercise, and medication to control their blood glucose levels and overcome insulin resistance. Oral antihyperglycemic agents are widely prescribed for T2D when onset is recent and often are prescribed individually or in combination to optimize glucose control (Gerich 2005, Krentz 2005, Phung 2010). Most individuals are overweight or obese at diagnosis and will be unable to achieve or sustain near normoglycemia without oral antidiabetic agents. Moreover, a sizeable proportion of these individuals eventually will require insulin therapy to maintain long-term glycemic control, either as monotherapy or in conjunction with oral antidiabetic therapy (Krentz 2005).

At present, oral and other injectable agents (besides insulin) are prescribed to target different areas of the body that affect blood glucose control, including the pancreas (causing insulin release), liver (lowering hepatic glucose production), gut (slowing absorption of carbohydrates), and muscles (improving insulin action). They vary in their relative risk of causing hypoglycemia, although most of them carry little or no risk (Phung 2010). Individuals with T2D, however, will benefit from self-monitoring of blood glucose (SMBG) to determine the effects of physical activity on their diabetes management even though they are much less likely to develop hypoglycemia or diabetic ketoacidosis (DKA) with exercise participation (Farmer 2008).

Case in Point: Blood Glucose and Weight Management in an Older Adult with T2D

BJ is a 74-year-old woman with T2D that was diagnosed when she turned 60 years old. Her blood glucose management was initially excellent with lifestyle changes alone (diet and exercise), but over time her control has worsened, particularly of late. Currently, she takes maximal daily doses of metformin and glyburide (a sulfonylurea) to manage her glycemic levels, along with a blood pressure medication for her elevated systolic blood pressure and a statin for her high cholesterol levels. She is scared to death of having to start taking insulin shots, which her doctor warned her may be necessary in the near future if her diabetes control fails to improve. She currently engages in almost daily walking for 20–30 min at a moderate pace, after which she occasionally develops hypoglycemia that she treats by eating cake icing. In addition, she takes a tai chi class once a week on Saturday mornings.

Resting Measurements

Height: 62 inches
Weight: 185 lb
BMI: 33.8 (obese)
Heart rate: 84 beats per minute (bpm)
Blood pressure: 125/78 mmHg (on medication for elevated systolic blood pressure)

Fasting Labs

Plasma glucose: 175 mg/dl (controlled with metformin and glyburide)
A1C: 8.0% (at her last visit, but in the 7.0–7.5% range previously)
Total cholesterol: 185 mg/dl (on medication)
Triglycerides: 215 mg/dl
High-density lipoprotein cholesterol: 55 mg/dl
Low-density lipoprotein cholesterol: 87 mg/dl

Questions to Consider

1. Are there any other lifestyle changes that BJ can make to avoid having to go on insulin?
2. Would BJ benefit from any other type of exercise training besides walking and tai chi?
3. Do any of the medications that BJ takes for diabetes affect her risk for hypoglycemia?
4. Should BJ be considering using any other diabetes medications instead of what she takes?
5. Do any of the other medications she takes for other conditions have any exercise effects?

(Continued on page 264.)

GENERAL CATEGORIES AND TYPES OF DIABETES MEDICATIONS

Traditional antihyperglycemic treatment strategies promote combination therapies that address the three major defects evident in T2D: impaired peripheral glucose uptake (liver, fat, and muscle), excessive hepatic glucose release (glucagon excess), and insufficient insulin secretion (pancreatic β-cells). Only recently has recognition of the critical role of the gastrointestinal system as a major culprit in glucose dysregulation been established (Kuritzky 2011). Newer strategies involve decreasing the rate of carbohydrate absorption from the gut (small intestine) to slow the increase in postprandial blood glucose levels as well as mimicking bodily peptides or increasing levels of peptides that prevent degradation of natural insulin-stimulating enzymes (Ratner 2004, Want 2008, Freeman 2009, Bergenstal 2010, Cuthbertson 2011).

A list of all the diabetes medications can be found in Table 15.1, along with their generic and trade names and general mechanisms of action. Insulin is not included in that list because it is covered fully in chapter 14. All of these medications are also included in appendix A.

Table 15.1 Oral and Other Diabetes Medications

Class of Drug	Brand Name Examples (Generic Names)	Mechanism of Action
Sulfonylureas	Diabinese (chlorpropamide) Amaryl (glimepiride) Glucotrol, Glucotrol XL (glipizide) DiaBeta, Micronase, Glynase, PresTab (glyburide)	Promote insulin secretion from the β-cells of the pancreas; some may increase insulin sensitivity
Biguanides	Glucophage, Glucophage XR (metformin)	Decrease liver glucose output; increase liver and muscle insulin sensitivity; no direct effect on β-cells
Thiazolidene-diones (glitazones or TZDs)	Avandia (rosiglitazone) Actos (pioglitazone)	Increase insulin sensitivity of peripheral tissues, such as muscle; however, Avandia has been associated with increased risk of heart attack and stroke, and now both medications in this class must carry an FDA "black box" warning on their labels; Avandia use is also now severely restricted by the FDA in the U.S.
Meglitinides	Prandin (repaglinide) Starlix (nateglinide) Glufast (mitiglinide)	Stimulate β-cells to increase insulin secretion but only for a very short duration (unlike sulfonylureas, which have a longer action)
α-Glucosidase inhibitors	Precose (acarbose) Glyset (miglitol)	Work in intestines to slow digestion of some carbohydrates to control postmeal blood glucose peaks
DPP-4 inhibitors (gliptins)	Januvia (sitagliptin) Galvus (vildagliptin) Onglyza (saxagliptin) Tradjenta (linagliptin)	Work by inhibiting DPP-4, an enzyme that breaks down glucagon-like peptide-1 (GLP-1) in the gut; delayed GLP-1 degradation extends the action of insulin while suppressing glucagon release
Amylin (injected)	Symlin (pramlintide)	Works in combination with insulin to control glycemic spikes for 3 h after meals
Incretins (injected)	Byetta (exenatide) Bydureon (exenatide XR) Victoza (liraglutide)	Stimulate insulin release; inhibit the liver's release of glucose by glucagon; delay the emptying of food from the stomach

Note: DPP-4, dipeptidyl peptidase-4; FDA, Food and Drug Administration; TZDs, thiazolidinediones.

MEDICATIONS TO IMPROVE INSULIN ACTION

Some diabetes medications improve insulin sensitivity in skeletal muscles, adipose tissue, and the liver, and others promote muscle glucose uptake and inhibit hepatic glucose output. The most widely prescribed diabetes medication, metformin, targets both hepatic glucose output (especially overnight while fasting) and peripheral insulin action (Nicholson 2009, Phung 2010, McIntosh 2011, Malin 2012). Initial treatment of T2D is usually with metformin alone, but often a second agent (like a sulfonylurea or nateglinide) is added for maximal glucose lowering for the first 2 years (Gerich 2005). In general, these medications mainly improve the action of insulin or lower hepatic glucose production at rest, not during exercise, so their risk of causing exercise-associated hypoglycemia is low (Krentz 2005, Boulé 2011).

PANCREATIC β-CELL STIMULANTS TO ENHANCE INSULIN RELEASE

Medications that stimulate insulin release (primarily sulfonylureas and meglitinides) are taken at mealtime to better manage postprandial glycemia (Larsen 1999, Krentz 2005, McIntosh 2011). Because of their effect on insulin release, these oral agents may lead to hypoglycemia with or without exercise (Larsen 1999, Rendell 2004). The prolonged length of action of some of these agents (most of the earlier generation sulfonylureas and some later ones) increases the risk for hypoglycemia, leading to a need for more frequent SMBG when individuals with T2D are regularly exercising (Larsen 1999). Moreover, sulfonylureas frequently contribute to weight gain, and a considerable proportion of individuals with T2D treated with sulfonylureas are not aware of the risks of hypoglycemia and weight gain associated with the treatment (Lund 2012).

MEDICATIONS TO SLOW INTESTINAL ABSORPTION OF CARBOHYDRATES

Another gastrointestinal-related phenomenon in diabetes is the absence of first-phase insulin secretion (Del Prato 2001). In healthy individuals, a dietary glucose load is met with an almost immediate insulin response known as first-phase insulin release; this prompt response by preformed insulin keeps pace with rapidly rising glycemia. Because of the absence of first-phase insulin release in individuals with T2D, rapidly rising glucose levels result in inappropriate tissue exposure during postprandial glucose peaks. α-Glucosidase inhibitors (e.g., acarbose) address this defect by slowing glucose absorption. Some newer peptide analogs that are injectable (e.g., exenatide and liraglutide) also delay gastric emptying (see more on these medications in the following section, Medications to Mimic the Effects of Gastric Peptides) (Polster 2011). Likewise, lifestyle modifications like choosing a low-glycemic index diet additionally produce a less rapid rise in glucose levels (Turner-McGrievy 2011).

MEDICATIONS TO MIMIC THE EFFECTS OF GASTRIC PEPTIDES

The gastrointestinal tract increasingly is recognized as a critical organ in blood glucose metabolism and regulation. Accordingly, some newer medications have been approved called incretin mimetics, which mimic the action of natural gut hormones that function as glucagon-like peptide-1 (GLP-1) receptor agonists, such as exenatide and liraglutide. These injectable medications help the pancreas release more insulin while slowing the rate of digestion so that glucose enters the blood more slowly (Polster 2011). It has been suggested that >50% of meal-stimulated insulin production is likely attributable to intestinal incretins (Freeman 2009). Although an extended-release, once-weekly injection of exenatide has been approved (as trade name Bydureon), clinical trials currently are under way to come up with alternate methods of delivery of this medication, such as orally or via a subcutaneous minipump that lasts 1 year, to increase patient compliance with treatment regimens.

Closely related to incretins are the dipeptidyl peptidase-4 (DPP-4) inhibitors, of which sitagliptin, vildagliptin, and linagliptin are examples (Del Prato 2011, Singh-Franco 2012). The mechanism of DPP-4 inhibitors is to increase levels of GLP-1 and gastric inhibitory peptide (GIP), both of which inhibit glucagon release. Once glucagon is blocked, increased insulin secretion and lower blood glucose levels are the result (Neumiller 2010). It is believed that DPP-4 inhibition lowers postprandial glucose concentrations via its effects on islet secretion rather than by delaying gastric emptying or reducing the rate at which ingested glucose enters the systemic circulation. Alterations in islet function, secondary to increased active GLP-1, are associated with the decreased postprandial glycemic excursion observed in the presence of vildagliptin, without differences in satiation or gastric volume despite these elevated levels of GLP-1 (Vella 2007, 2008).

DPP-4 inhibitors have become widely accepted in clinical practice because of their low risk of hypoglycemia, few adverse effects, and once-daily dosing. They are weight neutral (meaning that they do not cause weight gain or loss) and appear to decrease β-cell apoptosis and increase β-cell survival (Neumiller 2010). Metformin also inhibits DPP-4 activity and thus increases active GLP-1 concentrations after subcutaneous injection of exenatide, with the combination of the two medications being more effective in lowering glucose concentrations in adults with T2D compared with exenatide alone (Cuthbertson 2011).

EFFECTS OF DIABETES MEDICATIONS ON PHYSICAL ACTIVITY

Some diabetes medications increase the risk of hypoglycemia, whereas others do not. Table 15.2 lists all diabetes medications and their relative risk of causing both resting and exercise-associated decreases in blood glucose levels.

INSULIN

Medication adjustments to prevent hypoglycemia associated with physical activity are generally necessary only for individuals with T2D who use insulin or select insulin secretagogues (Larsen 1999, Rosenstock 2004). For anyone who is

Table 15.2 Hypoglycemia Risk with Use of Diabetes Medications

No or Minimal Risk	Higher Risk

Metformin (and combinations):
  Glucophage
  AvandaMet
    (metformin/rosiglitazone)
  JanuMet
    (metformin/sitagliptin)
  Jentadueto
    (metformin/linagliptin)
 	
α-Glucosidase inhibitors:
  Acarbose: Precose
  Miglitol: Glyset
 	
Thiazolidenediones:
  Pioglitazone: Actos
  Rosiglitizone: Avandia
 	
DPP-4 inhibitors:
  Sitagliptin: Januvia
  Vildagliptin: Galvus
  Saxagliptin: Onglyza
  Linagliptin: Tradjenta
 	
Amylin:
  Pramlintide: Symlin
 	
Incretins:
  Exenatide: Byetta
  Exenatide XR: Bydureon
  Liraglutide: Victoza
	Sulfonylureas (*highest risk):
	  Chlorpropamide: *Diabinese
	  Glyburide and combinations:
	    *DiaBeta
	    *Micronase
	    *Glynase
	    *PresTab
	    *Glucovance (glyburide/metformin)
	  Glimepiride:
	    Amaryl
	    Avandaryl
	    (glimepiride/rosiglitazone)
	  Glipizide and combinations:
	    Glucotrol, Glucotrol XL
	    MetaGlip (glipizide/metformin)
	
	Meglitindes:
	  Nateglinide: Starlix
	  Repaglinide: Prandin
	
	Insulin:
	  All types and delivery methods

Note: DPP-4, dipeptidyl peptidase-4.

an insulin user, short- or rapid-acting insulin doses may need to be reduced for exercise closely following its use to prevent hypoglycemia. (For a full discussion of insulin adjustments for physical activity, see chapter 14.) Newer, rapid-acting insulin analogs (i.e., lispro, aspart, and glulisine) induce more rapid decreases in blood glucose levels than regular human insulin. Thus, individuals who use these analogs need to monitor their blood glucose levels more frequently with physical activity to make compensatory dietary or medication regimen changes, particularly when exercising at insulin peak times. If only longer-acting insulins like glargine and detemir are being absorbed from subcutaneous depots during physical activity, exercise-induced hypoglycemia is not as likely (Plockinger 2008), although doses may need to be reduced to accommodate regular exercise participation.

INSULIN SECRETAGOGUES

The insulin secretagogues that carry the highest risk are the ones sold as generic glyburide (i.e., DiaBeta, Micronase, Glynase, and PresTab) or chlorprop-amide (Diabinese), all of which have a longer duration. (A full list of medications that increase hypoglycemia risk is included in Table 15.2.) Meglitinides also have a short-term effect on insulin secretion (intended to cover postprandial insulin needs) and may increase risk but generally to a lesser extent than sulfonylureas like glyburide because of their shorter duration (Rosenstock 2004, Bellomo Damato 2011, Kim 2011). Treatment with nateglinide or repaglinide may result in a higher incidence of hypoglycemia at the beginning of treatment (Vlckova 2009). To avoid hypoglycemia, individuals may need to reduce doses of any oral medications taken immediately before and possibly after exercise (Larsen 1999, Galbo 2007). Over-all, doses of select oral hypoglycemic agents (glyburide, glipizide, glimepiride, nateglinide, and repaglinide) also may need to be lowered in response to regular exercise training if an individual's frequency of hypoglycemic events increases (Larsen 1999, Rosenstock 2004).

OTHER DIABETES MEDICATIONS

Medications that decrease carbohydrate absorption rate and slow the increase in postprandial blood glucose levels have no direct effect on exercise responses. They can, however, possibly delay effective treatment of hypoglycemia during activities by slowing the absorption of carbohydrates ingested to treat this condi-tion (Krentz 2005). Some insulin users may take injections of a synthetic analog (i.e., pramlintide) to replace the hormone amylin that usually is cosecreted with insulin from the β-cells of the pancreas. The use of such an analog can complicate the treatment of exercise-induced hypoglycemia given that it slows the absorption of ingested carbohydrate from the gut and likely should not be taken before engaging in an acute bout of exercise (Want 2008).

Conversely, use of certain medications may instead lower hypoglycemia and even cardiovascular risk. For example, after 84 weeks, adults with T2D treated with exenatide just once a week continued to experience better glycemic control with sustained overall weight loss and a lower risk of hypoglycemia than those treated with insulin glargine (Diamant 2012). Similarly, when combined with life-style modification, exenatide treatment leads to significant weight loss, improved glycemic control, and decreased blood pressure compared with lifestyle modifica-tion alone in overweight or obese participants with T2D on metformin or sulfo-nylurea treatment (Apovian 2010). Moreover, saxagliptin may lower the risk of major adverse cardiovascular events in adults with T2D (Cobble 2012).

Other physiological responses to physical activity may or may not be affected by some diabetes medications. In one study, progressive exercise performed to exhaustion in the postprandial state did not worsen glucose control during and after exercise for people with T2D taking their usual dose of glyburide or metfor-min, and those medications had no impact on their cardiovascular, metabolic, and hormonal response to exercise (Cunha 2008). Along the same lines, in women with T2D, their usual dose of glibenclamide or metformin was taken before post-prandial exercise of moderate intensity without affecting their cardiovascular, metabolic, and hormonal responses. After exercise, these two medications prevent the normal rise in blood glucose, and metformin delays the fall in plasma lactate concentrations (Cunha 2007).

Certain diabetes medications also may affect assessment of other parameters, such as risk of falls or other adverse outcomes, potentially those associated with physical activity. For example, a recent study assessed whether any link exists between metformin and falls in older individuals with T2D (Berlie 2010). Long-term metformin use may result in peripheral neuropathy secondary to vitamin B_{12} deficiency, but its symptoms may be avoided or improved with supplementation of this vitamin in higher doses (Pflipsen 2009, Mizukami 2011, Solomon 2011, Reinstatler 2012). Insulin use additionally has been demonstrated to increase the risk of falls in the elderly, and thiazolidinediones increase fracture risk and may worsen fall-related outcomes. Thus, when creating a physical activity plan, the risk of falls and fall-related complications associated with these medications should not be ignored in certain populations.

Case in Point: Continued

BJ's blood glucose levels have continued to climb despite her best efforts, and she is afraid that she is going to have to revisit the insulin issue with her physician during her next visit. Because of her frequent hypoglycemic episodes (at least three times a week following walking), she also has been steadily gaining some extra weight, and she desperately wants to lose it to help with her diabetes control, plus her pants have been getting uncomfortably tight. She had started walking more after her last visit when her blood glucose levels were climbing; at that visit, her physician also increased her oral medication doses to maximal levels.

Additional Questions to Consider

1. Does BJ need to take lower doses of her current diabetes medications to prevent hypoglycemia, or is there another strategy that is more effective for reducing her risk?
2. Because weight gain from frequent hypoglycemia treatment is a concern, can she undertake any medication or lifestyle modifications to help her lose weight?

(Continued on page 267.)

EFFECT OF PHYSICAL ACTIVITY ON DIABETES MEDICATIONS

In many cases, regular participation in physical activity lowers the need for any diabetes medications. By way of example, one study examined older adults with T2D undertaking 16 weeks of progressive resistance training three times per week. Their participation resulted in lower A1C levels, increased muscle glycogen stores, and lower doses of all prescribed diabetes medication in 72% of participants (Castaneda 2002).

In other instances, physical activity may interfere with some medication effects. In one study, individuals with T2D performed a total of 35 min of exercise at three different submaximal intensities after taking metformin for 28 days. Metformin use increased heart rate and plasma lactate during exercise, along with fat oxidation. Although their glycemic response to a meal was reduced by metformin, exercise attenuated the reduction, likely because of the fact that glucagon levels were highest under those conditions. Thus, metformin and exercise therapies can affect each other, with exercise interfering with the glucose-lowering effect of metformin and increasing resting heart rate, thereby possibly leading to the prescription of lower exercise workloads based on heart rate (Boulé 2011). Similarly, in adults with prediabetes, although insulin sensitivity was considerably higher after 12 weeks of exercise training or metformin, adding this medication appeared to blunt the full beneficial effect of exercise training (Malin 2012).

OTHER DIABETES MEDICATION CONSIDERATIONS

The goal of most individuals with diabetes is to achieve optimum glucose control, along with weight loss and a minimum number of hypoglycemic events. All classes of antihyperglycemic medications used in combination with metformin demonstrate similar A1C reductions, but differences in weight gain and risk of hypoglycemia (Phung 2010). For instance, thiazolidinediones, sulfonylureas, and meglitinides are associated with weight gain, whereas GLP-1 agonists, α-glucosidase inhibitors, and DPP-4 inhibitors are associated with weight loss or no weight change. Other have found that the addition of exenatide once weekly to metformin also achieved these goals more often than did addition of maximum daily doses of either sitagliptin or pioglitazone (Bergenstal 2010). Moreover, pioglitazone results in weight gain, whereas sitagliptin caused some weight loss, but a lesser amount compared with exenatide once weekly or metformin (Russell-Jones 2012). Treatment with exenatide and liraglutide also leads to weight loss in overweight or obese patients with T2D (Vilsboll 2012). One study also reported that treatment with liraglutide in adults with type 1 diabetes (T1D) reduces their insulin requirements, with improved or unaltered glycemic control (Kielgast 2011).

Exenatide taken once weekly and metformin both result in similar improvements in glycemic control, along with weight reduction and no increased risk of hypoglycemia in a 26-week trial (Russell-Jones 2012). Hypoglycemia is uncommon using any of these medications, except when combined with a sulfonylurea (Shyangdan 2010); however, meglitinides also are associated with higher rates of hypoglycemia. The most common adverse events associated with all GLP-1 agonists are initial nausea and vomiting. GLP-1 agonists additionally have some effect on β-cell function that is not sustained after individuals stop taking them (Shyangdan 2010).

EFFECTS OF NONDIABETES MEDICATIONS ON PHYSICAL ACTIVITY

Diabetic individuals with comorbid health issues frequently are prescribed a variety of other medications, including β-blockers, diuretics, angiotensin converting enzyme inhibitors (ACE inhibitors), aspirin, lipid-lowering agents, and more. These medications generally do not affect exercise responses, with some notable exceptions that follow.

β-Receptor blocking medications. β-Blockers are known to blunt heart rate responses to exercise and lower maximal exercise capacity by 13% due to their negative inotropic and chronotropic effects (Sigal 1994). They also may block adrenergic symptoms of decreasing blood glucose levels, increasing the risk of experiencing an undetected hypoglycemic event during exercise. However, β-blockers may increase exercise capacity in individuals with coronary artery disease by reducing coronary ischemia during physical activity (de Muinck 1990).

Antihypertensive medications. Many individuals with T2D have hypertension. Although a nonpharmacologic approach is recommended as a first-line treatment for individuals with diabetes, if the main goal of lowering blood pressure to 135/85 mmHg is not attained, one or more medications may be prescribed (Grossman 2011). Patients at high risk for vascular disease, such as those with diabetes, have aggressive blood pressure targets because studies have shown that achieving these targets reduces events like acute coronary syndromes and stroke (Crawford 2009, Reboldi 2009). Of the possible prescribed medications, diuretics specifically may lower overall blood and fluid volumes and result in dehydration and electrolyte imbalances, particularly during exercise in the heat. Diuretics either should be potassium-sparing, or a potassium supplement should be given to prevent electrolyte imbalances that can affect exercise participation negatively (Caldwell 1987).

Cholesterol-lowering medication. The most commonly used medications for cholesterol reduction are currently several from the class of "statins," such as atorvastatin (Lipitor and Torvast), pravastatin (Pravachol and Selektine), and rosuvastatin (Crestar). They are actually HMG-CoA reductase inhibitors that work by inhibiting the enzyme HMG-CoA reductase, which plays a central role in the production of cholesterol in the liver. Although memory loss and T2D may be associated with statin use, the most common adverse side effects are raised liver enzymes and muscle problems that can affect the ability to exercise. Statin use has been associated with an elevated risk of myopathies (myalgia and myositis), particularly when combined with use of fibrates and niacin, although the risk of myopathy is very low (Nichols 2007). Statins, however, have been shown to increase exercise-related muscle injury, and susceptibility to such damage rises with advancing age (Parker 2012). In individuals unwilling or unable to change their diet and lifestyles sufficiently, the benefits of statins greatly exceed the risks, even with the potential for myotoxicity and an increase in the incidence of diabetes with their use (Kones 2010).

Case in Point: Wrap-Up

During her next visit, BJ's complaints about her frequent hypoglycemia and associated weight gain are taken seriously by her physician because he has wanted her to lose some weight to help manage her diabetes more effectively. He discusses two things with her: *1*) that she is having too many episodes of hypoglycemia associated with walking and her medication doses; and *2*) that it is time to rethink her medications. He decides to keep her on metformin but to replace glyburide with another medication less likely to cause hypoglycemia that also promotes weight loss.

Medication Regimen Changes: BJ really does not want to gain any more weight because of her medications or from frequent hypoglycemia treatment, so her physician agrees to forego switching her to insulin for the time being. Instead, he wants her to try a new medication, exenatide, once weekly (Bydureon). Even though it has to be injected, being able to do so only once a week significantly cuts down on the number of injections compared with using once-daily exenatide or daily injections of basal insulin. Exenatide is also well known to aid in weight loss given that it is a "weight-friendly" medication. She also will not have to worry about its causing her to develop hypoglycemia, as with glyburide.

Dietary Regimen Changes: BJ's physician suggests that she treat any hypoglycemic events with glucose (glucose tablets or candy containing dextrose, like Smarties) so that she takes in only a measured amount of carbohydrates and fewer calories (compared with an unknown quantity of cake icing). Also for the purposes of weight loss, she decides to cut back on her calorie intake by ~200–300 calories/day by focusing on taking in more natural, plant-based foods and fewer refined carbohydrates and red meats. She realizes that doing so may affect her blood glucose control, so she plans on using SMBG more often for a while to see the effects of her dietary (and medication) changes.

Physical Activity Regimen Changes: BJ now understands that moderate aerobic exercise is more likely to cause a decrease in her blood glucose levels (especially when taking a sulfonylurea) but that doing more intense activities may not have the same effect. She plans on trying to add in some faster intervals into her aerobic activities to use up more calories. In addition, she decides to add in some resistance training twice a week to see whether that will help her build muscle, lose body fat, and improve her overall diabetes control.

Use of oral antihyperglycemic agents, individually or as combination therapy, is common in individuals with T2D, together with improvements in lifestyle management. Oral and other injectable agents target different areas of the body that affect blood glucose control, including the pancreas, liver, gut, and muscles. Some of them can cause hypoglycemia, but most carry little or no risk. Individuals with T2D will benefit from using medications that allow safe physical activity participation and more effective weight management.

PROFESSIONAL PRACTICE PEARLS

- Oral and other antihyperglycemic agents, both individually and in combination, are widely prescribed for T2D when onset is recent and little or no insulin is taken.
- Oral and other injectable agents (besides insulin) are prescribed to target different areas of the body related to glycemic control, including the pancreas, liver, gut, and muscles.
- Medication dosage adjustments to prevent exercise-associated hypoglycemia may be required by individuals using insulin or certain insulin secretagogues.
- The insulin secretagogues that carry the highest risk are the ones sold as generic glyburide or chlorpropamide, which have a longer duration of action.
- Meglitinides also have a short-term effect on postprandial insulin secretion and may increase risk but generally to a lesser extent than sulfonylureas due to their short action.
- Overall doses of select oral hypoglycemic agents (glyburide, glipizide, glimepiride, nateglinide, and repaglinide) may need to be lowered for regular exercise participation.
- In other instances, physical activity may interfere with some medication effects; for example, metformin use may interfere with the full glucose-lowering effect of exercise.
- The goal of most individuals with diabetes is to achieve optimum glucose control, along with weight loss and a minimum number of hypoglycemic events.
- All classes of antihyperglycemic medications used in combination with metformin demonstrate similar A1C benefits but differences in weight gain and hypoglycemia risk.
- Most other medications prescribed for concomitant health problems do not affect exercise, with the exception of β-blockers, some diuretics, and statins.

REFERENCES

Apovian CM, Bergenstal RM, Cuddihy RM, Qu Y, Lenox S, Lewis MS, Glass LC: Effects of exenatide combined with lifestyle modification in patients with type 2 diabetes. *Am J Med* 123:468 e9–17, 2010

Bellomo Damato A, Stefanelli G, Laviola L, Giorgino R, Giorgino F: Nateglinide provides tighter glycaemic control than glyburide in patients with Type 2 diabetes with prevalent postprandial hyperglycaemia. *Diabet Med* 28:560–566, 2011

Bergenstal RM, Wysham C, Macconell L, Malloy J, Walsh B, Yan P, Wilhelm K, Malone J, Porter LE, Duration-Study Group: Efficacy and safety of exenatide once weekly versus sitagliptin or pioglitazone as an adjunct to metformin for treatment of type 2 diabetes (DURATION-2): a randomised trial. *Lancet* 376:431–439, 2010

Berlie HD, Garwood CL: Diabetes medications related to an increased risk of falls and fall-related morbidity in the elderly. *Ann Pharmacother* 44:712–717, 2010

Boulé NG, Robert C, Bell GJ, Johnson ST, Bell RC, Lewanczuk RZ, Gabr RQ, Brocks DR: Metformin and exercise in type 2 diabetes: examining treatment modality interactions. *Diabetes Care* 34:1469–1474, 2011

Caldwell JE: Diuretic therapy and exercise performance. *Sports Med* 4:290–304, 1987

Castaneda C, Layne JE, Munoz-Orians L, Gordon PL, Walsmith J, Foldvari M, Roubenoff R, Tucker KL, Nelson ME: A randomized controlled trial of resistance exercise training to improve glycemic control in older adults with type 2 diabetes. *Diabetes Care* 25:2335–2341, 2002

Cobble ME, Frederich R: Saxagliptin for the treatment of type 2 diabetes mellitus: assessing cardiovascular data. *Cardiovasc Diabetol* 11:6, 2012

Crawford MH: Combination therapy as first-line treatment for hypertension. *Am J Cardiovasc Drugs* 9:1–6, 2009

Cunha MR, da Silva ME, Machado HA, Fukui RT, Correa MR, Santos RF, Wajchenberg BL, Rondon MU, Negrao CE, Ursich MJ: The effects of metformin and glibenclamide on glucose metabolism, counter-regulatory hormones and cardiovascular responses in women with type 2 diabetes during exercise of moderate intensity. *Diabet Med* 24:592–599, 2007

Cunha MR, Silva ME, Machado HA, Fukui RT, Correia MR, Santos RF, Wajchenberg BL, Rocha DM, Rondon MU, Negrao CE, Ursich MJ: Cardiovascular, metabolic and hormonal responses to the progressive exercise performed to exhaustion in patients with type 2 diabetes treated with metformin or glyburide. *Diabetes Obes Metab* 10:238–245, 2008

Cuthbertson J, Patterson S, O'Harte FP, Bell PM: Addition of metformin to exogenous glucagon-like peptide-1 results in increased serum glucagon-like peptide-1 concentrations and greater glucose lowering in type 2 diabetes mellitus. *Metabolism* 60:52–56, 2011

de Muinck ED, Lie KI: Safety and efficacy of beta-blockers in the treatment of stable angina pectoris. *J Cardiovasc Pharmacol* 16 (Suppl. 5):S123–S128, 1990

Del Prato S, Barnett AH, Huisman H, Neubacher D, Woerle HJ, Dugi KA: Effect of linagliptin monotherapy on glycaemic control and markers of beta-cell function in patients with inadequately controlled type 2 diabetes: a randomized controlled trial. *Diabetes Obes Metab* 13:258–267, 2011

Del Prato S, Tiengo A: The importance of first-phase insulin secretion: implications for the therapy of type 2 diabetes mellitus. *Diabetes Metab Res Rev* 17:164–174, 2001

Diamant M, Van Gaal L, Stranks S, Guerci B, MacConell L, Haber H, Scism-Bacon J, Trautmann M: Safety and efficacy of once-weekly exenatide compared with insulin glargine titrated to target in patients with type 2 diabetes over 84 weeks. *Diabetes Care* 35:683–689, 2012

Farmer A, Balman E, Gadsby R, Moffatt J, Cradock S, McEwen L, Jameson K: Frequency of self-monitoring of blood glucose in patients with type 2 diabetes: association with hypoglycaemic events. *Curr Med Res Opin* 24:3097–3104, 2008

Freeman JS: Role of the incretin pathway in the pathogenesis of type 2 diabetes mellitus. *Cleve Clin J Med* 76 (Suppl. 5):S12–S19, 2009

Galbo H, Tobin L, van Loon LJ: Responses to acute exercise in type 2 diabetes, with an emphasis on metabolism and interaction with oral hypoglycemic agents and food intake. *Appl Physiol Nutr Metab* 32:567–575, 2007

Gerich J, Raskin P, Jean-Louis L, Purkayastha D, Baron MA: PRESERVE-beta: two-year efficacy and safety of initial combination therapy with nateglinide or glyburide plus metformin. *Diabetes Care* 28:2093–2099, 2005

Grossman E, Messerli FH: Management of blood pressure in patients with diabetes. *Am J Hypertens* 24:863–875, 2011

Kielgast U, Krarup T, Holst JJ, Madsbad S: Four weeks of treatment with liraglutide reduces insulin dose without loss of glycemic control in type 1 diabetic patients with and without residual beta-cell function. *Diabetes Care* 34:1463–1468, 2011

Kim MK, Suk JH, Kwon MJ, Chung HS, Yoon CS, Jun HJ, Ko JH, Kim TK, Lee SH, Oh MK, Rhee BD, Park JH: Nateglinide and acarbose for postprandial glucose control after optimizing fasting glucose with insulin glargine in patients with type 2 diabetes. *Diabetes Res Clin Pract* 92:322–328, 2011

Kones R: Rosuvastatin, inflammation, C-reactive protein, JUPITER, and primary prevention of cardiovascular disease—a perspective. *Drug Des Devel Ther* 4:383–413, 2010

Krentz AJ, Bailey CJ: Oral antidiabetic agents: current role in type 2 diabetes mellitus. *Drugs* 65:385–411, 2005

Kuritzky L, Samraj GP: Enhanced glycemic control with combination therapy for type 2 diabetes in primary care. *Diabetes Ther* 2:162–177, 2011

Larsen JJ, Dela F, Madsbad S, Vibe-Petersen J, Galbo H: Interaction of sulfonylureas and exercise on glucose homeostasis in type 2 diabetic patients. *Diabetes Care* 22:1647–1654, 1999

Lund A, Knop FK: Worry vs. knowledge about treatment-associated hypoglycaemia and weight gain in type 2 diabetic patients on metformin and/or sulphonylurea. *Curr Med Res Opin* 28:731–736, 2012

Malin SK, Gerber R, Chipkin SR, Braun B: Independent and combined effects of exercise training and metformin on insulin sensitivity in individuals with pre-diabetes. *Diabetes Care* 35:131–136, 2012

McIntosh B, Cameron C, Singh SR, Yu C, Ahuja T, Welton NJ, Dahl M: Second-line therapy in patients with type 2 diabetes inadequately controlled with met-formin monotherapy: a systematic review and mixed-treatment comparison meta-analysis. *Open Med* 5:e35–e48, 2011

Mizukami H, Ogasawara S, Yamagishi S, Takahashi K, Yagihashi S: Methylcobala-min effects on diabetic neuropathy and nerve protein kinase C in rats. *Eur J Clin Invest* 41:442–450, 2011

Neumiller JJ, Wood L, Campbell, RK: Dipeptidyl peptidase-4 inhibitors for the treatment of type 2 diabetes mellitus. *Pharmacotherapy* 30:463–484, 2010

Nichols GA, Koro CE: Does statin therapy initiation increase the risk for myopa-thy? An observational study of 32,225 diabetic and nondiabetic patients. *Clin Ther* 29:1761–1770, 2007

Nicholson W, Bolen S, Witkop CT, Neale D, Wilson L, Bass E: Benefits and risks of oral diabetes agents compared with insulin in women with gestational dia-betes: a systematic review. *Obstet Gynecol* 113:193–205, 2009

Parker BA, Augeri AL, Capizzi JA, Ballard KD, Troyanos C, Baggish AL, D'Hemecourt PA, Thompson PD: Effect of statins on creatine kinase levels before and after a marathon run. *Am J Cardiol* 109:282–287, 2012

Pflipsen MC, Oh RC, Saguil A, Seehusen DA, Seaquist D, Topolski R: The preva-lence of vitamin B(12) deficiency in patients with type 2 diabetes: a cross-sectional study. *J Am Board Fam Med* 22:528–534, 2009

Phung OJ, Scholle JM, Talwar M, Coleman CI: Effect of noninsulin antidiabetic drugs added to metformin therapy on glycemic control, weight gain, and hypoglycemia in type 2 diabetes. *JAMA* 303:1410–1418, 2010

Plockinger U, Topuz M, Riese B, Reuter T: Risk of exercise-induced hypoglycae-mia in patients with type 2 diabetes on intensive insulin therapy: comparison of insulin glargine with NPH insulin as basal insulin supplement. *Diabetes Res Clin Pract* 81:290–295, 2008

Polster M, Zanutto E, McDonald S, Conner C, Hammer M: A comparison of preferences for two GLP-1 products—liraglutide and exenatide—for the treatment of type 2 diabetes. *J Med Econ* 13:655–661, 2011

Ratner RE, Dickey R, Fineman M, Maggs DG, Shen L, Strobel SA, Weyer C, Kolterman OG: Amylin replacement with pramlintide as an adjunct to insulin therapy improves long-term glycaemic and weight control in type 1 diabetes mellitus: a 1-year, randomized controlled trial. *Diabet Med* 21:1204–1212, 2004

Reboldi G, Gentile G, Angeli F, Verdecchia P: Choice of ACE inhibitor combina-tions in hypertensive patients with type 2 diabetes: update after recent clinical trials. *Vasc Health Risk Manag* 5:411–427, 2009

Reinstatler L, Qi YP, Williamson RS, Garn JV, Oakley GP Jr: Association of biochemical B deficiency with metformin therapy and vitamin B supplements: the National Health and Nutrition Examination Survey, 1999–2006. *Diabetes Care* 35:327–333, 2012

Rendell M: The role of sulphonylureas in the management of type 2 diabetes mellitus. *Drugs* 64:1339–1358, 2004

Rosenstock J, Hassman DR, Madder RD, Brazinsky SA, Farrell J, Khutoryansky N, Hale PM, Repaglinide Versus Nateglinide Comparison Study Group: Repaglinide versus nateglinide monotherapy: a randomized, multicenter study. *Diabetes Care* 27:1265–1270, 2004

Russell-Jones D, Cuddihy RM, Hanefeld M, Kumar A, Gonzalez JG, Chan M, Wolka AM, Boardman MK, Duration-Study Group: Efficacy and safety of exenatide once weekly versus metformin, pioglitazone, and sitagliptin used as monotherapy in drug-naive patients with type 2 diabetes (DURATION-4): a 26-week double-blind study. *Diabetes Care* 35:252–258, 2012

Shyangdan DS, Royle PL, Clar C, Sharma P, Waugh NR: Glucagon-like peptide analogues for type 2 diabetes mellitus: systematic review and meta-analysis. *BMC Endocr Disord* 10:20, 2010

Sigal RJ, Purdon C, Bilinski D, Vranic M, Halter JB, Marliss EB: Glucoregulation during and after intense exercise: effects of beta-blockade. *J Clin Endocrinol Metab* 78:359–366, 1994

Singh-Franco D, McLaughlin-Middlekauff J, Elrod S, Harrington C: The effect of linagliptin on glycaemic control and tolerability in patients with type 2 diabetes mellitus: a systematic review and meta-analysis. *Diabetes Obes Metab* 14:694–708, 2012

Solomon LR: Diabetes as a cause of clinically significant functional cobalamin deficiency. *Diabetes Care* 34:1077–1080, 2011

Turner-McGrievy GM, Jenkins DJ, Barnard ND, Cohen J, Gloede L, Green AA: Decreases in dietary glycemic index are related to weight loss among individuals following therapeutic diets for type 2 diabetes. *J Nutr* 141:1469–1474, 2011

Vella A, Bock G, Giesler PD, Burton DB, Serra DB, Saylan ML, Deacon CF, Foley JE, Rizza RA, Camilleri M: The effect of dipeptidyl peptidase-4 inhibition on gastric volume, satiation and enteroendocrine secretion in type 2 diabetes: a double-blind, placebo-controlled crossover study. *Clin Endocrinol (Oxf)* 69:737–744, 2008

Vella A, Bock G, Giesler PD, Burton DB, Serra DB, Saylan ML, Dunning BE, Foley JE, Rizza RA, Camilleri M: Effects of dipeptidyl peptidase-4 inhibition on gastrointestinal function, meal appearance, and glucose metabolism in type 2 diabetes. *Diabetes* 56:1475–1480, 2007

Vilsboll T, Christensen M, Junker AE, Knop FK, Gluud LL: Effects of glucagon-like peptide-1 receptor agonists on weight loss: systematic review and meta-analyses of randomised controlled trials. *BMJ* 344:d7771, 2012

Vlckova V, Cornelius V, Kasliwal R, Wilton L, Shakir SA: Hypoglycaemia with oral antidiabetic drugs: results from prescription-event monitoring cohorts of rosiglitazone, pioglitazone, nateglinide and repaglinide. *Drug Saf* 32:409–418, 2009

Want LL: Optimizing treatment success with an amylin analogue. *Diabetes Educ* 34 (Suppl. 1):11S–17S, 2008

Chapter 16

Obesity, Orthopedic Limitations, and Osteoarthritis

Whereas body weight is more frequently normal or near normal at onset of type 1 diabetes (T1D) (Brown 2011), obesity and overweight are highly prevalent in both type 2 diabetes (T2D) and gestational diabetes (GDM) (American Diabetes Association 2013a). For individuals with any type of diabetes, however, body weight gain—specifically body fat excesses—remains a concern because it can affect insulin action and blood glucose management (Mourier 1997, Jacob 2006a, Amati 2009, Conway 2009). Fat stored deep in the abdominal area is also more associated with insulin resistance, hypertension, hyperlipidemias, and other metabolic dysfunction (O'Leary 2006, Koska 2008, Dubé 2011, Hill 2011, Amati 2012). Regular participation in physical activity, however, can lead to loss of metabolically active visceral fat and improve glycemic control (Stewart 2002, Cuff 2003, Ibanez 2005, Slentz 2005, O'Leary 2006, Delahanty 2008, Tsang 2008, Johnson 2009, Borel 2012).

Carrying excess body weight is a contributing factor in the development of orthopedic limitations that may affect an individual's ability to engage in physical activity. Such limitations include acute injuries, overtraining injuries, and osteoarthritis of the lower limb joints (Pollock 1991, Chumbley 2000, Messier 2000, Knapik 2011). With proper management and appropriate exercise prescription, individuals with orthopedic issues or osteoarthritis can safely and effectively participate in regular physical activity to better manage their diabetes and their overall health (Messier 2004, Foy 2011).

Case in Point: Exercise Rx for an Obese Adult with T2D and Hip Pain

DK is a 62-year-old mother of three children. She was diagnosed with GDM during her third pregnancy, which she learned would increase her risk of developing T2D later on. She had planned on taking off the extra 80 lb that she had accumulated over three pregnancies. As the years went by, however, she found that her days were full of working, being a wife, and raising her children. Instead of losing any weight, she ended up gaining 40 lb more. This past year, while she was happy to lose 20 lb without any effort on her part, she knew her thirst, fatigue, and blurry vision were not good signs, and she was not surprised when she was diagnosed with T2D when seeking treatment for recurrent vaginal yeast infections. A blood glucose value of 370 mg/dl confirmed her suspicions, and she was immediately started on metformin and told to lose some weight, improve her diet, and start exercising.

Resting Measurements

Height: 66 inches
Weight: 252 lb
BMI: 40.7 (morbid obesity)
Heart rate: 88 beats per minute (bpm)
Blood pressure: 130/82 mmHg (on medication)

Fasting Labs (1 Month after Diagnosis)

Plasma glucose: 145 mg/dl (controlled with metformin)
A1C: 7.2%
Total cholesterol: 205 mg/dl (on medication)
Triglycerides: 155 mg/dl
High-density lipoprotein cholesterol: 42 mg/dl
Low-density lipoprotein cholesterol: 132 mg/dl

Questions to Consider

1. What types of physical activity would be best for DK to control her blood glucose levels?
2. What steps should DK take to help her lose some weight?
3. Are there any precautions that DK needs to take to prevent exercise-related problems?

(Continued on page 280.)

OBESITY

Obesity and overweight are highly prevalent in both T2D and GDM (American Diabetes Association 2013a). BMI often exceeds 30 kg/m², and abdominal girth is large in those with T2D and GDM (prepregnancy), placing these individuals at high risk for cardiovascular disease and cancer (U.S. Department of Health and Human Services 2011). Therefore, weight loss is a primary treatment goal to improve insulin action and reduce disease risk in T2D, and a 7–10% reduction in body weight is recommended for important health outcomes related to blood pressure, glucose control, and cardiovascular disease risk (Ratner 2005a, American Diabetes Association 2013b).

For individuals with T1D, insulin use and intensive therapy can lead to weight gain and to the deposition of visceral (central) abdominal fat in particular (Kabadi 2000, Conway 2010, Brown 2011); in such cases, weight management goals should likely follow recommendations for T2D, and hypoglycemia should be prevented whenever possible to prevent additional weight gain resulting from treatment. In T2D, fear of weight gain, more frequent hypoglycemia, and other barriers to insulin use may limit its effectiveness in this population (Ross 2011).

WEIGHT GAIN, INSULIN RESISTANCE, VISCERAL FAT, AND CARDIOVASCULAR RISK

Medications and weight gain. Use of some oral antihyperglycemic agents for treatment of T2D contributes to weight gain. Although the use of thiazolidinediones, sulfonylureas, and glinides is associated with weight gain, GLP-1 analogs, α-glucosidase inhibitors, and DPP-4 inhibitors are associated with weight loss or no weight change (Phung 2010). Metformin, the most commonly prescribed medication for T2D, generally is considered to be weight neutral. As for insulin use, although weight gain in insulin users with T2D has been well documented (Action to Control Cardiovascular Risk in Diabetes Study Group 2008, Dailey 2010), the effects of its use have been less well studied in T1D. In a recent follow-up study (median follow-up time of 18 years), the prevalence of being overweight or obese was increasing among individuals with T1D, independent of age (Conway 2010). The percentage of individuals on intensive insulin therapy, however, increased nearly tenfold during follow-up, paralleling the increase of overweight or obesity and suggesting that tighter glucose control may be the cause. Others have reported that despite the initial weight loss at diagnosis, by 10–20 weeks after initiation of insulin treatment, almost one-third of diabetic children were overweight and obese (Newfield 2009). Likewise, in a 6-month trial in which adult individuals with T1D attempted to attain a normal A1C, the lipogenic effect of insulin with subsequent increase in fat mass was likely the primary cause of weight gain, but it was attenuated by increased levels of physical activity (Jacob 2006b).

Insulin and weight gain. The type of insulin used may modulate weight gain as well. For instance, in a 52-week study, including adults with both types of diabetes, use of insulin detemir improved glycemic control with no increase in the frequency of hypoglycemia or body weight (Marre 2009). Insulin detemir also is associated with a lower risk of nocturnal hypoglycemia (De Leeuw 2005) and severe hypoglycemia in children (Alemzadeh 2005). Weight gain may be less with detemir than with glargine for some (McAdam-Marx 2010), although the switch to using basal insulin analogs in place of insulin isophane alone reduces the risk of nocturnal and severe hypoglycemia (Monami 2009), which in turn may lead to less weight gain (Zachariah 2011). In T2D, although absolute weight gain was higher with glargine compared with detemir, weight gain per A1C change was similar given that a higher detemir dose was required to achieve a similar reduction (Dailey 2010).

In individuals with T1D, use of mealtime replacement with pramlintide in addition to insulin increases satiety and improves long-term glycemic and weight control (Ratner 2004) and does so without increasing the risk of severe hypoglycemia (Ratner 2005b). Frequent bouts of hypoglycemia require treatment and, consequently, can result in weight gain from the intake of excess calories. Intensive therapy has been associated with increased hypoglycemia, and physical activity raises the risk of hypoglycemia both during and following the activity (McMahon 2007). The key to prevention of exercise-related hypoglycemia and intake of excess calories remains effective adjustment of insulin and food regimens.

Effects of visceral fat. Excess visceral abdominal fat has been associated with insulin resistance across a range of middle-aged to older men and women, whereas more thigh subcutaneous fat is favorably related to improved insulin sensitivity and lower cardiometabolic risk (Koska 2008, Amati 2012). Fat stored deep in the abdominal area is also more associated with insulin resistance, hypertension, hyperlipidemias, and other metabolic dysfunction (Ibanez 2005, O'Leary 2006). The metabolic effects of reducing abdominal adiposity in T1D, however, have been studied only minimally. One group reported that 6 months of exercise training reduced visceral fat, but fat loss was not associated with A1C changes in adults with T1D (Jacob 2006a). A higher daily insulin dose and stricter glycemic goals appear to be related to increases in visceral adiposity, but it is unclear whether insulin therapy induces central fat deposition or if increased abdominal adiposity causes insulin resistance and higher insulin requirements (Dubé 2008).

Insulin resistance is associated with a more atherogenic lipid profile in both youth and adults with T1D (Maahs 2011), although insulin dose is a poor predictor of risk compared with levels of insulin resistance (Kilpatrick 2007). Although intensive treatment has been associated with a higher subsequent prevalence of metabolic syndrome (a cluster of cardiovascular risk factors that leads to "double diabetes" in individuals with T1D), the benefits of improved glycemic control still potentially outweigh the risks related to its possible development. Even in T1D, most established cardiovascular risk factors strongly predict total coronary artery disease (Orchard 2003), and weight management likely retards atherosclerosis progression (Costacou 2007). A worthy goal is to limit increases in visceral adiposity to lower the risk of cardiovascular complications without compromising glycemic control. Because daily exercise can lower both visceral fat and insulin resistance (Ingberg 2003, Slentz 2005, O'Leary 2006), it should be advocated for individuals with diabetes for that reason and many others.

PHYSICAL ACTIVITY IN THE MAINTENANCE AND LOSS OF BODY WEIGHT

Successful program elements. The most successful programs for long-term weight control have involved combinations of diet, exercise, and behavior modification (Catenacci 2011). Exercise interventions undertaken with the volumes typically recommended to improve glycemic control and lower cardiovascular risk (e.g., 150 min/week of brisk walking) usually are insufficient for major weight loss (Boulé 2001), likely because obese and older people frequently have difficulty performing sufficient exercise to create a large energy deficit and easily can counterbalance expenditures by additional food intake. About 1 h of daily moderate aerobic exercise produces at least as much fat loss as equivalent caloric restriction, with greater improvements in insulin action (Ross 2000, 2004). The optimal volume of exercise to achieve sustained major weight loss, however, is probably much larger than the amount required to achieve improved glycemic control and cardiovascular health (Boulé 2001, Physical Activity Guidelines Advisory Committee 2008). Individuals who successfully maintain large weight loss over at least 1 year typically engage in ~7 h/week of moderate- to vigorous-intensity exercise (Donnelly 2009), and higher exercise volumes (2,000–2,500 calories/week) produce greater and more sustained weight loss than 1,000 calories/week (Jakicic 2003, Jeffery 2003). Without concomitant changes in diet, a higher amount of activity is necessary for weight maintenance (Slentz 2004).

The National Weight Control Registry (NWCR) has examined characteristics of successful weight-loss maintainers, that is, individuals with a documented 30 lb or greater weight loss maintained for at least 1 year. Among other characteristics, this group consistently self-reports high levels of physical activity. People in the NWCR engaged in significantly more sustained bouts (~41 min on average) of moderate- to vigorous-intensity physical activity that were at least 10 min in duration than overweight controls, providing further evidence that physical activity, especially when sustained, is important for long-term maintenance of weight loss (Catenacci 2011).

Weight loss and medication use. Among overweight or obese patients with T2D, intentional weight loss of 7–14% typically is required for full discontinuation of at least one antidiabetic medication, whereas discontinuation of insulin requires closer to a mean weight reduction of 11% of initial body weight (Kumar 2012). Exercise is also critical for the loss of visceral fat (Ibanez 2005, Slentz 2005). In individuals with T1D, engaging in regular physical activity generally lowers overall insulin requirements and reduces the risk of weight gain associated with excess insulin use (Diabetes Control and Complications Trial Research Group 2001, Ferriss 2006, Jacob 2006b, Conway 2010, Brown 2011). In adults without diabetes, exercise has been shown to have consistent effects on body fatness in the absence of prescribed dietary change, with a progressive loss of body fat associated with higher exercise energy expenditures in both men and women (Elder 2007). Even energy expenditure from increased daily movement can aid in weight loss and weight maintenance (Weinsier 2002). Similarly, in individuals with T1D, physical activity can improve insulin action, albeit acutely, and potentially can lower insulin requirements and body weight. For example, in sedentary individuals with T1D (ages 13–30 years), engaging in either 12 weeks of aerobic or resistance exercise training lowered their insulin needs, waist circumference, and post-training blood glucose levels, although their A1C levels were not significantly improved (Ramalho 2006). Moreover, all T1D adolescents can benefit from combined aerobic and strength training undertaken twice weekly for 20 weeks, which results in lower daily insulin requirements, improved physical fitness, and an enhanced sense of well-being (D'Hooge 2011). Similar training also has been shown to reduce cardiovascular risk and insulin resistance risk factors in diabetic adolescent girls (Heyman 2007).

Weight loss and knee pain. Lifestyle interventions have resulted in weight loss and improved physical fitness among individuals with obesity. One recent investigation that was part of the Look AHEAD (Action for Health in Diabetes) trial investigated the effects of 12 months of intensive lifestyle intervention on reported knee pain at baseline in individuals with T2D (Foy 2011). It also examined whether changes in weight or fitness improved outcome measures, including pain, stiffness, and physical function. Lifestyle changes that included regular physical activity resulted in more favorable changes attributed to both greater weight loss and increased fitness. Severely obese participants in the intensive lifestyle intervention group also had similar adherence, percentage of weight loss, and improvement in cardiovascular risk compared with less obese participants (Unick 2011). In fact, regular physical activity prevents both the age-associated loss of muscle strength and the increase in muscle fat infiltration in older adults with moderate functional limitations (Goodpaster 2008), and even the combinations of circuit resistance training plus weight loss (Magrans-Courtney 2011) or moderate exercise plus modest weight loss (Messier 2004) improve symptoms of knee osteoarthritis more than either exercise or weight loss alone.

MODIFICATIONS FOR OBESITY

Combined programs of physical activity, dietary improvements, and behavior change are effective for obese individuals. Physical activity combined with dietary changes has been shown to be more effective for long-term weight loss than either done alone (Slentz 2004). Approaches that emphasize physical activity offer enhanced calorie expenditure and provide the benefits of improved fitness related to influencing blood lipids, blood glucose control, blood pressure, mood, and attitude (Garber 2011). Regular physical activity also helps maintain muscle mass while promoting fat loss during weight loss (Chomentowski 2009) and helps prevent weight regain after dieting (Wang 2008).

The optimal volume of exercise to achieve sustained major weight loss is likely much larger than that needed to achieve improved blood glucose control and cardiovascular health. Individuals who successfully maintain large weight loss over at least 1 year typically engage in ~7 h/week of moderate- to vigorous-intensity exercise (Donnelly 2009), although greater exercise volumes (2,000–2,500 calories/week) produce greater and more sustained weight loss than 1,000 calories/week (Jakicic 2003).

In all individuals with diabetes, both acute bouts of physical activity and regular exercise training favorably alter stress-related psychological factors like well-being (Kopp 2012), cognitive function (Colberg 2008), and mild to moderate depression (Lysy 2008). Moreover, regular physical activity improves quality of life in individuals with diabetes that other therapies frequently fail to fully achieve. Recommendations related to physical activity for individuals who are overweight or obese are given in Table 16.1.

Case in Point: Continued (Part 2)

DK was motivated to lose a lot of weight (the faster, the better), so she decided to cut back on her calorie intake and start exercising daily. Before her diagnosis, she was active and enjoyed dancing, exercise classes, and playing games with her children. She was cleared to exercise by her health-care provider who told her any weight loss would improve her hypertension and hyperlipidemia, too.

DK decided she would just have to walk longer to burn off calories and improve her blood glucose level. She decided to walk 60 min each day, most days of the week. She was sure this would work—until she tried it. After the first 40 min on the first day, she was not even sure she was going to make it home. When she walked into her house, she immediately went to the freezer and pulled out the ice cream. To top off her woes, her right hip was in severe pain for days afterward, and she was unable to do any walking.

Additional Questions to Consider

1. Is there anything DK can do to lessen her hip pain so that she can resume walking?
2. Because walking caused hip pain, does DK need to do another type of exercise instead?
3. Should DK consider going about losing weight in an alternate way?

(Continued on page 287.)

Table 16.1 Physical Activity Recommendations for Overweight and Obesity

When working with diabetic individuals who are overweight or obese, use the following guidelines to increase their physical activity level.

- An initial goal should be to simply increase the amount of daily physical movement from an inactive level.
- Engage in moderate aerobic exercise that uses large muscle groups, with an emphasis on increasing duration and frequency.
- Walking is an effective choice for continuous aerobic exercise; alternative types of exercise also include cycling and chair and water exercise.
- Non–weight-bearing activities may reduce the risk of orthopedic injury.
- Higher-intensity, weight-bearing activities like running and jogging are not recommended until body weight is reduced.
- Individuals should aim for 45 to 60 min of aerobic activity 5–7 days/week to maximize caloric expenditure.
- Individuals should aim for a target expenditure of 300–400 calories/day or 2,000 calories/week through physical activity.
- Individuals should additionally undertake recommended amounts of resistance training to build muscle strength and to retain muscle mass during weight loss.

ORTHOPEDIC INJURIES AND OTHER LIMITATIONS

Most people are not likely to develop an athletic injury from doing moderate-intensity activities in amounts that meet recommendations. Injuries and other adverse events, however, do sometimes occur, the most common being musculoskeletal injuries. Only one such injury occurs for every 1,000 h of walking for exercise, however, and fewer than four injuries occur for every 1,000 h of running in generally healthy adults (Physical Activity Guidelines Advisory Committee 2008).

Both physical fitness and total amount of physical activity affect the risk of musculoskeletal injuries. Individuals who are physically fit have a lower risk of injury than those who are not, although doing more activity generally raises the risk of injury (Knapik 2011, Bloemers 2012). The best strategy is for an individual to undertake regular physical activity to increase physical fitness and increase total activity gradually to minimize the injury risk from doing greater amounts of activity.

IMMEDIATE AND CHRONIC TREATMENT OF INJURIES

Treatment of acute injuries is best handled with RICE (Rest, Ice, Compression, and Elevation), as detailed in Table 16.2 (Wexler 1995, Chumbley 2000, Kannus 2000, Perryman 2002, Knapik 2011). Acute injuries should never be heated as doing so causes swelling, which is what RICE treatment is attempting to prevent.

REDUCING INFLAMMATION WITH MEDICATIONS

Nonsteroidal, anti-inflammatory drugs. Taking anti-inflammatory medications, otherwise known as nonsteroidal, anti-inflammatory drugs (NSAIDs), is often helpful when treating activity-related injuries (Paoloni 2009). Many of these NSAIDs are available in drugstores without a prescription. Aspirin, ibuprofen (sold as Advil or Nuprin), and naproxen (Aleve) all fight inflammation and reduce pain, but acetaminophen (commonly sold as Tylenol) is not anti-inflammatory and only limits pain. Prescription anti-inflammatory medications like Relafan, Celebrex, Daypro, and Naprosyn are also available. Follow RICE to treat both acute and overuse injuries (after workouts that aggravate the latter) and consider treating them with NSAIDs (Paoloni 2009).

Cortisone injection. If an affected area becomes inflamed enough that it does not improve with rest and NSAIDs or prescription pain medications, or if it is painful for several weeks without any improvement, a cortisone injection may be necessary to relieve pain and joint tenderness. Although it is localized to the affected area, cortisone can affect the whole body for days to weeks, and most preparations increase insulin resistance and hyperglycemia (Black 1989, Feldman-Billard 2006, Wang 2006, Gonzalez 2009, Jin 2009, Roh 2012, Simo 2012). Regardless of whether individuals use insulin or other medications for diabetes management, they may need to increase doses temporarily to cover these glycemic effects (Stephens 2008).

Table 16.2 Use of RICE for Injury Treatment

Individuals should follow these steps for immediate treatment of an acute injury:

- Rest: Immediately stop the physical activity.
- Ice: Apply ice (using a bag of crushed ice or even a bag of frozen vegetables) for 15 min, let the area warm back up, and reapply two or three times total, as tolerated.
- Compression: Wrap the injured area in a compression (ace) bandage.
- Elevation: Elevate the injured joint to reduce swelling (up higher than heart level).

See a physician for proper diagnosis and treatment of any serious, acute injury. For more chronic injuries from overtraining, RICE treatment is also effective, along with use of anti-inflammatory medications.

Furthermore, prolonged high-dose steroid treatment causes significant bone loss in patients with chronic kidney disease and is not advisable (Haris 2012).

Exercise therapy has shown to be a useful tool for the prevention of different diseases, including glucocorticoid myopathy and muscle unloading in the elderly. If cortisone is used, exercise can be prescribed to offset the potential loss of the myofibrillar apparatus, changes in the extracellular matrix, and a decrease in muscle strength and motor activity associated with its use, particularly in the elderly (Riso 2008, Seene 2012).

COMMON OVERUSE (CHRONIC) INJURIES

Typical overuse injuries in diabetes. Anyone with diabetes is more prone to developing overuse injuries with a slower onset that can limit movement around joints. Common injuries associated with a diabetic state are shoulder adhesive capsulitis ("frozen shoulder"), carpal tunnel syndrome (wrist pain), metatarsal fractures (foot bones), and neuropathy-related joint disorders (e.g., Charcot foot) in people with peripheral neuropathy (Graves 2003, Garcilazo 2010, Cakir 2011, Kiylioglu 2011, Plastino 2011, Ravindran Rajendran 2011, Rogers 2011, Roh 2012). Trigger fingers, which result in curled fingers because of shortening of ligaments, usually require cortisone injections or surgery to repair them (Wang 2006, Craig 2008, Rozental 2008, Plastino 2011). People with long-standing diabetes are additionally prone to nerve compression syndromes at the elbow and wrist that may be aggravated by repetitive activities, prolonged gripping, or direct nerve compression during weight training, cycling, and other activities (Chumbley 2000). In most cases, effective glycemic management reduces the risk for developing these injuries, which are largely the result of glycation of joint structures that increases rigidity (Basta 2002, Kang 2010, Abate 2011). Engaging in flexibility exercises done with resistance work that emphasizes and maintains a full range of motion around all the joints can also be beneficial (Herriott 2004). Common overuse injuries in people with diabetes and their symptoms, preventive measures, and treatments are given in Table 16.3.

Causes. In most sports and activities, overuse injuries are the most common and challenging to diagnose and treat, and they often worsen over time if neglected (Knobloch 2008, Zifchock 2008, Vleck 2010, Tenforde 2011). By definition, an overuse injury is caused by excessive use of a particular joint. Overuse injuries are more common in people with diabetes because of structural changes in their joints caused by long-term elevations in blood glucose levels and ensuing oxidative stress and damage (Basta 2002, Chen 2003, Kang 2010, Rechardt 2010, Abate 2011, Ko 2011). Regardless of the contributing cause, all overuse injuries are treated the same way. Moreover, their onset usually can be linked to changes in athletic endeavors or techniques, such as rapid progression in physical activity participation. To prevent such injuries, individuals should make only gradual increases in training duration, frequency, or intensity to allow the body time to adapt to minor traumas imposed by exercise, which can occur with adequate time for recovery and recuperation.

Some people are prone to developing overuse injuries, but their development is more often related to anatomical, biomechanical, or other considerations

Table 16.3 Common Overuse Injuries and Their Management

Injury	Area Affected	Symptoms	Treatment and Prevention
Carpal tunnel syndrome	Wrist	Pain, weakness, or numbness in hand and wrist; loss of grip strength	Rest, ice, NSAIDs, surgery if longer than 6 months
Tennis elbow	Outside of the elbow	Painful to touch or bump, pain when shaking hands or turning a doorknob	Rest, ice, NSAIDs, use of a strap around the upper forearm, using a two-handed backhand, exercises
Rotator cuff tendinitis	Shoulder	Pain when lifting arms, combing hair	Rest, ice, NSAIDs, stretching, and strengthening exercises
Chondromalacia patella	Knee	Knee pain made worse by bending the knees, doing full squats, or sitting for long periods with bent knees	Rest, ice, NSAIDs, strengthening the inner quads with weight training
Iliotibial band friction (ITBF) syndrome	Knee	Pain along the outside part of the knee or lower thigh	Rest, ice, gentle stretching (IT band and gluteal muscles), running on both sides of the road, wearing proper shoes
Shin splints	Front of lower legs, along the tibia bone	Generalized pain along the bones of lower leg	Rest, ice, NSAIDs, slow progression of training program, avoiding walking or running on hard surfaces
Plantar fasciitis	Heel, bottom of foot	Heel pain during first steps each morning and following periods of inactivity	Rest, ice, NSAIDs, stretching and massaging the plantar fascia, exercises
Achilles tendinitis	Heel and calves	Pain in the heels and tight calf muscles	Rest, ice, NSAIDs, frequent stretching of the calves and thighs, limited wearing of high-heeled shoes

Note: NSAIDs, nonsteroidal, anti-inflammatory drugs.

(Tweed 2008, Van Ginckel 2009). For instance, imbalances between strength and flexibility around joints (e.g., quads vs. hamstring strength) can predispose a person to hamstring pulls or other injuries (Zifchock 2008). Uneven body alignment, such as knock-knees, bowed legs, unequal leg lengths, and flat or high-arched feet, also can contribute (Collins 2009). Even old injuries lead to a greater likelihood of overuse injuries, as do factors like the type of running shoes an individual wears, the terrain (hilly, flat, or uneven), and whether exercise is done on hard surfaces like concrete roads or floors or softer ones like grass, dirt, or gravel trails, asphalt, and cushioned floors (Stiles 2009).

Role of inflammation. Many overuse injuries involve inflammation of an area, or redness, soreness, and swelling, designated as "–itis" at the end of its name. Tendinitis is inflammation of tendons, which attach muscles to bones; it is a common overuse injury that results from a tendon rubbing repeatedly against a bony structure, ligament, or another tendon or from being impinged (Rechardt 2010). Tennis elbow is a type of tendinitis on the outside of the elbow common in tennis players as well as rowers, carpenters, gardeners, golfers, and other exercisers who repeatedly bend their arms forcefully (Chumbley 2000). Swimmers often develop tendinitis and other impingement syndromes in the rotator cuff (shoulder) because of the overhead movement required by the sport (Chen 2003, Kang 2010, Rechardt 2010, Ko 2011). In sports that involve running and jumping, tendinitis often occurs in the knee, foot, and Achilles (heel) tendons.

PREVENTION OF OVERUSE INJURIES

Individuals who are experiencing nagging aches and pains that are only minor should simply cut back on the intensity, frequency, and duration of irritating activities to bring relief of symptoms (Fry 1991, Kuipers 1998, Roose 2009). One way to prevent problems in the first place is to adopt a hard–easy workout schedule in which workouts are alternated and varied by the day to avoid overstressing joints in the same way with every workout (Fry 1992). If problems are related to anatomical concerns, individuals should consider getting orthotics (e.g., to correct leg-length discrepancies) or do other activities that lower injury risk, such as working out on an elliptical trainer a few days a week instead of always running outdoors on asphalt. In addition, working with a coach or teacher or taking lessons can help improve training and technique. Engaging in proper warm-ups and cooldowns, icing inflamed joints after workouts, and using NSAIDs also can control inflammation and pain. Some key strategies associated with prevention of acute and chronic injuries are covered in Table 16.4.

Table 16.4 Prevention of Acute and Chronic Injuries Associated with Physical Activity

- Never bounce during stretches because doing so can cause injuries, although dynamic stretching is fine (movement stretches).
- If currently sedentary, start slowly and progress cautiously to avoid delayed-onset muscle soreness, an acute injury, or overtraining injuries.
- Warm up with stretches and easy aerobic work before undertaking vigorous exercise.
- Choose appropriate exercises, such as swimming if recovering from an ankle or knee injury.
- Vary the exercise program occasionally or try out new activities to emphasize different muscle groups and increase overall fitness.
- Cross-train to reduce the risk of injury by varying muscle and joint usage.
- Wear appropriate shoes and socks, and check feet after each exercise session.
- Avoid going back to normal activities until symptoms have almost completely gone away.
- For best results, include a warm-up and cooldown period with each exercise session.

Engaging in cross-training can help prevent and treat overuse injuries (Vleck 2010). Individuals should do other activities to maintain their overall fitness levels while the injured area recovers. For example, with lower leg pain, an individual can still work the upper body by doing activities that allow the legs to rest and recuperate. They also can alternate weight-bearing activities like walking or running with non–weight-bearing ones, such as swimming, upper-body work, and stationary cycling (Fry 1992). Strengthening the muscles around the previously injured joint to prevent recurrence, especially following tendinitis, is critical to preventing its recurrence. For example, following a shoulder joint injury like rotator cuff tendinitis and impingement, resistance work should include all sections of the deltoid muscle (in particular), along with exercises for the biceps, triceps, pectoral muscles, upper-back muscles, and neck muscles.

CHOOSING THE PROPER FOOTWEAR

Wearing proper shoes is critical to preventing many lower-extremity and foot problems. The best type of shoes to wear varies by activity. Walkers and runners generally need some cushioning, whereas tennis players require footwear with greater stability for side-to-side movements (Cheung 2008, Morio 2009). For most activities, however, shoes should be chosen based on whether an individual rotates on his or her feet toward the arch of the foot or toward the outside edge.

The wear pattern on the bottom of shoes indicates an individual's usual step pattern. For example, exercisers who overpronate (rotate their feet too far to the inside), have flat feet, or carry a lot of extra body weight wear out the insides of their soles first—in which case motion-control shoes may help (Ryan 2011). Generally heavy but durable, they are rigid, control-oriented running shoes that have firm midsoles designed to limit overpronation; they also come in varieties with more cushioning. When athletic shoes fail to compensate for overpronation, they place extra stress on the knees, hips, and ankles that can result in injuries.

Conversely, supinators usually have high arches and more rigid feet and thus wear out the soles of their shoes on the outside edge. These individuals will generally benefit from highly cushioned shoes with plenty of flexibility to encourage foot motion (Wolf 2008, Ryan 2011). Individuals with normal arches should choose shoes with moderate control, such as those with a two-density midsole. The type of arch a person has can be determined by having him or her walk with wet, bare feet, and examining the footprint to see how much of the arch region of the foot shows.

RECOGNIZING AND TREATING OVERTRAINING SYNDROME

Overtraining syndrome frequently occurs in individuals who are training for competition or a specific event without allowing adequate time for rest and recuperation (Fry 1991, Kuipers 1998, Cosca 2007, Roose 2009). Becoming more fit and improving performance is a balancing act between training and recovering from it (i.e., allowing recuperative time for repairing damage done with activity). Overloading the body excessively without enough recovery time can result in both physical and psychological symptoms.

The symptoms of overtraining include chronic tiredness, lethargy, soreness and aches, chronic pain in muscles and joints, an unexpected drop in performance, insomnia, an increased number of colds and upper-respiratory tract infections, mild depression, and general malaise (Hawley 2003, Purvis 2010). Another measure of overtraining syndrome is a gradual increase in resting heart rate. More frequent illnesses usually indicates that excessive training is compromising immune function, and because overtraining results in elevated levels of cortisol, blood glucose management may become more difficult as well. Cutting back on training should alleviate symptoms if the cause is truly overtraining (Hawley 2003, Purvis 2010). Engaging in cross-training that involves doing different activities may help if certain muscles or joints are being overworked, and doing so may improve psychological outlook. Total recovery from overtraining can take several weeks, during which time proper nutrition and stress reduction are important to the process.

Case in Point: Continued (Part 3)

DK called her health-care provider about the hip pain she had developed from walking. She was sure the diabetes was now causing some other problems and was afraid she was going to lose her leg. Once her health-care provider reassured her that was not so, DK was scheduled to have a few medical tests. She learned that diabetes was not the reason for her hip pain; rather, she had some arthritis in her hips that probably was exacerbated by her excess body weight and, more recently, by walking a long distance without working up to it slowly with shorter distances first. She was told that while the arthritis would cause some discomfort, weight loss could help decrease the pain, as could regular participation in moderate physical activity. Now exercise was more important for her than ever.

Additional Question to Consider

1. How should DK go about starting and progressing her activity in a way that will not exacerbate her osteoarthritis?

(Continued on page 293.)

OSTEOARTHRITIS

Arthritis is a common condition in older adults that is characterized by painful inflammation of a joint or joints. The most common type is osteoarthritis, which is associated with degeneration of bony joint surfaces, usually in the knees, hips, spine, hands, and toes. Often described as "wear and tear" arthritis, it is more common in joints that previously have been injured, particularly through traumatic, contact sports injuries. In addition, lower-extremity joints (i.e., the hip, knee, and ankle) are more likely to become arthritic in overweight individuals given that carrying extra weight puts additional stress on cartilage in hip and knee joints. Because most individuals with T2D and many with T1D are overweight or obese, they have a higher risk of developing this painful condition.

People with osteoarthritis generally are concerned that physical activity can make their condition worse. It undeniably can be painful during exercise and cause early fatigue, making it hard to begin or maintain regular physical activity. Anyone with this condition should become regularly active to lower the risk of other chronic diseases like heart disease and to help maintain a healthy body weight and lower blood glucose levels. When done safely, physical activity does not make the disease or the pain worse. In fact, adults with osteoarthritis can expect improvements in pain, physical function, quality of life, and mental health with regular activity.

PROGRESSION OF ARTHRITIS

Although arthritis can result from trauma or from repetitive use, often no single cause is identifiable. Joints, formed by the juxtaposition of two or more bones with cartilage coats on their ends, normally function to provide flexibility, stability, support, and protection to the skeleton, allowing movement of limbs. In a healthy joint, this coating maintains the separation between bones, allowing joints to move smoothly and without pain. In the early stages of osteoarthritis, however, the cartilage's surface becomes swollen, forming tiny crevices that hinder movement (Weinans 2012). A loss of elasticity in the cartilage also makes it more vulnerable to further damage, and outgrowths known as bone spurs often begin to form around its edges. Other associated joint structures, such as the synovial fluid in the middle, tendons, and ligaments, can become inflamed (Scanzello 2012). In advanced cases, the cartilage cushion is completely lost, limiting joint mobility. Glycation of joint surfaces, which occurs more readily during hyperglycemic excursions in anyone with diabetes, can contribute to faster deterioration of all joint structures (Basta 2002, Abate 2011).

SYMPTOMS OF ARTHRITIS

Arthritis is easily identifiable by its symptoms (Table 16.5), although their degree varies widely among individuals. It can cause pain in the affected joint or joints after repeated use, especially later in the day, or the individual may experience swelling, pain, and stiffness after long periods of inactivity (e.g., after sleep or sitting long periods) that subsides with activity. Symptoms vary with the affected joint. For instance, with knee arthritis, individuals may experience problems with that joint locking up, especially when stepping up or down. Hip problems usually make people limp, whereas affected finger joints often result in reduced strength and movement, making simple tasks such as buttoning clothes or opening jars difficult. An arthritic spine can cause neck and low-back pain, along with weakness and numbness, particularly if bony spurs have developed. Affected finger joints can result in hard, bony enlargements.

The pain associated with arthritis does not come from the joint cartilage surfaces as they contain no nerve endings, but rather it results from the irritated nerves in adjacent stretched or inflamed areas. Individuals may experience what is known as "referred pain," meaning that it is felt somewhere other than in the affected joint (Hoogeboom 2012). For example, an arthritic spine can cause pain

Table 16.5 Common Symptoms of Arthritis

- Pain, made worse by cool, damp weather
- Crackling or popping in the affected joints (most commonly knees)
- Enlarged, swollen joints, often tender when touched
- Stiffness and restricted movement in affected joints
- Unstable joints that move too far or in the wrong direction

in the neck, arms, or legs. Pain is continuous only when almost all of the cartilage surfaces of joints have been eroded, at which point it is indicative of advanced arthritis.

PHYSICAL ACTIVITY WITH ARTHRITIS

Participation in regular physical activity is possible with arthritis and should be encouraged given that it may actually improve joint symptoms in many cases (Vignon 2006). For instance, a 6-month weight-loss and walking program has been shown to result in lesser arthritic pain in overweight and obese older adults with knee arthritis (Messier 2000). Even long-distance running does not increase the risk of osteoarthritis of the knees and hips in healthy adults (Willick 2010) and engaging in most types of activity actually might have a protective effect against joint degeneration (Rogers 2002, Vignon 2006). Regular moderate aerobic or resistance activities will improve symptoms of arthritis, as long as the chosen exercise is not overly stressful to affected joints (Messier 2000, 2004; Magrans-Courtney 2011). Engaging long term in some types of intense exercise, however, may increase the risk of developing osteoarthritis (Michaelsson 2011). Switching to non–weight-bearing activities like cycling and aquatic exercise also may help, along with engaging in strength and full-range-of-movement exercises for painful joints (Vignon 2006).

In overweight and obese adults with T2D, the intensive lifestyle management associated with the Look AHEAD research program resulted in significant improvement in physical function and knee pain (Foy 2011). Lifestyle changes in that study also resulted in significant weight loss and improved fitness, along with improved physical function. Although diabetes does not increase the risk for arthritis, hip fractures are more common in people who do not regularly participate in weight-bearing exercise that strengthens the hips and lower-limb bones (Coupland 1999, Ilich 2008).

Individuals with osteoarthritis should match the type and amount of physical activity to their abilities and the severity of their condition (Vignon 2006). Most people usually can engage in moderate-intensity activity for ≥150 min/week and may choose to be active 3–5 days a week for 30–60 min/episode (Nelson 2007). Some individuals with arthritis can safely undertake >150 min of moderate-intensity activity each week and may be able to tolerate equivalent amounts of vigorous-intensity activity, but moderate activity should be a starting point. Both aerobic activity and muscle-strengthening activity provide therapeutic benefits for osteoarthritis (Nelson 2007, Magrans-Courtney 2011). Health-care providers typically counsel people with osteoarthritis to do activities that are low impact, not painful, and have low risk of joint injury, such as swimming, walking, and resistance training (Vignon 2006). Individuals should use pain as their guide in determining how much to do, and they likely should avoid sports with high risk of joint trauma, such as contact sports, racquetball, and others with frequent directional changes (Vignon 2006, Jones 2011).

Diabetic individuals are advised to start with range-of-motion exercises to increase joint mobility and light resistance work to increase the strength of the muscles surrounding any affected joints (Vignon 2006). For instance, for affected knees, individuals should work on strengthening both groups of muscles in the thigh that affect knee movement, including the quadriceps group in the front (knee extensors) and hamstrings in the back (flexors). In addition, non–weight-bearing ones like stationary cycling, aquatic activities, and light to moderate resistance work that put lower amounts of stress on joints should result in less pain and fewer arthritis-related problems. After activities, ice may need to be applied to arthritic joints (particularly knees) for 15–20 min to reduce swelling and help prevent soreness. NSAID medications may be beneficial in temporarily lessening exercise-associated discomfort.

NONMEDICAL TREATMENT OF ARTHRITIS

Much of the treatment for arthritis involves no prescriptions at all, focusing instead on ways to relieve painful joints through more practical changes or treatments, simply receiving massage therapy on muscles surrounding affected joints (Perlman 2012). Additional suggestions for ways to reduce joint pain associated with arthritis are given in Table 16.6.

MEDICATIONS TO MANAGE ARTHRITIC PAIN

NSAIDs. If additional relief for pain associated with arthritis is required, both prescription and nonprescription medications are available. Most individuals start

---

Table 16.6 Nonmedical Treatments for Osteoarthritis

Any or all of the suggestions pertaining to affected joints may help prevent and alleviate pain without the need for additional medications:

- Participate in regular, moderate aerobic or even resistance exercise.
- Perform strengthening and full-range-of-motion exercises for painful joints.
- Receive massage therapy on muscles surrounding affected joints.
- Use heat and cold packs whenever pain is bothersome and after exercise.
- Use special gadgets to open jars to reduce stress on finger joints.
- Use athletic tape around an arthritic knee to support and stabilize it.
- Wear wedged insoles in your shoes for hip or knee problems (or orthotics, particularly if you have one leg longer than the other).
- Lose weight (through exercise primarily) to alleviate lower-extremity arthritis pain.
- Use a cane or walking stick with painful hips or knees.

with an over-the-counter pain reliever, such as Tylenol, before moving on to NSAIDs like Advil and Nuprin, Aleve, or aspirin in recommended doses (Paoloni 2009, Verkleij 2011). The main problem with NSAIDs is that they can cause stomach problems and kidney damage over time, and the pain from arthritis may require an individual to use these medications for many years. Use of NSAIDs also generally is contraindicated in individuals with chronic kidney disease (Patel 2012). Moreover, to be effective, most painkillers must be taken regularly and frequently chronically.

Prescription painkillers. In rare cases of extreme pain, a physician can prescribe stronger pain medications, but they can be addictive and must be used with caution. Moreover, at least one anti-inflammatory prescription pain medication (Vioxx) already has been taken off the market because of concerns that it minimally doubled the risk of heart attacks and stroke compared with older, nonprescription pain medications like Aleve (Laine 2008). A mechanistically similar drug, Celebrex, is still available by prescription, however. Any pain medications, even over-the-counter ones, have the potential to interact with medications that an individual already is taking for diabetes management or other health issues. Individuals must let their health-care providers know what they are taking so that appropriate dosing and scheduling of all medications can be coordinated.

Dietary and herbal remedies. Finally, many individuals turn to dietary or herbal remedies for relief (Fouladbakhsh 2012, Lapane 2012). Dietary changes that can alleviate inflammation may help reduce arthritic pain, although many of these remedies remain unproven. For example, foods rich in omega-3 fatty acids (like fish and walnuts) and the spices ginger and turmeric may help reduce inflammation, whereas antioxidant-rich plant foods potentially can help reduce tissue damage from inflammation. For these and other health reasons, individuals with diabetes likely will benefit from the addition of oily fish and other sources of omega-3 fatty acids to their diet, along with plenty of antioxidant-rich vegetables, fruits, legumes, and nuts.

Supplementing with herbal remedies like glucosamine sulfate and chondroitin, two natural treatments for arthritis, generally is not backed by scientific studies (Scroggie 2003, Clegg 2006, Marshall 2006, Wandel 2010), although chondroitin sulfate may be somewhat effective for reducing the rate of decline in minimum joint space width in individuals with osteoarthritis of the knee (Hochberg 2008). In addition, certain natural herbs and spices, such as ginger, holy basil, turmeric, green tea, rosemary, scutlellaria, and huzhang, are thought to contain naturally occurring anti-inflammatory compounds known as COX-2 inhibitors (also found in prescription Celebrex and previously Vioxx). The benefit of any of these dietary supplements for arthritic pain, however, has yet to be proven in well-controlled research studies (Fouladbakhsh 2012, Lapane 2012).

SURGICAL TREATMENT OF ARTHRITIC JOINTS

When an individual reaches the point at which pain is severe and joint function is inadequate because of arthritis, he or she should consult with a health-care provider about the possibility of having corrective or joint replacement surgery.

This option has become an earlier, effective option for treating chronic arthritic pain, particularly of the knee. Many types of surgical procedures are available to treat different joints, with the most well-known being artificial joint replacement for completely destroyed joints, but other, less dramatic surgical procedures may treat arthritis in early stages and slow the progression of the disease (Wong 2011). Arthritis does not always worsen over time, however. If a person's symptoms stabilize, progression may be slow enough to leave plenty of time to explore other options. Technological advances in materials, operative procedures, product design, and manufacturing processes have brought joint replacement surgeries into the new millennium with a flourish (Brewster 2010). Surgical techniques are becoming more successful every day due to new bone substitutes, specialized alloys, and innovative designs for replacement joints (Wong 2011, Danisovic 2012). In the near future, minimally invasive joint replacement surgeries may

Table 16.7 Recommended Exercise Rx for Obesity, Orthopedic Limitations, and Arthritis

Mode	Aerobic: Walking, cycling, swimming, rowing, aquatic activities, seated exercises, dancing, conditioning machines, and more
	Resistance: All major muscle groups, using resistance bands, free weights, resistance training machines, isometric exercises, or calisthenics (using body weight); include four to five upper-body and four to five lower-body/core exercises
Intensity	Aerobic: 40–89% HRR (initial intensity may need to be lower for sedentary, deconditioned, and overweight individuals)
	Resistance: 50/60–80% 1 RM (starting on the low end)
	Both: Perceived exertion of "somewhat hard" to start; 5–7 (on 10 point scale)
Frequency	Aerobic: 5–7 days/week (including structured and lifestyle activity) to maximize caloric expenditure for weight loss; 3–7 days/week with orthopedic limitations or osteoarthritis
	Resistance: A minimum of 2 days/week (preferably 3), with at least 48 h of rest between sessions
Duration	Aerobic: 30–60 min daily, on the higher end for weight loss, the lower end for orthopedic issues; for a total of at least 150 min/week of moderate-intensity (or possibly higher) activity
	Resistance: 8–12 repetitions per exercise as a goal, but 10–15 repetitions initially; one to three sets per exercise
Progression	Aerobic: Start out on the "low" side and progress slowly over weeks to months; increase duration and frequency first for weight loss, intensity last
	Resistance: Start with one to two sets of 8–15 repetitions: one set of 10–15 repetitions to fatigue initially, progressing to 8–10 harder repetitions, and finally to two to three sets of 8–10 repetitions), although the presence of orthopedic limitations may require staying with higher repetitions and less resistance

Note: 1 RM, one-repetition maximum; HRR, heart rate reserve.

become available as a treatment option. If an individual undergoes knee or hip replacement surgery, however, he or she can plan on returning to regular physical activity afterward (Jones 2011, Wilson 2011).

Case in Point: Wrap-Up

In talking with her health-care provider, DK learned about other options for exercise. They decided it would be best for her to start with an activity other than walking because of the pain it caused in her hip. DK has a friend who does water aerobics, and she now thinks she may start with that activity first. She also set goals for how much time to spend exercising with the understanding that she will need to follow her plan for a few months to get her fitness level to where it should be, by starting with a small amount of exercise and adding more as tolerated. She now realizes that it may take her a while to lose all the weight she wants to, but she is determined to keep trying until she gets it done.

Exercise Program Goals

Mode of Activity: To start, given DK's hip pain issues, she should start with a mix of weight-bearing and non–weight-bearing activities, including water aerobics or other aquatic exercise (even some pool walking), stationary cycling, seated exercises, and use of conditioning machines that are lower impact (such as cross-trainers and elliptical machines). Varying her exercise from one day to the next (doing cross-training) will help to lessen the stress on her arthritic hips. As she becomes more conditioned, she can try both indoor treadmill walking and outdoor walking by starting with short bouts and working up from there. She also plans to add in some lower-body resistance training to help strengthen the muscles around her hips to prevent pain.

Intensity: DK should attempt to maintain a workout pace that feels "somewhat hard" on most days, using pain as her guide for exercise intensity on any given day. Her initial target heart rate should be in the range of 119–127 bpm (40–50% heart rate reserve, or HRR), with a later training goal of closer to 133 bpm (59% of HRR). In her case, however, doing any activity—even a very low-level one—can be beneficial for weight loss, diabetes management, and arthritis, so she plans to focus more on just being active than on her actual heart rate. She plans on approaching her resistance work the same way and may just use resistance bands to start.

Frequency: Because DK wants to lose weight through physical activity, exercising as many days a week as possible is best. She plans on being active 5 to 7 days a week, even if some days it just involves more daily movement. In any case, she plans to never take off >1 day in a row to better manage her blood glucose levels and to expend more calories. She should plan on doing resistance at least 2 days a week.

Duration: DK should engage in shorter bouts of exercise training to start, separated by a rest period, until she can train for 20–30 min continuously—whether doing aerobic or resistance workouts. Her training goal is 150 min of moderate physical activity spread throughout the week. Her eventual duration goal may be closer to 60 min a day to maximize her weight loss and maintenance.

Progression: DK should increase the duration of her planned workouts first to try to reach 150 min/week of moderate exercise. Once she is able to do that, she can either exercise more frequently or very slowly progress to a higher exercise intensity as long as the pain in her hip does not increase. Given that weight loss is a primary goal, focusing more on total energy expenditure should be her mode of progression, which she can accomplish by doing moderate activities for longer (≥60 min daily). Even as she progresses, her routine should continue to include various activities (cross-training) to help limit stress on her hip joint. In addition, she should plan on doing resistance training on at least two of her exercise training days, focusing in particular on strengthening the muscles around her hips joints to prevent pain recurrence.

Precautions: DK should not have to worry about exercise-associated hypoglycemia because she is only taking metformin. Her health-care provider already has cleared her to start exercising moderately, so she does not need to have an exercise stress test at this point. Her main precaution is simply to be careful to avoid overdoing her activities and exacerbating her hip pain that could cause her to revert to a more sedentary lifestyle.

Although excess body weight, orthopedic injuries and other issues, and osteoarthritis can make regular physical activity participation more challenging, the benefits of engaging in it far outweigh the risks. In fact, most arthritic pain can be improved with regular participation in moderate aerobic training and weight loss and should be encouraged for all individuals with diabetes. Care should be taken to prevent overuse injuries that can result from physical activity.

PROFESSIONAL PRACTICE PEARLS

- Whereas body weight is more frequently normal or near normal at onset of T1D, obesity and overweight are highly prevalent in both T2D and GDM.
- For individuals with any type of diabetes, body weight gain, especially when visceral fat, remains a concern because it can affect insulin action and blood glucose management.
- Use of insulin and some oral antihyperglycemic agents can contribute to weight gain (particularly visceral) and cardiovascular risk in individuals with T1D and T2D.
- The most successful programs for long-term weight control have involved combinations of diet, exercise, and behavior modification given that physical activity combined with dietary changes are more effective for long-term weight loss than either done alone.
- An initial goal for overweight or obese individuals should be to simply increase the amount of daily physical movement from an inactive level.
- For maximal weight loss, individuals should aim for a target expenditure of 300–400 calories/day or 2,000 calories/week through any type of physical activity.

- Excess body weight is a contributing factor in the development of orthopedic limitations like acute and overtraining injuries and osteoarthritis of the lower limb joints.
- To minimize risk of injury, an individual should exercise regularly to increase physical fitness and increase total activity gradually.
- Treatment of acute (and even chronic) athletic injuries is best handled with RICE (Rest, Ice, Compression, and Elevation).
- Taking anti-inflammatory medications, otherwise known as NSAIDs, is often helpful when treating activity-related injuries, but it may be contraindicated in individuals with chronic kidney disease.
- Individuals with diabetes are more prone to developing overuse injuries with a slower onset that can limit movement around joints, such as adhesive capsulitis.
- Individuals who are experiencing nagging aches and pains that are only minor should simply cut back on the intensity, frequency, and duration of irritating activities to bring relief of symptoms, along with engaging in hard and easy days and cross-training.
- Wearing proper shoes is critical to preventing many lower-extremity and foot problems, and the best type of shoes to wear varies by activity.
- Osteoarthritis is a common condition in older adults that is characterized by painful inflammation of a joint or joints, particularly hips, knees, hands, and toes.
- The pain associated with arthritis does not come from the joint cartilage surfaces themselves, but rather from the irritated nerves in adjacent stretched or inflamed areas.
- Participation in regular physical activity is possible with arthritis and should be encouraged given that it may actually improve joint symptoms in many cases.
- Individuals should start with range-of-motion exercises to increase joint mobility and resistance work to increase the strength of the muscles surrounding any affected joints.
- Although most can engage in moderate activity, individuals with osteoarthritis should match the type and amount of physical activity to their abilities and severity of their condition.
- Individuals may benefit from nonmedicinal methods like massage and dietary changes to alleviate pain from arthritis, followed by pain relievers and anti-inflammatory drugs.
- When pain is severe and joint function inadequate due to arthritis, corrective or joint replacement surgery may be necessary to restore physical function.

REFERENCES

Abate M, Schiavone C, Pelotti P, Salini V: Limited joint mobility in diabetes and ageing: recent advances in pathogenesis and therapy. *Int J Immunopathol Pharmacol* 23:997–1003, 2011

Action to Control Cardiovascular Risk in Diabetes Study Group, Gerstein HC, Miller ME, Byington RP, Goff DC Jr, Bigger JT, Buse JB, Cushman WC, Genuth S, Ismail-Beigi F, Grimm RH Jr, Probstfield JL, Simons-Morton DG, Friedewald WT: Effects of intensive glucose lowering in type 2 diabetes. *N Engl J Med* 358:2545–2559, 2008

Alemzadeh R, Berhe T, Wyatt DT: Flexible insulin therapy with glargine insulin improved glycemic control and reduced severe hypoglycemia among pre-school-aged children with type 1 diabetes mellitus. *Pediatrics* 115:1320–1324, 2005

Amati F, Dubé JJ, Coen PM, Stefanovic-Racic M, Toledo FG, Goodpaster BH: Physical inactivity and obesity underlie the insulin resistance of aging. *Diabetes Care* 32:1547–1549, 2009

Amati F, Pennant M, Azuma K, Dubé JJ, Toledo FG, Rossi AP, Kelley DE, Good-paster BH: Lower thigh subcutaneous and higher visceral abdominal adipose tissue content both contribute to insulin resistance. *Obesity (Silver Spring)* 20:1115–1117, 2012

American Diabetes Association: Diagnosis and classification of diabetes mellitus. *Diabetes Care* 36 (Suppl. 1):S67–S74, 2013a

American Diabetes Association: Standards of medical care in diabetes—2013. *Diabetes Care* 36 (Suppl. 1):S11–S66, 2013b

Basta G, Lazzerini G, Massaro M, Simoncini T, Tanganelli P, Fu C, Kislinger T, Stern DM, Schmidt AM, De Caterina R: Advanced glycation end products activate endothelium through signal-transduction receptor RAGE: a mechanism for amplification of inflammatory responses. *Circulation* 105:816–822, 2002

Black DM, Filak AT: Hyperglycemia with non-insulin-dependent diabetes following intraarticular steroid injection. *J Fam Pract* 28:462–463, 1989

Bloemers F, Collard D, Paw MC, Van Mechelen W, Twisk J, Verhagen E: Physical inactivity is a risk factor for physical activity-related injuries in children. *Br J Sports Med* 46:669-674, 2012

Borel AL, Nazare JA, Smith J, Almeras N, Tremblay A, Bergeron J, Poirier P, Despres JP: Visceral and not subcutaneous abdominal adiposity reduction drives the benefits of a 1-year lifestyle modification program. *Obesity (Silver Spring)* 20:1223–1233, 2012

Boulé NG, Haddad E, Kenny GP, Wells GA, Sigal RJ: Effects of exercise on glycemic control and body mass in type 2 diabetes mellitus: a meta-analysis of controlled clinical trials. *JAMA* 286:1218–1227, 2001

Brewster M: Does total joint replacement or arthrodesis of the first metatarsophalangeal joint yield better functional results? A systematic review of the literature. *J Foot Ankle Surg* 49:546–552, 2010

Brown RJ, Wijewickrama RC, Harlan DM, Rother KI: Uncoupling intensive insulin therapy from weight gain and hypoglycemia in type 1 diabetes. *Diabetes Technol Ther* 13:457–460, 2011

Cakir H, Van Vliet-Koppert ST, Van Lieshout EM, De Vries MR, Van Der Elst M, Schepers T: Demographics and outcome of metatarsal fractures. *Arch Orthop Trauma Surg* 131:241–245, 2011

Catenacci VA, Grunwald GK, Ingebrigtsen JP, Jakicic JM, McDermott MD, Phelan S, Wing RR, Hill JO, Wyatt HR: Physical activity patterns using accelerometry in the National Weight Control Registry. *Obesity (Silver Spring)* 19:1163–1170, 2011

Chen AL, Shapiro JA, Ahn AK, Zuckerman JD, Cuomo F: Rotator cuff repair in patients with type I diabetes mellitus. *J Shoulder Elbow Surg* 12:416–421, 2003

Cheung RT, Ng GY: Influence of different footwear on force of landing during running. *Phys Ther* 88:620–628, 2008

Chomentowski P, Dubé JJ, Amati F, Stefanovic-Racic M, Zhu S, Toledo FG, Goodpaster BH: Moderate exercise attenuates the loss of skeletal muscle mass that occurs with intentional caloric restriction-induced weight loss in older, overweight to obese adults. *J Gerontol A Biol Sci Med Sci* 64:575–580, 2009

Chumbley EM, O'Connor FG, Nirschl RP: Evaluation of overuse elbow injuries. *Am Fam Physician* 61:691–700, 2000

Clegg DO, Reda DJ, Harris CL, Klein MA, O'Dell JR, Hooper MM, Bradley JD, Bingham CO III, Weisman MH, Jackson CG, Lane NE, Cush JJ, Moreland LW, Schumacher HR Jr, Oddis CV, Wolfe F, Molitor JA, Yocum DE, Schnitzer TJ, Furst DE, Sawitzke AD, Shi H, Brandt KD, Moskowitz RW, Williams HJ: Glucosamine, chondroitin sulfate, and the two in combination for painful knee osteoarthritis. *N Engl J Med* 354:795–808, 2006

Colberg SR, Somma CT, Sechrist SR: Physical activity participation may offset some of the negative impact of diabetes on cognitive function. *J Am Med Dir Assoc* 9:434–438, 2008

Collins M, Raleigh SM: Genetic risk factors for musculoskeletal soft tissue injuries. *Med Sport Sci* 54:136–149, 2009

Conway B, Miller RG, Costacou T, Fried L, Kelsey S, Evans RW, Orchard TJ: Adiposity and mortality in type 1 diabetes. *Int J Obes (Lond)* 33:796–805, 2009

Conway B, Miller RG, Costacou T, Fried L, Kelsey S, Evans RW, Orchard TJ: Temporal patterns in overweight and obesity in type 1 diabetes. *Diabet Med* 27:398–404, 2010

Cosca DD, Navazio F: Common problems in endurance athletes. *Am Fam Physician* 76:237–244, 2007

Costacou T, Edmundowicz D, Prince C, Conway B, Orchard TJ: Progression of coronary artery calcium in type 1 diabetes mellitus. *Am J Cardiol* 100:1543–1547, 2007

Coupland CA, Cliffe SJ, Bassey EJ, Grainge MJ, Hosking DJ, Chilvers CE: Habitual physical activity and bone mineral density in postmenopausal women in England. *Int J Epidemiol* 28:241–246, 1999

Craig ME, Duffin AC, Gallego PH, Lam A, Cusumano J, Hing S, Donaghue KC: Plantar fascia thickness, a measure of tissue glycation, predicts the development of complications in adolescents with type 1 diabetes. *Diabetes Care* 31:1201–1206, 2008

Cuff DJ, Meneilly GS, Martin A, Ignaszewski A, Tildesley HD, Frohlich JJ: Effective exercise modality to reduce insulin resistance in women with type 2 diabetes. *Diabetes Care* 26:2977–2982, 2003

D'Hooge R, Hellinckx T, Van Laethem C, Stegen S, De Schepper J, Van Aken S, Dewolf D, Calders P: Influence of combined aerobic and resistance training on metabolic control, cardiovascular fitness and quality of life in adolescents with type 1 diabetes: a randomized controlled trial. *Clin Rehabil* 25:349–359, 2011

Dailey G, Admane K, Mercier F, Owens D: Relationship of insulin dose, A1C lowering, and weight in type 2 diabetes: comparing insulin glargine and insulin detemir. *Diabetes Technol Ther* 12:1019–1027, 2010

Danisovic L, Varga I, Zamborsky R, Bohmer D: The tissue engineering of articular cartilage: cells, scaffolds and stimulating factors. *Exp Biol Med (Maywood)* 237:10–17, 2012

De Leeuw I, Vague P, Selam JL, Skeie S, Lang H, Draeger E, Elte JW: Insulin detemir used in basal-bolus therapy in people with type 1 diabetes is associated with a lower risk of nocturnal hypoglycaemia and less weight gain over 12 months in comparison to NPH insulin. *Diabetes Obes Metab* 7:73–82, 2005

Delahanty LM, Nathan DM: Implications of the diabetes prevention program and Look AHEAD clinical trials for lifestyle interventions. *J Am Diet Assoc* 108 (4 Suppl. 1):S66–S72, 2008

Diabetes Control and Complications Trial Research Group: Influence of intensive diabetes treatment on body weight and composition of adults with type 1 diabetes in the Diabetes Control and Complications Trial. *Diabetes Care* 24:1711–1721, 2001

Donnelly JE, Blair SN, Jakicic JM, Manore MM, Rankin JW, Smith BK, American College of Sports Medicine: American College of Sports Medicine Position Stand. Appropriate physical activity intervention strategies for weight loss and prevention of weight regain for adults. *Med Sci Sports Exerc* 41:459–471, 2009

Dubé MC, Lemieux, Piche ME, Corneau L, Bergeron J, Riou ME, Weisnagel SJ: The contribution of visceral adiposity and mid-thigh fat-rich muscle to the metabolic profile in postmenopausal women. *Obesity (Silver Spring)* 19:953–959, 2011

Dubé MC, Prud'homme D, Lemieux S, Lavoie C, Weisnagel SJ: Body composition indices in women with well-controlled type 1 diabetes. *Diabetes Care* 31:e48, 2008

Elder SJ, Roberts SB: The effects of exercise on food intake and body fatness: a summary of published studies. *Nutr Rev* 65:1–19, 2007

Feldman-Billard S, Du Pasquier-Fediaevsky L, Heron E: Hyperglycemia after repeated periocular dexamethasone injections in patients with diabetes. *Ophthalmology* 113:1720–1723, 2006

Ferriss JB, Webb D, Chaturvedi N, Fuller JH, Idzior-Walus B, Eurodiab Prospective Complications Group: Weight gain is associated with improved glycaemic control but with adverse changes in plasma lipids and blood pressure in type 1 diabetes. *Diabet Med* 23:557–564, 2006

Fouladbakhsh J: Complementary and alternative modalities to relieve osteoarthritis symptoms. *Am J Nurs* 112 (3 Suppl. 1):S44–S51, 2012

Foy CG, Lewis CE, Hairston KG, Miller GD, Lang W, Jakicic JM, Rejeski WJ, Ribisl PM, Walkup MP, Wagenknecht LE, Look AHEAD Research Group: Intensive lifestyle intervention improves physical function among obese adults with knee pain: findings from the Look AHEAD trial. *Obesity (Silver Spring)* 19:83–93, 2011

Fry RW, Morton AR, Keast D: Overtraining in athletes. An update. *Sports Med* 12:32–65, 1991

Fry RW, Morton AR, Keast D: Periodisation and the prevention of overtraining. *Can J Sport Sci* 17:241–248, 1992

Garber CE, Blissmer B, Deschenes MR, Franklin BA, Lamonte MJ, Lee IM, Nieman DC, Swain DP, American College of Sports Medicine: American College of Sports Medicine position stand. Quantity and quality of exercise for developing and maintaining cardiorespiratory, musculoskeletal, and neuromotor fitness in apparently healthy adults: guidance for prescribing exercise. *Med Sci Sports Exerc* 43:1334–1359, 2011

Garcilazo C, Cavallasca JA, Musuruana JL: Shoulder manifestations of diabetes mellitus. *Curr Diabetes Rev* 6:334–340, 2010

Gonzalez P, Laker SR, Sullivan W, Harwood JE, Akuthota V: The effects of epidural betamethasone on blood glucose in patients with diabetes mellitus. *PMR* 1:340–345, 2009

Goodpaster BH, Chomentowski P, Ward BK, Rossi A, Glynn NW, Delmonico MJ, Kritchevsky SB, Pahor M, Newman AB: Effects of physical activity on strength and skeletal muscle fat infiltration in older adults: a randomized controlled trial. *J Appl Physiol* 105:1498–1503, 2008

Graves M, Tarquinio TA: Diabetic neuroarthropathy (Charcot joints): the importance of recognizing chronic sensory deficits in the treatment of acute foot and ankle fractures in diabetic patients. *Orthopedics* 26:415–418, 2003

Haris A, Szabo A, Lanyi E, Mucsi I, Polner K: Acute and long-term effects of corticosteroid therapy on bone metabolism in patients with kidney diseases. *Clin Nephrol* 78:17–23, 2012

Hawley CJ, Schoene RB: Overtraining syndrome: a guide to diagnosis, treatment, and prevention. *Phys Sportsmed* 31:25–31, 2003

Herriott MT, Colberg SR, Parson HK, Nunnold T, Vinik AI: Effects of 8 weeks of flexibility and resistance training in older adults with type 2 diabetes. *Diabetes Care* 27:2988–2989, 2004

Heyman E, Toutain C, Delamarche P, Berthon P, Briard D, Youssef H, Dekerdanet M, Gratas-Delamarche A: Exercise training and cardiovascular risk factors in type 1 diabetic adolescent girls. *Pediatr Exerc Sci* 19:408–419, 2007

Hill EE, Eisenmann JC, Gentile D, Holmes ME, Walsh D: The association between morning cortisol and adiposity in children varies by weight status. *J Pediatr Endocrinol Metab* 24:709–713, 2011

Hochberg MC, Zhan M, Langenberg P: The rate of decline of joint space width in patients with osteoarthritis of the knee: a systematic review and meta-analysis of randomized placebo-controlled trials of chondroitin sulfate. *Curr Med Res Opin* 24:3029–3035, 2008

Hoogeboom TJ, den Broeder AA, Swierstra BA, de Bie RA, van den Ende CH: Joint-pain comorbidity, health status, and medication use in hip and knee osteoarthritis: a cross-sectional study. *Arthritis Care Res (Hoboken)* 64:54–58, 2012

Ibanez J, Izquierdo M, Arguelles I, Forga L, Larrion JL, Garcia-Unciti M, Idoate F, Gorostiaga EM: Twice-weekly progressive resistance training decreases abdominal fat and improves insulin sensitivity in older men with type 2 diabetes. *Diabetes Care* 28:662–667, 2005

Ilich JZ, Brownbill RA: Habitual and low-impact activities are associated with better bone outcomes and lower body fat in older women. *Calcif Tissue Int* 83:260–271, 2008

Ingberg CM, Sarnblad S, Palmer M, Schvarcz E, Berne C, Aman J: Body composition in adolescent girls with type 1 diabetes. *Diabet Med* 20:1005–1011, 2003

Jacob AN, Adams-Huet B, Raskin P: The visceral and subcutaneous fat changes in type 1 diabetes: a pilot study. *Diabetes Obes Metab* 8:524–530, 2006a

Jacob AN, Salinas K, Adams-Huet B, Raskin P: Potential causes of weight gain in type 1 diabetes mellitus. *Diabetes Obes Metab* 8:404–411, 2006b

Jakicic JM, Marcus BH, Gallagher KI, Napolitano M, Lang W: Effect of exercise duration and intensity on weight loss in overweight, sedentary women: a randomized trial. *JAMA* 290:1323–1330, 2003

Jeffery RW, Wing RR, Sherwood NE, Tate DF: Physical activity and weight loss: does prescribing higher physical activity goals improve outcome? *Am J Clin Nutr* 78:684–689, 2003

Jin JY, Jusko WJ: Pharmacodynamics of glucose regulation by methylprednisolone. I. Adrenalectomized rats. *Biopharm Drug Dispos* 30:21–34, 2009

Johnson NA, Sachinwalla T, Walton DW, Smith K, Armstrong A, Thompson MW, George J: Aerobic exercise training reduces hepatic and visceral lipids in obese individuals without weight loss. *Hepatology* 50:1105–1112, 2009

Jones DL: A public health perspective on physical activity after total hip or knee arthroplasty for osteoarthritis. *Phys Sportsmed* 39:70–79, 2011

Kabadi UM, Vora A, Kabadi M: Hyperinsulinemia and central adiposity: influence of chronic insulin therapy in type 1 diabetes. *Diabetes Care* 23:1024–1025, 2000

Kang JH, Tseng SH, Jaw FS, Lai CH, Chen HC, Chen SC: Comparison of ultrasonographic findings of the rotator cuff between diabetic and nondiabetic patients with chronic shoulder pain: a retrospective study. *Ultrasound Med Biol* 36:1792–1796, 2010

Kannus P: Immobilization or early mobilization after an acute soft-tissue injury? *Phys Sportsmed* 28:55–63, 2000

Kilpatrick ES, Rigby AS, Atkin SL: Insulin resistance, the metabolic syndrome, and complication risk in type 1 diabetes: "double diabetes" in the Diabetes Control and Complications Trial. *Diabetes Care* 30:707–712, 2007

Kiylioglu N, Akyildiz UO, Ozkul A, Akyol A: Carpal tunnel syndrome and ulnar neuropathy at the wrist: comorbid disease or not? *J Clin Neurophysiol* 28:520–523, 2011

Knapik JJ, Spiess A, Swedler D, Grier T, Hauret K, Yoder J, Jones BH: Retrospective examination of injuries and physical fitness during Federal Bureau of Investigation new agent training. *J Occup Med Toxicol* 6:26, 2011

Knobloch K, Yoon U, Vogt PM: Acute and overuse injuries correlated to hours of training in master running athletes. *Foot Ankle Int* 29:671–676, 2008

Ko JY, Wang FS: Rotator cuff lesions with shoulder stiffness: updated pathomechanisms and management. *Chang Gung Med J* 34:331–340, 2011

Kopp M, Steinlechner M, Ruedl G, Ledochowski L, Rumpold G, Taylor AH: Acute effects of brisk walking on affect and psychological well-being in individuals with type 2 diabetes. *Diabetes Res Clin Pract* 95:25–29, 2012

Koska J, Stefan N, Permana PA, Weyer C, Sonoda M, Bogardus C, Smith SR, Joanisse DR, Funahashi T, Krakoff J, Bunt JC: Increased fat accumulation in liver may link insulin resistance with subcutaneous abdominal adipocyte enlargement, visceral adiposity, and hypoadiponectinemia in obese individuals. *Am J Clin Nutr* 87:295–302, 2008

Kuipers H: Training and overtraining: an introduction. *Med Sci Sports Exerc* 30:1137–1139, 2008

Kumar AA, Palamaner Subash Shantha G, Kahan S, Samson RJ, Boddu ND, Cheskin LJ: Intentional weight loss and dose reductions of anti-diabetic medications—a retrospective cohort study. *PLoS One* 7:e32395, 2012

Laine L, White WB, Rostom A, Hochberg M: COX-2 selective inhibitors in the treatment of osteoarthritis. *Semin Arthritis Rheum* 38:165–187, 2008

Lapane KL, Sands MR, Yang S, McAlindon TE, Eaton CB: Use of complementary and alternative medicine among patients with radiographic-confirmed knee osteoarthritis. *Osteoarthritis Cartilage* 20:22–28, 2012

Lysy Z, Da Costa D, Dasgupta K: The association of physical activity and depression in type 2 diabetes. *Diabet Med* 25:1133–1141, 2008

Maahs DM, Nadeau K, Snell-Bergeon JK, Schauer I, Bergman B, West NA, Rewers M, Daniels SR, Ogden LG, Hamman RF, Dabelea D: Association of insulin sensitivity to lipids across the lifespan in people with type 1 diabetes. *Diabet Med* 28:148–155, 2011

Magrans-Courtney T, Wilborn C, Rasmussen C, Ferreira M, Greenwood L, Campbell B, Kerksick CM, Nassar E, Li R, Iosia M, Cooke M, Dugan K, Willoughby D, Soliah L, Kreider RB: Effects of diet type and supplementation of glucosamine, chondroitin, and MSM on body composition, functional status, and markers of health in women with knee osteoarthritis initiating a resistance-based exercise and weight loss program. *J Int Soc Sports Nutr* 8:8, 2011

Marre M, Pinget M, Gin H, Thivolet C, Hanaire H, Robert JJ, Fontaine P: Insulin detemir improves glycaemic control with less hypoglycaemia and no weight gain: 52-week data from the PREDICTIVE study in a cohort of French patients with type 1 or type 2 diabetes. *Diabetes Metab* 35:469–475, 2009

Marshall PD, Poddar S, Tweed EM, Brandes L: Clinical inquiries: Do glucosamine and chondroitin worsen blood sugar control in diabetes? *J Fam Pract* 55:1091–1093, 2006

McAdam-Marx C, Bouchard J, Aagren M, Nelson R, Brixner D: Analysis of glycaemic control and weight change in patients initiated with human or analog insulin in an US ambulatory care setting. *Diabetes Obes Metab* 12:54–64, 2010

McMahon SK, Ferreira LD, Ratnam N, Davey RJ, Youngs LM, Davis EA, Fournier PA, Jones TW: Glucose requirements to maintain euglycemia after moderate-intensity afternoon exercise in adolescents with type 1 diabetes are increased in a biphasic manner. *J Clin Endocrinol Metab* 92:963–968, 2007

Messier SP, Loeser RF, Miller GD, Morgan TM, Rejeski WJ, Sevick MA, Ettinger WH Jr, Pahor M, Williamson JD: Exercise and dietary weight loss in overweight and obese older adults with knee osteoarthritis: the Arthritis, Diet, and Activity Promotion Trial. *Arthritis Rheum* 50:1501–1510, 2004

Messier SP, Loeser RF, Mitchell MN, Valle G, Morgan TP, Rejeski WJ, Ettinger WH: Exercise and weight loss in obese older adults with knee osteoarthritis: a preliminary study. *J Am Geriatr Soc* 48:1062–1072, 2000

Michaelsson K, Byberg L, Ahlbom A, Melhus H, Farahmand BY: Risk of severe knee and hip osteoarthritis in relation to level of physical exercise: a prospective cohort study of long-distance skiers in Sweden. *PLoS One* 6:e18339, 2011

Monami M, Marchionni N, Mannucci E: Long-acting insulin analogues vs. NPH human insulin in type 1 diabetes. A meta-analysis. *Diabetes Obes Metab* 11:372–378, 2009

Morio C, Lake MJ, Gueguen N, Rao G, Baly L: The influence of footwear on foot motion during walking and running. *J Biomech* 42:2081–2088, 2009

Mourier A, Gautier JF, De Kerviler E, Bigard AX, Villette JM, Garnier JP, Duvallet A, Guezennec CY, Cathelineau G: Mobilization of visceral adipose tissue related to the improvement in insulin sensitivity in response to physical training in NIDDM. Effects of branched-chain amino acid supplements. *Diabetes Care* 20:385–391, 1997

Nelson ME, Rejeski WJ, Blair SN, Duncan PW, Judge JO, King AC, Macera CA, Castaneda-Sceppa C: Physical activity and public health in older adults: recommendation from the American College of Sports Medicine and the American Heart Association. *Med Sci Sports Exerc* 39:1435–1445, 2007

Newfield RS, Cohen D, Capparelli EV, Shragg P: Rapid weight gain in children soon after diagnosis of type 1 diabetes: is there room for concern? *Pediatr Diabetes* 10:310–315, 2009

O'Leary VB, Marchetti CM, Krishnan RK, Stetzer BP, Gonzalez F, Kirwan JP: Exercise-induced reversal of insulin resistance in obese elderly is associated with reduced visceral fat. *J Appl Physiol* 100:1584–1589, 2006

Orchard TJ, Olson JC, Erbey JR, Williams K, Forrest KY, Smithline Kinder L, Ellis D, Becker DJ: Insulin resistance-related factors, but not glycemia, predict coronary artery disease in type 1 diabetes: 10-year follow-up data from the Pittsburgh Epidemiology of Diabetes Complications Study. *Diabetes Care* 26:1374–1379, 2003

Paoloni JA, Milne C, Orchard J, Hamilton B: Non-steroidal anti-inflammatory drugs in sports medicine: guidelines for practical but sensible use. *Br J Sports Med* 43:863–865, 2009

Patel K, Diamantidis C, Zhan M, Hsu VD, Walker LD, Gardner J, Weir MR, Fink JC: Influence of creatinine versus glomerular filtration rate on non-steroidal anti-inflammatory drug prescriptions in chronic kidney disease. *Am J Nephrol* 36:19–26, 2012

Perlman AI, Ali A, Njike VY, Hom D, Davidi A, Gould-Fogerite S, Milak C, Katz DL: Massage therapy for osteoarthritis of the knee: a randomized dose-finding trial. *PLoS One* 7:e30248, 2012

Perryman JR, Hershman EB: The acute management of soft tissue injuries of the knee. *Orthop Clin North Am* 33:575–585, 2002

Phung OJ, Scholle JM, Talwar M, Coleman CI: Effect of noninsulin antidiabetic drugs added to metformin therapy on glycemic control, weight gain, and hypoglycemia in type 2 diabetes. *JAMA* 303:1410–1418, 2010

Physical Activity Guidelines Advisory Committee: Physical Activity Guidelines Advisory Committee Report, 2008. Washington, DC, U.S. Department of Health and Human Services, 2008

Plastino M, Fava A, Carmela C, De Bartolo M, Ermio C, Cristiano D, Ettore M, Abenavoli L, Bosco D: Insulin resistance increases risk of carpal tunnel syndrome: a case-control study. *J Peripher Nerv Syst* 16:186–190, 2011

Pollock ML, Carroll JF, Graves JE, Leggett SH, Braith RW, Limacher M, Hagberg JM: Injuries and adherence to walk/jog and resistance training programs in the elderly. *Med Sci Sports Exerc* 23:1194–1200, 1991

Purvis D, Gonsalves S, Deuster PA: Physiological and psychological fatigue in extreme conditions: overtraining and elite athletes. *PMR* 2:442–450, 2010

Ramalho AC, de Lourdes Lima M, Nunes F, Cambui Z, Barbosa C, Andrade A, Viana A, Martins M, Abrantes V, Aragao C, Temistocles M: The effect of resistance versus aerobic training on metabolic control in patients with type-1 diabetes mellitus. *Diabetes Res Clin Pract* 72:271–276, 2006

Ratner RE, Dickey R, Fineman M, Maggs DG, Shen L, Strobel SA, Weyer C, Kolterman OG: Amylin replacement with pramlintide as an adjunct to insulin therapy improves long-term glycaemic and weight control in type 1 diabetes mellitus: a 1-year, randomized controlled trial. *Diabet Med* 21:1204–1212, 2004

Ratner R, Goldberg R, Haffner S, Marcovina S, Orchard T, Fowler S, Temprosa M, Diabetes Prevention Program Research Group: Impact of intensive lifestyle and metformin therapy on cardiovascular disease risk factors in the diabetes prevention program. *Diabetes Care* 28:888–894, 2005a

Ratner R, Whitehouse F, Fineman MS, Strobel S, Shen L, Maggs DG, Kolterman OG, Weyer C: Adjunctive therapy with pramlintide lowers HbA1c without concomitant weight gain and increased risk of severe hypoglycemia in patients with type 1 diabetes approaching glycemic targets. *Exp Clin Endocrinol Diabetes* 113:199–204, 2005b

Ravindran Rajendran S, Bhansali A, Walia R, Dutta P, Bansal V, Shanmugasundar G: Prevalence and pattern of hand soft-tissue changes in type 2 diabetes mellitus. *Diabetes Metab* 37:312–317, 2011

Rechardt M, Shiri R, Karppinen J, Jula A, Heliovaara M, Viikari-Juntura E: Lifestyle and metabolic factors in relation to shoulder pain and rotator cuff tendinitis: a population-based study. *BMC Musculoskelet Disord* 11:165, 2010

Riso EM, Ahtikoski A, Alev K, Kaasik P, Pehme A, Seene T: Relationship between extracellular matrix, contractile apparatus, muscle mass and strength in case of glucocorticoid myopathy. *J Steroid Biochem Mol Biol* 108:117–120, 2008

Rogers LC, Frykberg RG, Armstrong DG, Boulton AJ, Edmonds M, Van GH, Hartemann A, Game F, Jeffcoate W, Jirkovska A, Jude E, Morbach S, Morrison

WB, Pinzur M, Pitocco D, Sanders L, Wukich DK, Uccioli L: The Charcot foot in diabetes. *Diabetes Care* 34:2123–2129, 2011

Rogers LQ, Macera CA, Hootman JM, Ainsworth BE, Blairi SN: The association between joint stress from physical activity and self-reported osteoarthritis: an analysis of the Cooper Clinic data. *Osteoarthritis Cartilage* 10:617–622, 2002

Roh YH, Yi SR, Noh JH, Lee SY, Oh JH, Gong HS, Baek GH: Intra-articular corticosteroid injection in diabetic patients with adhesive capsulitis: a randomized controlled trial. *Knee Surg Sports Traumatol Arthrosc* 20:1943–1948, 2012

Roose J, de Vries WR, Schmikli SL, Backx FJ, van Doornen LJ: Evaluation and opportunities in overtraining approaches. *Res Q Exerc Sport* 80:756–764, 2009

Ross R, Janssen I, Dawson J, Kungl AM, Kuk JL, Wong SL, Nguyen-Duy TB, Lee S, Kilpatrick K, Hudson R: Exercise-induced reduction in obesity and insulin resistance in women: a randomized controlled trial. *Obesity Research* 12:789–798, 2004

Ross R, Dagnone D, Jones PJ, Smith H, Paddags A, Hudson R, Janssen I: Reduction in obesity and related comorbid conditions after diet-induced weight loss or exercise-induced weight loss in men. A randomized, controlled trial. *Ann Intern Med* 133:92–103, 2000

Ross SA, Tildesley HD, Ashkenas J: Barriers to effective insulin treatment: the persistence of poor glycemic control in type 2 diabetes. *Curr Med Res Opin* 27 (Suppl. 3):13–20, 2011

Rozental TD, Zurakowski D, Blazar PE: Trigger finger: prognostic indicators of recurrence following corticosteroid injection. *J Bone Joint Surg Am* 90:1665–1672, 2008

Ryan MB, Valiant GA, McDonald K, Taunton JE: The effect of three different levels of footwear stability on pain outcomes in women runners: a randomised control trial. *Br J Sports Med* 45:715–721, 2011

Scanzello CR, Goldring SR: The role of synovitis in osteoarthritis pathogenesis. *Bone* 51:249–257, 2012

Scroggie DA, Albright A, Harris MD: The effect of glucosamine-chondroitin supplementation on glycosylated hemoglobin levels in patients with type 2 diabetes mellitus: a placebo-controlled, double-blinded, randomized clinical trial. *Arch Intern Med* 163:1587–1590, 2003

Seene T, Kaasik P: Role of exercise therapy in prevention of decline in aging muscle function: glucocorticoid myopathy and unloading. *J Aging Res* 2012:172492, 2012

Simo R, Hernandez C: Prevention and treatment of diabetic retinopathy: evidence from large, randomized trials. The emerging role of fenofibrate. *Rev Recent Clin Trials* 7:71–80, 2012

Slentz CA, Aiken LB, Houmard JA, Bales CW, Johnson JL, Tanner CJ, Duscha BD, Kraus WE: Inactivity, exercise, and visceral fat. STRRIDE: a randomized, controlled study of exercise intensity and amount. *J Appl Physiol* 99:1613–1618, 2005

Slentz CA, Duscha BD, Johnson JL, Ketchum K, Aiken LB, Samsa GP, Houmard JA, Bales CW, Kraus WE: Effects of the amount of exercise on body weight, body composition, and measures of central obesity: STRRIDE—a randomized controlled study. *Arch Intern Med* 164:31–39, 2004

Stephens MB, Beutler AI, O'Connor FG: Musculoskeletal injections: a review of the evidence. *Am Fam Physician* 78:971–976, 2008

Stewart KJ: Exercise training and the cardiovascular consequences of type 2 diabetes and hypertension: plausible mechanisms for improving cardiovascular health. *JAMA* 288:1622–1631, 2002

Stiles VH, James IT, Dixon SJ, Guisasola IN: Natural turf surfaces: the case for continued research. *Sports Med* 39:65–84, 2009

Tenforde AS, Sayres LC, McCurdy ML, Collado H, Sainani KL, Fredericson M: Overuse injuries in high school runners: lifetime prevalence and prevention strategies. *PMR* 3:125–131, 2011

Tsang T, Orr R, Lam P, Comino E, Singh MF: Effects of Tai Chi on glucose homeostasis and insulin sensitivity in older adults with type 2 diabetes: a randomised double-blind sham-exercise-controlled trial. *Age Ageing* 37:64–71, 2008

Tweed JL, Campbell JA, Avil SJ: Biomechanical risk factors in the development of medial tibial stress syndrome in distance runners. *J Am Podiatr Med Assoc* 98:436–444, 2008

U.S. Department of Health and Human Services, Centers for Disease Control and Prevention: National diabetes fact sheet: national estimates and general information on diabetes and prediabetes in the United States, 2011, edited by Centers for Disease Control and Prevention. Atlanta, GA, U.S. Department of Health and Human Services, 2011

Unick JL, Beavers D, Jakicic JM, Kitabchi AE, Knowler WC, Wadden TA, Wing RR, Look AHEAD Research Group: Effectiveness of lifestyle interventions for individuals with severe obesity and type 2 diabetes: results from the Look AHEAD trial. *Diabetes Care* 34:2152–2157, 2011

Van Ginckel A, Thijs Y, Hesar NG, Mahieu N, De Clercq D, Roosen P, Witvrouw E: Intrinsic gait-related risk factors for Achilles tendinopathy in novice runners: a prospective study. *Gait Posture* 29:387–391, 2009

Verkleij SP, Luijsterburg PA, Bohnen AM, Koes BW, Bierma-Zeinstra SM: NSAIDs vs acetaminophen in knee and hip osteoarthritis: a systematic review regarding heterogeneity influencing the outcomes. *Osteoarthritis Cartilage* 19:921–929, 2011

Vignon E, Valat JP, Rossignol M, Avouac B, Rozenberg S, Thoumie, Avouac J, Nordin M, Hilliquin P: Osteoarthritis of the knee and hip and activity: a systematic international review and synthesis (OASIS). *Joint Bone Spine* 73:442–455, 2006

Vleck VE, Bentley DJ, Millet GP, Cochrane T: Triathlon event distance specialization: training and injury effects. *J Strength Cond Res* 24:30–36, 2010

Wandel S, Juni P, Tendal B, Nuesch E, Villiger PM, Welton NJ, Reichenbach S, Trelle S: Effects of glucosamine, chondroitin, or placebo in patients with osteoarthritis of hip or knee: network meta-analysis. *BMJ* 341:c4675, 2010

Wang AA, Hutchinson DT: The effect of corticosteroid injection for trigger finger on blood glucose level in diabetic patients. *J Hand Surg Am* 31:979–681, 2006

Wang X, Lyles MF, You T, Berry MJ, Rejeski WJ, Nicklas BJ: Weight regain is related to decreases in physical activity during weight loss. *Med Sci Sports Exerc* 40:1781–1788, 2008

Weinans H, Siebelt M, Agricola R, Botter SM, Piscaer TM, Waarsing JH: Pathophysiology of peri-articular bone changes in osteoarthritis. *Bone* 51:190–196, 2012

Weinsier RL, Hunter GR, Desmond RA, Byrne NM, Zuckerman PA, Darnell BE: Free-living activity energy expenditure in women successful and unsuccessful at maintaining a normal body weight. *Am J Clin Nutr* 75:499–504, 2002

Wexler RK: Lower extremity injuries in runners. Helping athletic patients return to form. *Postgrad Med* 98:185–187, 191–193, 1995

Willick SE, Hansen PA: Running and osteoarthritis. *Clin Sports Med* 29:417–428, 2010

Wilson MJ, Villar RN: Hip replacement in the athlete: is there a role? *Knee Surg Sports Traumatol Arthrosc* 19:1524–1530, 2011

Wolf S, Simon J, Patikas D, Schuster W, Armbrust P, Doderlein L: Foot motion in children shoes: a comparison of barefoot walking with shod walking in conventional and flexible shoes. *Gait Posture* 27:51–59, 2008

Wong JM, Khan WS, Chimutengwende-Gordon M, Dowd GS: Recent advances in designs, approaches and materials in total knee replacement: literature review and evidence today. *J Perioper Pract* 21:165–171, 2011

Zachariah S, Sheldon B, Shojaee-Moradie F, Jackson NC, Backhouse K, Johnsen S, Jones RH, Umpleby AM, Russell-Jones DL: Insulin detemir reduces weight gain as a result of reduced food intake in patients with type 1 diabetes. *Diabetes Care* 34:1487–1491, 2011

Zifchock RA, Davis I, Higginson J, McCaw S, Royer T: Side-to-side differences in overuse running injury susceptibility: a retrospective study. *Hum Mov Sci* 27:888–902, 2008

Chapter 17

Cardiovascular Diseases

Diabetes is a major risk factor for cardiovascular (or macrovascular) disease, as well as being a significant cause of premature mortality and morbidity (Booth 2006, Legato 2006, Fox 2008). In addition, diabetes increases an individual's risk of developing a number of microvascular problems, such as eye disease and blindness, kidney failure, nerve disease, and amputation (U.S. Department of Health and Human Services 2011). This chapter addresses possible macrovascular complications, while microvascular complications will be covered in upcoming chapters.

Any type of diabetes that is less than optimally controlled can accelerate the development of atherosclerosis (plaque formation in arteries around the body), and hyperglycemia is a major risk factor for all cardiovascular diseases. Individuals with type 2 diabetes (T2D) in particular have an exceedingly high lifetime risk of coronary artery disease (CAD) that is exacerbated by obesity (Booth 2006, Legato 2006, Fox 2008).

Although regular physical activity may prevent or delay cardiovascular and other diabetic complications (Howorka 1997, Loimaala 2003, Balducci 2006, Zoppini 2006, Cohen 2008, Pagkalos 2008), the majority of people with T2D are physically inactive (Morrato 2007). Blood glucose control usually is improved through exercise and weight loss in individuals with T2D and in some women with gestational diabetes (GDM), and improved glycemic control generally reduces disease risk (Ratner 2005, Snowling 2006, Buse 2007). A diagnosis of cardiovascular disease is not an absolute contraindication to exercise; rather, most individuals with varying conditions can and should participate in regular physical activity to improve their diabetes control and their health (Fletcher 1996, Kirk 2004, Cornelissen 2005a, Cauza 2006, Balady 2007, Gillison 2009, Hansen 2009, Heran 2011, Wise 2011).

Case in Point: Exercise Rx for an Adult with T2D and Cardiovascular Issues

IJ is a 64-year-old man who has T2D. His A1C value has never been below 7.5% since his diagnosis 7 years ago. He has a strong family history of heart disease (his mother and father both died from a heart attack in their 50s, and his younger brother just underwent angioplasty and stent placement) as well as many other cardiovascular risk factors that include inadequately controlled diabetes, marginally controlled hypertension, elevated blood lipids, a sedentary lifestyle, obesity, and former cigarette smoking (having quit 2 years ago after 40 years of smoking at least one pack daily). Following his latest checkup with his physician, he felt chastised enough to consider starting an exercise program with his wife of 42 years. His current medications include JanuMet (a combination agent with sitagliptin and metformin), a statin for cholesterol, and a blood pressure–lowering medication.

Resting Measurements

Height: 72 inches
Weight: 260 lb
BMI: 35.3 (obese)
Heart rate: 80 beats per minute (bpm)
Blood pressure: 140/88 mmHg (on medication)

Fasting Labs

Plasma glucose: 169 mg/dl (controlled with metformin and sitagliptin)
A1C: 7.6%
Total cholesterol: 182 mg/dl (on medication)
Triglycerides: 202 mg/dl
High-density lipoprotein cholesterol (HDL-C): 37 mg/dl
Low-density lipoprotein cholesterol (LDL-C): 105 mg/dl

Questions to Consider

1. What types of physical activity should IJ consider doing since he has been inactive?
2. How much activity should he do, how often, and how intensely?
3. Are there any precautions that IJ needs to take given his strong cardiovascular risk?

(Continued on page 317.)

COMMON CARDIOVASCULAR DISEASES AND TREATMENT IN DIABETES

CORONARY ARTERY DISEASE

Risk and prevalence. Many individuals who suffer from diabetes or prediabetes may also have cardiovascular disease. CAD is the major cause of mortality and morbidity in diabetes, and individuals with T2D have a lifetime risk of CAD that includes 67% of women and 78% of men (Booth 2006, Fox 2008). The relative risk of death related to CAD adjusted for other cardiac factors was reported to be 2.58 for women with diabetes and 1.85 for men in a meta-analysis of 10 research studies, suggesting that the impact of diabetes on the risk of coronary death actually may be significantly greater for older women than it is for men (Lee 2000).

Cardiac risk factors in adults with type 1 diabetes (T1D) include physical inactivity and smoking, both of which are significantly associated with the presence of coronary artery calcification, and T1D itself is independently associated with an increased risk (Bishop 2009). Even youth with T1D present early signs of athero-sclerosis, along with low physical activity levels and cardiorespiratory fitness (Tri-gona 2010).

Epidemiological studies generally have shown that improved blood glucose control may attenuate progression of cardiovascular disease processes (Stewart 2002, 2004). In the recent ACCORD (Action to Control Cardiovascular Risk in Diabetes) trial, however, the use of intensive therapy to reach normal A1C levels for 3.5 years compared with standard therapy (that had higher A1C goals) increased mortality and did not significantly reduce major cardiovascular events in high-risk individuals with T2D. Thus, there may be a previously unrecognized harm of intensive glucose lowering in these high-risk individuals (ACCORD Study Group 2008). In the Action in Diabetes and Vascular Disease: Preterax and Diamicron Modified Release Controlled Evaluation (ADVANCE) trial, A1C lev-els were associated with lower risks of macrovascular events and death down to a threshold of 7% and microvascular events down to a threshold of 6.5%, but no evidence of lower risks was found below these levels (or clear evidence of harm) (Zoungas 2012). In the Veterans Affairs Diabetes Trial (VADT), more frequent statin use (to lower LDL-C levels) was associated with accelerated coronary artery calcification in patients with T2D and advanced atherosclerosis (Saremi 2012).

Lifestyle management. Effective lifestyle management, including dietary improve-ments and regular physical activity, is an important strategy to lower risk of CAD (Look AHEAD Research Group 2010). Dietary approaches to primary and sec-ondary prevention include replacing saturated and trans fat intake with polyun-saturated fat to lower LDL-C and to raise HDL-C; eating fewer refined carbohydrates to avoid increases in triglycerides on a low-fat diet; consuming fish and fish oils to suppress cardiac arrhythmias and reduce triglycerides; and reducing intake of saturated fats, cholesterol, meats, and fatty dairy foods (Sacks 2002, Siri-Tarino 2010). Reductions in disease risk resulting from such dietary therapies com-pare favorably with drug treatments for hyperlipidemia and hypertension (Kones 2011). Reduction in central adiposity also has important effects on lowering circu-lating triglycerides and LDL-C levels, and weight loss that includes visceral fat loss also lowers cardiovascular disease risk (O'Leary 2006, Strasser 2012).

Engaging in home-based and other exercise programs is associated with a reduced incidence of cardiovascular disease in individuals with T2D (Shinji 2007, Marwick 2009) and improved lipids and cardiovascular risk factors in T1D (Laak-sonen 2000, Herbst 2007). Moreover, aerobic exercise training done alone or together with resistance training improves blood glucose control, systolic blood pressure, triglyceride levels, and waist circumference, all of which are significant risk factors. The benefits of resistance training in diabetic individuals with known coronary heart disease are well documented and can contribute to secondary pre-vention of heart disease and improve survival rates (Strasser 2010, Wise 2011).

To manage diagnosed disease, diet, exercise, and use of antihyperglycemic medications frequently are combined with other medications that target cardio-vascular disease risk factors, such as antihypertensive drugs, lipid-lowering agents, and antiplatelet medications (American Diabetes Association 2013). The use of HMG-CoA reductase inhibitors (statins) to correct lipid status may prevent major cardiovascular events independent of the baseline lipid or cardiovascular status;

smoking cessation and control of hypertension are also effective preventive measures (Coccheri 2007, Kones 2011). Statins also were found to be efficacious in preventing death and cardiovascular morbidity in people at low cardiovascular risk. Reductions in relative risk were similar to those seen in patients with a history of CAD (Tonelli 2011). Only limited evidence showed that primary prevention with statins may be cost-effective and improve quality of life, and caution is needed when prescribing statins for primary prevention among people with low cardiovascular risk (Taylor 2011).

Surgical treatments. With regard to treatment of diagnosed CAD, surgical treatments are the primary course of action. The efficacy and safety of coronary artery bypass grafts (CABG) have been compared to drug-eluting stent (DES) placement in individuals with diabetes and multivessel disease. CABG has been the preferred revascularization strategy in individuals with diabetes compared with DES, although DESs reduce the rate of target vessel revascularization compared with bare-metal stents (Lee 2010). CABG is associated with a lower risk for major adverse cardiac events compared with DES, mainly due to a lower risk for repeat revascularization despite a higher percentage of triple-vessel disease, although the incidence of death or myocardial infarction (MI) is similar between treatments (Lee 2010). Those undergoing CABG may have a higher risk for cerebrovascular events, however. Therefore, stent placement may be a viable alternative to CABG for selected patients with diabetes with multivessel coronary blockage (Takayama 2010). Early diagnosis of CAD and identification of high-risk subgroups, followed by appropriate therapy, may enhance survival.

PERIPHERAL ARTERY DISEASE

Diabetes also contributes to the development of peripheral artery disease (PAD), a cardiovascular condition that limits blood flow to the lower extremities. Its risk factors and micro- and macrovascular comorbidity are very similar in T1D and T2D (Zander 2002). Plaque can form in any artery around the body, but PAD usually occurs in peripheral arteries in the lower legs (Mohler 2012). People should be made aware that the presence of PAD may be a sign that they may have widespread plaque formation in other arteries around the body (Orchard 2003).

Symptoms and severity. The classic symptoms of PAD are pain, achiness, fatigue, burning, or discomfort in the muscles of the feet, calves, or thighs and usually appear during walking or exercise and go away after several minutes of rest. At first, these symptoms may appear only when individuals walk uphill, faster, or for longer distances, but as the disease progresses, symptoms can come on more quickly and with less activity (McDermott 2004, Mohler 2012). Some individuals also experience numbness in their legs or feet at rest, legs that feel cool to the touch, or pale skin in affected areas. Symptoms can progress to include impotence (in men), pain and cramps in the lower extremities at night, pain or tingling in the feet or toes so severe that even the weight of clothes or bed sheets is painful, pain that is worse when the leg is elevated and improves when it is dangled over the side of the bed, and nonhealing ulcers on the legs and feet (Alonso-Coello 2012, Mohler 2012).

While pain during walking due to intermittent claudication indicates a reduction in blood flow to that area (Mohler 2012), other symptoms may be indicative of more severe issues. For instance, a rupture of plaque formations in leg arteries can cause a blockage that limits or cuts off blood supply to the lower legs, resulting in pain, changes in skin color, sores or ulcers, difficulty walking, and even gangrene. If an individual experiences pain with walking or any of these other symptoms during or after physical activity and has not been diagnosed with PAD, he or she should confer with a health-care provider before proceeding with any exercise program.

Diagnosis. A provider can diagnose PAD by measuring leg blood pressure (ankle/brachial index) and comparing it to the arm pressure (McDermott 2004). If they are unequal, blockage in the lower limbs may be affecting the pressure there. Other discernible symptoms include possible loss of hair on the legs or feet, arterial bruits (a whooshing sound with the stethoscope over the leg artery), weak or absent pulses in the lower extremities, and more.

Treatment options. Along with physical activity, a healthy diet, and smoking cessation, certain medications can prevent clot formation (e.g., clopidogrel) or cause dilation of leg arteries (like cilostazil) (Alonso-Coello 2012). Treatment of PAD currently favors single antiplatelet therapy for primary and secondary prevention of cardiovascular events in most patients with PAD. In addition, surgical options to improve blood flow to the legs include angioplasty and stent placement or peripheral artery bypass surgery to circumvent blockages (Cvetanovski 2009, McQuade 2010). Additional therapies for relief of limb symptoms should be considered only after implementation of exercise therapy, smoking cessation, and evaluation for peripheral artery revascularization (Alonso-Coello 2012).

HYPERTENSION

Hypertension is a common comorbidity affecting >60% of individuals with T2D (National High Blood Pressure Education Program Working Group 1994, Stewart 2004). Moreover, the risk of vascular complications in hypertensive individuals with T2D is 66–100% higher than with either condition alone, meaning that the coexistence of both conditions is particularly damaging (Grossman 2000, Mourad 2008). Together they result in abnormalities in central and peripheral parameters of cardiovascular structure and function.

Blood pressure goals. A recent meta-analysis stated that the new recommended goal should be 130–135 mmHg systolic blood pressure for most adults with T2D (Nilsson 2011). Other risk factors should be controlled with a more ambitious strategy applied in the younger patients with shorter diabetes duration, but a more cautious approach should be taken in the elderly and frail patients with a number of vascular or nonvascular comorbidities (Crawford 2009).

Dietary treatment. The DASH (Dietary Approaches to Stop Hypertension) diet is well studied as an effective means to combat elevations in blood pressure. The diet is heavily focused on fruits, vegetables, whole grains, and low-fat dairy foods;

includes meat, fish, poultry, nuts, and beans; and is limited in sugar-sweetened foods and beverages, red meat, and added fats. In addition to its effect on blood pressure, it is considered a well-balanced approach to eating for the general public and is recommended as an ideal eating plan for all Americans. In individuals with T2D, one study reported that fruits and vegetables were the food groups in the DASH diet most associated with reduced blood pressure (de Paula 2011), whereas others have reported that following this diet reduces body weight and abdominal fat in adults with T2D (Azadbakht 2011). In youth with either type of diabetes, it improves LDL-C particle density, and in those with T2D, it also improves BMI (Liese 2011); tighter glycemic control ameliorates lipid profiles in both groups as well (Petitti 2007). Finally, although the DASH diet by itself lowers blood pressure in overweight individuals with elevated blood pressure, significant improvements in insulin sensitivity are found only when the diet is part of a more comprehensive lifestyle modification program that includes exercise and weight loss (Hinderliter 2011).

Treatment with exercise training alone. Most trials of exercise training for these conditions have focused on glycemic control and blood pressure reduction, whereas less is known about the effects of exercise on the cardiovascular consequences of diabetes and hypertension. Both aerobic and resistance training can lower BP in nondiabetic individuals, with slightly greater effects observed with the former (Kelley 2000, 2001a, 2001b; Cornelissen 2005a). Most studies show that both types of exercise lower blood pressure in diabetic individuals as well (Cauza 2005, Wagner 2006, Figueroa 2007, Cohen 2008, Pagkalos 2008). Systolic blood pressure is frequently lowered by 4–8 mmHg, with a lesser impact on diastolic values (Loimaala 2003, Kim 2006, Kadoglou 2007, Balducci 2008). The Look AHEAD (Action for Health in Diabetes) trial reported reductions in both systolic and diastolic blood pressure with exercise and weight loss (Pi-Sunyer 2007), but others have reported no changes with training in individuals with T2D (Sigal 2007, Wycherley 2008, Loimaala 2009). Similarly, carefully designed interventions utilizing increasing levels of physical activity also failed to show any change in blood pressure despite substantially increased activity levels (Tudor-Locke 2004, Araiza 2006).

Treatment with exercise plus weight loss. Reductions in blood pressure can, however, be accomplished with a combination of exercise and weight loss and may be partially explained by improvements in insulin sensitivity and loss of visceral fat (Stewart 2002). Exercise training reduces total and abdominal fat, which may mediate improvements in insulin sensitivity and blood pressure and improve endothelial vasodilator function (Wycherley 2008). Evidence for an exercise training benefit is strongest for improvements in endothelial vasodilator and left ventricular diastolic function. Thus, current evidence suggests that the benefits of exercise training go beyond the benefits of glycemic control and blood pressure reduction.

Pharmacological treatment. Individuals at high risk for vascular disease, such as anyone with diabetes, have aggressive blood pressure targets to reduce the risk of acute coronary events and stroke. The dual goals are to reduce blood pressure both quickly and to aggressively low targets; thus, the classic step therapy of a single medication at a time is likely inadequate (Crawford 2009). Combination therapies with at least two potent medications are becoming more commonplace and increase compliance with therapy. Angiotensin-converting enzyme (ACE) inhibitors that block the renin-angiotensin aldosterone system are the cornerstone of hypertension treatment in high-risk individuals; thus, newer combination pills include an ACE inhibitor with a diuretic or with a long-acting calcium channel antagonist (CCA). Using the latter may be superior to older diuretic-based combinations to prevent cardiovascular events (Crawford 2009). ACE inhibitor plus diuretic combination therapy improves blood pressure control, counterbalances renin-angiotensin system activation due to diuretic therapy, reduces the risk of electrolyte alterations, and has synergistic antiproteinuric effects. Combination ACE inhibitor and CCA therapy, however, provides a significant additive effect on blood pressure, may have favorable metabolic effects, and synergistically reduces proteinuria and the rate of decline in glomerular filtration rate, while also reducing cardiovascular outcomes in high-risk individuals (Reboldi 2009).

ENDOTHELIAL DYSFUNCTION

Endothelial dysfunction is a systemic, pathological state of the endothelium (the inner lining of blood vessels) characterized by a shift of the actions of the endothelium toward reduced vasodilation (a proinflammatory state) and prothrombic properties. It primarily reflects decreased availability of nitric oxide (NO), a critical endothelium-derived vasoactive factor with vasodilatory and anti-atherosclerotic properties (Woodman 2005). Endothelial changes are associated with most forms of cardiovascular disease, including CAD, PAD, hypertension, chronic heart failure, diabetes, and chronic renal failure. Mechanisms that participate in the reduced vasodilatory responses in endothelial dysfunction include reduced NO generation, oxidative excess, and reduced production of hyperpolarizing factor, along with a number of inflammatory substances. Endothelial dysfunction is an important early event in the pathogenesis of atherosclerosis, contributing to plaque initiation and progression, and its reversal may be associated with reduced cardiovascular risk (Woodman 2005).

Diabetes-related endothelial dysfunction. Vascular alterations are common in diabetes, even in the absence of overt vascular disease, and endothelial dysfunction may be an underlying cause of many of these problems (Deckert 1989, Coccheri 2007). Hyperglycemia, hyperinsulinemia, and oxidative stress all contribute to endothelial damage, leading to poor arterial function and greater susceptibility to atherogenesis (Gaede 2003, Woodman 2005, Zee 2006, Coccheri 2007). Elevated blood glucose levels drive production of reactive oxygen species (ROS) via multiple pathways, resulting in reduced NO availability and further generation of ROS. Hyperglycemia also accelerates arterial stiffening by increasing formation of advanced glycation end-products (AGEs) that alter vessel wall structure and function. Dyslipidemias common to T2D lead to accumulation of triglyceride-rich lipoproteins, small dense LDL-C, reduced HDL-C, and greater postprandial free fatty acid flux, all of which increase oxidative stress (Woodman 2005, Sena 2007). Even preadolescent youth with T1D and a mean diabetes duration of 4 years have displayed evidence of low-intensity vascular inflammation and attenuated flow-mediated dilation, suggesting that endothelial dysfunction and systemic inflammation, known harbingers of heightened future cardiovascular risk, are present even in preadolescent diabetic children (Babar 2011).

Treatment with diet and supplements. Dietary improvements may have a large impact on endothelial function. Diets rich in fruit, vegetables, fish, nuts, and olive oil appear to have beneficial effects on endothelial function; specific foods like cacao and green tea may as well because of their flavanol content (Heiss 2010, Westphal 2011). Recent studies have suggested beneficial effects of vitamin D and anthocyanins (Landberg 2012). Likewise, a less healthy diet directly impacts function: abnormal changes in oxidative–reductive balance parameters are paralleled by similar changes in markers of endothelial dysfunction and inflammation 4 h after ingestion of a fatty meal that induces endothelial changes (Neri 2010). Alterations in oxidation-reduction balance, NO bioavailability, and endothelial factors have been reported after a moderate-fat meal in individuals with T2D, but these post-prandial changes can be reversed by 15 days of standard antioxidant supplementation (i.e., vitamins C and E) (Neri 2005). α-Lipoic acid and resveratrol supplementation (and possibly red wine consumption) may improve endothelial function and reduce oxidative stress (Sena 2007).

Treatment with medications. Endothelial dysfunction may be improved with effective treatment of hyperlipidemias with statins and fenofibrate and improved glycemic control. The effects of various statins may be different, however. For instance, a recent study showed that in hyperlipidemic individuals with metabolic syndrome, atorvastatin is associated with a greater reduction in lipid markers of oxidation compared with pravastatin (Murrow 2012). Statins likely lower the oxidation of LDL-C in hyperlipidemic individuals (Thallinger 2005). Statin use, however, may significantly improve flow-mediated dilation only in people with better endothelial function to start (Zhang 2012).

A direct result of hyperglycemia, AGEs accumulate in poorly controlled diabetes and during aging, are proinflammatory, and negatively affect endothelial function (Basta 2002). Thus, tighter management of blood glucose levels and postprandial excursions lower oxidative stress and improve endothelial function. Interestingly, meals with higher AGEs (due to cooking temperature and time) induce a more pronounced acute impairment of vascular function than do otherwise identical meals with lower AGE content in individuals with T2D (Negrean 2007, Stirban 2008).

Treatment with exercise. Although both aerobic and resistance training have been shown to improve endothelial function in older individuals with T2D (Zoppini 2006, Cohen 2008), not all studies have shown post-training improvement (Wycherley 2008). In adults with T2D, aerobic exercise appears to be more beneficial than resistance exercise for improving endothelial function, although aerobic capacity may be a better predictor of changes in flow-mediated dilation than body weight, glycemic control, and insulin action (Kwon 2011). The beneficial effects of 3 months of training in reducing cardiovascular events persist for at least 24 months (Okada 2010).

Endothelial function has been shown to be enhanced in children and adolescents with T1D who undertake >60 min of daily moderate- to vigorous-intensity physical activity (Trigona 2010), and 18 weeks of training effectively reverses endothelial dysfunction (measured as brachial artery flow-mediated dilation) and improves physical fitness in children with diabetes (Seeger 2011). Others have reported that overweight youth participating in 12 weeks of training using active video gaming (Dance Dance Revolution) experience enhanced flow-mediated dilation, aerobic fitness, and mean arterial pressure, although improvements occurred without changes in inflammatory markers or NO production (Murphy 2009).

Case in Point: Continued (Part 2)

IJ was advised by his physician to first get an exercise stress test before starting any physical activity because of his heightened cardiovascular risk. During the test, IJ stopped relatively early complaining of muscle fatigue, but no electrocardiogram (ECG) abnormalities were noted during the testing, and he experienced no cardio-vascular symptoms. Consequently, IJ was cleared to start exercise training based on the results of this test and his prior checkup.

Additional Question to Consider

1. Is there still a risk that IJ could have underlying cardiovascular disease even though the exercise and other testing did not reveal any?

(Continued on page 321.)

MANIFESTATIONS OF CARDIOVASCULAR DISEASE

ANGINA AND SILENT ISCHEMIA

Angina. A symptom of an underlying cardiac problem, angina pectoris is a discomfort in the chest or adjacent areas caused by myocardial ischemia. It is most commonly caused by the inability of narrowed atherosclerotic coronary arteries to supply adequate oxygen to the heart under conditions of increased demand. Symptoms include pressure or squeezing sensations in the chest, pain in the shoulders, arms, neck, jaw, or back, or sensations like indigestion (Rodriguez-Ospina 2008, Kones 2010). Only a weak relationship exists between pain severity and degree of ischemia; however, worsening angina attacks, sudden-onset angina at rest, and angina lasting >15 min are symptoms of unstable angina (Aronow 2003). As these symptoms may herald an MI, they require urgent medical attention and generally are treated as a presumed heart attack.

Angina can be diagnosed with a resting ECG, exercise stress test, coronary angiography and cardiac catheterization, or computed tomography angiography. The main goals of treatment are to reduce pain and discomfort, limit recurrence, and prevent or lower an individual's risk for MI or death by treating the underlying condition. Treatments include lifestyle improvements, various medications (e.g., nitrates, β-blockers, and CCA), medical procedures (like angioplasty, stent placement, or CABG), cardiac rehabilitation, and other therapies, although sublingual nitroglycerin commonly is used to rapidly lessen the pain associated with acute events (Aronow 2003, Kones 2010).

Silent ischemia. Individuals with diabetes are more likely to experience a condition known as silent ischemia, which is a reduction in blood flow to the heart muscle through the coronary blood vessels that is painless and symptom free. Silent ischemia is an asymptomatic form of myocardial ischemia, which can be accompanied by changes in ECG, left ventricular function, myocardial perfusion, and metabolism. Silent myocardial ischemia is common in individuals with T2D; therefore, symptoms cannot be relied on for diagnosis and follow-up in these individuals. Adults with diabetes who experience an acute MI may not experience chest pain, and up to a third may have silent myocardial ischemia (Mamcarz 2004).

In the DIAD (Detection of Ischemia in Asymptomatic Diabetics) study, 1,123 individuals with T2D, ages 50–75 years, with no known or suspected CAD, were randomly assigned to either exercise stress testing and 5-year clinical follow-up or to follow-up only (Wackers 2004). In that population, silent myocardial ischemia was present in more than one in five asymptomatic people. Traditional and emerging cardiac risk factors, however, were not associated with abnormal exercise stress tests, although cardiac autonomic dysfunction was a strong predictor of ischemia. In those screened with adenosine-stress radionuclide myocardial perfusion imaging, the rate of cardiac events was low and the positive predictive value (for cardiac death or nonfatal MI) with moderate or large imaging defects was only 12%, suggesting that such events were not significantly reduced by this screening for myocardial ischemia over 4.8 years (Young 2009). Systematic attempts to detect silent ischemia in high-risk asymptomatic people with diabetes are unlikely to provide any major benefit on hard outcomes in those whose cardiovascular risk is controlled by an optimal medical treatment (Lievre 2011).

MYOCARDIAL INFARCTION

MI, commonly known as a heart attack, results from the interruption of blood supply to a part of the heart, causing heart cells to die, and most commonly is caused by occlusion (blockage) of a coronary artery following the rupture of a vulnerable atherosclerotic plaque (Wenaweser 2008). The usual symptoms of acute MI include sudden chest pain (typically radiating to the left arm or left side of the neck), shortness of breath, nausea, vomiting, heart palpitations, sweating, anxiety, weakness, a feeling of indigestion, and fatigue.

Many individuals with diabetes who have an acute MI fail to experience chest pain due to silent myocardial ischemia, or their first symptom of CAD may be sudden cardiac death (Mamcarz 2004, Coccheri 2007). Earlier detection of MI, however, results in better outcomes, whereas silent MI is associated with more adverse outcomes due to greater total ischemia with late detection (Cho 2012). In fact, a shorter symptom-to-balloon time has been associated with improved coronary flow, an increased likelihood of subsequent left ventricular systolic ejection fraction >40%, and higher 3-year survival in patients with MI who are treated with primary percutaneous coronary intervention (angioplasty) (Maeng 2010). The main predictors of silent MI are hypertension, history of cardiovascular diseases, and diabetes duration. Silent MI is associated with as poor a prognosis as symptomatic MI and frequently with a worse prognosis due to later detection (Valensi 2011).

Heart muscle damage can be detected with ECG, echocardiography, and various blood tests, usually creatine kinase and troponin levels (Chopra 2012). Acute treatment for MI includes oxygen, aspirin, and sublingual nitroglycerin. Many cases of MI with ST-segment elevation are treated with thrombolysis or percutaneous coronary intervention (Wenaweser 2008). If an MI occurs without ST-segment elevation, it usually can be managed with medications (Navarese 2011). In people who have multiple blockages and who are relatively stable, bypass surgery may be an option, especially in people with diabetes.

CONGESTIVE HEART FAILURE

Congestive heart failure is a common outcome of MI because of the weakening of the heart muscle by the infarcted area. Heart failure is a long-term (chronic) condition, but it sometimes can develop suddenly and may affect either or both sides of the heart (Parissis 2012). Systolic heart failure occurs when the heart cannot eject blood well, resulting in a lowered ejection fraction. Diastolic heart failure occurs when the heart muscle is still and does not fill easily with blood during diastole (rest) (Pecoits-Filho 2012). As the heart's pumping action is compromised, blood returning to the heart instead may back up in other areas of the body, causing fluid build-up in the lungs, liver, gastrointestinal tract, and arms and legs (Bagshaw 2010).

The most common cause of heart failure is CAD, but it also can be caused by emphysema, thyroid hormone imbalances, cardiomyopathies, and congenital heart diseases. Major risk factors for heart failure include CAD, diabetes, obesity, and hypertension, among others. In one study, individuals with diabetes who experienced acute heart failure more frequently had acute pulmonary edema, acute coronary syndrome (like ischemia or MI), and multiple comorbidities like renal dysfunction, anemia, hypertension, and PAD (Parissis 2012). Treatment options include diuresis, suppression of the overactive neurohormonal systems, augmentation of contractility, ventricular assist device implantation, heart transplantation, and other surgical procedures (Kemp 2012). Despite significant understanding of the underlying pathophysiological mechanisms, heart failure causes significant morbidity and conveys a 50% mortality rate in 5 years (Kemp 2012). Moreover, there is inverse association between glycemia and mortality in outpatients with chronic heart failure (Issa 2010).

STROKE

Another type of cardiovascular disease, carotid artery disease is a condition in which the carotid arteries become narrowed or blocked. When the arteries become narrowed, the condition is called carotid stenosis. If an artery is narrowed, a stroke can result from a thrombus, or clot, forming as the result of unstable plaque formations (Delgado-Mederos 2007). Carotid atherosclerosis is associated with CAD and highlights the importance of screening for ischemic heart disease in patients with asymptomatic carotid plaques (Ciccone 2011). Duration of diabetes is independently associated with ischemic stroke risk adjusting for risk factors;

the risk increases 3% each year, and triples with diabetes ≥10 years in duration (Banerjee 2012).

Although strokes can have different origins, flow blockages from clots cause ischemic strokes that account for ~83% of all cases (Higashida 2003). Less commonly, ruptured blood vessels that leak blood (hemorrhage) into the brain cause a hemorrhagic stroke. This second type of stroke usually is caused by either an aneurysm (a ballooning out of a vessel) or a vessel malformation. When a blood vessel that carries oxygen and nutrients to the brain is either blocked by a clot or bursts, part of the brain fails to get the blood and oxygen delivery that it requires, resulting in a stroke in the affected region. A stroke's impact can vary; only those functions normally controlled by the affected part of the brain will be impaired (Higashida 2003). A stroke that reduces blood flow to the back of the brain, for instance, is likely to negatively affect vision. Other areas of the brain control movement, speech, memory, and problem-solving ability.

TRANSIENT ISCHEMIC ATTACK

Transient ischemic attacks (TIAs) are minor or "warning" strokes that usually result in typical stroke symptoms. By definition, a TIA is a transient episode of neurological dysfunction caused by focal brain, spinal cord, or retinal ischemia, without acute infarction (Easton 2009). Normal brain blood flow is reduced for a short time and tends to resolve by itself. Even though the symptoms disappear after a short time, the occurrence of a TIA puts individuals at high risk of early stroke. They should heed the warning signs and take steps immediately to prevent an actual, more damaging stroke, including seeking medical care such as starting clot-preventing medications and controlling high blood pressure.

CARDIOVASCULAR DISEASE RISK FACTOR MANAGEMENT

Current recommendations focus on aggressive management of cardiovascular disease risk factors (Booth 2006, Smith 2006, Buse 2007). Blood pressure, cholesterol level, smoking status, and diabetes status are major risk factors for cardiovascular disease in adults. Among individuals 55 years old, those with an optimal risk-factor profile (total cholesterol level <180 mg/dl; blood pressure <120/80 mmHg; nonsmoker; no diabetes) had substantially lower risks of death from cardiovascular disease, nonfatal MI, or stroke through the age of 80 years than individuals with two or more major risk factors (Berry 2012). Smoking amplified the risk of mortality as well as cardiovascular events, and the effect size for CAD appeared to be higher than for other cardiac events in diabetic patients. Moreover, a trend of decreasing risk was observed among smoking quitters (Qin 2012).

Glucose-lowering agents used in diabetes control frequently are supplemented by medications that target cardiovascular disease, including ones used to lower blood pressure, blood lipids, and platelet clotting (American Diabetes Association 2013). Lifestyle management is also effective in lowering cardiovascular risk. Adherence to home-based and other exercise programs is associated with a reduced incidence of cardiovascular disease in people with T2D (Look AHEAD Research Group 2010) and lowered lipids and cardiovascular risk factors in T1D

(Laaksonen 2000, Herbst 2007). Aerobic exercise training done alone or combined with resistance training improves cardiovascular risk factors (i.e., glycemic control, systolic blood pressure, triglycerides, and waist circumference), although the impact of resistance exercise alone on these risk markers is likely significant in T2D as well (Strasser 2010). The impact is less well defined, however, given that a recent meta-analysis found that neither resistance training alone nor such training combined with any other form of exercise had any significant effects on cardiovascular risk markers (Chudyk 2011). Higher levels of physical fitness and activity are associated with lower cardiovascular risk and reduced early mortality in both healthy and diabetic populations (Blair 1995; Wei 2000; Lee 2001, 2009; Church 2004; McAuley 2007; Kokkinos 2009). All-cause and cardiac mortality risk was 1.7 to 6.6 times higher in low-fit compared with high-fit men with T2D, with the fittest men exhibiting the lowest risk (Church 2004, 2005). Having an exercise capacity above 10 metabolic equivalent (METs, for which 1 MET is resting) carries the lowest risk, independent of obesity (Church 2004, McAuley 2007, Kokkinos 2009). Exercise is an indispensable component in the medical treatment of patients with T1D as it improves glycemic control and decreases cardiovascular risk factors among those individuals as well (Salem 2010).

Individuals with T2D and ischemia had higher levels of total cholesterol, LDL-C, and triglycerides. HDL-C levels were significantly lower in these patients. The association of low HDL-C with high triglycerides was a strong indicator of myocardial ischemia in anyone without clinical cardiovascular signs (Pena 2012). A substantial proportion of youth with diabetes have abnormal serum lipids as well, with a greater prevalence among those with T2D than with T1D (Kershnar 2006).

Aerobic training also may decrease total cholesterol and LDL-C while raising HDL-C (Ronnemaa 1988, Kadoglou 2007). Some have reported only small decreases in total cholesterol with both aerobic and yoga training and no changes in HDL-C or LDL-C (Gordon 2008), although most report no effect of exercise training on lipids (Maiorana 2002, Tudor-Locke 2004, Araiza 2006, Wagner 2006, Sigal 2007, Loimaala 2009). A meta-analysis of training effects on blood lipids in adults with T2D found that LDL-C may be reduced by ~5% (Kelley 2007). Lipid profiles may benefit more from concomitant exercise training and weight reduction (Pi-Sunyer 2007). Most lifestyle interventions have been accompanied by a ~5 kg weight loss. Exercise, in combination with dietary improvements and weight loss, has been demonstrated to favorably modify lipids and lipoproteins, thereby lowering cardiovascular disease risk in people with T2D (Balady 2007).

Case in Point: Continued (Part 3)

IJ began his exercise program by walking with his wife around their neighborhood. On their first day out, he experienced some unusual chest discomfort that he tried to attribute to indigestion. His wife suspected otherwise and called for emergency medical services (EMS) using her cell phone. He was transported to the hospital by ambulance with a suspected acute coronary event of some type (acute coronary syndrome).

Additional Questions to Consider

1. Now that it appears that IJ has some type of cardiovascular disease ongoing, is it still safe for him to start an exercise program?
2. If so, when should he start training, and what activities is it safe for him to undertake?

(Continued on page 329.)

EXERCISE TRAINING BENEFITS FOR CARDIOVASCULAR DISEASES

AEROBIC TRAINING

Chronic low-grade systemic inflammation is a feature of chronic diseases like cardiovascular disease and T2D and may be involved in arterial plaque formation. In addition to increasing cardiorespiratory fitness, moderate physical exercise has marked anti-inflammatory effects and protects against insulin resistance and vascular complications (Belotto 2010). Physically fit individuals have a reduced risk of developing cardiovascular disease and other age-related chronic disorders. Following acute exercise, there is a transient increase in circulating levels of anti-inflammatory cytokines, whereas chronic exercise reduces basal levels of proinflammatory cytokines (Wilund 2007). This expression of antioxidant and anti-inflammatory mediators in the vascular wall may directly inhibit the development of atherosclerosis. These cytokines generated by muscle (i.e., myokines) may be involved in mediating the beneficial health effects against chronic diseases associated with low-grade inflammation (Pedersen 2006). Thus, physical activity is a useful weapon against local vascular and systemic inflammation in atherosclerosis (Pinto 2012).

RESISTANCE TRAINING

Because of the metabolic consequences of reduced muscle mass, normal aging or decreased physical activity may lead to a higher prevalence of metabolic disorders. Resistance training enhances muscular strength and endurance, functional capacity and independence, and quality of life while reducing disability in people with cardiovascular disease. It also alters visceral fat and levels of several proinflammatory cytokines produced in adipose tissue by promoting a negative energy balance, and that change in body fat distribution may lead to better metabolic control (Strasser 2012).

Resistance training done by individuals with diagnosed coronary heart disease can contribute to its secondary prevention with corresponding improvements in survival (Wise 2011). Previously, resistance training was not prescribed to adults with cardiovascular disease because it was believed that increased blood pressure during training would place them at increased risk for an adverse event. Now, however, this training is recommended for everyone, even those who have suffered a heart attack or stroke (McCartney 1999), given that it causes less ischemia than aerobic training (Featherstone 1993). The more dramatic increase in blood pressure results in greater blood flow through the coronary vessels—a comparable rise in systolic and diastolic blood pressures better maintains coronary perfusion, a lesser rise in cardiac output enhances flow, and more rest between resistance sets gives time for flow recovery compared with continuous aerobic exercise (Sigal 2004). In individuals with T2D, this training increases blood pressure more than aerobic training, but it decreases submaximal heart rate, resulting in greater blood flow to and less work performed by the heart (Maiorana 2002). Thus, for anyone with CAD, moderate resistance training actually may be a safer activity than most high-intensity aerobic ones, and these benefits have made it an accepted component of training programs (Williams 2007). Guidelines for safe and effective participation in resistance training for individuals with cardiovascular disease are included in Table 17.1.

CARDIAC REHABILITATION AND OTHER SUPERVISED TRAINING

Cardiac rehabilitation (rehab) is a medically supervised exercise program that helps to improve the health and well-being of people with coronary problems. Individuals at very high risk for cardiovascular disease (e.g., those with known CAD or exercise-induced ischemia) should exercise in a supervised cardiac rehabilitation program, at least initially (Smith 2006). Cardiac rehab has been shown to be safe and effective in many different populations. For example, no signs or symptoms of ischemia or abnormal heart rate or blood pressure responses were observed during the strength training program done by cardiac patients, suggesting that resistive training at up to 80% of a one-repetition maximum (1 RM) is both safe and efficacious in stable, aerobically trained individuals with diagnosed CAD (Ghilarducci 1989). For individuals who are postevent or postsurgery, supervision of exercise is recommended and frequently necessary for safe participation (Heran 2011). Other subjective rating scales used during exercise bouts (e.g., dyspnea, claudication, and angina scales) aid in ensuring the safety of physical activity

Table 17.1 Guidelines for Resistance Training with Cardiovascular Disease

- Breathe continually and avoid breath-holding during movements.
- Exhale during the exertion or lifting phase, and inhale while returning to starting position.
- Avoid sustained, tight gripping, and static lifts that may cause hypertensive responses.
- Lift weights with slow, controlled movements.
- Use a complete range of motion around each joint.
- Maintain good form and keep the body properly aligned throughout the lift, especially when using free weights or resistance bands.
- Adjust the resistance equipment to fit the body frame.
- Stop exercising if warning signs or symptoms occur, such as dizziness, unusual shortness of breath, or chest pain.

(Cullen 2002, Johnson 2010). Improvements in exercise capacity, obesity, and lipid levels are similar in older and younger patients who are enrolled in cardiac rehab and exercise training (Lavie 1993). Modest reductions in measures of obesity occur with this training, and obese individuals experience improvements in most coronary risk factors after rehab (Lavie 1996). Left ventricular function remains stable during moderate-intensity resistance exercise, even in individuals with congestive heart failure, suggesting that this form of exercise therapy can be used safely in rehabilitation programs (Karlsdottir 2002). It is even safe for individuals post-transplant: a lengthened set of single leg-press exercises at a moderate lifting intensity can be performed within safe and acceptable physiological limits following heart transplantation (Oliver 2001).

Most cardiac rehab programs have three phases (Balady 2007). The first phase is an inpatient one for the hospitalized patient who needs to gain the physical ability to minimally participate in self-care and other activities of daily living (Heran 2011). Phase II is part of the outpatient program following a heart attack, heart surgery, or other major heart problem and includes supervised exercise and a variety of measurements and assessments. Phase III is often referred to as the lifestyle maintenance phase of cardiac rehab because it emphasizes long-term lifestyle changes, such as a regular exercise program. Phase III programs usually are held at a community facility or at home with less monitoring (Balady 2007).

PHYSICAL ACTIVITY CONSIDERATIONS WITH CARDIOVASCULAR DISEASES

CORONARY ARTERY DISEASE

Individuals with chronic cardiovascular complications of diabetes often do not undertake regular physical activity. Yet, increasing physical activity levels is especially useful for this group to improve or maintain functional capacity, strength, balance, and flexibility. Their participation can be undertaken safely and effectively, as long as certain precautions are taken. It is recommended that physician approval be obtained before anyone with known cardiovascular disease begins a new exercise program, including a comprehensive assessment to determine the most appropriate physical activity parameters with regard to blood pressure and heart rate responses. Individuals should begin resistance training with lighter amounts to help decrease the myocardial oxygen demand on the heart (Smith 2006). Heart rate and blood pressure need to be monitored during training and remain within the limits established by an exercise stress test, keeping in mind that myocardial perfusion will be similar or enhanced during resistance training at heart rate limits established during aerobic exercise testing.

ANGINA AND SILENT ISCHEMIA

When prescribing exercise for individuals with diabetes, an exercise stress test may be of particular importance to determine whether any abnormalities such as angina or silent ischemia occur during exercise. Individuals should use the onset of angina as a guide to limit exercise intensity or duration. In general, if reaching

Table 17.2 Exercise Considerations for Coronary Artery Disease and Ischemia

- Assess cardiovascular risk with a physical activity history and/or an exercise test to guide safe and effective exercise prescription.
- High-risk individuals with established disease (e.g., recent acute coronary syndrome or revascularization) should be supervised in a cardiac rehabilitation or other medically supervised program, at least initially.
- For exercise-induced angina, keep exercise heart rate at least 10 bpm below the heart rate at which it occurs.
- Individuals should avoid activities that cause a hypertensive response (systolic blood pressure >260 mmHg, diastolic blood pressure >125 mmHg), including heavy lifting, straining, and Valsalva (breath-holding) maneuvers.
- Moderate resistance training actually may be a safer activity than most high-intensity aerobic activities because of increased myocardial perfusion during the former.
- Before starting a resistance exercise program, individuals should be instructed on proper weightlifting techniques to ensure that all exercises are performed safely and correctly.

a certain heart rate causes the development of chest pain during exercise, then exercise should be limited to an intensity with a heart rate at least 10 bpm below the pain threshold. For example, if jogging causes angina at a heart rate of 140 bpm, then exercise intensity should be lowered to a brisk walk or a slower jogging pace that keeps the heart rate at ≤130 bpm at all times. Individuals with angina and T2D classified as moderate or high risk preferably should exercise in a supervised cardiac rehabilitation program, at least initially (Smith 2006). These and other considerations are listed in Table 17.2.

PERIPHERAL ARTERY DISEASE

Older adults with PAD often report that leg pain while walking or standing limits their ability to exercise. For anyone with PAD, however, with and without intermittent claudication and pain during physical activity, low- to moderate-intensity walking, arm-crank, and cycling exercises all enhance mobility, functional capacity, exercise pain tolerance, and quality of life (Zwierska 2005, Pena 2009). Home-based walking interventions may not increase walking distance, but they can improve walking speed and quality of life in people with diabetes and PAD (Collins 2011). A low-intensity walking program for intermittent claudication may improve collateral circulation and muscle metabolism and, in turn, decrease pain (Pena 2009). A training program using intervals of walking and resting periods may result in improved tolerance for exercise, and even upper-body (arm-crank) training improves pain tolerance and exercise capacity (Zwierska 2005). Self-directed walking performed at least three times weekly is associated with significantly less functional decline and progression of PAD during the subsequent year whether individuals were symptomatic or asymptomatic (McDermott 2006). Moreover, self-efficacy is significantly associated with walking ability

Table 17.3 Exercise Considerations for Peripheral Artery Disease

- Daily physical activity sessions will maximize pain tolerance during movement and possibly slow the progression of PAD.
- A training program using intervals of walk and rest periods may result in improved tolerance for exercise and increased quality of life.
- Individuals with intermittent claudication during activity should determine their distance and duration for walking using a pain-limited threshold.
- Keep aerobic exercise intensity lower because higher intensity demands a greater blood supply and likely will cause claudication pain.
- Individuals should use conversation, music, and other elements to divert their attention from the discomfort and pain during physical activity.
- Stop activity when the discomfort or pain increases from moderate to intense discomfort and attention cannot be diverted from the pain.
- Undertake weight-bearing activities like walking; however, non–weight-bearing activities may be done if longer-duration and higher-intensity workouts are the goal.
- Seated resistance training can be done if leg pain during standing exercises is not tolerable.
- Monitor the extremities for any changes that may indicate a more severe problem, such as more intense pain, changes in skin color, sores or ulcers, and difficulty walking.

in individuals with diabetes and PAD (Collins 2010) Resistance training exercises also can be done seated to limit leg pain. Lower-body resistance training improves functional performance measured by treadmill walking, stair climbing ability, and quality-of-life measures (McDermott 2009). Thus, participation in walking or other daily exercise is critical to maintaining optimal circulation in the extremities when PAD is present (Table 17.3).

HYPERTENSION

Aerobic endurance training decreases resting blood pressure through a reduction of vascular resistance, in which the sympathetic nervous system and the renin-angiotensin system appear to be involved, and favorably affects insulin

Table 17.4 Exercise Considerations for Hypertension

- Assess cardiovascular risk with a physical activity history or an exercise test to guide safe and effective exercise prescription for hypertensive individuals.
- Individuals should avoid activities that cause an excessive hypertensive response (systolic blood pressure >260 mmHg, diastolic blood pressure >125 mmHg), including heavy lifting, straining, and Valsalva maneuvers.
- Resistance exercise actually may result in better myocardial perfusion than aerobic exercise of a similar intensity.
- Before starting a resistance exercise program, individuals should be instructed on proper weightlifting techniques to ensure that all exercises are performed safely and correctly.

action and concomitant cardiovascular risk factors in individuals with diabetes (Cornelissen 2005b). Endurance training should be included as part of a lifestyle treatment strategy. Resistance training also has been shown to result in reductions in resting blood pressure, suggesting that moderate-intensity resistance training should be part of the nonpharmacological intervention strategy to prevent and combat high blood pressure as well (Cornelissen 2005a). If individuals have pre-existing hypertension, they likely should avoid high-intensity aerobic work or heavy resistance exercises, which may cause blood pressures to rise dangerously high and precipitate a stroke or other cardiovascular event. As shown in Table 17.4, activities best avoided include near-maximal exercise of any type, heavy weight training, or any resistance exercise that results in holding the breath.

CONGESTIVE HEART FAILURE

For individuals with congestive heart failure (CHF), both aerobic and resistance training have been shown to be efficacious. Aerobic exercise may improve cardiorespiratory fitness, dyspnea, work capacity, and left ventricular function, whereas resistance exercise enhances left ventricular function, peak lactate levels, muscle strength, and muscle endurance (Bartlo 2007). Thus, both types of training should be included for these individuals as well. In addition, some studies have recommended the use of local muscle exercise (e.g., two-legged knee extensor and flexor exercises, handgrip strength) to improve skeletal muscle function, exercise capacity, quality of life, and ventilatory responses while decreasing sympathetic stress (Gordon 1996, 1997; Tyni-Lenne 1996, 1998; Izawa 2012). Handgrip strength may be an independent predictor of prognosis with congestive heart failure (Table 17.5) (Izawa 2009).

Table 17.5 Exercise Considerations for Congestive Heart Failure

- Assess risk with a physical activity history or an exercise test to guide safe and effective exercise prescription for individuals with CHF.
- Low- to moderate-intensity exercise can be undertaken by individuals with CHF, using dyspnea as a guide for exercise intensity.
- Doing local-muscle exercise, such as two-legged exercise training, may be a viable alternative to full body exercise.
- Low- to moderate-intensity resistance training can be undertaken given that left ventricular function remains stable during such exercise.
- Before starting a resistance exercise program, individuals should be instructed on proper weightlifting techniques to ensure that all exercises are performed safely and correctly.
- Handgrip strength may be an independent predictor of prognosis for individuals with CHF.

WARNING SIGNS AND TREATMENT OF HEART ATTACK OR STROKE

MYOCARDIAL INFARCTION

The most common symptom of MI is chest pain or discomfort, but women are somewhat more likely than men to experience other symptoms, including dyspnea, nausea and vomiting, and back or jaw pain (Cullen 2002, Aronow 2003, Wenaweser 2008, Johnson 2010). Individuals should stop whatever they are doing to determine the source of mild chest pain rather than potentially experience a more damaging heart attack; in other words, they should take any chest pain or discomfort seriously. When the heart is not receiving enough blood, lactic acid builds up, leading to pain or discomfort, and the lack of oxygen to the heart and other parts of the body can cause additional symptoms. People with diabetes often suffer from painless (symptom-free) heart attacks, so even a sudden onset of extreme fatigue is a symptom that needs to be considered (Wackers 2004, Ciccone 2011, Lievre 2011, Pena 2012). Heeding the warning signs and seeking medical attention immediately will lead to the best possible outcome. If detected early, blood clots often can be dissolved, resulting in less lasting damage to the heart or other areas of the body. Individuals should not wait more than 5 min after symptoms start to call for help. Using EMS by dialing 9-1-1 (in most areas of the U.S.) is the fastest and most effective way to get lifesaving medical attention.

If someone loses consciousness and stops breathing, he or she is experiencing cardiac arrest. Another person has to be present to activate EMS in that case. The individuals who are most likely to survive an out-of-hospital cardiac arrest are those who are witnessed to collapse by a bystander and found in a shockable rhythm (e.g., ventricular fibrillation or pulseless ventricular tachycardia) (McNally 2011). The national survival rate for full cardiac arrest not witnessed by EMS personnel is only 8.5% (McNally 2011). If an automated external defibrillator (AED) is available, it can be used to reset normal cardiac rhythm. Cardiopulmonary resuscitation (CPR) can be used after defibrillation to refill the heart or done

Table 17.6 Heart Attack Warning Signs

■ **Chest discomfort**
Discomfort in the center of the chest that lasts or is intermittent; it may feel like bad indigestion, uncomfortable pressure, squeezing, fullness, or acute and stabbing pain

■ **Discomfort elsewhere**
Pain or discomfort radiating down one or both arms, the back, neck, jaw, or stomach due to "referred pain," which is actually originating in the heart due to insufficient oxygen delivery

■ **Shortness of breath**
Dyspnea, particularly when it is unusual or unexpected, can occur along with or without chest discomfort

■ **Other symptoms**
Sudden sweating, nausea and vomiting, lightheadedness, or undue, unexplained fatigue

alone if an AED is not available. If CPR is performed, it may give an individual a few minutes of extended survival time while awaiting EMS services, but by itself it cannot restart a normal heart rhythm without external defibrillation. Common warning signs of heart attack are given in Table 17.6.

STROKE

For any type of stroke, the key word to describe its symptoms is "sudden" (Table 17.7). If someone experiences any or all of the symptoms of a stroke, such as sudden numbness down one side of the body or trouble speaking, immediately call 9-1-1 (or local EMS number) to summon an ambulance with advanced life support. Taking immediate action is critical because if given within 3 h of the start of symptoms, the clot-busting drug tPA (tissue-type plasminogen activator) given intravenously can improve the long-term outcomes for most individuals (Delgado-Mederos 2007).

Table 17.7 Stroke Warning Signs

- Sudden numbness or weakness, especially on one side of the body (e.g., legs, arms, face)
- Sudden confusion
- Sudden trouble with normal speaking or understanding
- Sudden loss of vision in one or both eyes
- Sudden trouble with walking, loss of balance, or lack of physical coordination
- Sudden onset, severe headache, and dizziness

Case in Point: Wrap-Up

During his hospitalization, it was determined that IJ had not suffered an MI, but rather that he had experienced unstable angina resulting from significant coronary artery occlusion in three vessels. His cardiologist recommended that he undergo CABG rather than placement of drug-eluting stents because of his diabetes status and significant cardiovascular risk factors. Post-CABG, IJ began doing some initial exercise therapy as part of the hospital's inpatient cardiac rehab program, and he was discharged with the recommendation that he continue with outpatient or community-based supervised training, at least for the first 8 weeks postsurgery.

Exercise Program Goals

Mode of Activity: IJ should begin his exercise program with walking exercise (indoor or outdoor) or stationary cycling to rebuild his endurance for participation in daily activities. Once his minimal cardiorespiratory fitness level has increased sufficiently, he can continue aerobic training by doing a variety of activities. Within 1–2 months, he should plan on adding in some light resistance training to improve his strength and better manage his blood glucose levels.

Intensity: During all phases of cardiac rehab, IJ should maintain a workout pace that does not exceed "somewhat hard." His initial target heart rate should be no higher than 113 bpm (40% heart rate reserve, or HRR), with a later training goal of closer to 122 bpm (50% of HRR) or possibly higher, as he is able. Doing any intensity activity will be beneficial to him for restoring endurance and strength lost because of cardiac issues and surgery. Beginning resistance training with light weights, elastic bands, or his own body weight may help him regain the physical strength to complete daily tasks.

Frequency: To help build aerobic fitness and manage diabetes, IJ should engage in aerobic exercise at least 3–5 days/week, with no more than 2 consecutive days without any activity. He should plan on adding resistance training at least 2 days a week.

Duration: IJ should engage in shorter bouts of exercise training to start, separated by a rest period, until he can train continuously for 15–30 min, with an ultimate training goal of 150 min of moderate aerobic activity spread throughout the week to aid with blood glucose control and secondary prevention of cardiovascular disease. Resistance training can start with as few as four to five exercises, with a goal of 8–10 exercises.

Progression: IJ should increase his exercise duration until he reaches a goal of at least 150 min/week of moderate exercise. Having achieved that, he can either exercise more frequently or very slowly progress to a higher exercise intensity. He should plan on doing resistance training at least 2 days/week, with 3 days being a better goal. The intensity of his resistance workouts can also progress once he reaches 2–3 days/week of training. Taking plenty of daily steps and standing more also should be lifestyle activity goals.

Precautions: IJ is still at high risk for other cardiovascular problems, so he should be aware of any new signs or symptoms that may develop over time that would indicate either a recurrence of his coronary blockage or another cardiac problem (like pain in his legs during walking from PAD or TIAs caused by carotid artery blockage).

Although diabetes itself is an independent and significant risk factor for cardiovascular disease, individuals with all types of cardiac conditions can still safely and effectively participate in physical activity. Both aerobic and resistance training is recommended, but resistance work actually may enhance myocardial perfusion during activity compared with more aerobic activities. During any activity, individuals should be cognizant of the development of any symptoms that could be related to ischemia, MI, or stroke, so that appropriate and timely medical treatment can be obtained.

PROFESSIONAL PRACTICE PEARLS

- Diabetes is a major risk factor for cardiovascular disease, as well as a significant cause of premature mortality and morbidity in individuals with both types of diabetes.

Table 17.8 General Exercise Rx for All Cardiovascular Diseases

Mode	Aerobic: Walking, jogging, cycling, swimming, rowing, aquatic activities, seated exercises, dancing, conditioning machines, and more
	Resistance: All major muscle groups, using resistance bands, free weights, resistance training machines, isometric exercises, and/or calisthenics (using body weight); include four to five upper body and four to five lower body/core exercises
Intensity	Aerobic: 30/40–89% HRR (initial intensity may need to be on the lower end for sedentary, deconditioned, and overweight individuals)
	Resistance: 50/60–80% 1 RM (low to moderate intensity, but starting on the lower end)
	Both: Perceived exertion of "somewhat hard," or 5–7 (on 10 point scale); use pain as a guide for angina (keeping heart rate 10 bpm below onset), or use a dyspnea scale for CHF
Frequency	Aerobic: 3–7 days/week (including structured and lifestyle activity)
	Resistance: A minimum of 2 days/week (preferably 3), with at least 48 hours of rest between sessions
Duration	Aerobic: 20–30 min most days, for a total of at least 150 min/week of moderate-intensity activity; minimum of 5–10 min/session, with rest periods in between as needed
	Resistance: 8–12 repetitions per exercise as a goal, but 10–15 repetitions initially; one to three sets per exercise
Progression	Aerobic: Start out on the "low" side and progress slowly over weeks to months; increase duration and frequency first for weight loss, intensity last
	Resistance: Start with one to two sets of 8–15 repetitions: one set of 10–15 repetitions to fatigue initially, progressing to 8–10 harder repetitions, and finally to two to three sets of 8–10 repetitions)

Note: 1 RM, one-repetition maximum; CHF, congestive heart failure; HRR, heart rate reserve.

■ A diagnosis of cardiovascular disease is not an absolute contraindication to exercise; rather, most individuals with varying conditions can and should participate in regular physical activity to improve their diabetes control and their health.

■ Individuals with T2D have a lifetime risk of developing CAD that includes 67% of women and 78% of men.

■ Effective lifestyle management, including dietary improvements and regular physical activity, is an important strategy to lower risk of all cardiovascular diseases.

■ Diabetes also contributes to the development of PAD, a condition that limits blood flow to the lower extremities and often causes pain during physical activity.

- The recommended goal is ≤130–135 mmHg systolic blood pressure for most adults with T2D, which can be achieved through lifestyle changes and medication use.
- Hyperglycemia, hyperinsulemia, and oxidative stress all contribute to endothelial dysfunction in all types of diabetes, leading to greater susceptibility to atherogenesis.
- Individuals with diabetes may experience angina pectoris (a sign of underlying cardiac disease), or reduced blood flow in the coronary arteries may be painless (silent ischemia).
- The usual symptoms of acute MI include sudden chest pain (typically radiating to the left arm or left side of the neck), shortness of breath, nausea, vomiting, heart palpitations, sweating, anxiety, weakness, a feeling of indigestion, and fatigue.
- Congestive heart failure is a common outcome of MI due to the weakening of the heart muscle and conveys a 50% mortality rate in 5 years.
- Carotid artery disease is caused by narrowing or blockage of the carotid arteries, which can result in stroke or "warning strokes" called transient ischemic attacks.
- Current recommendations focus on aggressive management of cardiovascular disease risk factors for primary prevention, which includes both aerobic and resistance training.
- Assess cardiovascular risk with a physical activity history or an exercise test to guide safe and effective exercise prescription.
- Individuals at very high risk for cardiovascular disease, postcardiac event, or surgery should exercise in a supervised cardiac rehabilitation program, at least initially.
- With coronary artery occlusion, moderate resistance training actually may be a safer activity than most high-intensity aerobic activities because of increased myocardial perfusion.
- For exercise-induced angina, individuals should keep their exercise heart rate at least 10 bpm below the heart rate at which pain occurs.
- Individuals should avoid activities that cause a hypertensive response (>260/125 mmHg), including heavy lifting, straining, and Valsalva (breathholding) maneuvers.
- Participation in walking or other daily exercise is critical to maintaining optimal circulation in the extremities when PAD is present.
- A training program using intervals of walk and rest periods may result in improved tolerance for exercise and increased quality of life in PAD.
- Individuals with intermittent claudication during activity should determine their distance and duration for walking using a pain-limited threshold.
- Activities best avoided by individuals with hypertension include near-maximal aerobic exercise, heavy weight training, or any resistance exercise that results in holding the breath.
- Low- to moderate-intensity exercise can be undertaken by individuals with congestive heart failure, using dyspnea as a guide for exercise intensity.
- Local muscle exercise, such as two-legged exercise training, may be a viable alternative to full-body exercise for individuals with congestive heart failure.

- Handgrip strength may be an independent predictor of prognosis for individuals with congestive heart failure.
- All individuals should be aware of the signs and symptoms of a heart attack or stroke during physical activity and activate EMS for the fastest response.

REFERENCES

Action to Control Cardiovascular Risk in Diabetes Study Group, Gerstein HC, Miller ME, Byington RP, Goff DC Jr, Bigger JT, Buse JB, Cushman WC, Genuth S, Ismail-Beigi F, Grimm RH Jr, Probstfield JL, Simons-Morton DG, Friedewald WT: Effects of intensive glucose lowering in type 2 diabetes. *N Engl J Med* 358:2545–2559, 2008

Alonso-Coello P, Bellmunt S, McGorrian C, Anand SS, Guzman R, Criqui MH, Akl EA, Olav Vandvik P, Lansberg MG, Guyatt GH, Spencer FA: Antithrombotic therapy in peripheral artery disease: antithrombotic therapy and prevention of thrombosis, 9th ed: American College of Chest Physicians Evidence-Based Clinical Practice Guidelines. *Chest* 141 (2 Suppl.):e669S–e690S, 2012

American Diabetes Association: Standards of medical care in diabetes—2013. *Diabetes Care* 36 (Suppl. 1):S11–S66, 2013

Araiza P, Hewes H, Gashetewa C, Vella CA, Burge MR: Efficacy of a pedometer-based physical activity program on parameters of diabetes control in type 2 diabetes mellitus. *Metabolism* 55:1382–1387, 2006

Aronow WS: Treatment of unstable angina pectoris/non-ST-segment elevation myocardial infarction in elderly patients. *J Gerontol A Biol Sci Med Sci* 58:M927–M933, 2003

Azadbakht L, Fard NR, Karimi M, Baghaei MH, Surkan PJ, Rahimi M, Esmaillzadeh A, Willett WC: Effects of the Dietary Approaches to Stop Hypertension (DASH) eating plan on cardiovascular risks among type 2 diabetic patients: a randomized crossover clinical trial. *Diabetes Care* 34:55–57, 2011

Babar GS, Zidan H, Widlansky ME, Das E, Hoffmann RG, Daoud M, Alemzadeh R: Impaired endothelial function in preadolescent children with type 1 diabetes. *Diabetes Care* 34:681–685, 2011

Bagshaw SM, Cruz DN: Fluid overload as a biomarker of heart failure and acute kidney injury. *Contrib Nephrol* 164:54–68, 2010

Balady GJ, Williams MA, Ades PA, Bittner V, Comoss P, Foody JM, Franklin B, Sanderson B, Southard D, Cardiac Rehabilitation American Heart Association Exercise, the Council on Clinical Cardiology Prevention Committee, Nursing American Heart Association Council on Cardiovascular, Epidemiology American Heart Association Council on Prevention, Physical Activity American Heart Association Council on Nutrition, Metabolism, American Association of Cardiovascular and Pulmonary Rehabilitation: Core components of cardiac rehabilitation/secondary prevention programs: 2007 update: a scientific statement from the American Heart Association Exercise, Cardiac Rehabilitation, and Prevention Committee, the Council on Clinical Cardiology; the Councils on Cardiovascular Nursing, Epidemiology and Prevention, and Nutrition, Physical Activity, and Metabolism; and the American Association of Cardiovascular and Pulmonary Rehabilitation. *Circulation* 115:2675–2682, 2007

Balducci S, Zanuso S, Fernando F, Nicolucci A, Cardelli P, Cavallo S, Fallucca S, Alessi E, Pugliese G, Fallucca F: The Italian diabetes and exercise study. *Diabetes* 57 (Suppl. 1):A306–A307, 2008

Balducci S, Iacobellis G, Parisi L, Di Biase N, Calandriello E, Leonetti F, Fallucca R: Exercise training can modify the natural history of diabetic peripheral neuropathy. *J Diabetes Complications* 20:216–223, 2006

Banerjee C, Moon YP, Paik MC, Rundek T, Mora-McLaughlin C, Vieira JR, Sacco RL, Elkind MS: Duration of diabetes and risk of ischemic stroke: the Northern Manhattan Study. *Stroke* 43:1212–1217, 2012

Bartlo P: Evidence-based application of aerobic and resistance training in patients with congestive heart failure. *J Cardiopulm Rehabil Prev* 27:368–375, 2007

Basta G, Lazzerini G, Massaro M, Simoncini T, Tanganelli P, Fu C, Kislinger T, Stern DM, Schmidt AM, De Caterina R: Advanced glycation end products activate endothelium through signal-transduction receptor RAGE: a mechanism for amplification of inflammatory responses. *Circulation* 105:816–822, 2002

Belotto MF, Magdalon J, Rodrigues HG, Vinolo MA, Curi R, Pithon-Curi TC, Hatanaka E: Moderate exercise improves leucocyte function and decreases inflammation in diabetes. *Clin Exp Immunol* 162:237–243, 2010

Berry JD, Dyer A, Cai X, Garside DB, Ning H, Thomas A, Greenland P, Van Horn L, Tracy RP, Lloyd-Jones DM: Lifetime risks of cardiovascular disease. *N Engl J Med* 366:321–329, 2012

Bishop FK, Maahs DM, Snell-Bergeon JK, Ogden LG, Kinney GL, Rewers M: Lifestyle risk factors for atherosclerosis in adults with type 1 diabetes. *Diab Vasc Dis Res* 6:269–275, 2009

Blair SN, Kohl HW III, Barlow CE, Paffenbarger RS Jr, Gibbons LW, Macera CA: Changes in physical fitness and all-cause mortality. A prospective study of healthy and unhealthy men. *JAMA* 273:1093–1098, 1995

Booth GL, Kapral MK, Fung K, Tu JV: Recent trends in cardiovascular complications among men and women with and without diabetes. *Diabetes Care* 29:32–37, 2006

Buse JB, Ginsberg HN, Bakris GL, Clark NG, Costa F, Eckel R, Fonseca V, Gerstein HC, Grundy S, Nesto RW, Pignone MP, Plutzky J, Porte D, Redberg R, Stitzel KF, Stone NJ, American Heart Association, American Diabetes Association: Primary prevention of cardiovascular diseases in people with diabetes mellitus: a scientific statement from the American Heart Association and the American Diabetes Association. *Circulation* 115:114–126, 2007

Cauza E, Hanusch-Enserer U, Strasser B, Kostner K, Dunky A, Haber P: The metabolic effects of long term exercise in type 2 diabetes patients. *Wien Med Wochenschr* 156:515–519, 2006

Cauza E, Hanusch-Enserer U, Strasser B, Ludvik B, Metz-Schimmerl S, Pacini G, Wagner O, Georg P, Prager R, Kostner K, Dunky A, Haber P: The relative benefits of endurance and strength training on the metabolic factors and muscle function of people with type 2 diabetes mellitus. *Arch Phys Med Rehabil* 86:1527–1533, 2005

Cho JY, Jeong MH, Ahn YK, Kim JH, Chae SC, Kim YJ, Hur SH, Seong IW, Hong TJ, Choi DH, Cho MC, Kim CJ, Seung KB, Chung WS, Jang YS, Cho SY, Rha SW, Bae JH, Cho JG, Park SJ, Investigators Korea Acute Myocardial Infarction Registry: Comparison of outcomes of patients with painless versus painful ST-segment elevation myocardial infarction undergoing percutaneous coronary intervention. *Am J Cardiol* 109:337–343, 2012

Chopra S, Peter S: Screening for coronary artery disease in patients with type 2 diabetes mellitus: an evidence-based review. *Indian J Endocrinol Metab* 16:94–101, 2012

Chudyk A, Petrella RJ: Effects of exercise on cardiovascular risk factors in type 2 diabetes: a meta-analysis. *Diabetes Care* 34:1228–1237, 2011

Church TS, Cheng YJ, Earnest CP, Barlow CE, Gibbons LW, Priest EL, Blair SN: Exercise capacity and body composition as predictors of mortality among men with diabetes. *Diabetes Care* 27:83–88, 2004

Church TS, LaMonte MJ, Barlow CE, Blair SN: Cardiorespiratory fitness and body mass index as predictors of cardiovascular disease mortality among men with diabetes. *Arch Intern Med* 165:2114–2120, 2005

Ciccone MM, Niccoli-Asabella A, Scicchitano P, Gesualdo M, Notaristefano A, Chieppa D, Carbonara S, Ricci G, Sassara M, Altini C, Quistelli G, Lepera ME, Favale S, Rubini G: Cardiovascular risk evaluation and prevalence of silent myocardial ischemia in subjects with asymptomatic carotid artery disease. *Vasc Health Risk Manag* 7:129–134, 2011

Coccheri S: Approaches to prevention of cardiovascular complications and events in diabetes mellitus. *Drugs* 67:997–1026, 2007

Cohen ND, Dunstan DW, Robinson C, Vulikh E, Zimmet PZ, Shaw JE: Improved endothelial function following a 14-month resistance exercise training program in adults with type 2 diabetes. *Diabetes Res Clin Pract* 79:405–411, 2008

Collins TC, Lunos S, Ahluwalia JS: Self-efficacy is associated with walking ability in persons with diabetes mellitus and peripheral arterial disease. *Vasc Med* 15:189–195, 2010

Collins TC, Lunos S, Carlson T, Henderson K, Lightbourne M, Nelson B, Hodges JS: Effects of a home-based walking intervention on mobility and quality of life in people with diabetes and peripheral arterial disease: a randomized controlled trial. *Diabetes Care* 34:2174–2179, 2011

Cornelissen VA, Fagard RH: Effect of resistance training on resting blood pressure: a meta-analysis of randomized controlled trials. *J Hypertens* 23:251–259, 2005a

Cornelissen VA, Fagard RH: Effects of endurance training on blood pressure, blood pressure-regulating mechanisms, and cardiovascular risk factors. *Hypertension* 46:667–675, 2005b

Crawford MH: Combination therapy as first-line treatment for hypertension. *Am J Cardiovasc Drugs* 9:1–6, 2009

Cullen DL, Rodak B: Clinical utility of measures of breathlessness. *Respir Care* 47:986–993, 2002

Cvetanovski MV, Jovev S, Cvetanovska M, Blazevski B, Colanceski R, Andreevska T, Gramatnikovski N, Kartalov A: Femoropopliteal bypass vs percutaneous transluminal angioplasty and stenting in treatment of peripheral artery diseases of infrainquinal segment—short-term results. *Prilozi* 30:105–118, 2009

de Paula TP, Steemburgo T, de Almeida JC, Dall'alba V, Gross JL, de Azevedo MJ: The role of Dietary Approaches to Stop Hypertension (DASH) diet food groups in blood pressure in type 2 diabetes. *Br J Nutr* 108:155–162, 2012

Deckert T, Feldt-Rasmussen B, Borch-Johnsen K, Jensen T, Kofoed-Enevoldsen A: Albuminuria reflects widespread vascular damage. The Steno hypothesis. *Diabetologia* 32:219–226, 1989

Delgado-Mederos R, Rovira A, Alvarez-Sabin J, Ribo M, Munuera J, Rubiera M, Santamarina E, Maisterra O, Delgado P, Montaner J, Molina CA: Speed of tPA-induced clot lysis predicts DWI lesion evolution in acute stroke. *Stroke* 38:955–960, 2007

Easton JD, Saver JL, Albers GW, Alberts MJ, Chaturvedi S, Feldmann E, Hatsukami TS, Higashida RT, Johnston SC, Kidwell CS, Lutsep HL, Miller E, Sacco RL, American Heart Association, American Stroke Association Stroke Council, Council on Cardiovascular Surgery and Anesthesia, Council on Cardiovascular Radiology and Intervention, Council on Cardiovascular Nursing, Interdisciplinary Council on Peripheral Vascular Disease: Definition and evaluation of transient ischemic attack: a scientific statement for healthcare professionals from the American Heart Association/American Stroke Association Stroke Council; Council on Cardiovascular Surgery and Anesthesia; Council on Cardiovascular Radiology and Intervention; Council on Cardiovascular Nursing; and the Interdisciplinary Council on Peripheral Vascular Disease. The American Academy of Neurology affirms the value of this statement as an educational tool for neurologists. *Stroke* 40:2276–2293, 2009

Featherstone JF, Holly RG, Amsterdam EA: Physiologic responses to weight lifting in coronary artery disease. *Am J Cardiol* 71:287–292, 1993

Figueroa A, Baynard T, Fernhall B, Carhart R, Kanaley JA: Endurance training improves post-exercise cardiac autonomic modulation in obese women with and without type 2 diabetes. *Eur J Appl Physiol* 100:437–444, 2007

Fletcher GF, Balady G, Blair SN, Blumenthal J, Caspersen C, Chaitman B, Epstein S, Sivarajan Froelicher ES, Froelicher VF, Pina IL, Pollock ML: Statement on exercise: benefits and recommendations for physical activity programs for all Americans. A statement for health professionals by the Committee on Exercise and Cardiac Rehabilitation of the Council on Clinical Cardiology, American Heart Association. *Circulation* 94:857–862, 1996

Fox CS, Pencina MJ, Wilson PW, Paynter NP, Vasan RS, D'Agostino RB Sr: Lifetime risk of cardiovascular disease among individuals with and without diabetes stratified by obesity status in the Framingham heart study. *Diabetes Care* 31:1582–1584, 2008

Gaede P, Vedel P, Larsen N, Jensen GV, Parving HH, Pedersen O: Multifactorial intervention and cardiovascular disease in patients with type 2 diabetes. *N Engl J Med* 348:383–393, 2003

Ghilarducci LE, Holly RG, Amsterdam EA: Effects of high resistance training in coronary artery disease. *Am J Cardiol* 64:866–870, 1989

Gillison FB, Skevington SM, Sato A, Standage M, Evangelidou S: The effects of exercise interventions on quality of life in clinical and healthy populations; a meta-analysis. *Soc Sci Med* 68:1700–1710, 2009

Gordon A, Tyni-Lenne R, Jansson E, Kaijser L, Theodorsson-Norheim E, Sylven C: Improved ventilation and decreased sympathetic stress in chronic heart failure patients following local endurance training with leg muscles. *J Card Fail* 3:3–12, 1997

Gordon A, Tyni-Lenne R, Persson H, Kaijser L, Hultman E, Sylven C: Markedly improved skeletal muscle function with local muscle training in patients with chronic heart failure. *Clin Cardiol* 19:568–574, 1996

Gordon LA, Morrison EY, McGrowder DA, Young R, Fraser YT, Zamora EM, Alexander-Lindo RL, Irving RR: Effect of exercise therapy on lipid profile and oxidative stress indicators in patients with type 2 diabetes. *BMC Complement Altern Med* 8:21, 2008

Grossman E, Messerli FH, Goldbourt U: High blood pressure and diabetes mellitus: are all antihypertensive drugs created equal? *Arch Intern Med* 160:2447–2452, 2000

Hansen D, Dendale P, Jonkers RA, Beelen M, Manders RJ, Corluy L, Mullens A, Berger J, Meeusen R, van Loon LJ: Continuous low- to moderate-intensity exercise training is as effective as moderate- to high-intensity exercise training at lowering blood HbA(1c) in obese type 2 diabetes patients. *Diabetologia* 52:1789–1797, 2009

Heiss C, Keen CL, Kelm M: Flavanols and cardiovascular disease prevention. *Eur Heart J* 31:2583–2592, 2010

Heran BS, Chen JM, Ebrahim S, Moxham T, Oldridge N, Rees K, Thompson DR, Taylor RS: Exercise-based cardiac rehabilitation for coronary heart disease. *Cochrane Database Syst Rev*:CD001800, 2011

Herbst A, Kordonouri O, Schwab KO, Schmidt F, Holl RW, DPV Initiative of the German Working Group for Pediatric Diabetology Germany: Impact of physical activity on cardiovascular risk factors in children with type 1 diabetes: a multicenter study of 23,251 patients. *Diabetes Care* 30:2098–2100, 2007

Higashida RT, Furlan AJ, Roberts H, Tomsick T, Connors B, Barr J, Dillon W, Warach S, Broderick J, Tilley B, Sacks D, Technology Assessment Committee of the American Society of Interventional and Therapeutic Neuroradiology, Technology Assessment Committee of the Society of Interventional Radiology: Trial design and reporting standards for intra-arterial cerebral thrombolysis for acute ischemic stroke. *Stroke* 34:e109–e137, 2003

Hinderliter AL, Babyak MA, Sherwood A, Blumenthal JA: The DASH diet and insulin sensitivity. *Curr Hypertens Rep* 13:67–73, 2011

Howorka K, Pumprla J, Haber P, Koller-Strametz J, Mondrzyk J, Schabmann A: Effects of physical training on heart rate variability in diabetic patients with various degrees of cardiovascular autonomic neuropathy. *Cardiovasc Res* 34:206–214, 1997

Issa VS, Amaral AF, Cruz FD, Ayub-Ferreira SM, Guimaraes GV, Chizzola PR, Souza GE, Bocchi EA: Glycemia and prognosis of patients with chronic heart failure—subanalysis of the Long-Term Prospective Randomized Controlled Study Using Repetitive Education at Six-Month Intervals and Monitoring for Adherence in Heart Failure Outpatients (REMADHE) trial. *Am Heart J* 159:90–97, 2010

Izawa KP, Watanabe S, Oka K, Hiraki K, Morio Y, Kasahara Y, Watanabe Y, Katata H, Osada N, Omiya K: Upper and lower extremity muscle strength levels associated with an exercise capacity of 5 metabolic equivalents in male patients with heart failure. *J Cardiopulm Rehabil Prev* 32:85–91, 2012

Izawa KP, Watanabe S, Osada N, Kasahara Y, Yokoyama H, Hiraki K, Morio Y, Yoshioka S, Oka K, Omiya K: Handgrip strength as a predictor of prognosis in Japanese patients with congestive heart failure. *Eur J Cardiovasc Prev Rehabil* 16:21–27, 2009

Johnson MJ, Oxberry SG, Cleland JG, Clark AL: Measurement of breathlessness in clinical trials in patients with chronic heart failure: the need for a standardized approach: a systematic review. *Eur J Heart Fail* 12:137–147, 2010

Kadoglou NP, Iliadis F, Angelopoulou N, Perrea D, Ampatzidis G, Liapis CD, Alevizos M: The anti-inflammatory effects of exercise training in patients with type 2 diabetes mellitus. *Eur J Cardiovasc Prev Rehabil* 14:837–843, 2007

Karlsdottir AE, Foster C, Porcari JP, Palmer-McLean K, White-Kube R, Backes RC: Hemodynamic responses during aerobic and resistance exercise. *J Cardiopulm Rehabil* 22:170–177, 2002

Kelley GA, Kelley KA, Tran ZV: Aerobic exercise and resting blood pressure: a meta-analytic review of randomized, controlled trials. *Prev Cardiol* 4:73–80, 2001a

Kelley GA, Kelley KS: Effects of aerobic exercise on lipids and lipoproteins in adults with type 2 diabetes: a meta-analysis of randomized-controlled trials. *Public Health* 121:643–655, 2007

Kelley GA, Kelley KS: Progressive resistance exercise and resting blood pressure: a meta-analysis of randomized controlled trials. *Hypertension* 35:838–843, 2000

Kelley GA, Sharpe Kelley K: Aerobic exercise and resting blood pressure in older adults: a meta-analytic review of randomized controlled trials. *J Gerontol A Biol Sci Med Sci* 56:M298–M303, 2001b

Kemp CD, Conte JV: The pathophysiology of heart failure. *Cardiovasc Pathol* 21:365–371, 2012

Kershnar AK, Daniels SR, Imperatore G, Palla SL, Petitti DB, Pettitt DJ, Marcovina S, Dolan LM, Hamman RF, Liese AD, Pihoker C, Rodriguez BL: Lipid abnormalities are prevalent in youth with type 1 and type 2 diabetes: the SEARCH for Diabetes in Youth Study. *J Pediatr* 149:314–319, 2006

Kim SH, Lee SL, Kang ES, Kang S, Hur KY, Lee HJ, Ahn CW, Cha BS, Yoo JS, Lee HC: Effects of lifestyle modification on metabolic parameters and carotid intima-media thickness in patients with type 2 diabetes mellitus. *Metabolism* 55:1053–1059, 2006

Kirk A, Mutrie N, MacIntyre P, Fisher M: Effects of a 12-month physical activity counselling intervention on glycaemic control and on the status of cardiovascular risk factors in people with type 2 diabetes. *Diabetologia* 47:821–832, 2004

Kokkinos P, Myers J, Nylen E, Panagiotakos DB, Manolis A, Pittaras A, Blackman MR, Jacob-Issac R, Faselis C, Abella J, Singh S: Exercise capacity and all-cause mortality in African American and Caucasian men with type 2 diabetes. *Diabetes Care* 32:623–628, 2009

Kones R: Recent advances in the management of chronic stable angina II. Antiischemic therapy, options for refractory angina, risk factor reduction, and revascularization. *Vasc Health Risk Manag* 6:749–774, 2010

Kones R: Primary prevention of coronary heart disease: integration of new data, evolving views, revised goals, and role of rosuvastatin in management. A comprehensive survey. *Drug Des Devel Ther* 5:325–380, 2011

Kwon HR, Min KW, Ahn HJ, Seok HG, Lee JH, Park GS, Han KA: Effects of aerobic exercise vs. resistance training on endothelial function in women with type 2 diabetes mellitus. *Diabetes Metab J* 35:364–373, 2011

Laaksonen DE, Atalay M, Niskanen LK, Mustonen J, Sen CK, Lakka TA, Uusitupa MI: Aerobic exercise and the lipid profile in type 1 diabetic men: a randomized controlled trial. *Med Sci Sports Exerc* 32:1541–1548, 2000

Landberg R, Naidoo N, van Dam RM: Diet and endothelial function: from individual components to dietary patterns. *Curr Opin Lipidol* 23:147–155, 2012

Lavie CJ, Milani RV: Effects of cardiac rehabilitation and exercise training in obese patients with coronary artery disease. *Chest* 109:52–56, 1996

Lavie CJ, Milani RV, Littman AB: Benefits of cardiac rehabilitation and exercise training in secondary coronary prevention in the elderly. *J Am Coll Cardiol* 22:678–683, 1993

Lee DC, Sui X, Church TS, Lee IM, Blair SN: Associations of cardiorespiratory fitness and obesity with risks of impaired fasting glucose and type 2 diabetes in men. *Diabetes Care* 32:257–262, 2009

Lee IM, Skerrett PJ: Physical activity and all-cause mortality: what is the dose-response relation? *Med Sci Sports Exerc* 33 (6 Suppl.):S459–S471; discussion S493–S494, 2001

Lee MS, Yang T, Dhoot J, Iqbal Z, Liao H: Meta-analysis of studies comparing coronary artery bypass grafting with drug-eluting stenting in patients with diabetes mellitus and multivessel coronary artery disease. *Am J Cardiol* 105:1540–1544, 2010

Lee WL, Cheung AM, Cape D, Zinman B: Impact of diabetes on coronary artery disease in women and men: a meta-analysis of prospective studies. *Diabetes Care* 23:962–968, 2000

Legato MJ, Gelzer A, Goland R, Ebner SA, Rajan S, Villagra V, Kosowski M: Gender-specific care of the patient with diabetes: review and recommendations. *Gend Med* 3:131–158, 2006

Liese AD, Bortsov A, Gunther AL, Dabelea D, Reynolds K, Standiford DA, Liu L, Williams DE, Mayer-Davis EJ, D'Agostino RB Jr, Bell R, Marcovina S: Association of DASH diet with cardiovascular risk factors in youth with diabetes mellitus: the SEARCH for Diabetes in Youth study. *Circulation* 123:1410–1417, 2011

Lievre MM, Moulin P, Thivolet C, Rodier M, Rigalleau V, Penfornis A, Pradignac A, Ovize M, Dynamit Investigators: Detection of silent myocardial ischemia in asymptomatic patients with diabetes: results of a randomized trial and meta-analysis assessing the effectiveness of systematic screening. *Trials* 12:23, 2011

Loimaala A, Groundstroem K, Rinne M, Nenonen A, Huhtala H, Parkkari J, Vuori I: Effect of long-term endurance and strength training on metabolic control and arterial elasticity in patients with type 2 diabetes mellitus. *Am J Cardiol* 103:972–977, 2009

Loimaala A, Huikuri HV, Koobi T, Rinne M, Nenonen A, Vuori I: Exercise training improves baroreflex sensitivity in type 2 diabetes. *Diabetes* 52:1837–1842, 2003

Look AHEAD Research Group, Wing RR: Long-term effects of a lifestyle intervention on weight and cardiovascular risk factors in individuals with type 2 diabetes mellitus: four-year results of the Look AHEAD trial. *Arch Intern Med* 170:1566–1575, 2010

Maeng M, Nielsen PH, Busk M, Mortensen LS, Kristensen SD, Nielsen TT, Andersen HR, Danami Investigators: Time to treatment and three-year mortality after primary percutaneous coronary intervention for ST-segment elevation myocardial infarction—a DANish Trial in Acute Myocardial Infarction-2 (DANAMI-2) substudy. *Am J Cardiol* 105:1528–1534, 2010

Maiorana A, O'Driscoll G, Goodman C, Taylor R, Green D: Combined aerobic and resistance exercise improves glycemic control and fitness in type 2 diabetes. *Diabetes Res Clin Pract* 56:115–123, 2002

Mamcarz A, Chmielewski M, Braksator W, Syska-Sumnska J, Janiszewski M, Krol J, Kuch M, Kuch J, Dluiniewski M: Factors influencing cardiac complications in patients with type-2 diabetes mellitus and silent myocardial ischaemia: five-year follow-up. *Pol Arch Med Wewn* 112:1433–1443, 2004

Marwick TH, Hordern MD, Miller T, Chyun DA, Bertoni AG, Blumenthal RS, Philippides G, Rocchini A, Council on Clinical Cardiology, American Heart Association Exercise, Cardiac Rehabilitation, and Prevention Committee, Council on Cardiovascular Disease in the Young, Council on Cardiovascular Nursing, Council on Nutrition, Physical Activity, and Metabolism, Interdisciplinary Council on Quality of Care and Outcomes Research: Exercise training for type 2 diabetes mellitus: impact on cardiovascular risk: a scientific statement from the American Heart Association. *Circulation* 119:3244–3262, 2009

McAuley PA, Myers JN, Abella JP, Tan SY, Froelicher VF: Exercise capacity and body mass as predictors of mortality among male veterans with type 2 diabetes. *Diabetes Care* 30:1539–1543, 2007

McCartney N: Acute responses to resistance training and safety. *Med Sci Sports Exerc* 31:31–37, 1999

McDermott MM, Ades P, Guralnik JM, Dyer A, Ferrucci L, Liu K, Nelson M, Lloyd-Jones D, Van Horn L, Garside D, Kibbe M, Domanchuk K, Stein JH, Liao Y, Tao H, Green D, Pearce WH, Schneider JR, McPherson D, Laing ST, McCarthy WJ, Shroff A, Criqui MH: Treadmill exercise and resistance training in patients with peripheral arterial disease with and without intermittent claudication: a randomized controlled trial. *JAMA* 301:165–174, 2009

McDermott MM, Liu K, Ferrucci L, Criqui MH, Greenland P, Guralnik JM, Tian L, Schneider JR, Pearce WH, Tan J, Martin GJ: Physical performance in peripheral arterial disease: a slower rate of decline in patients who walk more. *Ann Intern Med* 144:10–20, 2006

McDermott MM, Liu K, Greenland P, Guralnik JM, Criqui MH, Chan C, Pearce WH, Schneider JR, Ferrucci L, Celic L, Taylor LM, Vonesh E, Martin GJ, Clark E: Functional decline in peripheral arterial disease: associations with the ankle brachial index and leg symptoms. *JAMA* 292:453–461, 2004

McNally B, Robb R, Mehta M, Vellano K, Valderrama AL, Yoon PW, Sasson C, Crouch A, Perez AB, Merritt R, Kellermann A, Centers for Disease Control and Prevention: Out-of-hospital cardiac arrest surveillance—Cardiac Arrest

Registry to Enhance Survival (CARES), United States, October 1, 2005– December 31, 2010. *MMWR Surveill Summ* 60:1–19, 2011

McQuade K, Gable D, Pearl G, Theune B, Black S: Four-year randomized prospective comparison of percutaneous ePTFE/nitinol self-expanding stent graft versus prosthetic femoral-popliteal bypass in the treatment of superficial femoral artery occlusive disease. *J Vasc Surg* 52:584–590; discussion 590–591, 591 e1–591 e7, 2010

Mohler ER III, Bundens W, Denenberg J, Medenilla E, Hiatt WR, Criqui MH: Progression of asymptomatic peripheral artery disease over 1 year. *Vasc Med* 17:10–16, 2012

Morrato EH, Hill JO, Wyatt HR, Ghushchyan V, Sullivan PW: Physical activity in U.S. adults with diabetes and at risk for developing diabetes, 2003. *Diabetes Care* 30:203–209, 2007

Mourad JJ, Le Jeune S: Blood pressure control, risk factors and cardiovascular prognosis in patients with diabetes: 30 years of progress. *J Hypertens* 26 (Suppl. 3):S7–S13, 2008

Murphy EC, Carson L, Neal W, Baylis C, Donley D, Yeater R: Effects of an exercise intervention using Dance Dance Revolution on endothelial function and other risk factors in overweight children. *Int J Pediatr Obes* 4:205–214, 2009

Murrow JR, Sher S, Ali S, Uphoff I, Patel R, Porkert M, Le NA, Jones D, Quyyumi AA: The differential effect of statins on oxidative stress and endothelial function: atorvastatin versus pravastatin. *J Clin Lipidol* 6:42–49, 2012

National High Blood Pressure Education Program Working Group: National High Blood Pressure Education Program Working Group report on hypertension in diabetes. *Hypertension* 23:145–158; discussion 159–160, 1994

Navarese EP, De Servi S, Gibson CM, Buffon A, Castriota F, Kubica J, Petronio AS, Andreotti F, De Luca G: Early vs. delayed invasive strategy in patients with acute coronary syndromes without ST-segment elevation: a meta-analysis of randomized studies. *QJM* 104:193–200, 2011

Negrean M, Stirban A, Stratmann B, Gawlowski T, Horstmann T, Gotting C, Kleesiek K, Mueller-Roesel M, Koschinsky T, Uribarri J, Vlassara H, Tschoepe D: Effects of low- and high-advanced glycation endproduct meals on macro- and microvascular endothelial function and oxidative stress in patients with type 2 diabetes mellitus. *Am J Clin Nutr* 85:1236–1243, 2007

Neri S, Calvagno S, Mauceri B, Misseri M, Tsami A, Vecchio C, Mastrosimone G, Di Pino A, Maiorca D, Judica A, Romano G, Rizzotto A, Signorelli SS: Effects of antioxidants on postprandial oxidative stress and endothelial dysfunction in subjects with impaired glucose tolerance and type 2 diabetes. *Eur J Nutr* 49:409–416, 2010

Neri S, Signorelli SS, Torrisi B, Pulvirenti D, Mauceri B, Abate G, Ignaccolo L, Bordonaro F, Cilio D, Calvagno S, Leotta C: Effects of antioxidant supplementation on postprandial oxidative stress and endothelial dysfunction: a single-blind, 15-day clinical trial in patients with untreated type 2 diabetes, subjects with impaired glucose tolerance, and healthy controls. *Clin Ther* 27:1764–1773, 2005

Nilsson PM: Target blood pressure in diabetes patients with hypertension—what is the accumulated evidence in 2011? *J Zhejiang Univ Sci B* 12:611–623, 2011

O'Leary VB, Marchetti CM, Krishnan RK, Stetzer BP, Gonzalez F, Kirwan JP: Exercise-induced reversal of insulin resistance in obese elderly is associated with reduced visceral fat. *J Appl Physiol* 100:1584–1589, 2006

Okada S, Hiuge A, Makino H, Nagumo A, Takaki H, Konishi H, Goto Y, Yoshimasa Y, Miyamoto Y: Effect of exercise intervention on endothelial function and incidence of cardiovascular disease in patients with type 2 diabetes. *J Atheroscler Thromb* 17:828–833, 2010

Oliver D, Pflugfelder PW, McCartney N, McKelvie RS, Suskin N, Kostuk WJ: Acute cardiovascular responses to leg-press resistance exercise in heart transplant recipients. *Int J Cardiol* 81:61–74, 2001

Orchard TJ, Olson JC, Erbey JR, Williams K, Forrest KY, Smithline Kinder L, Ellis D, Becker DJ: Insulin resistance-related factors, but not glycemia, predict coronary artery disease in type 1 diabetes: 10-year follow-up data from the Pittsburgh Epidemiology of Diabetes Complications Study. *Diabetes Care* 26:1374–1379, 2003

Pagkalos M, Koutlianos N, Kouidi E, Pagkalos E, Mandroukas K, Deligiannis A: Heart rate variability modifications following exercise training in type 2 diabetic patients with definite cardiac autonomic neuropathy. *Br J Sports Med* 42:47–54, 2008

Parissis JT, Rafouli-Stergiou P, Mebazaa A, Ikonomidis I, Bistola V, Nikolaou M, Meas T, Delgado J, Vilas-Boas F, Paraskevaidis I, Anastasiou-Nana M, Follath F: Acute heart failure in patients with diabetes mellitus: clinical characteristics and predictors of in-hospital mortality. *Int J Cardiol* 157:108–113, 2012

Pecoits-Filho R, Bucharles S, Barberato SH: Diastolic heart failure in dialysis patients: mechanisms, diagnostic approach, and treatment. *Semin Dial* 25:35–41, 2012

Pedersen BK: The anti-inflammatory effect of exercise: its role in diabetes and cardiovascular disease control. *Essays Biochem* 42:105–117, 2006

Pena KE, Stopka CB, Barak S, Gertner HR Jr, Carmeli E: Effects of low-intensity exercise on patients with peripheral artery disease. *Phys Sportsmed* 37:106–110, 2009

Pena Y, Fernandez-Britto JE, Bacallao J, Batista JF, de Leon ML: Lipid levels as predictors of silent myocardial ischemia in a type 2 diabetic population in havana. *MEDICC Rev* 14:18–24, 2012

Petitti DB, Imperatore G, Palla SL, Daniels SR, Dolan LM, Kershnar AK, Marcovina S, Pettitt DJ, Pihoker C, Search for Diabetes in Youth Study Group:

Serum lipids and glucose control: the SEARCH for Diabetes in Youth study. *Arch Pediatr Adolesc Med* 161:159–165, 2007

Pi-Sunyer X, Blackburn G, Brancati FL, Bray GA, Bright R, Clark JM, Curtis JM, Espeland MA, Foreyt JP, Graves K, Haffner SM, Harrison B, Hill JO, Horton ES, Jakicic J, Jeffery RW, Johnson KC, Kahn S, Kelley DE, Kitabchi AE, Knowler WC, Lewis CE, Maschak-Carey BJ, Montgomery B, Nathan DM, Patricio J, Peters A, Redmon JB, Reeves RS, Ryan DH, Safford M, Van Dorsten B, Wadden TA, Wagenknecht L, Wesche-Thobaben J, Wing RR, Yanovski SZ: Reduction in weight and cardiovascular disease risk factors in individuals with type 2 diabetes: one-year results of the Look AHEAD trial. *Diabetes Care* 30:1374–1383, 2007

Pinto A, Di Raimondo D, Tuttolomondo A, Butta C, Milio G, Licata G: Effects of physical exercise on inflammatory markers of atherosclerosis. *Curr Pharm Des* 18:4326-4349, 2012

Qin R, Chen T, Lou Q, Yu D: Excess risk of mortality and cardiovascular events associated with smoking among patients with diabetes: meta-analysis of observational prospective studies. *Int J Cardiol*, 2012

Ratner R, Goldberg R, Haffner S, Marcovina S, Orchard T, Fowler S, Temprosa M, Group Diabetes Prevention Program Research: Impact of intensive lifestyle and metformin therapy on cardiovascular disease risk factors in the Diabetes Prevention Program. *Diabetes Care* 28:888–894, 2005

Reboldi G, Gentile G, Angeli F, Verdecchia P: Choice of ACE inhibitor combinations in hypertensive patients with type 2 diabetes: update after recent clinical trials. *Vasc Health Risk Manag* 5:411–427, 2009

Rodriguez-Ospina L, Montano-Soto L: Management of chronic stable angina pectoris. *Bol Asoc Med P R* 100:39–47, 2008

Ronnemaa T, Marniemi J, Puukka P, Kuusi T: Effects of long-term physical exercise on serum lipids, lipoproteins and lipid metabolizing enzymes in type 2 (non-insulin-dependent) diabetic patients. *Diabetes Res* 7:79–84, 1988

Sacks FM, Katan M: Randomized clinical trials on the effects of dietary fat and carbohydrate on plasma lipoproteins and cardiovascular disease. *Am J Med* 113 (Suppl. 9B):13S–24S, 2002

Salem MA, Aboelasrar MA, Elbarbary NS, Elhilaly RA, Refaat YM: Is exercise a therapeutic tool for improvement of cardiovascular risk factors in adolescents with type 1 diabetes mellitus? A randomised controlled trial. *Diabetol Metab Syndr* 2:47, 2010

Saremi A, Bahn G, Reaven PD: Progression of vascular calcification is increased with statin use in the Veterans Affairs Diabetes Trial (VADT). *Diabetes Care* 35:2390–2392, 2012

Seeger JP, Thijssen DH, Noordam K, Cranen ME, Hopman MT, Nijhuis-van der Sanden MW: Exercise training improves physical fitness and vascular function in children with type 1 diabetes. *Diabetes Obes Metab* 13:382–384, 2011

Sena CM, Nunes E, Louro T, Proenca T, Seica RM: Endothelial dysfunction in type 2 diabetes: effect of antioxidants. *Rev Port Cardiol* 26:609–619, 2007

Shinji S, Shigeru M, Ryusei U, Mitsuru M, Shigehiro K: Adherence to a home-based exercise program and incidence of cardiovascular disease in type 2 diabetes patients. *Int J Sports Med* 28:877–879, 2007

Sigal RJ, Kenny GP, Wasserman DH, Castaneda-Sceppa C: Physical activity/exercise and type 2 diabetes. *Diabetes Care* 27:2518–2539, 2004

Sigal RJ, Kenny GP, Boulé NG, Wells GA, Prud'homme D, Fortier M, Reid RD, Tulloch H, Coyle D, Phillips P, Jennings A, Jaffey J: Effects of aerobic training, resistance training, or both on glycemic control in type 2 diabetes: a randomized trial. *Ann Intern Med* 147:357–369, 2007

Siri-Tarino PW, Sun Q, Hu FB, Krauss RM: Saturated fat, carbohydrate, and cardiovascular disease. *Am J Clin Nutr* 91:502–509, 2010

Smith SC Jr, Allen J, Blair SN, Bonow RO, Brass LM, Fonarow GC, Grundy SM, Hiratzka L, Jones D, Krumholz HM, Mosca L, Pasternak RC, Pearson T, Pfeffer MA, Taubert KA: AHA/ACC guidelines for secondary prevention for patients with coronary and other atherosclerotic vascular disease: 2006 update: endorsed by the National Heart, Lung, and Blood Institute. *Circulation* 113:2363–2372, 2006

Snowling NJ, Hopkins WG: Effects of different modes of exercise training on glucose control and risk factors for complications in type 2 diabetic patients: a meta-analysis. *Diabetes Care* 29:2518–2527, 2006

Stewart KJ: Exercise training and the cardiovascular consequences of type 2 diabetes and hypertension: plausible mechanisms for improving cardiovascular health. *JAMA* 288:1622–1631, 2002

Stewart KJ: Role of exercise training on cardiovascular disease in persons who have type 2 diabetes and hypertension. *Cardiol Clin* 22:569–586, 2004

Stirban A, Negrean M, Gotting C, Uribarri J, Gawlowski T, Stratmann B, Kleesiek K, Koschinsky T, Vlassara H, Tschoepe D: Dietary advanced glycation endproducts and oxidative stress: in vivo effects on endothelial function and adipokines. *Ann N Y Acad Sci* 1126:276–279, 2008

Strasser B, Arvandi M, Siebert U: Resistance training, visceral obesity and inflammatory response: a review of the evidence. *Obes Rev* 13:578–591, 2012

Strasser B, Siebert U, Schobersberger W: Resistance training in the treatment of the metabolic syndrome: a systematic review and meta-analysis of the effect of resistance training on metabolic clustering in patients with abnormal glucose metabolism. *Sports Med* 40:397–415, 2010

Takayama T, Hiro T, Hirayama A: Is angioplasty able to become the gold standard of treatment beyond bypass surgery for patients with multivessel coronary artery disease? Therapeutic strategies for 3-vessel coronary artery disease: OPCAB vs PCI(PCI-Side). *Circ J* 74:2744–2749, 2010

Taylor F, Ward K, Moore TH, Burke M, Davey Smith G, Casas JP, Ebrahim S: Statins for the primary prevention of cardiovascular disease. *Cochrane Database Syst Rev* 19:CD004816, 2011

Thallinger C, Urbauer E, Lackner E, Graselli U, Kostner K, Wolzt M, Joukhadar C: The ability of statins to protect low density lipoprotein from oxidation in hypercholesterolemic patients. *Int J Clin Pharmacol Ther* 43:551–557, 2005

Tonelli M, Lloyd A, Clement F, Conly J, Husereau D, Hemmelgarn B, Klarenbach S, McAlister FA, Wiebe N, Manns B, Alberta Kidney Disease Network: Efficacy of statins for primary prevention in people at low cardiovascular risk: a meta-analysis. *CMAJ* 183:E1189–E1202, 2011

Trigona B, Aggoun Y, Maggio A, Martin XE, Marchand LM, Beghetti M, Farpour-Lambert NJ: Preclinical noninvasive markers of atherosclerosis in children and adolescents with type 1 diabetes are influenced by physical activity. *J Pediatr* 157:533–539, 2010

Tudor-Locke C, Bell RC, Myers AM, Harris SB, Ecclestone NA, Lauzon N, Rodger NW: Controlled outcome evaluation of the First Step Program: a daily physical activity intervention for individuals with type II diabetes. *Int J Obes Relat Metab Disord* 28:113–119, 2004

Tyni-Lenne R, Gordon A, Europe E, Jansson E, Sylven C: Exercise-based rehabilitation improves skeletal muscle capacity, exercise tolerance, and quality of life in both women and men with chronic heart failure. *J Card Fail* 4:9–17, 1998

Tyni-Lenne R, Gordon A, Sylven C: Improved quality of life in chronic heart failure patients following local endurance training with leg muscles. *J Card Fail* 2:111–117, 1996

U.S. Department of Health and Human Services, Centers for Disease Control and Prevention: National diabetes fact sheet: national estimates and general information on diabetes and prediabetes in the United States, 2011, edited by Centers for Disease Control and Prevention. Atlanta, GA, U.S. Department of Health and Human Services, 2011

Valensi P, Lorgis L, Cottin Y: Prevalence, incidence, predictive factors and prognosis of silent myocardial infarction: a review of the literature. *Arch Cardiovasc Dis* 104:178–188, 2011

Wackers FJ, Young LH, Inzucchi SE, Chyun DA, Davey JA, Barrett EJ, Taillefer R, Wittlin SD, Heller GV, Filipchuk N, Engel S, Ratner RE, Iskandrian AE, Detection of Ischemia in Asymptomatic Diabetics Investigators: Detection of silent myocardial ischemia in asymptomatic diabetic subjects: the DIAD study. *Diabetes Care* 27:1954–1961, 2004

Wagner H, Degerblad M, Thorell A, Nygren J, Stahle A, Kuhl J, Brismar TB, Ohrvik J, Efendic S, Bavenholm PN: Combined treatment with exercise training and acarbose improves metabolic control and cardiovascular risk factor profile in subjects with mild type 2 diabetes. *Diabetes Care* 29:1471–1477, 2006

Wei M, Gibbons LW, Kampert JB, Nichaman MZ, Blair SN: Low cardiorespiratory fitness and physical inactivity as predictors of mortality in men with type 2 diabetes. *Ann Intern Med* 132:605–611, 2000

Wenaweser P, Windecker S: Acute coronary syndromes: management and secondary prevention. *Herz* 33:25–37, 2008

Westphal S, Luley C: Flavanol-rich cocoa ameliorates lipemia-induced endothelial dysfunction. *Heart Vessels* 26:511–515, 2011

Williams MA, Haskell WL, Ades PA, Amsterdam EA, Bittner V, Franklin BA, Gulanick M, Laing ST, Stewart KJ, American Heart Association Council on Clinical Cardiology, American Heart Association Council on Nutrition, Physical Activity, and Metabolism: Resistance exercise in individuals with and without cardiovascular disease: 2007 update: a scientific statement from the American Heart Association Council on Clinical Cardiology and Council on Nutrition, Physical Activity, and Metabolism. *Circulation* 116:572–584, 2007

Wilund KR: Is the anti-inflammatory effect of regular exercise responsible for reduced cardiovascular disease? *Clin Sci (Lond)* 112:543–555, 2007

Wise FM, Patrick JM: Resistance exercise in cardiac rehabilitation. *Clin Rehabil* 25:1059–1065, 2011

Woodman RJ, Chew GT, Watts GF: Mechanisms, significance and treatment of vascular dysfunction in type 2 diabetes mellitus: focus on lipid-regulating therapy. *Drugs* 65:31–74, 2005

Wycherley TP, Brinkworth GD, Noakes M, Buckley JD, Clifton PM: Effect of caloric restriction with and without exercise training on oxidative stress and endothelial function in obese subjects with type 2 diabetes. *Diabetes Obes Metab* 10:1062–1073, 2008

Young LH, Wackers FJ, Chyun DA, Davey JA, Barrett EJ, Taillefer R, Heller GV, Iskandrian AE, Wittlin SD, Filipchuk N, Ratner RE, Inzucchi SE: Cardiac outcomes after screening for asymptomatic coronary artery disease in patients with type 2 diabetes: the DIAD study: a randomized controlled trial. *JAMA* 301:1547–1555, 2009

Zander E, Heinke P, Reindel J, Kohnert KD, Kairies U, Braun J, Eckel L, Kerner W: Peripheral arterial disease in diabetes mellitus type 1 and type 2: are there different risk factors? *Vasa* 31:249–254, 2002

Zee RY, Romero JR, Gould JL, Ricupero DA, Ridker PM: Polymorphisms in the advanced glycosylation end product-specific receptor gene and risk of incident myocardial infarction or ischemic stroke. *Stroke* 37:1686–1690, 2006

Zhang L, Gong D, Li S, Zhou X: Meta-analysis of the effects of statin therapy on endothelial function in patients with diabetes mellitus. *Atherosclerosis* 223:78–85, 2012

Zoppini G, Targher G, Zamboni C, Venturi C, Cacciatori V, Moghetti P, Muggeo M: Effects of moderate-intensity exercise training on plasma biomarkers of inflammation and endothelial dysfunction in older patients with type 2 diabetes. *Nutr Metab Cardiovasc Dis* 16:543–549, 2006

Zoungas S, Chalmers J, Ninomiya T, Li Q, Cooper ME, Colagiuri S, Fulcher G, de Galan BE, Harrap S, Hamet P, Heller S, MacMahon S, Marre M, Poulter N, Travert F, Patel A, Neal B, Woodward M: Association of HbA1c levels with vascular complications and death in patients with type 2 diabetes: evidence of glycaemic thresholds. *Diabetologia* 55:636–643, 2012

Zwierska I, Walker RD, Choksy SA, Male JS, Pockley AG, Saxton JM: Upper- vs lower-limb aerobic exercise rehabilitation in patients with symptomatic peripheral arterial disease: a randomized controlled trial. *J Vasc Surg* 42:1122–1130, 2005

Chapter 18

Peripheral Neuropathy, Ulcers, and Amputations

T
he main manifestations of diabetic neuropathy are peripheral and autonomic in nature (Vinik 2003a, 2003b, 2007). The former topic is discussed in this chapter, and the latter is included in chapter 19. Up to 40% of individuals with diabetes may experience peripheral neuropathy, and 60% of lower-extremity amputations are related to suboptimal blood glucose control (Lemaster 2003, 2008; Narayan 2006). Pain or loss of sensation in the feet or hands, known as peripheral neuropathy, is nerve damage that is common in individuals with type 1 diabetes (T1D) and type 2 diabetes (T2D) (Lipsky 2006, Smith 2008). Its presence increases the likelihood of developing nonhealing ulcers on the feet and lower legs, as well as having a lower-limb amputation (Singh 2005, Lipsky 2006, Alvarsson 2012). Although certain precautions must be taken when physical activity is undertaken with any of these health issues, in most cases it is possible and recommended for improving diabetes management and lowering cardiovascular and amputation risk.

Case in Point: Exercise Management for an Adult with T2D and Peripheral Neuropathy

NP is a 66-year-old man with T2D for >20 years. For the better part of those two decades, his glycemic management has been marginal, and lately he has noticed that he has lost a good portion of the feeling in his feet, leaving them numb on the soles and unable to feel the ground below him well when he walks. His diabetes is managed with three mediations at this point: metformin, a sulfonylurea, and sitagliptin (Januvia). He also takes a lipid-lowering agent and two blood pressure medications, as well as a supplement with α-lipoic acid, to try to improve his loss of sensation in his feet. He used to be more physically active than he is now, but he has slacked off lately and rarely does any planned exercise. His job in construction does keep him on his feet a lot, however, and he thinks that counts for something.

Resting Measurements

Height: 69 inches
Weight: 210 lb
BMI: 31.0 (obese)
Heart rate: 82 beats per minute (bpm)
Blood pressure: 130/85 mmHg (on medication)

Fasting Labs

Plasma glucose: 158 mg/dl (controlled with three medications)
A1C: 7.8%
Total cholesterol: 205 mg/dl (on medication)
Triglycerides: 178 mg/dl
High-density lipoprotein cholesterol: 41 mg/dl
Low-density lipoprotein cholesterol: 129 mg/dl

Questions to Consider

1. What type of exercise can NP safely do with insensate feet?
2. Are any precautions needed for NP when he exercises?

(Continued on page 358.)

PERIPHERAL NEUROPATHY

Neuropathies are characterized by a progressive loss of nerve fiber function. Most peripheral neuropathy affects the extremities, particularly the lower legs and feet, but also the hands. Hyperglycemia causes nerve toxicity, leading to nerve damage and apoptosis (Singleton 2003, Smith 2008), which causes microvascular damage and perfusion loss. Symptoms manifest as neuropathic pain or loss of sensation that, coupled with poor blood flow, increase the risk of foot injury and ulceration (Coccheri 2007, Smith 2008). A widely accepted definition of diabetic peripheral neuropathy is the presence of symptoms and/or signs of peripheral nerve dysfunction in people with diabetes after exclusion of other causes.

Although non–diabetes-related causes exist (Lozeron 2002), neuropathies are the most common complication of diabetes, affecting up to 50% of individuals with diabetes. In T1D, distal polyneuropathy typically becomes symptomatic after many years of chronic, prolonged hyperglycemia. Conversely, those with T2D may develop it after only a few years of known poor glycemic control, or they already may have it at the time of diabetes diagnosis (Casellini 2007). In either type, enhanced glucose control significantly prevents the development of clinical neuropathy and reduces nerve conduction and vibration threshold abnormalities (Callaghan 2012).

Of interest, plantar fascia thickness determined via ultrasound has been shown to be an alternative index of tissue glycation, a marker of microvascular disease, and a significant predictor of the subsequent development of microvascular complications in T1D (Craig 2008). This finding suggests that glycation and oxidation of collagen in soft tissues may be independent risk factors for microvascular issues like peripheral neuropathy.

TYPES OF PERIPHERAL NEUROPATHY

The most common type of diabetic neuropathy, distal symmetrical polyneuropathy (DSP), typically involves both small and large nerve fibers (Casellini

2007), as detailed in Table 18.1. The small nerve fiber neuropathies generally are considered to be a component of metabolic syndrome and impaired glucose tolerance; these often begin painfully and present with a loss of intraepidermal nerve fibers. They may show no objective signs or evidence of nerve damage, however. Regrettably, small-fiber neuropathy frequently leads to foot ulceration, subsequent gangrene, and lower extremity amputations (U.S. Department of Health and Human Services 2011). On the other hand, large nerve-fiber neuropathy generally results in numbness in the feet and hands and ataxia (lack of coordination during gross motor movements), impairing activities of daily living and causing falls and fractures (Casellini 2007). The presence of pain in DSP is associated with its clinical severity and presence of "burning" symptoms, but it is not associated with the degree of involvement of large-diameter sensory fibers or diabetes severity (Mondelli 2012).

Table 18.1 Common Types of Peripheral Neuropathy

Type	Characteristics
Distal symmetrical polyneuropathy (DSP)	■ Affects sensory, motor, and autonomic functions in varying degrees, with sensory abnormalities predominating ■ Affects peripheral nerves in a length-dependent pattern, with the longest nerves affected first ■ Painful paresthesias (a "pins and needles" sensation) and numbness, starting in the toes and ascending like stockings over months and years ■ When ascended above the knees, then similar symptoms occur in the hands, progressing up the arm like gloves ■ When severe, affects anterior aspect of the trunk, vertex of the head ■ Mild weakness of foot muscles and decreased ankle and knee reflexes ■ With impaired proprioception and vibratory perception, gait affected (sensory ataxia)
Small-fiber neuropathy	■ Distal symmetrical neuropathy primarily affecting small-diameter sensory fibers (i.e., A delta and C fibers) ■ Painful paresthesias perceived as burning, stabbing, crushing, aching, or cramp-like, with increased severity at night ■ Loss of pain and temperature sensation with relative sparing of distal reflexes and proprioception
Asymmetrical neuropathies	■ Single or multiple cranial or somatic mononeuropathies, including the following: ■ Median neuropathy of the wrist (carpal tunnel syndrome) ■ Other single or multiple limb mononeuropathies ■ Thoracic radiculoneuropathy ■ Lumbosacral radiculoplexus neuropathy ■ Cervical radiculoplexus neuropathy
Focal and multifocal neuropathies	■ Cranial neuropathy ■ Proximal motor neuropathy (diabetic amyotrophy) ■ Thoracic or lumbar radiculopathies ■ Focal limb neuropathies (entrapment neuropathies)

Symptoms alone have relatively poor diagnostic accuracy in predicting the presence of DSP, but signs are better predictors than symptoms. Moreover, the presence of a single abnormality is less sensitive for its diagnosis than multiple abnormalities. The combination of neuropathic symptoms, signs, and electrodiagnostic findings provides the most accurate diagnosis of this type of peripheral neuropathy (England 2005).

SYMPTOMS OF PERIPHERAL NEUROPATHY

Sensory symptoms. Sensory symptoms associated with peripheral neuropathy may be negative or positive, diffuse or focal. Negative sensory symptoms include feelings of numbness or deadness (like wearing gloves or socks). Loss of balance, especially with eyes closed, and painless injuries due to loss of sensation are common. Positive symptoms may be described as burning, prickling pain, tingling, electric shock–like feelings, aching, tightness, or hypersensitivity to touch (Ametov 2003, Pittenger 2005, Casellini 2007).

Motor symptoms. Motor changes may include distal, proximal, or more focal weakness. In upper extremities, distal symptoms may include impaired fine hand coordination and difficulty with tasks (e.g., opening jars or turning keys). Early symptoms of foot weakness include foot slapping, toe scuffing, or frequent tripping, whereas proximal limb weakness may result in difficulty climbing and descending stairs, getting up from a seated or supine position, and raising the arms above the shoulders, as well as more frequent falls (due to the knees giving way). In DSP, minor weakness of the toes and feet is possible, but severe weakness is unlikely, although possible, in asymmetrical neuropathies. Motor neuropathy may occur along with sensory neuropathy, resulting in sensorimotor neuropathy (Ametov 2003, Balducci 2006).

DETECTION OF PERIPHERAL NEUROPATHY

Testing for peripheral neuropathy begins with an assessment of gross light touch and pinprick sensation (Table 18.2). The first clinical sign that usually develops in DSP is a decrease in or loss of vibratory and pinprick sensation over the toes. As it progresses, decreased sensation may move upward into the legs and then from the hands into the arms, a pattern often referred to as "stocking and glove" sensory loss. Severely affected patients may lose sensation in a "shield" distribution on the chest. The inability to perceive the tuning fork (vibration) or the monofilament (light touch test) identifies individuals with a 60% risk of developing a foot ulcer in the next 3 years (Pham 2000).

TREATMENT OF PERIPHERAL NEUROPATHY

Pharmacological treatment. Successful treatment of diabetic neuropathy requires addressing the underlying pathogenic mechanisms, treating symptoms to improve quality of life, and preventing progression and complications of diabetes. Pharmacological agents with proven efficacy for painful peripheral neuropathies include the tricyclic antidepressants, the selective serotonin and noradrenaline reuptake

Table 18.2 Tests for Peripheral Neuropathy

- **Vibration (Tuning Fork)**
  Test vibratory sense in the feet with a 128 Hz tuning fork placed at the base of the great toenail.
- **Monofilament (Light Touch) Sensation**
  Test protective sensation with 10 g monofilament, briefly applying the tip perpendicular to the plantar surface of the foot, using sufficient force to buckle the monofilament.
- **Deep Tendon Reflexes**
  With neuropathy, commonly hypoactive or absent. Perform strength testing and examine for distal intrinsic extremity muscle atrophy, since weakness of small foot muscles may develop; also check dorsal pedal and posterior tibial pulses.
- **Skin Examination**
  Examine the skin for dryness, tinea pedis, cracks, onychomycoses, acute erythema and tenderness, and fluctuance under calluses.
- **Tinel Test**
  Tap the volar aspect of the wrist. Tingling, paresthesia, or pain in the area of the thumb, index finger, middle finger, and radial one-half of the ring finger suggests compression of the median nerve in the carpal tunnel, carpal tunnel syndrome, or median nerve injury.
- **Cranial Nerve Test**
  Walk on the heels and toes; heel-toe walking tests not only distal lower-extremity strength but balance as well.

inhibitors, anticonvulsants, opiates, membrane stabilizers, α-lipoic acid, and topical agents including capsaicin, although most of these are not approved by the U.S. Food and Drug Administration for use in the treatment of neuropathy (Tesfaye 2011). Pregabalin recently has been established as effective for relief of pain (Bril 2011), along with duloxetine hydrochloride (Casellini 2007).

Treatment with supplements. The development of peripheral neuropathy may be affected by micronutrient status. Long-term metformin use may cause vitamin B12 deficiencies, which can result in symptoms of peripheral nerve damage (Pongchaidecha 2004, Pflipsen 2009, Farvid 2011, Mizukami 2011, Solomon 2011, Reinstatler 2012). Two individuals with isolated sensory axonal neuropathy secondary to vitamin B12 deficiency had complete recovery of nerve function after cyanocobalamin replacement. In another study, among adults with T2D, 22% exhibited a vitamin B12 deficiency from metformin use (Pflipsen 2009). Thus, testing levels of serum vitamin B12 and its metabolites should be done in the case of any distal symmetric neuropathy (Torre 2012).

Supplementation with other micronutrients may ameliorate its symptoms (Farvid 2011), particularly intake of vitamins B_1, B_6, B_{12}, folate, and biotin (Pongchaidecha 2004, Farvid 2011, Solomon 2011). Vitamin D deficiency is an independent risk factor for diabetic peripheral neuropathy, and its supplementation may prevent or delay the onset (Shehab 2012). In fact, lack of adequate levels of vitamin D is associated with self-reported peripheral neuropathy symptoms even after adjusting for obesity, comorbidities, use of medications for neuropathy, and diabetes duration and level of control (Soderstrom 2012). Vitamin D deficiency is an independent risk factor for diabetic peripheral neuropathy, and its supplementation could prevent or delay neuropathy onset (Shehab 2012). Finally, strong antioxidants, such as α-lipoic acid, have been shown to improve nerve blood flow, reduce oxidative stress, and improve distal nerve conduction in individuals with diabetic neuropathy (Nagamatsu 1995, Ziegler 1997, Ametov 2003, Sena 2007, Papanas 2012). When intravenous racemic α-lipoic acid was used in one study, it rapidly led to improvements in sensory symptoms that were attributed to a reduction in nerve pathophysiology. Thus, this supplement appears to be a useful ancillary treatment for the symptoms of diabetic polyneuropathy (Ametov 2003).

LOWER-LIMB ULCERS

PREVENTION AND DETECTION

The loss of sensation in the feet predisposes individuals to the development of foot ulcers and gangrene without proper care of the feet (Abbott 1998). Peripheral nerve damage blunts the usual symptoms of pain resulting from high impact on feet or friction and pressure from footwear, making it easy to develop a blister or sore on the feet without being aware of it. In some cases, a simple blister can progress to a full-blown infected abscess or ulcer and ultimately result in a lower-limb amputation if not properly cared for in a timely manner (Hunt 2009).

Substantial evidence supports screening all patients with diabetes to identify those at risk for foot ulceration. Prevention of diabetic foot ulcers begins with screening for loss of protective sensation, which is best accomplished using a monofilament touch test. In addition, health-care providers may quantify neuropathy with biothesiometry, measure plantar foot pressure, and assess lower-extremity vascular status with Doppler ultrasound and ankle–brachial blood pressure indices (Hunt 2009). These measurements, along with the medical history and physical examination, enable clinicians to stratify individuals by risk and determine the best intervention.

Peripheral vascular disease and peripheral neuropathy together with lack of foot self-examination, poor glycemic control, and anemia are main significant risk factors for diabetic foot ulceration (Hokkam 2009). Thus, individuals should be educated about proper foot care and the need for periodic foot examinations to prevent ulceration or to catch it early. Other effective interventions include optimizing glycemic control, smoking cessation, intensive podiatric care, debridement of calluses, and certain types of prophylactic foot surgery (Singh 2005, Hunt 2009).

TREATMENT

Because it is impractical and unnecessary to ask individuals not to weight-bear at all (Lemaster 2008), relief of plantar pressure through the use of offloading casting devices remains the mainstay for management of unhealed neuropathic ulcers, and providing appropriate footwear is essential in ulcer prevention. Simple nonsurgical debridement and application of hydrogels are both effective in preparing the ulceration for healthy granulation and, therefore, enhancing healing. Initial antibiotic therapy for infected ulcers should cover the most common bacterial flora. Limited evidence supports the use of adjunctive therapies, such as hyperbaric oxygen and cytokines or growth factors. In selected cases, recombinant human platelet–derived growth factor has been shown to enhance healing; however, its widespread use cannot be advised because of the availability of more cost-effective approaches. Overall, the best management of foot ulcers is achieved by what is taken out of the foot (such as pressure, callus, infection, and slough) rather than what is put on the foot (adjuvant treatment) (Hunt 2009, Ndip 2012).

FOOTWEAR

In general, individuals should use silica gel or air midsoles in their shoes along with polyester or polyester-blend (cotton-polyester) socks to prevent the formation of blisters and to keep feet dry during physical activities (Colberg 2010). To promote effective ulcer healing, plantar pressures can be reduced with casts, walkers, and therapeutic footwear (Bus 2008a, 2008b). Individuals with neuropathy and foot deformity commonly are prescribed with custom footwear, in particular after ulcer healing. The goal of this footwear is to redistribute and reduce plantar foot pressures and to prevent ulcer recurrence (Bus 2008a, 2008b). Careful attention to foot care by health-care professionals may be more important than therapeutic footwear, but special footwear is likely beneficial in people with diabetes who do not receive such close attention to foot care and in anyone with severe foot deformities (Reiber 2002).

AMPUTATIONS

CAUSE OF AMPUTATIONS

Foot infections cause substantial morbidity and frequent visits to health-care professionals and may lead to amputation of a lower extremity (Lipsky 2006). For people with diabetes, elevated blood glucose levels adversely affect the ability to heal. Slow-healing wounds invite hard-to-treat infections that eventually can lead to amputation. In fact, individuals with diabetes are 15 times more likely to undergo limb amputations than those without diabetes. In one study, individuals with diabetes who underwent amputations were more commonly affected by foot infections and kidney disorders. Women with diabetes were 10 years older than men when amputated, and men underwent more multiple amputations and had more foot infections than women. Of all diabetes-related amputations, however, 88% were preceded by foot ulcers (Alvarsson 2012).

PROSTHESIS USE

With a prosthetic limb after amputation, younger individuals may progress more quickly in gait training and walk more than older individuals. The extent of walking in most amputees is compared with the minimal levels required for them to function in different living environments. At the time of discharge from the inpatient gait-training program, however, older unilateral amputees and transfemoral amputees in one study were not able to walk the 600 steps a day necessary to manage with a moderate level of support in a one-level apartment or home (Holden 1987). Others have reported that mobility rates 1 year after prosthetic provision for unilateral transtibial and transfemoral amputees worsen with increasing age at amputation and a higher level of amputation (up the leg) (Davies 2003). In above-knee amputees, good stump quality is one of the major determinants of mobility outcome. Efforts should be made to minimize stump complications. In particular, incorrect positioning of the stump, which is responsible for hip flexor retraction, should be avoided after surgery (Traballesi 2007).

PHYSICAL ACTIVITY PARTICIPATION WITH PERIPHERAL NEUROPATHY, ULCERS, OR AMPUTATION

Mild to moderate exercise may help prevent the onset of peripheral neuropathy (Balducci 2006). At least one small study has shown that 10 weeks of supervised aerobic and strengthening exercise training improves neuropathic and cutaneous nerve fiber branching undertaken by adults with T2D and peripheral neuropathy (Kluding 2012). Although physical activity likely cannot fully reverse the symptoms of peripheral neuropathy, it can prevent further loss of muscle strength and flexibility commonly experienced by individuals with DSP. Peripheral neuropathy, with the associated decrease in sensation, carries with it an increased risk of injury, along with greater discomfort associated with painful types of neuropathy during physical activity. The individual with insensate feet may not have the pain sensation needed to recognize that an injury has occurred, and a blister or repeated trauma may go unnoticed.

DAILY FOOT CARE

Engaging in physical activity with peripheral issues, however, does increase the risk of foot problems like ulcers. Comprehensive foot care, including daily inspection of feet and use of proper footwear, is recommended for prevention and early detection of sores or ulcers (Singh 2005, Hunt 2009). All individuals should closely examine their feet on a daily basis (or have someone else inspect them) to detect sores or ulcers early and should follow recommendations for the use of proper footwear and appropriate socks (synthetic-cotton blends that keep feet drier) (Reiber 2002).

RISK OF ULCERATION (OR REULCERATION) WITH WEIGHT-BEARING ACTIVITY

Individuals without acute foot ulcers can undertake moderate weight-bearing exercise, although anyone with a foot injury or open sore or ulcer should be restricted to non–weight-bearing physical activity until the ulceration has fully healed. Prior guidelines stated that people with severe peripheral neuropathy should avoid weight-bearing activities to reduce the risk of foot ulcerations (Graham 1990). Moderate walking, however, does not appear to increase the risk of foot ulcers or reulceration in individuals with peripheral neuropathy and fully healed or no ulcerations (Lemaster 2003, 2008). In fact, over a 12-month period, promoting weight-bearing activity in individuals with T2D did not lead to any increase in foot ulcers. In another study, individuals with T2D and peripheral neuropathy participated in walking on a treadmill, balance exercises, and strengthening exercises for the lower extremities using body-weight resistance. Close monitoring of the plantar surface of the feet indicated that the exercise program was well tolerated with no adverse events (Tuttle 2012). Thus, weight-bearing activity can be considered following adequate assessment and counseling of patients with peripheral neuropathy (Lemaster 2008). Of note, a study also demonstrated the effectiveness of 6 months of weekly tai chi training in improving plantar sensation and balance in elderly adults and elderly adults with diabetes with a large plantar sensation loss (Richerson 2007).

GAIT ALTERATIONS

With peripheral neuropathy, sensations connected to balance and strength can be diminished. Gait can be altered, contributing to the development of orthopedic issues and a greater risk of falling. Individuals may become fearful of falling and avoid physical activity. Walking, standing, or getting out of a chair can be difficult. Furthermore, diabetes may affect gait mechanics even before the onset of peripheral neuropathy and other associated threats to mobility. By way of example, individuals with diabetes have a shorter stride length for fast walking and a longer percentage of the gait cycle with the knee in first flexion for both fast and usual walking, even without diagnosed peripheral neuropathy. They exhibit a smaller hip range of motion in the sagittal plane during usual walking, and during fast walking, they use lower ankle and higher knee generative mechanical work expenditure compared with controls (Ko 2011). These findings suggest that even individuals with T2D without overt peripheral neuropathy exhibit altered and less efficient gait patterns that are more apparent during walking at a maximum speed.

Additionally, walking capacity and performance decrease with the progression of foot complications. Although walking is recommended to improve fitness, it cannot be prescribed in isolation considering the increased risk of plantar injury. Walking exercise should be supplemented by partial or non–weight-bearing exercises to improve physical fitness in populations with diabetes who have, or are at high risk of developing peripheral neuropathy (Table 18.3) (Kanade 2006). In all cases, safety must be the prime consideration of the exercise prescription.

Table 18.3 Exercise Recommendations for Peripheral Neuropathy

- Daily range-of-motion exercises to help minimize shortening of connective tissue
- Individuals without acute foot ulcers can engage in mild or moderate weight-bearing exercise, although low-impact activities like cycling, swimming, and aquatic and chair exercise are viable options as well
- Individuals with a foot injury or open sore should avoid or limit weight-bearing activities because of an increased chance of soft tissue and joint injury
- Individuals should wear proper footwear and inspect their feet after physical activity to prevent blisters and detect injuries
- Avoid jogging because it places a threefold increase in pressure on the foot compared with walking
- Chair exercises for individuals with limited mobility to improve flexibility and strength

SPORTS PARTICIPATION BY AMPUTEES

In general, sports participation is associated with a beneficial effect on the cardiopulmonary system, psychological well-being, social reintegration, and physical functioning in amputees as well. Younger individuals with unilateral transtibial amputations achieve better athletic performance and encounter fewer problems when participating in sports compared with older individuals with bilateral transfemoral amputations (Bragaru 2011). Regardless of their amputation level, individuals with limb amputations can participate in a wide range of recreational activities. Sport prosthetic devices are used mostly by competitive athletes. Individuals with limb amputations, however, appear to benefit both physically and psychologically from participation in sports or regular physical activity. Therefore, sports should be included in rehabilitation programs, and individuals with limb amputations should be encouraged to pursue a physically active life (Bragaru 2011). Proper stump care, however, is critical to being able to continue physical activity and to preventing additional problems related to possible stump skin infection or debridement (Traballesi 2007).

Table 18.4 Additional Physical Activity Considerations with Peripheral Neuropathy

Safety Concerns	Actions
Discomfort or pain with physical activity	■ Limit weight-bearing options based on level of tolerance ■ Engage in more non–weight-bearing activities
Foot injury, infection, or ulceration	■ Monitor feet daily for blisters, cuts, scrapes ■ Use proper hygiene for foot and skin care ■ Choose appropriate footwear (shoes and socks) ■ Consider the need for orthotics or orthopedic shoes
Use of a prosthetic device (post–lower-limb amputation)	■ Check the stump every day for redness, blisters, soreness, or swelling (and treat promptly) ■ Clean the inside of the stump socket daily and dry it well before using replacing it on the stump

Case in Point: Wrap-Up

When NP starts doing more planned physical activity, he will need to worry about prevention of injury to his insensate feet. He states that he mostly likes to walk, but his health-care provider advises him that he should consider engaging in a variety of activities, including some that are not weight-bearing, to limit his risk for foot trauma and subsequent ulceration. He agrees to have his wife inspect his feet for him daily, or he will use a mirror to examine the plantar surfaces of his feet on his own.

Exercise Program Goals

Mode of Activity: Because of NP's peripheral neuropathy, he should consider engaging in a variety of activities from the start, including both weight-bearing and non–weight-bearing ones. Stationary cycling, walking on a treadmill or out-doors, and use of other conditioning machines that are lower impact (such as cross-trainers and elliptical machines) are all good choices for him (because he stated that he does not like aquatic activities). Seated activities are another option, both for aerobic and resistance training. Using resistance training machines is also less weight-bearing that using free weights and should be rec-ommended.

Intensity: Given that mild to moderate activity has been found to be safe for indi-viduals with DSP (which is what he has), NP should keep his workouts in the "somewhat hard" range to minimize the possibility for undetected trauma to his feet. On the conditioning machines, however, he can choose "interval" pro-grams that intersperse harder intervals with easier ones to gain more fitness. His initial target heart rate should be in the range of 111–118 bpm (40–50%, heart rate reserve, or HRR), with a later training goal of no more than 125 bpm (59% of HRR). For resistance work, his intensity should be similar, although he can do heavier lifting while seated on upper-body resistance machines without potentially affecting his feet.

Frequency: Ideally, NP should engage in at least 3–5 days of aerobic training weekly, and he should not let more than 2 days lapse between workout ses-sions to optimize his blood glucose and blood pressure control to help prevent additional peripheral (or other) nerve damage. Resistance training can be done 2 days a week to start, with a goal of 3 days eventually.

Duration: At the start of his training program, NP should engage in shorter bouts of exercise training, separated by a rest period, until he can train for 20–30 min continuously. His ultimate training goal is 150 min of physical activity spread throughout the week. On most training days, he can engage in longer durations of non–weight-bearing activity because those activities have a lesser potential for causing foot trauma.

Progression: With peripheral neuropathy as a concern, NP should primarily focus on increasing the duration of his structured workouts to achieve at least 150 min of moderate exercise spread throughout the week. His resistance train-ing should progress from 2 days/week to 3 days/week, and he may choose to add additional resistance exercises.

Possible Precautions: Walking is an appropriate weight-bearing activity for NP, but if he should develop an acute infection or ulcer on the plantar surface of his foot, he should avoid weight-bearing activities until it has fully healed. Daily inspections of his feet for signs of trauma are also critical, along with use of proper footwear and socks that keep his feet as dry as possible. His use of a sulfonylurea also increases his risk for exercise-associated hypoglycemia, so he should use self-monitoring and keep some readily absorbed carbohydrates with him during exercise.

The development of peripheral nerve damage is common in individuals with both T1D and T2D. The most common type, DSP, includes sensorimotor symptoms reflective of both small- and large-fiber damage. Having peripheral neuropathy increases the risk of developing an ulcer and having a lower limb amputation. With proper care and preventive measures, individuals with peripheral neuropathy can benefit from regular participation in mild to moderate aerobic and resistance activities.

PROFESSIONAL PRACTICE PEARLS

- Pain or loss of sensation in the feet or hands, known as peripheral neuropathy, is nerve damage that is common in individuals with T1D and T2D.
- Diabetic peripheral neuropathy is the presence of symptoms and/or signs of peripheral nerve dysfunction in people with diabetes after exclusion of other causes.
- Up to 40% of individuals with diabetes may experience peripheral neuropathy, and 60% of lower-extremity amputations are related to suboptimal glycemic control.
- The most common type of diabetic neuropathy, DSP, typically involves both small and large nerve fibers.
- Small-fiber neuropathy often begins painfully and frequently leads to foot ulceration, subsequent gangrene, and lower-extremity amputations.
- Large-nerve fiber neuropathy generally results in numbness in the feet and hands and ataxia, impairing activities of daily living and causing possible falls and fractures.
- Sensory symptoms due to peripheral neuropathy may be negative or positive, diffuse or focal, whereas motor changes may include distal, proximal, or more focal weakness.
- The first clinical sign that usually develops in DSP is a decrease in or loss of vibratory and pinprick sensation around the big toe.
- Decreased sensation may move upward into the legs and then from the hands into the arms, a pattern often referred to as "stocking and glove" sensory loss.
- The inability to perceive vibration or light touch identifies individuals with a 60% risk of developing a foot ulcer in the next 3 years.
- Treatment for peripheral neuropathy includes both pharmacological and supplement interventions (like B vitamins, vitamin D, and α-lipoic acid).
- The loss of sensation in the feet predisposes individuals to development of foot ulcers and gangrene and the need for lower-limb amputation without proper care of the feet.
- Individuals with diabetes are 15 times more likely to undergo limb amputations than those without diabetes.
- Comprehensive foot care, including daily inspection of feet and use of proper footwear, is recommended for prevention and early detection of sores or ulcers.

- Individuals without acute foot ulcers can undertake moderate weight-bearing exercise, and moderate walking does not increase the risk of foot ulcers or reulceration.
- Anyone with a foot injury or open sore or ulcer should be restricted to non–weight-bearing physical activity until the ulceration has fully healed.
- Gait can be altered by the presence of peripheral neuropathy, contributing to development of orthopedic issues and a greater risk of falling.
- Walking exercise should be supplemented by partial or non–weight-bearing exercises to improve physical fitness in diabetic populations with peripheral neuropathy.
- Using a prosthetic device, individuals with limb amputations can participate in a wide range of recreational activities.

REFERENCES

Abbott CA, Vileikyte L, Williamson S, Carrington AL, Boulton AJ: Multicenter study of the incidence of and predictive risk factors for diabetic neuropathic foot ulceration. *Diabetes Care* 21:1071–1075, 1998

Alvarsson A, Sandgren B, Wendel C, Alvarsson M, Brismar K: A retrospective analysis of amputation rates in diabetic patients: can lower extremity amputations be further prevented? *Cardiovasc Diabetol* 11:18, 2012

Ametov AS, Barinov A, Dyck PJ, Hermann R, Kozlova N, Litchy WJ, Low PA, Nehrdich D, Novosadova M, O'Brien PC, Reljanovic M, Samigullin R, Schuette K, Strokov I, Tritschler HJ, Wessel K, Yakhno N, Ziegler D, Sydney Trial Study Group: The sensory symptoms of diabetic polyneuropathy are improved with alpha-lipoic acid: the SYDNEY trial. *Diabetes Care* 26:770–776, 2003

Balducci S, Iacobellis G, Parisi L, Di Biase N, Calandriello E, Leonetti F, Fallucca F: Exercise training can modify the natural history of diabetic peripheral neuropathy. *J Diabetes Complications* 20:216–223, 2006

Bragaru M, Dekker R, Geertzen JH, Dijkstra PU: Amputees and sports: a systematic review. *Sports Med* 41:721–740, 2011

Bril V, England JD, Franklin GM, Backonja M, Cohen JA, Del Toro DR, Feldman EL, Iverson DJ, Perkins B, Russell JW, Zochodne DW, American Academy of Neurology, American Asociation of Neuromuscular and Electrodiagnostic Medicine, American Academy of Physical and Rehabilitation Medicine: Evidence-based guideline: treatment of painful diabetic neuropathy—report of the American Association of Neuromuscular and Electrodiagnostic Medicine, the American Academy of Neurology, and the American Academy of Physical Medicine and Rehabilitation. *Muscle Nerve* 43:910–917, 2011

Bus SA: Foot structure and footwear prescription in diabetes mellitus. *Diabetes Metab Res Rev* 24 (Suppl. 1):S90–S95, 2008a

Bus SA, Valk GD, van Deursen RW, Armstrong DG, Caravaggi C, Hlavacek P, Bakker K, Cavanagh PR: The effectiveness of footwear and offloading interventions to prevent and heal foot ulcers and reduce plantar pressure in diabetes: a systematic review. *Diabetes Metab Res Rev* 24 (Suppl. 1):S162–S180, 2008b

Callaghan BC, Little AA, Feldman EL, Hughes RA: Enhanced glucose control for preventing and treating diabetic neuropathy. *Cochrane Database Syst Rev* 6:CD007543, 2012

Casellini CM, Vinik AI: Clinical manifestations and current treatment options for diabetic neuropathies. *Endocr Pract* 13:550–566, 2007

Coccheri S: Approaches to prevention of cardiovascular complications and events in diabetes mellitus. *Drugs* 67:997–1026, 2007

Colberg SR, Sigal RJ, Fernhall B, Regensteiner JG, Blissmer BJ, Rubin RR, Chasan-Taber L, Albright AL, Braun B, American College of Sports Medicine, American Diabetes Association: Exercise and type 2 diabetes: the American College of Sports Medicine and the American Diabetes Association: joint position statement. *Diabetes Care* 33:e147–e167, 2010

Craig ME, Duffin AC, Gallego PH, Lam A, Cusumano J, Hing S, Donaghue KC: Plantar fascia thickness, a measure of tissue glycation, predicts the development of complications in adolescents with type 1 diabetes. *Diabetes Care* 31:1201–1206, 2008

Davies B, Datta D: Mobility outcome following unilateral lower limb amputation. *Prosthet Orthot Int* 27:186–190, 2003

England JD, Gronseth GS, Franklin G, Miller RG, Asbury AK, Carter GT, Cohen JA, Fisher MA, Howard JF, Kinsella LJ, Latov N, Lewis RA, Low PA, Sumner AJ, American Academy of Neurology, American Association of Electrodiagnostic Medicine, American Academy of Physical Medicine and Rehabilitation: Distal symmetric polyneuropathy: a definition for clinical research: report of the American Academy of Neurology, the American Association of Electrodiagnostic Medicine, and the American Academy of Physical Medicine and Rehabilitation. *Neurology* 64:199–207, 2005

Farvid MS, Homayouni F, Amiri Z, Adelmanesh F: Improving neuropathy scores in type 2 diabetic patients using micronutrients supplementation. *Diabetes Res Clin Pract* 93:86–94, 2011

Graham C, Lasko-McCarthey P: Exercise options for persons with diabetic complications. *Diabetes Educ* 16:212–320, 1990

Hokkam EN: Assessment of risk factors in diabetic foot ulceration and their impact on the outcome of the disease. *Prim Care Diabetes* 3:219–224, 2009

Holden JM, Fernie GR: Extent of artificial limb use following rehabilitation. *J Orthop Res* 5:562–568, 1987

Hunt D: Diabetes: foot ulcers and amputations. *Clin Evid (Online)* pii: 0602 12 Jan 2009

Kanade RV, van Deursen RW, Harding K, Price P: Walking performance in people with diabetic neuropathy: benefits and threats. *Diabetologia* 49:1747–1754, 2006

Kluding PM, Pasnoor M, Singh R, Jernigan S, Farmer K, Rucker J, Sharma NK, Wright DE: The effect of exercise on neuropathic symptoms, nerve function, and cutaneous innervation in people with diabetic peripheral neuropathy. *J Diabetes Complications* 26:424–429, 2012

Ko SU, Stenholm S, Chia CW, Simonsick EM, Ferrucci L: Gait pattern alterations in older adults associated with type 2 diabetes in the absence of peripheral neuropathy—results from the Baltimore Longitudinal Study of Aging. *Gait Posture* 34:548–552, 2011

Lemaster JW, Mueller MJ, Reiber GE, Mehr DR, Madsen RW, Conn VS: Effect of weight-bearing activity on foot ulcer incidence in people with diabetic peripheral neuropathy: feet first randomized controlled trial. *Phys Ther* 88:1385–1398, 2008

Lemaster JW, Reiber GE, Smith DG, Heagerty PJ, Wallace C: Daily weight-bearing activity does not increase the risk of diabetic foot ulcers. *Med Sci Sports Exerc* 35:1093–1099, 2003

Lipsky BA, Berendt AR, Deery HG, Embil JM, Joseph WS, Karchmer AW, LeFrock JL, Lew DP, Mader JT, Norden C, Tan JS, Infectious Diseases Society of America: Diagnosis and treatment of diabetic foot infections. *Plast Reconstr Surg* 117 (7 Suppl.):212S–238S, 2006

Lozeron P, Nahum L, Lacroix C, Ropert A, Guglielmi JM, Said G: Symptomatic diabetic and non-diabetic neuropathies in a series of 100 diabetic patients. *J Neurol* 249:569–575, 2002

Mizukami H, Ogasawara S, Yamagishi S, Takahashi K, Yagihashi S: Methylcobalamin effects on diabetic neuropathy and nerve protein kinase C in rats. *Eur J Clin Invest* 41:442–450, 2011

Mondelli M, Aretini A, Baldasseroni A: Distal symmetric polyneuropathy in diabetes. Differences between patients with and without neuropathic pain. *Exp Clin Endocrinol Diabetes* 120:45–50, 2012

Nagamatsu M, Nickander KK, Schmelzer JD, Raya A, Wittrock DA, Tritschler H, Low PA: Lipoic acid improves nerve blood flow, reduces oxidative stress, and improves distal nerve conduction in experimental diabetic neuropathy. *Diabetes Care* 18:1160–1167, 1995

Narayan KM, Boyle JP, Geiss LS, Saaddine JB, Thompson TJ: Impact of recent increase in incidence on future diabetes burden: U.S., 2005–2050. *Diabetes Care* 29:2114–2116, 2006

Ndip A, Ebah L, Mbako A: Neuropathic diabetic foot ulcers—evidence-to-practice. *Int J Gen Med* 5:129–134, 2012

Papanas N, Maltezos E: Alpha-lipoic acid, diabetic neuropathy, and Nathan's prophecy. *Angiology* 63:81–83, 2012

Pflipsen MC, Oh RC, Saguil A, Seehusen DA, Seaquist D, Topolski R: The prevalence of vitamin B(12) deficiency in patients with type 2 diabetes: a cross-sectional study. *J Am Board Fam Med* 22:528–534, 2009

Pham H, Armstrong DG, Harvey C, Harkless LB, Giurini JM, Veves A: Screening techniques to identify people at high risk for diabetic foot ulceration: a prospective multicenter trial. *Diabetes Care* 23:606–611, 2000

Pittenger GL, Mehrabyan A, Simmons K, Amandarice, Dublin C, Barlow P, Vinik AI: Small fiber neuropathy is associated with the metabolic syndrome. *Metab Syndr Relat Disord* 3:113–121, 2005

Pongchaidecha M, Srikusalanukul V, Chattananon A, Tanjariyaporn S: Effect of metformin on plasma homocysteine, vitamin B12 and folic acid: a cross-sectional study in patients with type 2 diabetes mellitus. *J Med Assoc Thai* 87:780–787, 2004

Reiber GE, Smith DG, Wallace C, Sullivan K, Hayes S, Vath C, Maciejewski ML, Yu O, Heagerty PJ, LeMaster J: Effect of therapeutic footwear on foot reulceration in patients with diabetes: a randomized controlled trial. *JAMA* 287:2552–2558, 2002

Reinstatler L, Qi YP, Williamson RS, Garn JV, Oakley GP Jr: Association of biochemical B deficiency with metformin therapy and vitamin B supplements: the National Health and Nutrition Examination Survey, 1999–2006. *Diabetes Care* 35:327–333, 2012

Richerson S, Rosendale: Does tai chi improve plantar sensory ability? A pilot study. *Diabetes Technol Ther* 9:276–286, 2007

Sena CM, Nunes E, Louro T, Proenca T, Seica RM: Endothelial dysfunction in type 2 diabetes: effect of antioxidants. *Rev Port Cardiol* 26:609–619, 2007

Shehab D, Al-Jarallah K, Mojiminiyi OA, Al Mohamedy H, Abdella NA: Does vitamin D deficiency play a role in peripheral neuropathy in type 2 diabetes? *Diabet Med* 29:43–49, 2012

Singh N, Armstrong DG, Lipsky BA: Preventing foot ulcers in patients with diabetes. *JAMA* 293:217–228, 2005

Singleton JR, Smith AG, Russell JW, Feldman EL: Microvascular complications of impaired glucose tolerance. *Diabetes* 52:2867–2873, 2003

Smith AG, Singleton JR: Impaired glucose tolerance and neuropathy. *Neurologist* 14:23–29, 2008

Soderstrom LH, Johnson SP, Diaz VA, Mainous AG III: Association between vitamin D and diabetic neuropathy in a nationally representative sample: results from 2001–2004 NHANES. *Diabet Med* 29:50–55, 2012

Solomon LR: Diabetes as a cause of clinically significant functional cobalamin deficiency. *Diabetes Care* 34:1077–1080, 2011

Tesfaye S, Vileikyte L, Rayman G, Sindrup S, Perkins B, Baconja M, Vinik A, Boulton A, on Behalf of the Toronto Expert Panel on Diabetic Neuropathy:

Painful diabetic peripheral neuropathy: consensus recommendations on diagnosis, assessment and management. *Diabetes Metab Res Rev* [epub ahead of print] 21 Jun 2011

Torre CD, Lucchetta M, Cacciavillani M, Campagnolo M, Manara R, Briani C: Reversible isolated sensory axonal neuropathy due to cobalamin deficiency. *Muscle Nerve* 45:428–430, 2012

Traballesi M, Porcacchia P, Averna T, Angioni C, Lubich S, Di Meo F, Brunelli S: Prognostic factors in prosthetic rehabilitation of bilateral dysvascular above-knee amputee: is the stump condition an influencing factor? *Eura Medicophys* 43:1–6, 2007

Tuttle LJ, Hastings MK, Mueller MJ: A moderate-intensity weight-bearing exercise program for a person with type 2 diabetes and peripheral neuropathy. *Phys Ther* 92:133–141, 2012

U.S. Department of Health and Human Services, Centers for Disease Control and Prevention: National diabetes fact sheet: national estimates and general information on diabetes and prediabetes in the United States, 2011, edited by Centers for Disease Control and Prevention. Atlanta, GA, U.S. Department of Health and Human Services, 2011

Vinik AI, Freeman R, Erbas T: Diabetic autonomic neuropathy. *Semin Neurol* 23:365–372, 2003a

Vinik AI, Vinik E: Prevention of the complications of diabetes. *Am J Manag Care* 9 (3 Suppl.):S63–S80; quiz S81–S84, 2003b

Vinik AI, Ziegler D: Diabetic cardiovascular autonomic neuropathy. *Circulation* 115:387–397, 2007

Ziegler D, Schatz H, Conrad F, Gries FA, Ulrich H, Reichel G: Effects of treatment with the antioxidant alpha-lipoic acid on cardiac autonomic neuropathy in NIDDM patients. A 4-month randomized controlled multicenter trial (DEKAN Study). Deutsche Kardiale Autonome Neuropathie. *Diabetes Care* 20:369–373, 1997

Chapter 19
Autonomic Neuropathy

A utonomic and peripheral are the main types of diabetic neuropathy (Vinik 2003a, 2003b, 2007). Peripheral neuropathies are covered in chapter 18, and this chapter focuses on autonomic neuropathies. Diabetes-related damage to the central nervous system (autonomic neuropathy) can result in silent ischemia, hyperthermia, or lightheadedness with standing and during exercise.

In fact, severe autonomic neuropathy may make it difficult for an individual to change body position (e.g., going from sitting to standing or from lying to sitting) without experiencing orthostatic hypotension, which can result in dizziness or fainting (Purewal 1995, Maser 2005, Vinik 2011). Other exercise concerns are related to hyperthermia during physical activity, which is more common in autonomic neuropaths and can lead to severe dehydration, along with gastroparesis (a lesser ability to digest and absorb carbohydrates and food), which may increase the incidence and severity of hypoglycemia (Ma 2009, Parkman 2010). Last, the presence of autonomic neuropathy may cause an elevated heart rate at rest (e.g., >100 beats per minute [bpm] instead of the normal 72), as well as a lesser rise in heart rate during physical exertion (Vinik 2007, 2011). In spite of these possible consequences, physical activity can be undertaken safely when appropriate caution is used.

Case in Point: Exercise Management for an Adult with T2D and Autonomic Neuropathy

NA is an 82-year-old woman who has had type 2 diabetes (T2D) for 25 years. Although she has some loss of sensation in her feet (that started a few years ago), her bigger concern is that she easily gets dizzy when she stands up and walks around. On her last visit with her physician, she was diagnosed with orthostatic hypotension, a type of autonomic neuropathy caused by central nerve damage, and resting tachycardia. Due to her dizziness, she is rarely venturing outside her house these days and is leading a mostly sedentary lifestyle. She controls her diabetes with metformin and a daily injection of basal insulin (glargine), and she takes two blood pressure medications (a diuretic and another), a lipid-lowering agent, and an antiarrhythmic medication for chronic atrial fibrillation. So far, she has not been prescribed any medications to treat her orthostatic hypotension.

Resting Measurements

Height: 62 inches
Weight: 162 lb
BMI: 29.6 (high end of "overweight" category)
Heart rate: 102 bpm
Blood pressure: 155/88 mmHg (on medication)

Fasting Labs

Plasma glucose: 122 mg/dl (controlled with metformin and basal insulin)
A1C: 6.5%
Total cholesterol: 145 mg/dl (on medication)
Triglycerides: 122 mg/dl
High-density lipoprotein cholesterol: 38 mg/dl
Low-density lipoprotein cholesterol: 83 mg/dl

Questions to Consider

1. What type of physical activity would be safe for NA to do given her diagnosed autonomic neuropathy (orthostatic hypotension and resting tachycardia)?
2. Are any precautions needed for NA when she exercises?

(Continued on page 376.)

MANIFESTATIONS OF AUTONOMIC NEUROPATHY

Autonomic neuropathy broadly affects the involuntary functions of the body and may involve the cardiovascular, gastrointestinal, and genitourinary systems and the sweat glands (Table 19.1) (Vinik 2007). Individuals with generalized autonomic neuropathies may report ataxia, gait instability, or near syncope and syncope. In addition, autonomic neuropathies have further symptoms that relate specifically to the anatomic site of nerve damage (Casellini 2007, Parkman 2010).

Table 19.1 Typical Symptoms of Autonomic Neuropathy

Cardiac	Sinus tachycardia, orthostatic hypotension, sinus arrhythmia, decreased heart rate variability with deep breathing, and near syncope upon changing positions from recumbent to standing
Gastrointestinal	Dysphagia, abdominal pain, nausea and vomiting, malabsorption, fecal incontinence, diarrhea, and constipation
Bladder	Poor urinary stream, feeling of incomplete bladder emptying, and straining to void
Sudomotor	Heat intolerance, heavy sweating of head, neck, and trunk with anhidrosis of lower trunk and extremities, and gustatory sweating

Although some degree of autonomic involvement is present in most patients with distal symmetrical polyneuropathy (DSP), individuals may or may not be aware of autonomic problems, and pure autonomic neuropathy due to diabetes is rare. Manifestations of autonomic neuropathy, however, may include orthostatic hypotension, resting tachycardia, loss of normal sinus arrhythmia ratio, anhidrosis (lack of normal sweating), bowel or bladder dysfunction, and small pupils sluggishly reactive to light, among other symptoms (Casellini 2007, Vinik 2007, Parkman 2010).

Some forms of autonomic dysfunction with the greatest impact on the ability to engage in physical activity are discussed in the sections that follow, that is, cardiac autonomic neuropathy (CAN), orthostatic hypotension, and gastroparesis. Although heat intolerance and dehydration are also potential exercise concerns, they are not discussed separately.

CARDIAC AUTONOMIC NEUROPATHY

When neuropathy affects the innervation of the heart, it is referred to as CAN, and its presence is linked with poor prognosis and premature mortality (Vinik 2007). Although only a quarter of people with diabetes have CAN, most exhibit some alterations in autonomic function, and incidence increases up to as high as 65% with advancing age and diabetes duration (Ziegler 1992).

Defined by abnormalities of the parasympathetic (PNS) and sympathetic nervous systems (SNS), vagal (PNS) dysfunction usually occurs earlier, although dysfunction of both can be present. The presence of CAN doubles mortality risk and results in a greater frequency of silent myocardial ischemia (Vinik 2007), orthostatic hypotension, or resting tachycardia (Low 1975, Ewing 1986). The importance of recognizing autonomic dysfunction as a predictor of morbidity and mortality with intensification of treatment suggests that all individuals with T2D at onset and those with type 1 diabetes (T1D) after 5 years should be screened for autonomic imbalance (Vinik 2012).

A small set of variables, including glycemic control (A1C), hypertension, DSP, and retinopathy, have been shown to predict the risk of CAN in individuals with T1D (Witte 2005). In addition, cardiac autonomic imbalance and inflammation occur early in diabetes and are interrelated as this imbalance correlates with the adipose tissue-derived inflammation seen early in T2D (Lieb 2012). Clinical features of CAN include silent ischemia (ST depression) and infarction (Q waves), tachycardia at rest and early in exercise, reduced maximal heart rate and exercise intolerance, exercise-induced hypotension after strenuous activity, thermoregulatory dysfunction, a tendency to dehydrate, and reduced heart rate variability, which is due to a shift in cardiac autonomic balance toward SNS dominance (Vinik 2011).

Detection. Screening for CAN should include a battery of autonomic tests (including heart rate variability) that evaluate both branches of the autonomic nervous system (ANS), as shown in Table 19.2. Analysis of heart rate variability is a noninvasive method using electrocardiogram (ECG) to assess overall autonomic activity, along with a prolonged QTc interval (i.e., the QT interval on the ECG corrected for heart rate) and postural hypotension (Khoharo 2012). Combined with respiratory activity, it independently and simultaneously measures PNS and SNS activity and defines autonomic balance, which involves complex interactions and mechanisms that maintain heart rate and blood pressure. Others have found that reduced postexercise heart rate variability with an exaggerated exercise blood pressure response suggest preclinical autonomic dysfunction characterized by impaired vagal modulation (Weston 2012).

Autonomic dysfunction is characterized by heightened activity of the SNS, suppressed activity of the PNS, and an impaired ability of the ANS to regulate the cardiovascular system (Vinik 2011). Reduced heart rate variability has dire consequences in terms of morbidity and mortality, independent of cardiovascular risk factors (Maser 2005), and it also predicts coronary artery calcium progression in adults with T1D, suggesting that autonomic neuropathy may be associated with atherosclerosis (Rodrigues 2010).

Treatment. Once CAN has been diagnosed, health-care providers may consider altering prescribed exercise, increasing surveillance for cardiac ischemia, carefully

Table 19.2 Noninvasive Tests for Autonomic Neuropathy

- Heart rate response to deep breathing (heart rate variability)
  - ☐ To perform this test, an individual lies quietly and breathes at a rate of six breaths per minute to elicit maximum variation in heart rate
  - ☐ An abnormal expiration-to-inspiration ratio based on age norms indicates PNS dysfunction
  - ☐ Beat-to-beat heart rate variation measured during deep breathing is indicative of PNS innervation only
- Heart rate response to standing
  - ☐ For this test, an individual is connected to ECG while lying down before going to a full, upright standing position
  - ☐ In healthy individuals, heart rate increases are maximal by the 15th beat after standing, followed by a relative slowing of heart rate by the 30th beat, whereas in individuals with autonomic neuropathy only a gradual increase in heart rate occurs
  - ☐ ECG tracings are used to determine the 30:15 ratio, which compares the longest R-R interval (at 30 beats) to the shortest (at 15 beats)
  - ☐ Tests cardiovascular response to going from a horizontal position to a vertical one, which elicits both PNS withdrawal and SNS activation
- Valsalva maneuver
  - ☐ To do this maneuver, an individual tries to forcibly exhale while keeping the mouth and nose closed for 15 sec
  - ☐ Those with autonomic issues may have a blunted heart rate response and a slow recovery from strain
  - ☐ ECG tracings are used to calculate the ratio of the longest R-R interval after the maneuver (bradycardia from blood pressure overshoot) to the shortest interval during it (tachycardia)
  - ☐ Influenced by alternating PNS and SNS control that elicits tachycardia and peripheral vasoconstriction during strain, followed by a reflex overshoot in blood pressure and bradycardia after its release
- Systolic blood pressure response to standing
  - ☐ This test can be completed during testing of heart rate response to standing with concomitant blood pressure monitoring

reexamining the list of medications, and aggressively treating cardiovascular risk factors (e.g., hypertension) that may be associated with the development of CAN (Maser 2005). Tighter glycemic control, possible supplementation with antioxidants like α-lipoic acid, use of select medications (e.g., angiotensin converting enzyme inhibitors, angiotensin type 1 receptor blockers, aldosterone blockers, calcium channel blockers, β-blockers, and metformin, among others), and strict management of hypertension are all possible treatments to assist in controlling it (Witte 2005, Vinik 2006, Spallone 2011). In individuals with T2D, intensive treatment simultaneously targeting hyperglycemia, hypertension, dyslipidemia, and microalbuminuria has been shown to reduce the risk of developing autonomic neuropathy (Vinik 2003a, 2007).

ORTHOSTATIC HYPOTENSION

A change from lying to standing normally results in activation of a baroreceptor-initiated, centrally mediated sympathetic reflex, resulting in an increase

---

- □ Results are considered abnormal if diastolic pressure drops more than 10 mmHg or systolic decreases by 30 within 2 min
- □ In normal subjects, a rapid fall in blood pressure that follows standing (less than 10 mmHg in less than 2 min) is quickly counterbalanced by baroreflex-mediated vasoconstriction and bradycardia
- □ Primarily determined by SNS-mediated baroreceptor response to standing; blood pressure usually changes minimally when standing from a supine or sitting position
- ■ Diastolic blood pressure response to sustained handgrip
  - □ For this test, a hand dynamometer is gripped to maximal isometric contraction and then held at 30% of maximum for five minutes
  - □ An increase of less than 10 mmHg is considered abnormal because a usual response elicits a diastolic rise of 16 mmHg or more
  - □ Indicative of SNS response elicited by local, sustained isometric muscle contraction
- ■ Power spectral analysis (heart rate variability)
  - □ Analysis of heart rate variation can be performed on short R-R sequences (such as 7-min ECG tracings) or on 24-h ECG recordings
  - □ Individuals with advance autonomic dysfunction may have alterations in all measures taken from intervals (low frequency, high frequency, or the ratio)
  - □ Power spectrum is reported as low-frequency (LF: SNS and PNS) and high-frequency bands (HF: vagal activity only) or as LF:HF ratio (autonomic balance)
- ■ Prolonged QTc interval
  - □ For this test, the QTc interval and QT dispersion (difference between longest and shortest intervals) can be determined from an ECG tracing
  - □ Prolonged measures of either QTc interval or QT dispersion are indicative of an imbalance between right and left heart SNS innervation
  - □ Abnormalities may be indicative of autonomic dysfunction, increased risk of sudden death, CAD, or other diabetic complications

---

Note: CAD, coronary artery disease; CNS, central nervous system; ECG, electrocardiogram; PNS, parasympathetic nervous systems; QTc, corrected QT interval; SNS, sympathetic nervous systems.

in peripheral vascular resistance and cardiac acceleration. Orthostatic hypotension, another sign of autonomic neuropathy, is characterized by a defect in this reflex arc, resulting in signs and symptoms like weakness, faintness, dizziness, visual impairment, and syncope. The main factors producing hypotension are a blunted catecholamine response to standing and failure of lower-limb vascular resistance to increase adequately (Purewal 1995). Although the absolute fall in blood pressure is arbitrary, this condition usually is defined as a fall in systolic blood pressure that is >30 mmHg in response to postural change (i.e., lying down to standing) (Maser 2005) and frequently results from damage to the efferent sympathetic vasomotor nerve fibers (Vinik 2006).

Other causes of occasional dizziness or lightheadedness may be relatively minor, including mild dehydration, hypoglycemia, or prolonged hot tub or sun exposure. Occasional symptoms may not be indicative of orthostatic hypotension. Even in individuals with diabetes, such symptoms may be caused by dehydration secondary to hyperglycemia and excessive urination rather than nerve damage. Advanced age, use of certain medications (e.g., diuretics and β-blockers), heat exposure, bed rest, and pregnancy are other possible causes of symptomology (Caldwell 1987).

Although heart rate and blood pressure responses to postural change can be used to diagnose this condition, more recently, another "squatting" test has been suggested as an alternative to study the natural history of this disorder with regard to baroreceptor sensitivity in individuals with diabetes (Philips 2010, 2011; Scheen 2012). This test involves an original squat test (1 min standing, 1 min squatting, 1 min standing) with continuous monitoring of heart rate and blood pressure, which are blunted when CAN is present (Scheen 2012).

When diagnosed as resulting from autonomic damage, orthostatic hypotension can benefit from both nonpharmacological and pharmacological treatments. Treatment is focused on increasing blood volume, decreasing venous pooling, and increasing vasoconstriction while minimizing supine hypertension. The nonpharmacological approaches, such as increased water intake, adequate salt intake, and use of lower-extremity stockings or abdominal compression, can reduce symptoms like dizziness and dyspnea (Purewal 1995, Figueroa 2010). Most medications taken to treat CAN are also effective for this condition, but some medications prescribed to treat painful peripheral neuropathy may aggravate it.

GASTROPARESIS

Gastroparesis, or chronic delayed gastric emptying without mechanical obstruction, is another manifestation of autonomic nerve dysfunction that affects ~40% of individuals with T1D and up to 30% of individuals with T2D (Parkman 2010). Gastroparesis typically causes nausea, vomiting, early satiety, bloating, postprandial fullness, intestinal pain, alternating bouts of constipation and diarrhea, and lack of appetite. These symptoms can be extremely troubling for individuals with this condition chronically. Anyone with gastroparesis is also at risk for malnutrition, weight loss, impaired drug absorption, disordered glycemic control (due to slower absorption of food and delayed treatment of hypoglycemia), and poor quality of life.

The diagnosis of diabetes-related gastroparesis is made by documenting the presence of chronic upper gastrointestinal symptoms, ruling out mechanical obstruction, and demonstrating delayed gastric emptying. Treatment options include dietary modifications, prokinetic agents, and antiemetic agents (Parkman 2010). Although often attributed to the presence of irreversible nerve damage, acute hyperglycemia represents a potentially reversible cause of gastric dysfunction in diabetes (Ma 2009).

PHYSICAL ACTIVITY PARTICIPATION WITH AUTONOMIC NEUROPATHY

TRAINING EFFECTS

The presence of CAN impairs exercise tolerance and lowers maximal heart rate (Kahn 1986, Vinik 2007). Slower heart rate recovery after physical exertion is associated with greater mortality risk (Cheng 2003, Vinik 2007). Moderate-intensity aerobic training can improve autonomic function and shift the autonomic balance back toward more balance between the sympathetic and parasympathetic function in individuals with and without CAN (Howorka 1997, Loimaala 2003, Pagkalos 2008, Vinik 2011). In fact, regular exercise training increases heart rate variability, suggesting that there is a shift in the cardiac sympathovagal balance in favor of parasympathetic dominance in individuals with diabetes. Long-term physical training may be an effective means to reverse the autonomic dysregulation seen in T2D (Howorka 1997, Loimaala 2003, Pagkalos 2008, Sridhar 2010). However, improvements may be evident only following acute submaximal exercise (Figueroa 2007).

PHYSICAL ACTIVITY PRECAUTIONS AND RECOMMENDATIONS

When autonomic dysfunction in any form is present, a conservative approach to exercise is recommended. Given the likelihood of silent ischemia, resting and exercise heart rate alterations, and blood pressure abnormalities, individuals with CAN should have physician approval and possibly undergo stress testing to screen for cardiovascular abnormalities before commencing exercise (Vinik 2007).

RECOMMENDED ACTIVITIES

Although most aerobic and resistance activities are suitable for individuals with autonomic dysfunction, they are advised, when certain symptoms are present, to avoid rapid changes in movement that may result in fainting and to engage in longer warm-up and cooldown periods, especially for more intense resistance or aerobic training. If postural hypotension is present, inadequate heart rate and blood pressure and responses may occur with incremental work; therefore, these individuals should focus on lower-intensity activities in which mild changes in both are more easily tolerated and that lessen ventricular ectopy.

EXERCISE INTENSITY AND DURATION

For individuals with autonomic neuropathy, increases in physical activity levels must be approached with caution because of the role of the ANS in hormonal and cardiovascular regulation during exercise. Furthermore, exercise intensity should be monitored by means other than heart rate alone (such as subjective ratings of perceived exertion), because it may no longer rise as much as expected or be the best way to monitor intensity unless maximal heart rate is determined (Colberg 2003). Intensity may be accurately prescribed using the HR reserve method (a percentage of the difference between maximal and resting HR, added to the resting value) to approximate oxygen consumption during submaximal exercise, with maximal HR directly measured, rather than estimated, for better accuracy (Colberg 2003, Vinik 2007). In addition, perceived exertion ratings may be used (Colberg 2003). Physical stamina required to engage in longer-duration activities may be compromised; therefore, duration of physical activity should progress slowly.

EXERCISE WITH CARDIAC SYMPTOMS

When CAN is present, the heart rate response is abnormal at rest, when standing, and during strain related to holding the breath (Valsalva maneuver) (Colberg 2003). Blood pressure responses can be abnormal when changing positions or performing isometric exercise. Moreover, the potential for exercise-related dehydration is a concern, as is impaired thermoregulation during activities in environmental extremes, and extra fluids may need to be consumed to protect against both dehydration and hyperthermia. Care must be taken with all components of the exercise prescription.

EXERCISE WITH ORTHOSTATIC HYPOTENSION

When orthostatic hypotension is present, individuals may experience more erratic blood pressure responses to physical activity. Accordingly, they would benefit from monitoring their blood pressure during physical activity to determine whether different postures (e.g., sitting, standing, reclining, supine) affect their symptoms and

Table 19.3 Exercise Recommendations for Autonomic Neuropathy

- Individuals with autonomic neuropathy (particularly CAN) should avoid high-intensity physical activities unless they have been cleared by a physician to participate
- They should avoid physical exertion in hot or cold environments because dehydration may be a risk for those who have difficulty with thermoregulation
- Individuals must be made aware that hypotension may occur after vigorous activities
- Recumbent cycling or water aerobics may be safer activities for individuals with orthostatic hypotension
- For better accuracy, individuals should monitor exercise intensity with the heart rate reserve (HRR) method using a measured maximal heart rate, if possible, or use perceived exertion
- If gastroparesis is an issue, individuals should carefully plan when to undertake physical activity (to avoid potential hypoglycemia during exercise done after meals)

ability to exercise (Figueroa 2010). Dehydration may exacerbate symptoms, particularly with sweating and fluid losses during exercise, so ensuring adequate hydration at all times is critical as well (American College of Sports Medicine 2007).

EXERCISE WITH GASTROPARESIS

The presence of any of the symptoms of gastroparesis can make physical activity more difficult to perform. Medications and foods must be balanced as part of the exercise prescription to minimize the impact of these symptoms (Ma 2009, Parkman 2010). Eating large meals before exercise should be avoided, as it could result in delayed emptying of food; therefore, only small food portions before exercise are recommended. Individuals should use rapidly absorbed glucose tablets to treat hypoglycemia and when blood glucose levels decrease to 100 mg/dl to prevent severe hyperglycemia.

ALTERED HORMONAL RESPONSES

Of interest, in individuals with T1D, autonomic neuropathy further reduces counterregulatory catecholamine responses, which increases the risk for severe hypoglycemia associated with exercise (Meyer 1998). Intensive therapy, however, with an emphasis on preventing hypoglycemia, reverses hypoglycemia unawareness

Table 19.4 Additional Physical Activity Considerations with Autonomic Neuropathy

Safety Concerns	Actions
Altered ability to recognize signs and symptoms of hypoglycemia	■ Monitor blood glucose during physical activity ■ Set higher blood glucose goals
Blunted heart rate responses to physical activity	■ Monitor intensity with perceived exertion, heart rate reserve (HRR), or "talk" test
Erratic blood pressure response during exercise, along with increased risk of postural hypotension	■ Monitor blood pressure during physical activity ■ Determine if different positions (sitting, standing, reclining, supine) affect results ■ Ensure adequate hydration
Lack of effective thermoregulation for hot and cold environments	■ Monitor environment ■ Drink fluids to prevent dehydration ■ Wear proper clothing
Erratic emptying rate of stomach and digestion of food	■ Monitor blood glucose as needed ■ Use foods partially absorbed in the mouth to treat hypoglycemia (e.g., glucose tabs, glucose gels, and hard candies) ■ Delay injection of rapid-acting insulin until after activity
Discomfort following consumption of a meal or specific type of food	■ Determine if physical activity impedes or promotes food mobility ■ Plan timing of physical activity as symptoms tolerate

in individuals with autonomic dysfunction despite marginal improvement in adrenaline responses; prevention of hypoglycemia also results in a lower occurrence despite impaired counterregulation (Fanelli 1997). Thus, autonomic neuropathy, long diabetes duration, and antecedent recent hypoglycemia contribute to varying extents to impaired adrenaline responses and hypoglycemia unawareness (which is largely a reversible condition with prevention of hypoglycemia) (Realsen 2011).

Case in Point: Wrap-Up

Because NA's biggest concern is related to orthostatic hypotension, she should attempt to limit any risk associated with exercising with that condition. First, however, she needs to address any other factors that could be causing or exacerbating her blood pressure responses, such as dehydration or use of certain medications. Moreover, she should consider engaging in physical activities that do not require rapid directional changes or postural changes. Before starting her exercise sessions, she should drink plenty of fluids to ensure that she is beginning with adequate hydration levels, and she should avoid exercising in hot environments.

Exercise Program Goals

Mode of Activity: The recommended activities for NA include recumbent stationary cycling and aquatic exercises. She also can choose to participate in seated aerobic workouts and seated resistance training exercises.

Intensity: For NA, intensity is not as big a concern as simply finding ways to be active doing anything. If she should desire to monitor her exercise intensity, however, she should do it using either the heart rate reserve (HRR) method with results from a maximal cycle ergometer test to determine her actual maximal heart rate, which may be blunted by autonomic neuropathy, or she can use her perceived exertion as a guide to work up to doing activities that feel "somewhat hard" to her.

Frequency: For better blood glucose management, NA should plan on exercising at least 3–5 days/week, and she should avoid letting >2 days lapse without engaging in some activity.

Duration: NA should start with exercise bouts of at least 10 min/session and attempt to work up to doing 30 min continuously, whether aerobic or resistance work, with a goal of 150 min of physical activity spread throughout the week.

Progression: NA should slowly work up to doing aerobic exercise more continuously as her fitness level increases, and she should plan to do seated resistance training at least 2 days/week, possibly 3 days/week. She should not focus as much on increasing her exercise intensity, but rather should focus on conservatively increasing duration and frequency due to her autonomic issues.

Possible Precautions: NA may need to have her medications checked to see whether any of them are contributing to her dizziness (as some medications can). If she is taking any that may be making that condition worse (such as a diuretic that may cause dehydration that she is not sensing well because of autonomic dysfunction), she may need to cut back on her doses or try an alternate medication. In addition, maintaining adequate hydration should be a major focus for her, especially whenever she participates in physical activities that could increase her sweat losses of water (especially during hotter conditions) and when her blood glucose levels are elevated.

Many individuals with T1D and T2D develop some autonomic nerve dysfunction as a result of diabetes and its associated hyperglycemia and oxidative stress. Any type of autonomic neuropathy potentially can affect the ability to exercise and alter normal exercise responses (such as heart rate and blood pressure). Once autonomic neuropathy has been diagnosed, individuals should take these alterations into account to be able to exercise safely and effectively with this diabetic complication.

PROFESSIONAL PRACTICE PEARLS

- Autonomic neuropathy is diabetes-related damage to the central nervous system that rarely occurs without other (peripheral) nerve damage.
- It broadly affects the involuntary functions of the body and may involve he cardiovascular, gastrointestinal, and genitourinary systems and the sweat glands.
- Manifestations may include orthostatic hypotension, resting tachycardia, loss of normal sinus arrhythmia ratio, anhidrosis, bowel or bladder dysfunction, and small pupils sluggishly reactive to light.
- CAN affects the innervation of the heart, and its presence is linked with poor prognosis and premature mortality.
- Abnormalities of the PNS, SNS, or both may be present, but parasympathetic (vagal) dysfunction usually occurs earlier.
- Screening for cardiac involvement should include a battery of autonomic tests (including heart rate variability) that evaluate both branches of the ANS.
- Tighter glycemic control, use of select medications, α-lipoic acid supplements, and strict management of hypertension may be used to treat cardiac autonomic neuropathy.
- Orthostatic hypotension is characterized by signs and symptoms like weakness, faintness, dizziness, visual impairment, and syncope.
- Treatment for orthostatic hypotension is directed at increasing blood volume, decreasing venous pooling, and increasing vasoconstriction while minimizing supine hypertension.
- Gastroparesis affects ~40% of individuals with T1D and up to 30% of individuals with T2D and typically causes nausea, vomiting, early satiety, bloating, postprandial fullness, intestinal pain, bouts of constipation and diarrhea, and lack of appetite.
- Treatment options for gastroparesis include dietary modifications, prokinetic agents, and antiemetic agents.
- Regular exercise training increases heart rate variability with a shift in the cardiac sympathovagal balance in favor of parasympathetic dominance in diabetes.

■ Individuals with CAN should have physician approval and possibly undergo stress testing before commencing exercise.

■ Abnormal heart rate and blood pressure responses, along with impaired thermoregulation and hydration status, may affect an individual's exercise responses.

■ Physical activities that involve rapid changes in movement that may result in fainting may need to be avoided, and individuals should engage in longer warm-up and cooldown periods, especially for more intense resistance or aerobic training.

■ Intensity may be accurately prescribed using HRR with maximal HR directly measured rather than estimated; other options include use of perceived exertion and the talk test.

■ Increases in exercise duration should progress slowly when autonomic dysfunction of any type is present as they may be less well tolerated.

■ With cardiac dysfunction, blood pressure responses may be abnormal when changing positions or performing isometric exercise.

■ Particularly with orthostatic hypotension, extra fluids may need to be consumed to protect against both dehydration and hyperthermia.

■ With gastroparesis, eating large meals before exercise should be avoided as doing so could result in delayed emptying of food and raise hypoglycemia risk.

REFERENCES

American College of Sports Medicine, Sawka MN, Burke LM, Eichner ER, Maughan RJ, Montain SJ, Stachenfeld NS: American College of Sports Medicine position stand. Exercise and fluid replacement. *Med Sci Sports Exerc* 39:377–390, 2007

Caldwell JE: Diuretic therapy and exercise performance. *Sports Med* 4:290–304, 1987

Casellini CM, Vinik AI: Clinical manifestations and current treatment options for diabetic neuropathies. *Endocr Pract* 13:550–566, 2007

Cheng YJ, Lauer MS, Earnest CP, Church TS, Kampert JB, Gibbons LW, Blair SN: Heart rate recovery following maximal exercise testing as a predictor of cardiovascular disease and all-cause mortality in men with diabetes. *Diabetes Care* 26:2052–2057, 2003

Colberg SR, Swain DP, Vinik AI: Use of heart rate reserve and rating of perceived exertion to prescribe exercise intensity in diabetic autonomic neuropathy. *Diabetes Care* 26:986–990, 2003

Ewing DJ, Clarke BF: Diabetic autonomic neuropathy: present insights and future prospects. *Diabetes Care* 9:648–665, 1986

Fanelli C, Pampanelli S, Lalli C, Del Sindaco P, Ciofetta M, Lepore M, Porcellati F, Bottini P, Di Vincenzo A, Brunetti P, Bolli GB: Long-term intensive therapy of IDDM patients with clinically overt autonomic neuropathy: effects on hypoglycemia awareness and counterregulation. *Diabetes* 46:1172–1181, 1997

Figueroa A, Baynard T, Fernhall B, Carhart R, Kanaley JA: Endurance training improves post-exercise cardiac autonomic modulation in obese women with and without type 2 diabetes. *Eur J Appl Physiol* 100:437–444, 2007

Figueroa JJ, Basford JR, Low PA: Preventing and treating orthostatic hypotension: as easy as A, B, C. *Cleve Clin J Med* 77:298–306, 2010

Howorka K, Pumprla J, Haber P, Koller-Strametz J, Mondrzyk J, Schabmann A: Effects of physical training on heart rate variability in diabetic patients with various degrees of cardiovascular autonomic neuropathy. *Cardiovasc Res* 34:206–214, 1997

Kahn JK, Zola B, Juni JE, Vinik AI: Decreased exercise heart rate and blood pressure response in diabetic subjects with cardiac autonomic neuropathy. *Diabetes Care* 9:389–394, 1986

Khoharo HK, Halepoto AW: QTc-interval, heart rate variability and postural hypotension as an indicator of cardiac autonomic neuropathy in type 2 diabetic patients. *J Pak Med Assoc* 62:328–331, 2012

Lieb DC, Parson HK, Mamikunian G, Vinik AI: Cardiac autonomic imbalance in newly diagnosed and established diabetes is associated with markers of adipose tissue inflammation. *Exp Diabetes Res* 2012:878760, 2012

Loimaala A, Huikuri HV, Koobi T, Rinne M, Nenonen A, Vuori I: Exercise training improves baroreflex sensitivity in type 2 diabetes. *Diabetes* 52:1837–1842, 2003

Low PA, Walsh JC, Huang CY, McLeod JG: The sympathetic nervous system in diabetic neuropathy. A clinical and pathological study. *Brain* 98:341–356, 1975

Ma J, Rayner CK, Jones KL, Horowitz M: Diabetic gastroparesis: diagnosis and management. *Drugs* 69:971–986, 2009

Maser RE, Lenhard MJ: Cardiovascular autonomic neuropathy due to diabetes mellitus: clinical manifestations, consequences, and treatment. *J Clin Endocrinol Metab* 90:5896–5903, 2005

Meyer C, Grossmann R, Mitrakou A, Mahler R, Veneman T, Gerich J, Bretzel RG: Effects of autonomic neuropathy on counterregulation and awareness of hypoglycemia in type 1 diabetic patients. *Diabetes Care* 21:1960–1966, 1998

Pagkalos M, Koutlianos N, Kouidi E, Pagkalos E, Mandroukas K, Deligiannis A: Heart rate variability modifications following exercise training in type 2 diabetic patients with definite cardiac autonomic neuropathy. *Br J Sports Med* 42:47–54, 2008

Parkman HP, Fass R, Foxx-Orenstein AE: Treatment of patients with diabetic gastroparesis. *Gastroenterol Hepatol (N Y)* 6:1–16, 2010

Philips JC, Marchand M, Scheen AJ: Changes in pulse pressure, heart rate and the pulse pressure x heart rate product during squatting in type 1 diabetes according to age. *Diabet Med* 27:753–761, 2010

Philips JC, Marchand M, Scheen AJ: Squatting, a posture test for studying cardiovascular autonomic neuropathy in diabetes. *Diabetes Metab* 37:489–496, 2011

Purewal TS, Watkins PJ: Postural hypotension in diabetic autonomic neuropathy: a review. *Diabet Med* 12:192–200, 1995

Realsen JM, Chase HP: Recent advances in the prevention of hypoglycemia in type 1 diabetes. *Diabetes Technol Ther* 13:1177–1186, 2011

Rodrigues TC, Ehrlich J, Hunter CM, Kinney GJ, Rewers M, Snell-Bergeon JK: Reduced heart rate variability predicts progression of coronary artery calcification in adults with type 1 diabetes and controls without diabetes. *Diabetes Technol Ther* 12:963–969, 2010

Scheen AJ, Philips JC: Squatting test: a dynamic postural manoeuvre to study baroreflex sensitivity. *Clin Auton Res* 22:35–41, 2012

Spallone V, Ziegler D, Freeman R, Bernardi L, Frontoni S, Pop-Busui R, Stevens M, Kempler P, Hilsted J, Tesfaye S, Low P, Valensi P, on behalf of the Toronto Consensus Panel on Diabetic Neuropathy: Cardiovascular autonomic neuropathy in diabetes: clinical impact, assessment, diagnosis, and management. *Diabetes Metab Res Rev* [epub ahead of print] 22 Jun 2011

Sridhar B, Haleagrahara N, Bhat R, Kulur AB, Avabratha S, Adhikary P: Increase in the heart rate variability with deep breathing in diabetic patients after 12-month exercise training. *Tohoku J Exp Med* 220:107–113, 2010

Vinik AI: The conductor of the autonomic orchestra. *Front Endocrinol (Lausanne)* 3:71, 2012

Vinik AI, Erbas T: Cardiovascular autonomic neuropathy: diagnosis and management. *Curr Diab Rep* 6:424–430, 2006

Vinik AI, Freeman R, Erbas T: Diabetic autonomic neuropathy. *Semin Neurol* 23:365–372, 2003a

Vinik AI, Maser RE, Ziegler D: Autonomic imbalance: prophet of doom or scope for hope? *Diabet Med* 28:643–651, 2011

Vinik AI, Vinik E: Prevention of the complications of diabetes. *Am J Manag Care* 9 (3 Suppl.):S63–S80; quiz S81–S84, 2003b

Vinik AI, Ziegler D: Diabetic cardiovascular autonomic neuropathy. *Circulation* 115:387–397, 2007

Weston KS, Sacre JW, Jellis CL, Coombes JS: Contribution of autonomic dysfunction to abnormal exercise blood pressure in type 2 diabetes mellitus. *J Sci Med Sport* 16:8-12, 2012

Witte DR, Tesfaye S, Chaturvedi N, Eaton SE, Kempler P, Fuller JH, Eurodiab Prospective Complications Study Group: Risk factors for cardiac autonomic neuropathy in type 1 diabetes mellitus. *Diabetologia* 48:164–171, 2005

Ziegler D, Gries FA, Spuler M, Lessmann F: The epidemiology of diabetic neuropathy. Diabetic Cardiovascular Autonomic Neuropathy Multicenter Study Group. *J Diabetes Complications* 6:49–57, 1992

Chapter 20

Retinopathy and Other Diabetic Eye Diseases

Individuals with diabetes are prone to developing a variety of eye complications related to hyperglycemia and hypertension, including retinopathy, macular edema, cataracts, and glaucoma. Proliferative diabetic retinopathy (PDR) is the main cause of blindness in developed countries and is associated with increased cardiovascular mortality (Klein 1992, Juutilainen 2007). The presence of any eye disease may or may not require physical activity limitations based on its severity. In all cases in which exercise participation will not aggravate eye disease, engaging in regular physical activity is recommended for glycemic control and overall health. Modifications to the type or intensity of exercise done may be necessary to prevent exercise-associated exacerbation.

Case in Point: Exercise Management for an Adult with T1D and Retinopathy

SO is a 24-year-old woman who has had type 1 diabetes (T1D) since she was 4 years old. Her only medication is insulin, taken as a basal-bolus regimen of glargine (twice a day in a split dose) and lispro (with meals and for correction of hyperglycemia). She has been in good health overall and very physically active. On her last visit to her ophthalmologist, however, she was diagnosed with severe non-proliferative retinopathy, likely the result of suboptimal control of her blood glucose levels throughout most of her teenage years and a rapid reduction in her A1C levels when switching to intensive insulin therapy within the past 2 years. She is concerned about how the diagnosis will affect her ability to engage in her usual physical activities (i.e., swimming, running, racquetball, and resistance training), which she does daily on a rotating basis to help manage her glycemic levels.

Resting Measurements

Height: 66 inches
Weight: 125 lb
BMI: 20.2 (normal)
Heart rate: 72 beats per minute (bpm)
Blood pressure: 110/65 mmHg

Fasting Labs

Plasma glucose: 45–175 (controlled with insulin)
A1C: 6.2%
Total cholesterol: 115 mg/dl
Triglycerides: 28 mg/dl
High-density lipoprotein cholesterol: 55 mg/dl
Low-density lipoprotein cholesterol: 54 mg/dl

Questions to Consider

1. What type of physical activities are safe for SO to do with severe nonproliferative retinopathy?
2. Are any precautions needed for NA when she exercises?

(Continued on page 385.)

DIABETES-RELATED EYE DISEASES

Diabetes is the leading cause of new blindness in adults ages 20 to 74 years. As of 2004, ~4.1 million Americans 40 years and older had developed diabetic retinopathy, and 1 in 12 of those individuals had advanced, vision-threatening retinopathy (Kempen 2004). Another study estimated that retinopathy resulting from T1D affects 1 in 300 adults with this type of diabetes and that half of those cases are advanced and vision-threatening (Roy 2004). Elderly individuals with diabetes are 1.5 times more likely to develop vision loss and blindness, and 12,000 to 24,000 Americans with diabetes become legally blind each year due to complications associated with diabetic retinopathy (Tumosa 2008). The incidence of retinopathy and vision-threatening retinopathy among Americans 40 years and older with diabetes is projected to triple (to a total of 19.4 million) by 2050, whereas increases among older individuals (≥65 years) are expected to be even more pronounced. Cataract cases are likely to increase by 235%, and the number of glaucoma cases among Hispanics with diabetes ≥65 years will increase 12-fold (Saaddine 2008). These projections portend a staggering number of cases of eye disease resulting from both T1D and type 2 diabetes (T2D) in the next 30 years.

RETINOPATHY

Diabetic retinopathy is the most common eye disease among individuals with both T1D and T2D and a leading cause of blindness in American adults. It also has a significant association with mortality risk from cardiovascular causes (Klein 1992, Juutilainen 2007). Advanced glycation end-products (AGEs) are important in the development of retinal abnormalities in PDR (Gunduz 2007). In some individuals with retinopathy, blood vessels swell and leak fluid, or abnormal new blood vessels may grow on the surface of the retina in the back of the eye. Tight control of blood glucose levels and effective blood pressure management are essential for preventing or arresting the development of diabetic retinopathy, but they are

Table 20.1 Stages of Diabetic Retinopathy

- Mild nonproliferative retinopathy: At this earliest stage, small areas of balloon-like swelling in the retina's tiny blood vessels (microaneurysms) are present.
- Moderate nonproliferative retinopathy: At this stage, some blood vessels that nourish the retina may be blocked.
- Severe nonproliferative retinopathy: More blood vessels are blocked, depriving several areas of the retina of their blood supply, which leads to these areas sending signals that stimulate the growth of new blood vessels.
- Proliferative retinopathy: The new blood vessels that grow along the retina and the surface of the clear, vitreous fluid inside the eye are abnormal and fragile. Although these blood vessels themselves do not cause symptoms or vision loss, if they hemorrhage, severe vision loss and even blindness can result. Retinal detachment is also common at this stage.

often difficult to achieve, and diabetic retinopathy develops in a high proportion of people with diabetes over time (Kempen 2004).

Stages. Diabetic retinopathy occurs in four stages that correspond to degrees of severity (Table 20.1): nonproliferative diabetic retinopathy (NPDR) that is mild, moderate, or severe, and PDR (Klein 1992). Specific alterations in the retina characterize the early stages: microaneurysms and hemorrhages, alteration of the blood–retinal barrier, capillary closure, and alterations in the neuronal and glial cells of the retina (Cunha-Vaz 2005). The last stage (PDR) involves the growth of new, abnormal vessels via neovascularization. The majority of the neovascular membranes are adherent to the posterior vitreous cortex; when the posterior hyaloid exerts traction, the edges of the neovascular complex are pulled forward, resulting in vitreous hemorrhage (Gunduz 2007). With PDR, scar tissue also may form near the retina, detaching it from the back of the eye and resulting in blindness from retinal detachment. Significant loss of vision is also possible, either acutely or chronically, due to visual field blockage by blood from hemorrhages that remains in the vitreous fluid of the eye.

Prevention of retinopathy. Both blood pressure and glycemic management are essential in limiting progression of retinopathy. Nonproliferative stages require no treatment; however, despite advances in diabetes care, PDR remains a leading cause of preventable vision loss. As this eye disease is symptomless until the final stage, the best prevention is to have a comprehensive, dilated eye exam annually to detect retinal changes early in the disease.

Prevention with medication has also been studied. The ACCORD (Action to Control Cardiovascular Risk in Diabetes) trial included a lipid management arm in which individuals meeting a certain atherogenic dyslipidemia phenotype were assigned randomly to treatment with fenofibrate or placebo, each with a statin drug. Use of fenofibrate was associated with a significant reduction in the risk of progression of retinopathy and may be beneficial in its prevention alongside intensive management of traditional risk factors, such as hyperglycemia and high blood pressure (Simo 2012).

Treatment of retinopathy. At present, no pharmaceutical therapies are available that halt the progression of diabetic retinopathy by treating the underlying progress of microvascular damage. Current treatments for PDR, such as laser photocoagulation, intravitreous injections of corticosteroids, or anti-vascular endothelial growth factor (anti-VEGF) agents, are used only for advanced PDR (Montero 2011). Use of steroids potentially may increase intraocular pressure and cause progression of cataracts, however (Boscia 2010).

Surgical treatment consisting of laser burns done in scatter patterns on the peripheral retina (panretinal photocoagulation) is used to cause shrinkage of the abnormal vessels to stabilize them (Chappelow 2012). In one study, individuals who had undergone that treatment were followed for 10 years (Dogru 1999). Although vision was preserved in most, progression of cataracts, macular edema, vitreous hemorrhage, macular traction, and neovascular glaucoma were the main causes of visual loss. More recently, intravitreal use of triamcinolone acetonide as an adjunctive therapy for individuals with both PDR and macular edema has been added to photocoagulation with promising results (Zein 2006, Aydin 2009). This surgical procedure, however, results in some loss of night, peripheral, and color vision; when a greater number of laser treatments is required to stabilize and shrink the abnormal vessels, the result is more extensive loss of peripheral retinal tissue and noncentral vision.

If an individual's vision is blocked by retinal hemorrhaging that does not clear out on its own, a surgical procedure called a vitrectomy may be undertaken to remove the blood-filled, gel-like vitreous fluid from the eye and replace it with a clear saline solution to restore vision (Yeoh 2008, Boscia 2010). Intravitreal injection of bevacizumab (Avastin) before vitrectomy surgery may help manage tractional retinal detachment or vitreous hemorrhage due to severe PDR (Yeoh 2008).

MACULAR EDEMA

Because of blockage of existing vessels, the fluid from new, abnormal ones may leak into the center of the macula where sharp, central vision is regulated. The fluid makes the macula swell, blurring vision and resulting in clinically significant macular edema (CSME) (Watkinson 2008). Although it can occur at any stage of diabetic retinopathy, it is more likely to manifest as retinopathy progresses to more severe stages (Boscia 2010). About half of the people with proliferative retinopathy also have CSME, although it is the most common cause of visual impairment in those who also have NPDR. The development of CSME correlated most strongly with the duration of diabetes in one study (Patel 2012).

Use of steroids placed inside the eye by either intravitreal injection or surgical implantation may improve visual outcomes in eyes with persistent or refractory CSME (Grover 2008), although intravitreal steroids do have some potential adverse effects, such as contributing to the progression of cataracts and elevating intraocular pressure (Boscia 2010). Like PDR, CSME can be treated with laser surgery; it uses a focal laser procedure to place several hundred small laser burns in the areas of retinal leakage surrounding the macula. These burns slow the leakage of fluid and reduce the amount of fluid in the retina, which reduces swelling there and restores vision.

In older adults, macular changes also can result in age-related macular degeneration (AMD), which shares common risk factors with cardiovascular disease (Knudtson 2006). Physical activity participation reduces the risk of AMD, suggesting a lifestyle behavior that might be protective against its development (Knudtson 2006). In addition, specifically targeting mitochondria with pharmacological agents to protect against oxidative stress or promote repair of mitochondrial DNA damage may offer potential alternatives for the treatment of retinal degenerative diseases like AMD (Jarrett 2008).

CATARACTS

A cataract, a clouding or fogging of the normally clear lens of the eye, is more common in people with diabetes and may result from fluctuations in blood glucose levels. Having a cataract means that the eye cannot focus light properly and vision is impaired (Watkinson 2008). Although anyone can develop cataracts, individuals with diabetes frequently experience this condition at an earlier age, and they progress over a shorter time period, possibly because of an increase in aldose reductase activity. In fact, diabetes is associated with a fivefold higher prevalence of cataracts, which remains a major cause of blindness throughout the world (Obrosova 2010). Treatment usually involves surgical removal of the cloudy lens and its replacement with a clear lens implant that may be able to correct visual acuity without the need for glasses or contact lenses.

GLAUCOMA

When fluid inside the eye fails to drain properly due to a buildup of pressure there, it results in glaucoma. The elevated intraocular pressure damages the optic nerve and eye vasculature over time, causing changes in vision. In the most common form, no symptoms are present until the disease is advanced and causes significant vision loss. Less commonly, symptoms can include headaches, eye aches or pain, blurred vision, watering eyes, halos around lights, and loss of vision. The most common diseases responsible for development of neovascular glaucoma are diabetic retinopathy, ischemic central retinal vein occlusion (the second most common retinal disease behind retinopathy), and ocular ischemic syndrome (Hayreh 2007).

Usual treatment of glaucoma involves the use of pressure-reducing eye drops, laser procedures, other medications, or surgery. In neovascular glaucoma, anti-VEGF drugs can facilitate filtrating surgery (Figueroa 2009). For this type of eye disease related to diabetes, an annual glaucoma screening to detect problems early is the best prevention. Maintaining adequate hydration may have a positive effect on glaucoma (Manz 2007).

Case in Point: Continued

While window-shopping in the mall one afternoon, SO began to notice what appeared to be a flag waving in the periphery of her vision off to her right. After a few moments, she realized that the movement was inside, rather than outside, her eye. When she covered her left eye with her hand, she realized that she was seeing the "flag" in her right eye only. Petrified, she called for an emergency appointment with her ophthalmologist and worried all evening and through the next day before she was seen by him. At the next-day appointment, her worst fears were confirmed: her retinopathy had progressed to the proliferative stage, and what she had seen inside her eye (and could still see to a lesser extent) was blood hemorrhaging into the vitreous fluid from a leaky vessel. He advised her to undergo laser therapy to stabilize her eyes, and he warned her that exercise was going to be an issue until her eyes stabilized somewhat (as abnormal vessels had grown in both).

Additional Questions to Consider

1. Are there any safe exercises for SO to do during her laser treatments for PDR?
2. How will she know when her eye disease has stabilized enough for her to be able to return to her normal exercise routines?

(Continued on page 389.)

PHYSICAL ACTIVITY PARTICIPATION WITH RETINOPATHY AND OTHER EYE DISEASES

RETINOPATHY

The presence of retinopathy should be evaluated annually based on established clinical guidelines. People without diabetic retinopathy or who have mild NPDR have no eye-related activity limitations. Those with moderate, severe, and very severe NPDR and those with PDR should be educated on the limitations during exercise and even routine physical activities. In individuals with NPDR, PDR, or CSME, careful optical screening and physician approval are recommended before initiating an exercise program.

Even though an acute bout of exercise increases systemic and retinal blood pressure during the activity, no studies have shown a worsening of retinopathy with physical activity participation. In the absence of active retinal hemorrhaging, low-intensity training may be undertaken in most individuals with T1D or T2D and may improve cardiovascular function by 15% without adverse retinal outcomes (Bernbaum 1989a, 1989b).

In general, the stage of retinopathy determines which activities are appropriate and which activities should be avoided, as shown in Table 20.2. Although exercise itself has not been shown to accelerate the proliferative process, certain exercise precautions may be needed to prevent new retinal hemorrhages or detachment. The mild nonproliferative stage requires no precautions, but individuals who have progressing NPDR or unstable proliferative disease will have significant restrictions in their level of physical exertion and activity options.

For example, if NPDR is moderate, individuals should avoid activities that dramatically increase intraocular blood pressure, such as heavy weightlifting or head-down (head lower than the heart) activities. For more severe diabetic eye

Table 20.2 Physical Activity Considerations with Retinopathy

Stage of Retinopathy	Physical Activity and Exercise Recommendations
None	No physical activity or exercise limitations
Mild nonproliferative	No physical activity or exercise limitations
Moderate nonproliferative	Avoid activities that dramatically elevate systemic or intraocular blood pressure, such as power lifting and breath-holding (Valsalva maneuver)
Severe nonproliferative	Limit increases in systemic or intraocular blood pressure (Valsalva maneuver) and avoid activities that jar the head like boxing and intense competitive sports Heart rate should not exceed that which elicits a systolic blood pressure response >170 mmHg
Proliferative	Avoid strenuous activity, high-impact activities, Valsalva maneuvers, and activities that potentially can jar the head or raise intraocular pressures, including high-impact aerobic dance, all weightlifting, jogging, competitive sports, boxing, kickboxing, racquet sports, scuba diving, waterskiing, trumpet playing, rollercoasters, head-down activities, or any done during an active retinal hemorrhage Encourage activities that are low-impact and aerobic and stress cardiovascular conditioning (e.g., swimming without diving, walking, low-impact aerobic dance, stationary cycling, and endurance exercise)

disease, they should avoid all jumping, jarring, or breath-holding activities that can cause intraocular bleeding and increase the risk of retinal tears or retinal detachment, including heavy weightlifting and other intense aerobic activities.

If an individual has a retinal hemorrhage or notices dramatic, sudden changes in sight, he or she should either forego exercise or immediately stop any ongoing activity and consult an eye specialist for further guidance about resuming activity. Activities that greatly increase intraocular pressure are never advised with uncontrolled proliferation of neovascularization, nor are jumping or jarring activities, all of which increase hemorrhage risk (Colberg 2010). Moreover, the risk for retinal detachment in such cases is increased by participation in vigorous-intensity exercise.

OTHER EYE DISEASES

Macular edema and glaucoma should be evaluated by an ophthalmologist or optometrist and activity guidelines should be determined by the results of the examination. In general, neither disease is a contraindication to physical activity, but those with CSME usually have some retinopathy that may require accommodation during exercise (to lower concomitant risk of hemorrhage or retinal detachment). Anyone with glaucoma may need to avoid high-intensity activities that increase further intraocular pressures.

Table 20.3 Exercise Recommendations for Retinopathy and Other Eye Diseases

- Individuals with NPDR, PDR, or CSME should undergo careful optical screening and obtain physician approval before initiating an exercise program.
- Physical activity recommendations should be based on the severity and stage of diabetic retinopathy or other eye diseases.
- Individuals with unstable proliferative disease should receive medical clearance for exercise from an ophthalmologist before participating because of their increased risk of hemorrhage or retinal detachment.
- Individuals with unstable, advanced PDR should avoid activities that can produce large increases in blood pressure, such as high-intensity aerobic exercise, heavy resistance training, jumping or jarring activities, or exercises in a head-down position.
- With visual impairment, individuals should choose appropriate options for physical activity, such as swimming using lane guides, stationary cycling, treadmill walking, tandem cycling, and dancing, using a sighted person as a guide when necessary.

Note: CSME, clinically significant macular edema; NPDR, nonproliferative diabetic retinopathy; PDR, proliferative diabetic retinopathy.

Finally, although cataracts can obscure vision and make specific activities more dangerous (such as cycling outdoors or using free weights) (Obrosova 2010), their presence does not preclude participation in most types of aerobic or resistance training, although these activities may need to be curtailed for a day or two following cataract surgery. Exercise recommendations for individuals with retinopathy and other eye diseases are given in Table 20.3.

VISUAL IMPAIRMENT

Any level of visual impairment resulting from diabetes-related or other eye disease should not be considered to be a contraindication to exercise. Physical activities should be chosen to accommodate the level of impairment, however. Some examples of more appropriate exercise for individuals with significant loss of vision or visual acuity include swimming using lane guides, stationary cycling, treadmill walking, tandem cycling, and dancing with a partner. In some cases, using a sighted person as a guide will be required. In cases in which PDR results in total blindness, the perceived loss of independence and mobility may result in a need for support in managing the lifestyle changes necessary for good blood glucose control, particularly with regard to continued exercise participation (Devenney 2011).

A higher incidence of falls related to vision loss remains a problem among older individuals and should be addressed adequately by exercise strategies (Dhital 2010). Visual field loss has been shown to be the primary vision component that increases the risk of falls, and individuals with this loss may benefit from mobility training to reduce the risk of falling (Freeman 2007). Both central and peripheral visual impairment are independently associated with increased risk for falls and falls with injury, suggesting that targeting both the central and peripheral compo-

nents may be necessary to effectively reduce the risk of falling caused by significant vision loss (Patino 2010).

Case in Point: Wrap-Up

Since SO may not have any visual signs or symptoms that her condition is stabilizing
(other than a lack of active hemorrhages) and wants to be able to continue exercising regularly, she will simply have to modify the types of activities that she is doing
until her retinopathy appears to stabilize following laser treatments. Doing any activity during a period of active hemorrhaging is contraindicated, but after the bleeding
stops, she can engage in mild to moderate activities that do not excessively increase
her intraocular pressure or jar her head. Slow walking and other activities of daily living should not contribute to hemorrhage risk and are encouraged.

Exercise Program Goals

Mode of Activity: Low- to moderate-intensity activities that are not jarring can be
included in SO's workout regimen, including conditioning machines (like cross-
trainers and elliptical machines), lap swimming, and spinning (cycling) classes.
She should avoid high-impact aerobics, jogging or running, and racquet sports,
all of which have a greater potential to cause retinal hemorrhages. Intense resistance training also is contraindicated at present.

Intensity: SO will need to moderate her exercise intensity for the time being. She
is already well conditioned, but her biggest concern now is the stability of the
abnormal vessels in her retina. Accordingly, she should engage in no harder
than moderate-intensity activities ("somewhat hard" or 5–6 on a 10-point scale)
and avoid ones that feel "hard." She can do interval or hill workouts on the conditioning machines as long as she monitors her heart rate and stays below recommended levels. Her heart rate should stay in a low- to moderate-intensity
range, which is 109–145 bpm (30–59% heart rate reserve, or HRR). Her intensity during each training session can vary, however, and she may choose to do
relatively harder and easier training days to vary her routine.

Frequency: Training frequency for SO is not as big a concern as intensity. She can
follow recommendations for active adults to engage in ≥5 days/week of moderate training, with more frequent exercise making her diabetic regimen changes
easier to manage.

Duration: SO should aim to do at least 30 min/session of moderate training, with a
target training goal of 150 min/week of moderate exercise to meet minimal recommendations for active adults with T1D. If she does lower-intensity work, she
can do it for 30–60 min instead.

Progression: Given her initial fitness status and prior sports history, SO qualifies to
be in the "maintenance" phase of training. However, her exercise intensity will
have to be moderated for the present time, which she can offset somewhat with
longer-duration training. Once her eye disease stabilizes, she can progress to
adding in some low or moderate (but not intense) resistance training at least 2
days/week. For now, she should continue to vary her activities or add in new ones
for variety, fitness gains, injury prevention, and motivation to continue her training.

Daily Movement: Given that most daily movement is low intensity, SO can and should engage in as much as possible to help her keep her blood glucose levels at a lower level.

Possible Precautions: SO has been active for most of her life, and she has no risk factors for cardiovascular disease other than T1D for 20 years. Moreover, a graded exercise test is intense by design, so she should not be required to do one before starting an exercise program, given her PDR. She should, however, continue to monitor for any signs or symptoms of cardiovascular disease and contact her health-care providers should any occur. As far as her retinopathy goes, in addition to avoiding head-jarring and overly intense activities, any time that she has an active retinal bleed (if she has any more), she needs to avoid all exercise of any intensity and rest until the hemorrhaging has stopped and the eye has stabilized enough to prevent additional bleeding into the vitreous caused by exercise-related elevations in systolic blood pressure. Once she has completed all laser surgery and her eyes have been stable for a period of 6–12 months, she can consider returning to doing more intense physical activities upon the advice of her optical health-care provider.

Diabetic eye diseases are prevalent among individuals with both T1D and T2D and can impose restrictions on physical activity participation. In particular, when proliferative diabetic retinopathy is present and not fully stabilized by laser surgery or other treatment, individuals should be careful to avoid activities that cause large increases in intraocular pressure or that jar the head as both can increase the risk of retinal hemorrhage or detachment. Once eye diseases have been stabilized, no physical activity is contraindicated at that point, but caution should be taken in making accommodations to activities when any lasting vision loss is present.

PROFESSIONAL PRACTICE PEARLS

- Individuals with diabetes are prone to developing a variety of eye diseases, including retinopathy, macular edema, cataracts, and glaucoma.
- PDR, the most severe type of diabetic retinopathy, is the main cause of blindness in industrialized countries and is associated with increased cardiovascular mortality.
- Tight control of both glycemic levels and blood pressure is essential for preventing or arresting the development of diabetic retinopathy, but often it is difficult to achieve.
- Current treatments for PDR include laser photocoagulation, intravitreous injections of corticosteroids, or anti-VEGF agents.
- If an individual's vision is blocked by retinal hemorrhaging, a vitrectomy may be needed to replace the vitreous fluid with a clear saline solution to restore vision.
- About half of the people with proliferative retinopathy also have CSME, a swelling of that area of the eye that results in blurred central vision.
- In older adults, macular changes can result in AMD, which shares common risk factors with cardiovascular disease.

- When fluid inside the eye fails to drain properly due to a buildup of pressure, it results in glaucoma, which can be treated with pressure-reducing eye drops or by other means.
- The presence of any eye disease may or may not require physical activity limitations based on its severity.
- Individuals with NPDR, PDR, or CSME should undergo careful optical screening and obtain physician approval before initiating an exercise program.
- People without diabetic retinopathy or who have only the mild nonproliferative type have no eye-related physical activity limitations.
- In the absence of active retinal hemorrhaging, low-intensity training may be undertaken in most individuals who have T1D or T2D.
- Individuals with uncontrolled PDR should avoid activities that greatly raise intraocular pressure or jar the head, both of which increase hemorrhage risk.
- If an individual has a retinal hemorrhage or notices dramatic, sudden changes in vision, he or she should either forego exercise or immediately stop any ongoing activity.
- Any level of visual impairment should not be considered a contraindication to exercise, but physical activities should accommodate the level of impairment.
- A higher incidence of falls related to vision loss remains a problem among older individuals and should be addressed adequately by exercise strategies as well.

REFERENCES

Aydin E, Demir HD, Yardim H, Erkorkmaz U: Efficacy of intravitreal triamcinolone after or concomitant with laser photocoagulation in nonproliferative diabetic retinopathy with macular edema. *Eur J Ophthalmol* 19:630–637, 2009

Bernbaum M, Albert SG, Cohen JD: Exercise training in individuals with diabetic retinopathy and blindness. *Arch Phys Med Rehabil* 70:605–611, 1989a

Bernbaum M, Albert SG, Cohen JD, Drimmer A: Cardiovascular conditioning in individuals with diabetic retinopathy. *Diabetes Care* 12:740–742, 1989b

Boscia F: Current approaches to the management of diabetic retinopathy and diabetic macular oedema. *Drugs* 70:2171–2200, 2010

Chappelow AV, Tan K, Waheed NK, Kaiser PK: Panretinal photocoagulation for proliferative diabetic retinopathy: pattern scan laser versus argon laser. *Am J Ophthalmol* 153:137–142 e2, 2012

Colberg SR, Sigal RJ, Fernhall B, Regensteiner JG, Blissmer BJ, Rubin RR, Chasan-Taber L, Albright AL, Braun B, American College of Sports Medicine, American Diabetes Association: Exercise and type 2 diabetes: the American College of Sports Medicine and the American Diabetes Association: joint position statement. *Diabetes Care* 33:e147–e167, 2010

Cunha-Vaz J, Bernardes R: Nonproliferative retinopathy in diabetes type 2: initial stages and characterization of phenotypes. *Prog Retin Eye Res* 24:355–377, 2005

Devenney R, O'Neill S: The experience of diabetic retinopathy: a qualitative study. *Br J Health Psychol* 16:707–721, 2011

Dhital A, Pey T, Stanford MR: Visual loss and falls: a review. *Eye (Lond)* 24:1437–1446, 2010

Dogru M, Nakamura M, Inoue M, Yamamoto M: Long-term visual outcome in proliferative diabetic retinopathy patients after panretinal photocoagulation. *Jpn J Ophthalmol* 43:217–224, 1999

Figueroa MS, Contreras I, Noval S: Anti-angiogenic drugs as an adjunctive therapy in the surgical treatment of diabetic retinopathy. *Curr Diabetes Rev* 5:52–56, 2009

Freeman EE, Munoz B, Rubin G, West SK: Visual field loss increases the risk of falls in older adults: the Salisbury eye evaluation. *Invest Ophthalmol Vis Sci* 48:4445–4450, 2007

Grover D, Li TJ, Chong CC: Intravitreal steroids for macular edema in diabetes. *Cochrane Database Syst Rev* (1):CD005656, 2008

Gunduz K, Bakri SJ: Management of proliferative diabetic retinopathy. *Compr Ophthalmol Update* 8:245–256, 2007

Hayreh SS: Neovascular glaucoma. *Prog Retin Eye Res* 26:470–485, 2007

Jarrett SG, Lin H, Godley BF, Boulton ME: Mitochondrial DNA damage and its potential role in retinal degeneration. *Prog Retin Eye Res* 27:596–607, 2008

Juutilainen A, Lehto S, Ronnemaa T, Pyorala K, Laakso M: Retinopathy predicts cardiovascular mortality in type 2 diabetic men and women. *Diabetes Care* 30:292–299, 2007

Kempen JH, O'Colmain BJ, Leske MC, Haffner SM, Klein R, Moss SE, Taylor HR, Hamman RF, Eye Diseases Prevalence Research Group: The prevalence of diabetic retinopathy among adults in the United States. *Arch Ophthalmol* 122:552–563, 2004

Klein R, Klein BE, Moss SE: Epidemiology of proliferative diabetic retinopathy. *Diabetes Care* 15:1875–1891, 1992

Knudtson MD, Klein R, Klein BE: Physical activity and the 15-year cumulative incidence of age-related macular degeneration: the Beaver Dam Eye Study. *Br J Ophthalmol* 90:1461–1463, 2006

Manz F: Hydration and disease. *J Am Coll Nutr* 26 (5 Suppl.):535S–541S, 2007

Montero JA, Ruiz-Moreno JM, Correa ME: Intravitreal anti-VEGF drugs as adjuvant therapy in diabetic retinopathy surgery. *Curr Diabetes Rev* 7:176–184, 2011

Obrosova IG, Chung SS, Kador PF: Diabetic cataracts: mechanisms and management. *Diabetes Metab Res Rev* 26:172–180, 2010

Patel AS, Patel CC, Goyal A, Anchala A, Adrean S, Hughes B, Mahmoud TH: Impact of ocular hypotensive lipids on clinically significant diabetic macular edema. *Eur J Ophthalmol* 22:709–713, 2012

Patino CM, McKean-Cowdin R, Azen SP, Allison JC, Choudhury F, Varma R, Los Angeles Latino Eye Study Group: Central and peripheral visual impairment and the risk of falls and falls with injury. *Ophthalmology* 117:199–206 e1, 2010

Roy MS, Klein R, O'Colmain BJ, Klein BE, Moss SE, Kempen JH: The prevalence of diabetic retinopathy among adult type 1 diabetic persons in the United States. *Arch Ophthalmol* 122:546–551, 2004

Saaddine JB, Honeycutt AA, Narayan KM, Zhang X, Klein R, Boyle JP: Projection of diabetic retinopathy and other major eye diseases among people with diabetes mellitus: United States, 2005–2050. *Arch Ophthalmol* 126:1740–1747, 2008

Simo R, Hernandez C: Prevention and treatment of diabetic retinopathy: evidence from large, randomized trials: the emerging role of fenofibrate. *Rev Recent Clin Trials* 7:71–80, 2012

Tumosa N: Eye disease and the older diabetic. *Clin Geriatr Med* 24:515–527, vii, 2008

Watkinson S, Seewoodhary R: Ocular complications associated with diabetes mellitus. *Nurs Stand* 22:51–57; quiz 58, 60, 2008

Yeoh J, Williams C, Allen P, Buttery R, Chiu D, Clark B, Essex R, McCombe M, Qureshi S, Campbell WG: Avastin as an adjunct to vitrectomy in the management of severe proliferative diabetic retinopathy: a prospective case series. *Clin Experiment Ophthalmol* 36:449–454, 2008

Zein WM, Noureddin BN, Jurdi FA, Schakal A, Bashshur ZF: Panretinal photocoagulation and intravitreal triamcinolone acetonide for the management of proliferative diabetic retinopathy with macular edema. *Retina* 26:137–142, 2006

Chapter 21

Microalbuminuria, Nephropathy, and End-Stage Renal Disease

Chronic hyperglycemia remains the primary cause of the metabolic, biochemical, and vascular abnormalities in diabetic nephropathy, and the risk for developing specific comorbidities increases as nephropathy progresses. Diabetic nephropathy develops in ~30% of individuals with diabetes and is a major risk factor for death (Bo 2005, Coccheri 2007). Kidney disease is highly prevalent in type 2 diabetes (T2D), and moderate to severe renal functional impairment occurs in ~20–30% of those individuals (Koro 2009).

Individuals with overt nephropathy frequently exhibit a diminished capacity for exercise, resulting in a self-limitation of physical activity. Yet, people at all stages of nephropathy can benefit from staying physically active, and physical activity during dialysis sessions is possible and often recommended to increase functional capacity. Given that both aerobic and resistance training can improve physical function and quality of life in individuals with kidney disease, both are recommended and can be undertaken safely with certain precautions.

Case in Point: Exercise Management for an Adult with T2D and End-Stage Renal Disease

PD is a 70-year-old woman who has had T2D for 25 years. Her diabetes is pretty well managed at this point and currently is controlled with a daily injection of basal insulin (glargine). She also takes a lipid-lowering agent and two renal-protective medications (an angiotensin-converting enzyme [ACE] inhibitor and an angiotensin II receptor blocker [ARB]), both of which also help lower her blood pressure. She has been undergoing thrice-weekly dialysis treatments for the past 2 months since progressing to stage 5 chronic kidney disease, and she is suffering from a general tiredness that makes her unwilling (and unable) to participate in any regular physical activity. She is finding it hard to do basic things like grocery shopping and laundry as well. Her quality of life has greatly diminished since her kidney disease progressed to the point at which she needed dialysis treatments, but she wants to start feeling better and lose some weight, and her health-care provider has advised her to start doing more physical activity.

Resting Measurements

Height: 64 inches
Weight: 255 lb
BMI: 43.8 (morbidly obese)

Heart rate: 92 beats per minute (bpm)
Blood pressure: 140/90 mmHg (on medication)

Fasting Labs

Plasma glucose: 108 mg/dl (controlled with Jentadueto and basal insulin)
A1C: 6.8%
Total cholesterol: 175 mg/dl (on medication)
Triglycerides: 78 mg/dl
High-density lipoprotein cholesterol: 38 mg/dl
Low-density lipoprotein cholesterol: 125 mg/dl

Questions to Consider

1. What type of exercise can PD safely do with end-stage renal disease?
2. Is it possible for her to exercise while undergoing dialysis treatments?
3. Are any precautions needed for PD when she exercises?

(Continued on page 402.)

MICROABUMINURIA AND NEPHROPATHY

Many individuals who suffer from diabetes develop varying degrees of kidney disease, from microalbuminuria to end-stage renal failure (Mogensen 2003). Promotion of excessive oxidative stress in the vascular and cellular milieu results in endothelial cell dysfunction, which is one of the earliest and most pivotal metabolic consequences of chronic hyperglycemia (Negrean 2007). These derangements are caused by excessive production of advanced glycation end products and free radicals and by the suppression of antioxidants and antioxidant mechanisms (Singh 2011). Microalbuminuria and gross proteinuria are significantly associated with subsequent mortality from all causes and from cardiovascular, cerebrovascular, and coronary heart diseases, independent of known cardiovascular risk factors and diabetes-related variables (Valmadrid 2000, Astrup 2008). Individuals of both sexes with impaired kidney function are at increased risk of bone loss, even with minimal reduction in kidney function (Ishani 2008; Jamal 2010).

Both aerobic and resistance training improve physical function and quality of life in individuals with kidney disease (Painter 2000a, 2000b; Johansen 2005). Exercise training delays the progression of diabetic nephropathy in animals (Tufescu 2008, Ghosh 2009), but little evidence is available in humans.

MICROALBUMINURIA

The kidneys process ~200 quarts of blood a day to sift out 2 quarts of waste products and extra water that is removed as urine (Bagshaw 2010). Blood enters the kidneys through arteries that branch into tiny clusters of looping blood vessels, each one a glomerulus. In total, each kidney has ~1 million glomeruli. Diabetic nephropathy is the leading cause of glomerular disease and of total kidney failure in the U.S. Chronic hyperglycemia appears to scar the glomeruli and increase their speed of blood flow, putting a strain on the filtering glomeruli and raising blood pressure; such damage is considered irreversible (Mogensen 2003).

Minute amounts of albumin in the urine is the main characteristic of microalbuminuria and is a common risk factor for overt nephropathy (Coccheri 2007) and cardiovascular mortality (Gimeno Orna 2003). It usually is defined as urinary albumin excretion rates of >20 and up to 200 mcg/min, whereas normoalbuminuric individuals have excretion rates of ≤20 mcg/min. Early albuminuria reflects vascular endothelial dysfunction, which may be mediated in part by chronic inflammation (Lin 2008).

Detection. Until recently, microalbuminuria generally was detected using overnight or 24-h urine collection methods. A systematic review suggested, however, that the marginal benefit of using a timed urine collection over a spot albumin-to-creatinine ratio to detect microalbuminuria for screening in individuals with diabetes is small and not worth the cost and inconvenience of collecting a timed sample (Ewald 2004). Early renal damage may not always be detected because diabetes-induced nephron hypertrophy maintains the glomerular filtration rate and an elevated plasma creatinine concentration is a relatively late manifestation of diabetic nephropathy. Anemia occurs more frequently, however, in individuals with diabetes and may be an early sign (Ritz 2005, Khoshdel 2008).

Treatment. Tight glycemic and blood pressure management may delay progression of microalbuminuria (Klein 1993, John 1994), along with exercise and dietary changes (Fredrickson 2004, Lazarevic 2007). Smoking cessation in newly diagnosed individuals with T2D also has been shown to ameliorate metabolic parameters, blood pressure, and levels of microalbuminuria (Voulgari 2011). Accordingly, use of current therapies to maintain good glycemic control, strict blood pressure management, and adequate blood lipid levels, along with adoption of lifestyle measures like regular exercise, optimization of diet, and smoking cessation, may help to reduce oxidative stress and endothelial cell dysfunction and retard the progression of microalbuminuria to diabetic nephropathy (Singh 2011). In fact, it has been suggested that individuals with microalbuminuria receive antihypertensive treatment, even those with normal blood pressure (Mogensen 2008). In addition, inhibition of the renal angiotensin aldosterone system with use of ACE inhibitors and ARBs is considered to be renal protective for many with diabetes, even before the onset of microalbuminuria (Mogensen 2003, Newman 2005, Sarafidis 2008).

NEPHROPATHY

Progressive nephropathy represents a substantial source of morbidity and mortality in people with diabetes. Increasing albuminuria is a strong predictor of progressive renal dysfunction and heightened cardiovascular risk (Lin 2008). Overt nephropathy is defined by gross proteinuria, or >200 mcg/min of albumin in urine. It is the next stage in progression of diabetic kidney disease and is considered more severe than microalbuminuria. In individuals with type 1 diabetes (T1D), inflammation and endothelial dysfunction are both considered to play a role in the development of gross proteinuria and diabetic nephropathy (Sahakyan 2010).

Treatment. Use of ACE inhibitors and ARBs is recommended to preserve kidney function at this stage of progression (Sarafidis 2008). ARBs reduce proteinuria, independent of the degree of proteinuria and of underlying disease. Reduction in proteinuria from either ARBs or ACE inhibitors is similar, and their combination has been shown to be more effective in reducing daily proteinuria, at least in the short term, but without always resulting in concomitant improvement in glomerular filtration rates (Cheng 2012, Jennings 2007). Some evidence suggests that the combination also may increase the risk of hyperkalemia (elevated potassium levels). On an alternative note, there is growing evidence that lipid abnormalities may be a risk factor for renal disease and that statin use may confer a renoprotective effect by reducing proteinuria and the rate of decline of renal function (Kshirsagar 2000, Agarwal 2005, Cases 2005).

Other combinations of treatments may reduce kidney stress as well. They may include a salt- or protein-restrictive diet, use of diuretics (furosemide, spironolactone), additional antihypertensives (besides ACE inhibitors and ARBs), body weight reduction, and cessation of cigarette smoking. In individuals with more advanced kidney dysfunction, correction of hyperkalaemia and metabolic acidosis may be necessary, along with intake of vitamin D supplements and erythropoietin for the correction of mineral metabolism disorders and anemia, respectively (Schena 2011).

END-STAGE RENAL DISEASE

Once an individual reaches the stage at which the kidneys can no longer function properly, fluids and waste products begin to build up in the body, causing swelling in the hands, feet, abdomen, or face. The body's production of red blood cells can be compromised due to a lesser release of erythropoietin, a hormone normally produced by the kidney that promotes the formation of red blood cells in the bone marrow. Anemia is a frequent complication of diabetic nephropathy; however, it only recently has been recognized that anemia is seen not only in preterminal renal failure, but also frequently when only minor derangement of renal function is present (Ritz 2005). In reality, at any level of glomerular filtration, anemia is more frequent and severe in diabetic compared with nondiabetic individuals. A major cause of anemia is an inappropriate release of erythropoietin by the kidney, combined with iron deficiency and the use of ACE inhibitors (Ritz 2005).

Upon progressing to end-stage renal disease (i.e., stage 5 chronic kidney disease), people must go on dialysis, either hemodialysis or peritoneal dialysis, or receive a new kidney through transplantation to stay alive. Some individuals with T1D or T2D undergoing kidney transplantation may elect to receive a new pancreas at the same time that can reverse their diabetic state (Wiseman 2012a, 2012b). Other short-term treatments to reduce stress on the kidneys are the same as those advised for less severe kidney dysfunction (Schena 2011).

PHYSICAL ACTIVITY PARTICIPATION WITH NEPHROPATHY AND END-STAGE RENAL DISEASE

Individuals with progressive renal dysfunction are at increased risk for hypoglycemia for multifactorial reasons. Insulin and, to some degree, the incretin hormones are eliminated more slowly, as are antihyperglycemic drugs with renal excretion (such as metformin, all DPP-4 inhibitors except for linagliptin, and most insulin secretagogues) (Inzucchi 2012). In addition, individuals with greater kidney dysfunction likely will be taking insulin in place of other medications (e.g., metformin, glyburide) that are contraindicated in such cases, and more severe renal functional impairment is associated with slower elimination of all insulins. Thus, dose reductions of insulin may be necessary, especially with exercise as an added variable affecting blood glucose levels, and more frequent self-monitoring of blood glucose likely is warranted.

MICROALBUMINURIA AND NEPHROPATHY

Although an acute bout of exercise has been shown to transiently increase postexercise levels of urinary albumin even in normoalbuminuric individuals with diabetes and no evidence of kidney disease (with a possible greater effect in women than in men) (Newman 2000), physical activity does not appear to otherwise worsen kidney function (Koh 2011). The presence of microabuminuria per se does not necessitate exercise restrictions.

Pre-exercise screening. Before initiation of physical activity participation, individuals with overt nephropathy should be screened carefully, have physician approval, and possibly undergo stress testing to detect coronary artery disease (CAD) and abnormal heart rate and blood pressure responses (Colberg 2010).

Exercise type. Both aerobic and resistance training improve physical function and quality of life in individuals with kidney disease (Painter 2000a, 2000b; Johansen 2005). Resistance exercise training is especially effective in improving muscle function and activities of daily living, which normally are affected severely by late-stage kidney disease (Johansen 2005).

Exercise intensity. The intensity of physical activity is the main consideration of the exercise prescription when nephropathy is present because of the linear association of the blood pressure response to intensity. As the workload being performed increases, the blood pressure response also rises. Light to moderate physical activity, with an acceptable blood pressure response, generally is considered safe and beneficial in those who have nephropathy or microalbuminuria. For anyone with overt nephropathy or gross proteinuria, strenuous physical activity is not prudent because of the exaggerated blood pressure response usually experienced by such individuals.

Individuals with nephropathy should begin physical activity at a low intensity and volume because their aerobic capacity and muscle function are substantially reduced (Colberg 2010). If an individual is in the later stages of kidney disease, intense exercise usually is not recommended because of limited exercise capacity. Avoidance of the Valsalva maneuver or high-intensity exercise to prevent excessive increases in blood pressure is advised (Colberg 2010).

Anemia considerations. Moreover, anemia is more common in individuals at any stage of kidney disease and may result in symptoms of chronic tiredness and a lim-

Table 21.1 Physical Activity Considerations with Nephropathy

Increased Risk of	Physical Activity	Points to Consider
Bone disease	Strength training program	■ Promote bone strength ■ Improve balance and gait ■ Reduce risk of falls and fractures
Hypertension or exaggerated blood pressure response to physical activity	Avoid or modify physical activities that cause extreme increases in systolic blood pressure	■ Monitor blood pressure ■ Adjust medications as needed to keep resting and exercise blood pressure in desired ranges
Edema	As tolerated	■ Provide instruction for dietary and fluid intake to minimize peripheral edema ■ Foot elevation or use of compression stockings may help
Anemia	As tolerated	■ Treat as needed with erythropoietin and iron supplementation ■ Keep hematocrit levels between 33% and 36%
Loss of independence	Promote physically active lifestyle	■ Increase ability to maintain activities of daily living ■ May limit dependence on others as disease progresses
Depression	Promote physically active lifestyle	■ Provide a level of protection from depression, hopelessness, and feelings of doom associated with more severe stages of kidney disease

ited ability to participate in physical activities. Its treatment with administration of erythropoietin and iron supplementation may be necessary to reverse anemia and optimize physical activity participation (Ritz 2005, Khoshdel 2008).

END-STAGE RENAL DISEASE

Individuals in the final stage of chronic kidney disease usually have low functional and aerobic capacity. Aerobic activities are preferred, but the individual's degree of kidney impairment dictates his or her ability to perform aerobic activity. Individuals who are weak can benefit from strength-training interventions. Resistance and aerobic exercise programs should be initiated at relatively low intensity and progressed slowly as tolerated to avoid injury and discontinuation of exercise.

Exercise and dialysis. Light to moderate exercise is recommended even for patients on dialysis (Table 21.2). Exercise training increases physical function and quality of life in individuals with kidney disease and may even be undertaken during dialysis sessions. Supervised, moderate aerobic exercise undertaken during dialysis sessions is as effective as home-based exercise and may improve compliance (Johansen 2005, Koh 2010). A yoga-based exercise program has been shown to improve measures of pain, fatigue, sleep disturbance, and biochemical markers in hemodialysis patients (Yurtkuran 2007).

If an individual requires dialysis, exercise is contraindicated if the blood levels of hematocrit, calcium, potassium, or magnesium become unbalanced as a result of the treatments. Certain treatments have been shown to decrease serum magnesium levels and result in hypotension (Pakfetrat 2010), particularly when acetate dialysate is used instead of bicarbonate dialysate, indicating that care must be taken to avoid such occurrences if exercise is undertaken (Thaha 2005, Elsharkawy 2006).

In a recent study involving 8 weeks of intradialysis exercise consisting of 15 min of low-intensity aerobic exercise undertaken during the first 2 hours of dialysis, significant and beneficial decreases were found in serum phosphate and potassium levels while serum calcium and hemoglobin levels did not change significantly. Thus, aerobic exercise is a complementary, safe, and effective clinical treatment modality in individuals with end-stage renal disease undergoing dialysis treatments (Makhlough 2012).

Exercise post–kidney transplant surgery. Individuals who have undergone kidney transplants can safely restart exercise training 6–8 weeks after surgery, once they are stable and free of signs of rejection of the new kidney.

Table 21.2 Exercise Recommendations for End-Stage Renal Disease

- Individuals should begin aerobic activity at a low level, perhaps using interval work, followed by gradual increases in their activity plan
- Have individuals progress over time to brisk walking, swimming, and cycling activities, as well as resistance training to improve strength
- Individuals on dialysis may incorporate low or moderate aerobic exercise into the dialysis session to increase participation and tolerance
- Post–kidney transplant, individuals may restart exercise 6–8 weeks following surgery, as long as no signs of rejection of the new kidney are present

EXERCISE-INDUCED MICROALBUMINURIA

Acute exercise, particularly when more intense, has been shown to transiently increase postexercise levels of urinary albumin even in normoalbuminuric individuals with no evidence of kidney disease (Newman 2000). In one study on youth with T1D ages 10 to 18 years, postexercise microalbuminuria exceeded normal values in nine individuals exercising at 100% of maximum, but only in seven and three undergoing exercise at 80% or 60% of maximum, respectively. Thus, it appears that postexercise microalbuminuria increases with exercise intensity; it is also associated with sex, body composition, and fitness levels. The prognostic significance of transient microalbuminuria induced by intense exercise in youth with T1D is not known, however (Kornhauser 2010).

Case in Point: Wrap-Up

To begin doing more planned activities, PD met with her health-care provider to get her input on where to start. Because PD exhibits signs of anemia, her provider started her on an appropriate treatment to raise her red blood cell count. The provider also suggested that she partake in the intradialysis exercise training program that is available in the dialysis center that PD uses.

Exercise Program Goals

Mode of Activity: PD's current low fitness level and general fatigue necessitate that she start with low-level aerobic activities, such as treadmill walking, stationary cycling, seated exercises, or possibly aquatic walking or other activities. Doing some light resistance training with bands, hand weights, or household items is also recommended for her as a place to start building her strength. PD plans to start by doing either walking or cycling in the dialysis center during her treatments.

Intensity: Given that mild to moderate activity can be done by anyone with kidney disease, PD should avoid going over the "somewhat hard" range of training. Her heart rate likely will go higher until her anemia is under control, so using heart rate as a guide is not important at this point. Similarly, her resistance work should feel light at this point.

Frequency: Ideally, PD should engage in at least 3–5 days of aerobic training weekly and not let >2 days lapse between workout sessions to optimize both her blood glucose and blood pressure management. Once she is feeling stronger as a result of anemia treatment, she can start with light resistance work 2 days/week using resistance bands or hand weights at home.

Duration: To start, PD can engage in shorter bouts of exercise training (i.e., 5–10 min at a time), separated by rest periods, with a goal of being able to train continuously for 20–30 min/session. Although an ideal training goal is 150 min of physical activity spread throughout the week, PD should focus more on doing what she can at this point, given her need for dialysis. Any activity is better than none, and everything she does will benefit her.

Progression: With end-stage renal disease and dialysis as major limiting factors, PD should focus primarily on increasing the duration of her structured workouts to increase her endurance capacity, physical function, and quality of life. Increases in intensity are not likely to be well tolerated and are not advised, although an increase in training frequency is a possible goal. She may progress to doing resistance exercise three times per week.

Possible Precautions: DP's use of even just basal insulin requires that she be made aware of the possibility of exercise-induced hypoglycemia and have readily absorbed carbohydrates available. In addition, she should be aware that there is a possibility of dialysis-induced hypotension; her fluid intake restrictions may need to be monitored carefully to avoid dehydration and hypotension. In addition, she should continue having her hematocrit levels tested and anemia treated while on dialysis. She should have her electrolyte levels monitored and treated if they should become unbalanced by dialysis treatments.

The development of kidney problems related to long-standing diabetes is fairly prevalent in individuals with both main types of diabetes. Physical activity participation is possible—even when undergoing dialysis treatments—and should be encouraged for individuals with any level of diagnosed kidney disease to help manage blood glucose and blood pressure level to possibly prevent or delay disease progression.

PROFESSIONAL PRACTICE PEARLS

- Diabetic nephropathy, varying from microalbuminuria to end-stage renal failure, develops in ~30% of individuals with diabetes and is a major mortality risk factor.
- Minute amounts of albumin in the urine is the main characteristic of microalbuminuria and is a common risk factor for overt nephropathy (gross proteinuria).
- Use of blockers of the renin-angiontensin system, including ACE inhibitors and ARBs, is also recommended to preserve kidney function at all stages of disease progression.
- Anemia occurs more frequently in individuals with diabetes and may be an early sign of kidney damage; in more severe disease, it requires treatment to restore hematocrit levels.
- Upon progressing to stage 5 chronic kidney disease, people must go on hemodialysis or peritoneal dialysis or receive a new kidney through transplantation to stay alive.
- Individuals with overt nephropathy frequently exhibit a diminished capacity for exercise, resulting in a self-limitation from physical activity.
- Both aerobic and resistance training improve physical function and quality of life in individuals with kidney disease and are recommended for all stages of disease.
- The presence of microalbuminuria does not require physical activity restrictions; however, individuals with overt nephropathy should be screened carefully, have physician approval, and possibly undergo stress testing before starting exercise.
- Light to moderate physical activity, with an acceptable blood pressure response, generally is considered safe and beneficial in those with nephropathy or microalbuminuria.
- Avoidance of the Valsalva maneuver or high-intensity exercise to prevent excessive increases in blood pressure is advised.
- Light to moderate exercise is recommended even for patients on dialysis and can be undertaken during dialysis treatments to increase compliance.
- Exercise is contraindicated if the blood levels of hematocrit, calcium, potassium, or magnesium become unbalanced as a result of dialysis treatments.

REFERENCES

Agarwal R, Curley TM: The role of statins in chronic kidney disease. *Am J Med Sci* 330:69–81, 2005

Astrup AS, Tarnow L, Pietraszek L, Schalkwijk CG, Stehouwer CD, Parving HH, Rossing P: Markers of endothelial dysfunction and inflammation in type 1 diabetic patients with or without diabetic nephropathy followed for 10 years: association with mortality and decline of glomerular filtration rate. *Diabetes Care* 31:1170–1176, 2008

Bagshaw SM, Cruz DN: Fluid overload as a biomarker of heart failure and acute kidney injury. *Contrib Nephrol* 164:54–68, 2010

Bo S, Ciccone G, Rosato R, Gancia R, Grassi G, Merletti F, Pagano GF: Renal damage in patients with type 2 diabetes: a strong predictor of mortality. *Diabet Med* 22:258–265, 2005

Cases A, Coll E: Dyslipidemia and the progression of renal disease in chronic renal failure patients. *Kidney Int Suppl* 99:S87–S93, 2005

Cheng J, Zhang X, Tian J, Li Q, Chen J: Combination therapy an ACE inhibitor and an angiotensin receptor blocker for IgA nephropathy: a meta-analysis. *Int J Clin Pract* 66:917–923, 2012

Coccheri S: Approaches to prevention of cardiovascular complications and events in diabetes mellitus. *Drugs* 67:997–1026, 2007

Colberg SR, Sigal RJ, Fernhall B, Regensteiner JG, Blissmer BJ, Rubin RR, Chasan-Taber L, Albright AL, Braun B, American College of Sports Medicine, American Diabetes Association: Exercise and type 2 diabetes: the American College of Sports Medicine and the American Diabetes Association: joint position statement. *Diabetes Care* 33:e147–e167, 2010

Elsharkawy MM, Youssef AM, Zayoon MY: Intradialytic changes of serum magnesium and their relation to hypotensive episodes in hemodialysis patients on different dialysates. *Hemodial Int* 10 (Suppl. 2):S16–S23, 2006

Ewald B, Attia J: Which test to detect microalbuminuria in diabetic patients? A systematic review. *Aust Fam Physician* 33:565–567, 571, 2004

Fredrickson SK, Ferro TJ, Schutrumpf AC: Disappearance of microalbuminuria in a patient with type 2 diabetes and the metabolic syndrome in the setting of an intense exercise and dietary program with sustained weight reduction. *Diabetes Care* 27:1754–1755, 2004

Ghosh S, Khazaei M, Moien-Afshari F, Ang LS, Granville DJ, Verchere CB, Dunn SR, McCue P, Mizisin A, Sharma K, Laher I: Moderate exercise attenuates caspase-3 activity, oxidative stress, and inhibits progression of diabetic renal disease in db/db mice. *Am J Physiol Renal Physiol* 296:F700–F708, 2009

Gimeno Orna JA, Boned Juliani B, Lou Arnal LM, Castro Alonso FJ: Microalbuminuria and clinical proteinuria as the main predictive factors of cardiovascular morbidity and mortality in patients with type 2 diabetes. *Rev Clin Esp* 203:526–531, 2003

Inzucchi SE, Bergenstal RM, Buse JB, Diamant M, Ferrannini E, Nauck M, Peters AL, Tsapas A, Wender R, Matthews DR: Management of hyperglycaemia in type 2 diabetes: a patient-centered approach. Position statement of the American Diabetes Association (ADA) and the European Association for the Study of Diabetes (EASD). *Diabetologia* 55:1577–1596, 2012

Ishani A, Paudel M, Taylor BC, Barrett-Connor E, Jamal S, Canales M, Steffes M, Fink HA, Orwoll E, Cummings SR, Ensrud KE, Osteoporotic Fractures in Men Study Group: Renal function and rate of hip bone loss in older men: the Osteoporotic Fractures in Men Study. *Osteoporos Int* 19:1549–1556, 2008

Jamal SA, Swan VJ, Brown JP, Hanley DA, Prior JC, Papaioannou A, Langsetmo L, Josse RG, Canadian Multicentre Osteoporosis Study Research Group: Kidney function and rate of bone loss at the hip and spine: the Canadian Multicentre Osteoporosis Study. *Am J Kidney Dis* 55:291–299, 2010

Jennings DL, Kalus JS, Coleman CI, Manierski C, Yee J: Combination therapy with an ACE inhibitor and an angiotensin receptor blocker for diabetic nephropathy: a meta-analysis. *Diabet Med* 24:486–493, 2007

Johansen KL: Exercise and chronic kidney disease: current recommendations. *Sports Med* 35:485–499, 2005

John L, Rao PS, Kanagasabapathy AS: Rate of progression of albuminuria in type II diabetes: five-year prospective study from south India. *Diabetes Care* 17:888–890, 1994

Khoshdel A, Carney S, Gillies A, Mourad A, Jones B, Nanra R, Trevillian P: Potential roles of erythropoietin in the management of anaemia and other complications diabetes. *Diabetes Obes Metab* 10:1–9, 2008

Klein R, Klein BE, Moss SE: Prevalence of microalbuminuria in older-onset diabetes. *Diabetes Care* 16:1325–1330, 1993

Koh KH, Dayanath B, Doery JC, Polkinghorne KR, Teede H, Kerr PG: Effect of exercise on albuminuria in people with diabetes. *Nephrology (Carlton)* 16:704–709, 2011

Koh KP, Fassett RG, Sharman JE, Coombes JS, Williams AD: Effect of intradialytic versus home-based aerobic exercise training on physical function and vascular parameters in hemodialysis patients: a randomized pilot study. *Am J Kidney Dis* 55:88–99, 2010

Kornhauser C, Malacara JM, Macias-Cervantes MH, Rivera-Cisneros AE: Effect of exercise intensity on albuminuria in adolescents with type 1 diabetes mellitus. *Diabet Med* 29:70–73, 2010

Koro CE, Lee BH, Bowlin SJ: Antidiabetic medication use and prevalence of chronic kidney disease among patients with type 2 diabetes mellitus in the United States. *Clin Ther* 31:2608–2617, 2009

Kshirsagar AV, Joy MS, Hogan SL, Falk RJ, Colindres RE: Effect of ACE inhibitors in diabetic and nondiabetic chronic renal disease: a systematic overview of randomized placebo-controlled trials. *Am J Kidney Dis* 35:695–707, 2000

Lazarevic G, Antic S, Vlahovic P, Djordjevic V, Zvezdanovic L, Stefanovic V: Effects of aerobic exercise on microalbuminuria and enzymuria in type 2 diabetic patients. *Ren Fail* 29:199–205, 2007

Lin J, Glynn RJ, Rifai N, Manson JE, Ridker PM, Nathan DM, Schaumberg DA: Inflammation and progressive nephropathy in type 1 diabetes in the Diabetes Control and Complications Trial. *Diabetes Care* 31:2338–2343, 2008

Makhlough A, Ilali E, Mohseni R, Shahmohammadi S: Effect of intradialytic aerobic exercise on serum electrolytes levels in hemodialysis patients. *Iran J Kidney Dis* 6:119–123, 2012

Mogensen CE: Microalbuminuria and hypertension with focus on type 1 and type 2 diabetes. *J Intern Med* 254:45–66, 2003

Mogensen CE: Twelve shifting paradigms in diabetic renal disease and hypertension. *Diabetes Res Clin Pract* 82 (Suppl. 1):S2–S9, 2008

Negrean M, Stirban A, Stratmann B, Gawlowski T, Horstmann T, Gotting C, Kleesiek K, Mueller-Roesel M, Koschinsky T, Uribarri J, Vlassara H, Tschoepe D: Effects of low- and high-advanced glycation endproduct meals on macro- and microvascular endothelial function and oxidative stress in patients with type 2 diabetes mellitus. *Am J Clin Nutr* 85:1236–1243, 2007

Newman DJ, Mattock MB, Dawnay AB, Kerry S, McGuire A, Yaqoob M, Hitman GA, Hawke C: Systematic review on urine albumin testing for early detection of diabetic complications. *Health Technol Assess* 9:iii–vi, xiii–163, 2005

Newman DJ, Pugia MJ, Lott JA, Wallace JF, Hiar AM: Urinary protein and albumin excretion corrected by creatinine and specific gravity. *Clin Chim Acta* 294:139–155, 2000

Painter P, Carlson L, Carey S, Paul SM, Myll J: Low-functioning hemodialysis patients improve with exercise training. *Am J Kidney Dis* 36:600–608, 2000a

Painter P, Carlson L, Carey S, Paul SM, Myll J: Physical functioning and health-related quality-of-life changes with exercise training in hemodialysis patients. *Am J Kidney Dis* 35:482–492, 2000b

Pakfetrat M, Roozbeh Shahroodi J, Malekmakan L, Zare N, Hashemi Nasab M, Hossein Nikoo M: Is there an association between intradialytic hypotension and serum magnesium changes? *Hemodial Int* 14:492–497, 2010

Ritz E, Haxsen V: Diabetic nephropathy and anaemia. *Eur J Clin Invest* 35 (Suppl. 3):66–74, 2005

Sahakyan K, Klein BE, Lee KE, Tsai MY, Klein R: Inflammatory and endothelial dysfunction markers and proteinuria in persons with type 1 diabetes mellitus. *Eur J Endocrinol* 162:1101–1105, 2010

Sarafidis PA, Stafylas PC, Kanaki AI, Lasaridis AN: Effects of renin-angiotensin system blockers on renal outcomes and all-cause mortality in patients with diabetic nephropathy: an updated meta-analysis. *Am J Hypertens* 21:922–929, 2008

Schena FP: Management of patients with chronic kidney disease. *Intern Emerg Med* 6 (Suppl. 1):77–83, 2011

Singh DK, Winocour P, Farrington K: Oxidative stress in early diabetic nephropathy: fueling the fire. *Nat Rev Endocrinol* 7:176–184, 2011

Thaha M, Yogiantoro M, Soewanto, Pranawa: Correlation between intradialytic hypotension in patients undergoing routine hemodialysis and use of acetate compared in bicarbonate dialysate. *Acta Med Indones* 37:145–148, 2005

Tufescu A, Kanazawa M, Ishida A, Lu H, Sasaki Y, Ootaka T, Sato T, Kohzuki M: Combination of exercise and losartan enhances renoprotective and peripheral effects in spontaneously type 2 diabetes mellitus rats with nephropathy. *J Hypertens* 26:312–321, 2008

Valmadrid CT, Klein R, Moss SE, Klein BE: The risk of cardiovascular disease mortality associated with microalbuminuria and gross proteinuria in persons with older-onset diabetes mellitus. *Arch Intern Med* 160:1093–1100, 2000

Voulgari C, Katsilambros N, Tentolouris N: Smoking cessation predicts amelioration of microalbuminuria in newly diagnosed type 2 diabetes mellitus: a 1-year prospective study. *Metabolism* 60:1456–1464, 2011

Wiseman AC: Pancreas transplant options for patients with type 1 diabetes mellitus and chronic kidney disease: simultaneous pancreas kidney or pancreas after kidney? *Curr Opin Organ Transplant* 17:80–86, 2012a

Wiseman AC, Gralla J: Simultaneous pancreas kidney transplant versus other kidney transplant options in patients with type 2 diabetes. *Clin J Am Soc Nephrol* 7:656–664, 2012b

Yurtkuran M, Alp A, Dilek K: A modified yoga-based exercise program in hemodialysis patients: a randomized controlled study. *Complement Ther Med* 15:164–171, 2007

Chapter 22

Female-Only Concerns and Pregnancy with Preexisting Diabetes

W omen with type 1 diabetes (T1D) or type 2 diabetes (T2D) have to deal with hormonal fluctuations resulting from their monthly menstrual cycles, and during pregnancy, that can make diabetes management more challenging (Yeung 2010). Even use of oral contraceptives can alter the normal hormonal changes in diabetic women (Sacerdote 1982, Cheang 2011). For any women with preexisting diabetes, optimizing blood glucose levels before and during early pregnancy can reduce the risks of fetal and maternal complications dramatically (Kinsley 2007). Being physically active throughout pregnancy both enhances insulin action in the mother (Young 1992, Wolfe 2003a) and limits her possible weight gain (Negrato 2009) and is recommended, with some adjustments to prevent injury or complications.

Case in Point: Exercise Rx for a Pregnant Woman with T1D

OS is a 29-year-old woman who has had T1D for 11 years and is planning to get pregnant for the first time. She has heard stories and worries about the possibility of having a baby with a birth defect due to her diabetes, and she is concerned that she may give her child T1D. She considers herself normally active—working out maybe 3 days/week doing aerobic dance classes—but she is not sure what type of activities she will be allowed to do during pregnancy with her diabetes; besides, everyone she knows stopped working out while pregnant. Her current medications include insulin lispro (Humalog) delivered via insulin pump.

Resting Measurements

Height: 66 inches
Weight: 132 lb (prepregnancy)
BMI: 21.3 (normal)
Heart rate: 77 beats per minute (bpm)
Blood pressure: 115/75 mmHg

Fasting Labs

Plasma glucose: variable (65–240 mg/dl; controlled with an insulin pump)
A1C: 6.6%
Cholesterol: good when last checked (2–3 years previously)

Questions to Consider

1. What type of exercise can OS safely engage in before getting pregnant and during her pregnancy?
2. What are an appropriate exercise frequency, intensity, and duration?
3. How should her exercise training progress during her pregnancy and after giving birth?
4. What precautions should OS take, and does she have any exercise limitations?

(Continued on page 416.)

FEMALE-ONLY CONCERNS

Changes in fluxes of female hormones in nonpregnant women and, additionally, placental hormones during pregnancy can have a large impact on insulin action (Wolfe 2003a, Yeung 2010, Newbern 2011). Such changes lead to difficulties in regulating glycemia, particularly in women who require insulin. A better understanding of the effects of these hormones, however, can make diabetes management less challenging for diabetic women.

MENSTRUAL CYCLE EFFECTS ON INSULIN ACTION

The normal female menstrual cycle has a follicular phase, which goes from the start of menses up to ovulation at midcycle, and a luteal phase, spanning the time from ovulation to the next menses. Women are more insulin resistant during the luteal phase because of greater release of certain female hormones (estradiol and progesterone in particular) during that time (Yeung 2010). Given that menstrual cycles in a given woman may vary in length and the fact that it may take several days for individuals using long-acting basal insulin to achieve a steady state with regard to any dosage adjustment, it is difficult to design an insulin regimen that maintains euglycemia throughout the menstrual cycle, particularly in labile patients (Sacerdote 1982). Such changes can particularly affect women with T1D and introduce an additional factor to balance in achieving balanced blood glucose levels with an active lifestyle.

CONTRACEPTIVE EFFECTS ON GLYCEMIC CONTROL

Use of oral contraceptives can alter the normal hormonal changes in diabetic women as well. Most of these pills or treatments currently are formulated with low-dose estrogen and progestin and may have divergent effects on insulin action in lean versus obese women (Cheang 2011). Even if their effect is to elevate insulin resistance as has been reported (Spellacy 1988), because they prevent ovulation and modulate hormone release, their effect on glycemic control may be more consistent over the monthly cycle, leading to greater predictability and easier glucose control. In fact, such contraceptive use has been reported to abolish luteal phase exacerbation of hyperglycemia in young women with T1D (Sacerdote 1982).

PREGNANCY CONSIDERATIONS WITH PREEXISTING DIABETES

Women with diabetes that predates the pregnancy may have either T1D or T2D. The prevalence of pregestational diabetes of either type is rising rapidly, mostly due to increases in T2D among younger women (Bell 2008). Having diabetes before and throughout pregnancy requires that individuals place their emphasis on maintaining blood glucose control throughout the entire process, optimally starting well before conception. Because gestational diabetes mellitus (GDM) usually is diagnosed at 24–28 weeks of gestation with an oral glucose challenge (American Diabetes Association 2013a, 2013b), it is addressed separately in chapter 7.

CONSEQUENCES OF POOR GLYCEMIC CONTROL DURING PREGNANCY

Poorly controlled diabetes before conception and during pregnancy among women with preexisting diabetes can cause major birth defects in offspring and spontaneous abortions, as well as abnormal fetal growth and development (e.g., macrosomia, or "big baby syndrome"). In one study in the U.K., ethnicity was found to have a significant impact on the outcome of diabetic pregnancies, with worse outcomes for babies born to Asian mothers compared with Caucasian, although the use of insulin prepregnancy rather than type of diabetes appeared to predict adverse outcomes (Verheijen 2005). In a meta-analysis, however, women with T2D had no better perinatal outcomes despite lower glycemic levels than T1D, indicating that T2D in pregnancy should still be considered a serious condition worthy of frequent glucose monitoring and maintenance of strict glycemic control (Balsells 2009).

BENEFITS OF OPTIMIZATION OF BLOOD GLUCOSE LEVELS

Optimal glycemic control from preconception through pregnancy can reduce the risk of maternal and fetal complications in women with diabetes (Kinsley 2007). The risk of fetal congenital abnormalities in pregnant women with diabetes of any type is related intricately to the level of glycemic control in early pregnancy; thus, attainment of strict glycemic targets as close to normal as possible throughout pregnancy should be attempted (Kinsley 2007). Moreover, regular physical activity has been proven to result in marked benefits for mother and fetus. Maternal benefits include improved cardiovascular function, limited pregnancy weight gain, decreased musculoskeletal discomfort, reduced incidence of muscle cramps and lower limb edema, mood stability, and attenuation of GDM and gestational hypertension (Melzer 2010). Fetal benefits include decreased fat mass, improved stress tolerance, and advanced neurobehavioral maturation. In addition, physical activity throughout pregnancy usually results in shorter active labor and decreased incidence of operative delivery (Melzer 2010).

A substantial proportion of women stop exercising after they discover they are pregnant, however, and only few begin participating in exercise activities during pregnancy. The adoption or continuation of a sedentary lifestyle during pregnancy may contribute to the development of certain disorders during and after pregnancy, such as preeclampsia, dyspnea, hypertension, and maternal and childhood obesity. The exaggerated release of placental hormones during pregnancy, including placental growth hormone and others, results in insulin resistance and causes overall insulin requirements to increase during pregnancy (Newbern 2011). A greater release of these hormones during the third trimester, in particular, spares the mother's blood glucose for the fetus by increasing her insulin resistance. Fortunately, physical activity conveys similar benefits to insulin action in pregnant and nonpregnant women (Gradmark 2011).

AVOIDANCE OF SEVERE HYPOGLYCEMIA DURING PREGNANCY

Avoidance of severe hyperglycemia is essential in optimizing pregnancy outcomes in mothers with diabetes; however, for women using insulin, tight control increases their risk for experiencing severe hypoglycemia that requires outside assistance to treat. Blood glucose treatment targets differ considerably between clinics, with some advocating lower glycemic limits in the range of 60 mg/dl (3.33 mmol/l). Women, however, need to be aware that such vastly improved glycemic control or recurrent hypoglycemia may impair glucose counterregulatory responses and that those responses may be altered by pregnancy itself (ter Braak 2002).

In results from three trials with 223 women and their babies (i.e., limited data), few differences in outcomes were seen between very tight (60–90 mg/dl, or 3.33–5.0 mmol/L) and tight-moderate (80–115 mg/dl, or 4.45–6.38 mmol/l) glycemic control targets in pregnant women with preexisting T1D, including actual glycemic control achieved. Some evidence of harm (such as increased preeclampsia, cesarean deliveries, and birth weights >90th percentile) was found for looser control (fasting blood glucose >126 mg/dl, or 7 mmol/l) (Middleton 2012). Increased rates of macrosomia continue to be observed despite near-normal A1C levels, possibly in part because of rebound hyperglycemia elicited by hypoglycemia (ter Braak 2002). Furthermore, for women with T1D, the risk of severe hypoglycemia already is increased before pregnancy and increases during the first trimester. The most predictive factors of an episode during that time are prior severe hypoglycemia before pregnancy, longer duration of diabetes, an A1C level ≤6.5%, and a higher total daily insulin dose (Evers 2002).

PHYSICAL ACTIVITY PARTICIPATION BY PREGNANT WOMEN WITH PREEXISTING DIABETES

PHYSICAL ACTIVITY DURING PREGNANCY

Being physically active will minimize insulin requirements during pregnancy, even during the last trimester and regardless of the type of diabetes a woman has (Young 1992, Wolfe 2003a). Being active while pregnant also will prevent excessive weight gain, lower risk of new-onset hypertension (particularly preeclampsia) (Negrato 2009), and help maintain fitness levels (Wolfe 2003b). Increased total physical activity is associated with reduced fasting insulin levels in overweight or obese pregnant women (Liu 2010), and they can achieve and maintain recommended levels of physical activity throughout pregnancy. Interventions to promote activity should target changes in habitual activities at work and at home, in particular walking (McParlin 2010). If regular physical activity has been an integral part of a woman's diabetes regimen during pregnancy and she is forced to reduce or terminate participation, her insulin needs will increase, likely dramatically, both from the action of placental hormones that enhance insulin resistance and the decrease in insulin action with physical inactivity (Wolfe 2003a).

The energy expenditure required for any physical activity, especially weight-bearing activity, is increased during pregnancy (Melzer 2009). Regimen adjustments will be needed to maintain euglycemia despite an altered use of fuels during activity. Exercise intensity usually decreases naturally during the later stages of pregnancy as well, which may necessitate additional alterations in insulin or food intake for activities (Wolfe 2003b, Melzer 2009). For women using insulin, either before or just during pregnancy, insulin pump therapy is a viable option for insulin delivery. Pumps have the added advantage of allowing for rapid changes in basal insulin delivery compared with longer-acting basal insulin injections (Castorino 2012).

PHYSICAL ACTIVITY AFTER PREGNANCY

Postpartum exercise of any intensity should be encouraged as it can greatly reduce a new mother's risk for a whole host of chronic health problems, including obesity, cardiovascular disease, and metabolic syndrome (Davenport 2010). Moreover, moderate exercise during lactation does not affect the quantity or composition of breast milk or affect infant growth and should be encouraged to provide multiple positive health benefits to both mother and child (Davies 2003).

EXERCISE PRESCRIPTION FOR PREGNANT WOMEN

Women with preexisting diabetes during pregnancy are encouraged to engage in regular physical activity to help enhance insulin action. Pregnant women with diabetes generally can follow recommendations made for all pregnant women by the American College of Obstetricians and Gynecologists (Committee on Obstetric Practice 2002).

Frequency and intensity. Engaging in physical activity consistently makes blood glucose management easier in pregnant women with any type of diabetes. Engaging in 30 min of moderate-intensity exercise (e.g., brisk walking) during most days of the week (with a target of 2.5 h/week) has been adopted as a recommendation for pregnant women without medical or obstetrical complications (Committee on Obstetric Practice 2002). Women also can benefit from engaging in mild activities, although vigorous ones generally are not recommended during pregnancy unless women have already been engaging in them regularly. Recommended activities include moderate walking, indoor cycling, swimming and aquatic activities, low-impact aerobics, seated exercise routines, and mild or moderate resistance training (Physical Activity Guidelines Advisory Committee 2008). Women who habitually

Table 22.1 Exercise Intensity Guidelines for Women During Pregnancy and Postpartum

- Healthy women who are not already highly active or doing vigorous-intensity activity should get at least 150 min/week of moderate-intensity aerobic activity during pregnancy and the postpartum period, preferably spread throughout the week.
- Pregnant women who habitually engage in vigorous-intensity aerobic activity or who are highly active can continue physical activity during pregnancy and the postpartum period, provided that they remain healthy and discuss with their health-care provider how and when activity should be adjusted over time.

engage in vigorous or high amounts of activity or strength training preconception can continue these activities during pregnancy and after giving birth (Table 22.1).

EXERCISE MODIFICATIONS FOR PREGNANCY

Activities to limit or avoid. Most types of exercise are safe during pregnancy, although some involve positions and movements that may be uncomfortable, tiring, or harmful. After the first trimester of pregnancy, women should not engage in exercise that requires them to lie flat on their backs as doing so can reduce blood flow to the fetus (Committee on Obstetric Practice 2002). Standing still for long

Table 22.2 Physical Activity Modifications and Considerations for Pregnancy

- Women should engage in 30 min of moderate exercise most days of the week, aiming for a total of 150 min, starting out slowly if sedentary prepregnancy
- Running, certain racquet sports, and resistance training can be continued by women doing them before becoming pregnant, but they are not advisable as new activities during pregnancy
- Pregnant women should avoid contact sports, downhill skiing, scuba diving, and sports requiring quick directional changes, among others
- After the first trimester of pregnancy, individuals should avoid doing any exercise lying flat on their backs that can reduce blood flow to the fetus
- Individuals should wear comfortable clothing that will help them remain cool, along with a bra that fits well and provides adequate support
- All pregnant women should drink plenty of water during physical activities to help keep from overheating and dehydrating
- Individuals need to consume enough daily calories to replace those used during exercise
- Exercise done in hot, humid weather or with a fever should be avoided
- Women should stop exercising and call their health care provider if they develop symptoms during physical activity, including vaginal bleeding, dizziness, increased shortness of breath, chest pain, headache, muscle weakness, calf pain or swelling, uterine contractions, decreased fetal movement, or fluid leaking from the vagina

periods of time also should be avoided. They are advised to avoid certain activities, such as contact sports, activities requiring many directional changes (like racquetball), water skiing, scuba diving, and cycling outdoors (when balance becomes an issue) (Davies 2003). During the third trimester, women should consider substituting non–weight-bearing activities like aquatics and stationary cycling for running and jogging or excessive amounts of walking. Additional modifications and considerations are included in Table 22.2.

Safety considerations. Safety concerns for pregnant women revolve around prevention of falls, blows to the abdomen, or reduction of blood flow through the placenta. Physical activities that are done in environmental extremes are best

Table 22.3 Recommended Exercise Rx for Pregnant Women with Preexisting Diabetes

Mode	Aerobic: Walk, stationary cycle, swim, aquatic activities, conditioning machines, prenatal exercise classes, prenatal yoga, seated exercises, and possibly jogging/running (but only if already highly active prior to pregnancy)
	Resistance: Light to moderate resistance exercises
	Exercises to Avoid: Activities lying flat on the back and any that increase the risk of falling or abdominal trauma (e.g., contact or collision sports, horseback riding, downhill skiing, water skiing, soccer, outdoor cycling, basketball, most racquet sports, and scuba diving)
Intensity	Aerobic: If inactive: moderate-intensity aerobic activity (40–59% heart rate reserve [HRR] or "somewhat hard") during pregnancy and postpartum
	If already active or doing vigorous aerobic activity: moderate- to vigorous-intensity activity (40–89% HRR, or "somewhat hard" to "hard")
	Resistance: Start with light weights or lower resistance unless already doing moderate exercises prior to conception
Frequency	3–7 days, spread throughout the week
	Better done on most, if not all, days of the week for easier blood glucose management
	Can include aerobic training, resistance work, or a combination of both on any given day
Duration	30 min/session (range of 20–45 min)
	At least 150 min of moderate-intensity physical activity spread throughout the week (or possibly a lesser duration when exercise intensity is higher)
Progression	If just starting, increase duration of moderate exercise slowly; if already more active, maintain or lower intensity during pregnancy rather than attempting to progress to higher levels
	Resistance training will have to be modified to avoid any exercises lying flat on the back after the first trimester of pregnancy or that could cause loss of balance

avoided during pregnancy (Committee on Obstetric Practice 2002). Finally, the precautions to avoid hypoglycemia or hyperglycemia resulting from exercise are similar for pregnant and nonpregnant women, although insulin users will have to be more diligent about monitoring blood glucose levels and making appropriate changes in food intake or insulin when engaging in physical activities.

Case in Point: Wrap-Up

OS is able to talk with her endocrinologist about her prepregnancy concerns. She learns that most studies indicate that offspring of women with T1D have a ~2% risk of developing the disease. Getting her blood glucose into immaculate control *before* getting pregnant is also the best policy, given that most birth defects form in the very early stages of pregnancy (the first 4–6 weeks) when she may not even know she is pregnant. Her health-care provider encourages OS to join a diabetes preconception program at a local hospital, where she will go for weekly consultations and group discussions until she conceives. She also plans to increase her exercise to a daily routine to help her better manage her diabetes control, including physical activity as an integral part of this routine.

Exercise Program Goals

Mode of Activity: Because OS is somewhat physically active, she can continue doing the same activities she likes, including aerobic dance, but also broadening her choices to include brisk walking, swimming, stationary cycling, and conditioning machines. She should start doing some light resistance training (both lower- and upper-body exercises) before she conceives, if possible.

Intensity: OS should plan on doing moderate-intensity exercise that feels "somewhat hard" (5–7 on a 10-point scale) and not progress beyond that during pregnancy. Her target heart rate should be around 40–59% heart rate reserve (HRR) (123–144 bpm) to receive maximal glycemic and fitness benefits from her training, although engaging in lower intensities later in pregnancy is acceptable because of the increased energy costs associated with exercising late in pregnancy with a heavier body weight. Because she is new to resistance training, she should start with doing more repetitions with lighter weights until her strength begins to improve.

Frequency: Because it is easier to manage blood glucose levels with more frequent and consistent exercise patterns, OS should aim to do some type of training least 5–7 days/week, although some days may involve only aerobic training, others may include resistance training, or she may engage in a combination on any given day.

Duration: OS should try to do at least 20–30 min of activity daily, with a target goal of a minimum of 150 min of moderate physical activity spread throughout the week.

Progression: Although OS can engage in some harder intervals, for the majority of her pregnancy, she will need to limit herself to doing moderate physical activity. She should plan on progressing her exercise training after delivery, however, to including a mix of moderate and vigorous training of various types to lower her cardiovascular risk. In her case, she can do intense training for less time or moderate work for a longer duration.

Daily Movement: OS should engage in as much daily movement as possible to maximize her energy expenditure (to prevent excess weight gain during pregnancy) and to minimize the excursions in her blood glucose levels after eating. She should stand and take more daily steps throughout the day.

Possible Precautions: Other than having T1D for just over 10 years, OS has no other risk factors for cardiovascular issues. Also, she has been physically active, so doing a maximal exercise test at this point is unnecessary and would be contraindicated during pregnancy anyway. She will need to closely monitor her blood glucose levels, not only with exercise but at all times of the day to keep her postprandial values as low as possible. Learning how to do that before pregnancy is critical to effective management early in pregnancy (when she may not know she is pregnant). Most pregnant women with T1D experience at least one severe hypoglycemic event during pregnancy, so she should be prepared by having a glucagon kit available, and for treatment of other hypoglycemia, she should always be prepared with glucose or another readily absorbed carbohydrate source. Her basal insulin requirements may double or triple by the end of her pregnancy, meaning that she and her health-care provider will need to stay on top of her insulin needs throughout her pregnancy. She should be advised that immediately after giving birth, her insulin requirements may drop precipitously and will need to be adjusted back down. Breastfeeding her baby—which is best for both mother and child—will keep her caloric needs up and her insulin needs lower during the postpartum period.

Diabetes poses additional considerations for women, including the effects of normal menstrual cycle fluctuations and hormonal changes during pregnancy. Physical activity is beneficial in both cases, however, for managing insulin resistance and keeping insulin requirements lower. Exercise done during pregnancy bestows additional benefits related to management of body weight and avoidance of fitness declines with inactivity. Certain modifications for pregnancy likely will be necessary to ensure that participation is safe for the woman and her developing fetus.

PROFESSIONAL PRACTICE PEARLS

- Fluxes of female hormones in nonpregnant women and also of placental ones during pregnancy can have a large impact on insulin action.
- Having diabetes before and throughout pregnancy requires that individuals maintain blood glucose control throughout, optimally starting well before conception.
- The risk of fetal congenital defects born to women with diabetes is related to glycemic control in early pregnancy, although macrosomia and other problems can arise later.
- The energy expenditure required for any physical activity, especially weight-bearing activity, is increased during pregnancy.

■ Being physically active will minimize insulin requirements during pregnancy, even during the last trimester and regardless of the type of diabetes a woman has.

■ For women using insulin, either before or just during pregnancy, insulin pump therapy is a viable option for insulin delivery.

■ If a pregnant women has been engaging in regular physical activity during pregnancy and is forced to limit or stop her participation, her insulin needs will increase dramatically.

■ Postpartum exercise of any intensity should be encouraged as it can greatly reduce a new mother's risk for a host of chronic health problems.

■ Engaging in 30 min of moderate intensity physical activity on most days of the week, with a target of ≥150 min/week, is recommended.

■ Most moderate aerobic exercise is acceptable during pregnancy with pre-existing diabetes, although ones that increase risk of falls and traumatic injury should be avoided.

■ Women can benefit from engaging in mild activities, although vigorous ones generally are not recommended as a new endeavor during pregnancy.

■ Women who habitually engage in vigorous or high amounts of activity or strength training can continue these activities during pregnancy and after giving birth.

REFERENCES

American Diabetes Association: Diagnosis and classification of diabetes mellitus. *Diabetes Care* 36 (Suppl. 1):S67–S74, 2013a

American Diabetes Association: Standards of medical care in diabetes—2013. *Diabetes Care* 36 (Suppl. 1):S11–S66, 2013b

Balsells M, Garcia-Patterson A, Gich I, Corcoy R: Maternal and fetal outcome in women with type 2 versus type 1 diabetes mellitus: a systematic review and metaanalysis. *J Clin Endocrinol Metab* 94:4284–4291, 2009

Bell R, Bailey K, Cresswell T, Hawthorne G, Critchley J, Lewis-Barned N, Northern Diabetic Pregnancy Survey Steering Group: Trends in prevalence and outcomes of pregnancy in women with pre-existing type I and type II diabetes. *BJOG* 115:445–452, 2008

Castorino K, Paband R, Zisser H, Jovanovic L: Insulin pumps in pregnancy: using technology to achieve normoglycemia in women with diabetes. *Curr Diab Rep* 12:53–59, 2012

Cheang KI, Essah PA, Sharma S, Wickham EP III, Nestler JE: Divergent effects of a combined hormonal oral contraceptive on insulin sensitivity in lean versus obese women. *Fertil Steril* 96:353–359 e1, 2011

Committee on Obstetric Practice, American College of Obstetricians and Gynecologists.: ACOG committee opinion: exercise during pregnancy and the postpartum period. *Int J Gynaecol Obstet* 77:79–81, 2002

Davenport MH, Giroux I, Sopper MM, Mottola MF: Postpartum exercise regardless of intensity improves chronic disease risk factors. *Med Sci Sports Exerc* 43:951–958, 2010

Davies GA, Wolfe LA, Mottola MF, MacKinnon C, Arsenault MY, Bartellas E, Cargill Y, Gleason T, Iglesias S, Klein M, Martel MJ, Roggensack A, Wilson K, Gardiner P, Graham T, Haennel R, Hughson R, MacDougall D, McDermott J, Ross R, Tiidus P, Trudeau F, Canadian Society for Exercise Physiology Board of Directors SOGC Clinical Practice Obstetrics Committee: Exercise in pregnancy and the postpartum period. *J Obstet Gynaecol Can* 25:516–529, 2003

Evers IM, ter Braak EW, de Valk HW, van Der Schoot B, Janssen N, Visser GH: Risk indicators predictive for severe hypoglycemia during the first trimester of type 1 diabetic pregnancy. *Diabetes Care* 25:554–559, 2002

Gradmark A, Pomeroy J, Renstrom F, Steiginga S, Persson M, Wright A, Bluck L, Domellof M, Kahn SE, Mogren I, Franks PW: Physical activity, sedentary behaviors, and estimated insulin sensitivity and secretion in pregnant and nonpregnant women. *BMC Pregnancy Childbirth* 11:44, 2011

Kinsley B: Achieving better outcomes in pregnancies complicated by type 1 and type 2 diabetes mellitus. *Clin Ther* 29 (Suppl. D):S153–S160, 2007

Liu JH, Mayer-Davis EJ, Pate RR, Gallagher AE, Bacon JL: Physical activity during pregnancy is associated with reduced fasting insulin—the Pilot Pregnancy and Active Living Study. *J Matern Fetal Neonatal Med* 23:1249–1252, 2010

McParlin C, Robson SC, Tennant PW, Besson H, Rankin J, Adamson AJ, Pearce MS, Bell R: Objectively measured physical activity during pregnancy: a study in obese and overweight women. *BMC Pregnancy Childbirth* 10:76, 2010

Melzer K, Schutz Y, Boulvain M, Kayser B: Physical activity and pregnancy: cardiovascular adaptations, recommendations and pregnancy outcomes. *Sports Med* 40:493–507, 2010

Melzer K, Schutz Y, Boulvain M, Kayser B: Pregnancy-related changes in activity energy expenditure and resting metabolic rate in Switzerland. *Eur J Clin Nutr* 63:1185–1191, 2009

Middleton P, Crowther CA, Simmonds L: Different intensities of glycaemic control for pregnant women with pre-existing diabetes. *Cochrane Database Syst Rev* 8:CD008540, 2012

Negrato CA, Jovanovic L, Tambascia MA, Geloneze B, Dias A, Calderon Ide M, Rudge MV: Association between insulin resistance, glucose intolerance, and hypertension in pregnancy. *Metab Syndr Relat Disord* 7:53–59, 2009

Newbern D, Freemark M: Placental hormones and the control of maternal metabolism and fetal growth. *Curr Opin Endocrinol Diabetes Obes* 18:409–416, 2011

Physical Activity Guidelines Advisory Committee: Physical Activity Guidelines Advisory Committee Report, 2008. Washington, DC, U.S. Department of Health and Human Services, 2008

Sacerdote A, Bleicher SJ: Oral contraceptives abolish luteal phase exacerbation of hyperglycemia in type I diabetes. *Diabetes Care* 5:651–652, 1982

Spellacy WN, Ellingson AB, Kotlik A, Tsibris JC: Plasma glucose and insulin levels in women using a levonorgestrel-containing triphasic oral contraceptive for three months. *Contraception* 38:27–35, 1988

ter Braak EW, Evers IM, Willem Erkelens D, Visser GH: Maternal hypoglycemia during pregnancy in type 1 diabetes: maternal and fetal consequences. *Diabetes Metab Res Rev* 18:96–105, 2002

Verheijen EC, Critchley JA, Whitelaw DC, Tuffnell DJ: Outcomes of pregnancies in women with pre-existing type 1 or type 2 diabetes, in an ethnically mixed population. *BJOG* 112:1500–1503, 2005

Wolfe LA, Heenan AP, Bonen A: Aerobic conditioning effects on substrate responses during graded cycling in pregnancy. *Can J Physiol Pharmacol* 81:696–703, 2003a

Wolfe LA, Weissgerber TL: Clinical physiology of exercise in pregnancy: a literature review. *J Obstet Gynaecol Can* 25:473–483, 2003b

Yeung EH, Zhang C, Mumford SL, Ye A, Trevisan M, Chen L, Browne RW, Wactawski-Wende J, Schisterman EF: Longitudinal study of insulin resistance and sex hormones over the menstrual cycle: the BioCycle Study. *J Clin Endocrinol Metab* 95:5435–5442, 2010

Young JC, Treadway JL: The effect of prior exercise on oral glucose tolerance in late gestational women. *Eur J Appl Physiol Occup Physiol* 64:430–433, 1992

Chapter 23

Older Adults

Aging results in a slow decline in maximal heart rate, aerobic capacity, lung function, and nerve function (unrelated to diabetes), regardless of physical activity levels, and some of these processes can be accelerated by the presence of diabetes (Basta 2002, Anton 2004, Abate 2011). The usual declines in insulin action with aging (Clevenger 2002), however, actually may be more associated with obesity and physical activity than with aging itself (Amati 2009). Elderly individuals face unique challenges related to continued physical activity participation, including joint injuries, arthritis, osteoporosis and fracture risk, falls, and frailty (Coupland 1999; Trappe 2001; McCabe 2007; Morrison 2010, 2012; Scott 2012). Regular physical activity is critical to managing many of these conditions, however, and in many cases may actually prevent or possibly reverse them.

Case in Point: Exercise Rx for an Elderly Adult with T2D

BA is an 82-year-old man with type 2 diabetes (T2D) for 15 years. He exhibits some systolic hypertension common among older individuals but is not taking any blood pressure medications. His diabetes treatment includes metformin and pioglitazone (Actos). He also controls his blood cholesterol levels with a statin medication. He is a fairly healthy and active individual, although he does have some arthritic pain in his left knee that is sometimes limiting to his exercise participation. He tries to do some walking or stationary cycling most days of the week for 20–30 min at a time.

Resting Measurements

Height: 64 inches
Weight: 172 lb
BMI: 29.5 (overweight)
Heart rate: 82 beats per minute (bpm)
Blood pressure: 145/75 mmHg

Fasting Labs (1 Month after Diagnosis)

Plasma glucose: 125 mg/dl (controlled with metformin)
A1C: 7.2%
Total cholesterol: 178 mg/dl (on medication)

Triglycerides: 85 mg/dl
High-density lipoprotein cholesterol: 45 mg/dl
Low-density lipoprotein cholesterol: 116 mg/dl

Questions to Consider

1. What types of physical activity should BA focus on doing at this point in his life?
2. Are there any precautions for him related to exercise or other health issues?

(Continued on page 436.)

PHYSICAL CHANGES AND CONCERNS IN OLDER INDIVIDUALS

Getting older causes changes in physical function and exercise performance. For instance, the world record in the clean-and-jerk power lift is 20% lower in men and 40% lower in women in individuals >50 years of age. The rate of decline (~1% per year) in power with advancing age is similar for world record holders, other master athletes, and healthy untrained individuals, suggesting the importance of the aging process over physical activity history (Thé 2003). The overall magnitude of decline in peak muscular power is even greater in tasks requiring more complex and powerful movements, although upper- and lower-body muscular power demonstrate similar rate of decline with age (Anton 2004). The decrease in performance also seen in master swimmers is due to both decrease in the metabolic power available and to an increase in the energy cost of swimming with age (Zamparo 2012).

There has been a continued increase in the number of older participants in sporting events like running, swimming, cycling, rowing, and weightlifting. Some master athletes come from a background with years of training and competition experience, whereas others have only begun to compete as they approach middle-age and older (Trappe 2001). Elderly individuals are both past their peak for most activities and more prone to developing acute and overuse injuries related to sports and physical activity participation (Cosca 2007, Knobloch 2008). For a fuller discussion of physical activity issues related specifically to obesity, orthopedic limitations, acute and overuse injuries, or osteoarthritis, please refer to chapter 16.

PHYSICAL CHANGES THAT AFFECT MOVEMENT

Aging results in a slow decline in maximal heart rate, aerobic capacity, lung function, and nerve function (unrelated to diabetes) (Hollenberg 2006). These changes result in lower overall strength and endurance, in part resulting from selective loss of the fast-twitch muscle fibers used for power and speed, although using those fibers will slow their loss. Regardless of age, athletes have been shown to be more insulin sensitive than normal-weight sedentary subjects, who in turn were more insulin sensitive than obese subjects. Thus, insulin resistance is more likely the result of obesity and physical inactivity rather than aging per se (Amati 2009).

In addition, loss of calcium and other minerals from bones accelerates with age, particularly in postmenopausal women, but weight-bearing and resistance exercise can slow and reverse those losses to some extent (Bemben 2000). Moreover, training will keep ventilatory muscles stronger. Although the body's maximal ability to use oxygen during exercise typically declines at least 1% per year (Hollenberg 2006), highly trained older athletes show a slower, but steady, rate of decline of only 0.5% annually. Although runners of any age who exercise moderately tend to be physically better off than less active people their age, extensive training for marathons, ultramarathons, and triathlons can increase the risk of injury (Vleck 2010) and osteoarthritis (Michaelsson 2011).

JOINT INJURIES WITH AGING

Overuse joint injuries. Older exercisers also face some general physical problems that make overuse injuries more common. For instance, joints become less flexible with age, and changes in body's connective tissues combined with arthritis and hyperglycemia mean that knees, hips, and other joints must bear greater stress during exercise than muscles. Older age, previous joint injury and surgery, and higher BMI are independent risk factors for hip and knee osteoarthritis, although participation in physical activity does not appear to increase these risks and no threshold of increasing risk exists with increased training among walkers and runners engaging in recommended levels of activity (Hootman 2003). Stretching regularly can help slow the loss of flexibility but is not able to prevent it completely (Herriott 2004), and diabetes also can hasten the loss of flexibility due to glycation of joint surfaces, particularly when glycemic levels are not well controlled (Abate 2011).

Exercise modifications to prevent injury. Participation in other activities besides running may require adjustments with aging to prevent injuries. For instance, swimming increases the likelihood of experiencing rotator cuff tears; thus, older swimmers should avoid excessive use of hand paddles (which increase stress on the shoulders) and swim fins (which aggravate knee problems), and they should increase swimming distances gradually (Richardson 1991). Older cyclists are more likely to suffer from compressive or inflammatory syndromes involving nerves in the upper body. These problems are largely preventable by reducing training (McLennan 1991). Older cyclists should use the correct seat height, wear padded gloves, use a padded seat (like a gel pad), wear padded cycling shorts, and avoid resting on their hands on the handlebars (Cosca 2007). Older golfers can develop shoulder problems; neck, lower back, and wrist pain; and golf or tennis elbow. Golfers should warm up properly, stretch, and do strengthening exercises, especially for the lower back muscles (Jobe 1991).

OSTEOARTHRITIS MANAGEMENT

The most common type of arthritis, osteoarthritis, can result from trauma or from repetitive use, which makes it extremely common in elderly individuals with decades of wear and tear on joints from excessive body weight and general joint use (Vignon 2006). Glycation of joint surfaces, which occurs with hyperglycemia in individuals with diabetes, can contribute to faster deterioration of all joint structures, including those affected by osteoarthritic changes (Basta 2002, Abate 2011). Pain is only continuous when almost all of the cartilage surfaces of joints have been eroded, at which point it is indicative of advanced arthritis and results in a lower quality of life (Hoogeboom 2012). In older adults, performing few or no muscle strengthening activities or engaging in activities that cause a high mechanical strain lead to an increased risk of knee osteoarthritis over time (Verweij 2009). In addition, knee and hip arthritic pain may directly contribute to the progression of sarcopenia and increased falls risk in older women (Scott 2012).

Physical activity with osteoarthritis. Regular physical activity should be encouraged for individuals with osteoarthritis and may improve joint symptoms in many cases (Rogers 2002, Vignon 2006), along with causing weight loss (Messier 2000). Even running does not increase the risk of osteoarthritis of the knees and hips in healthy adults (Willick 2010), and engaging in most types of activity is protective against further joint degeneration (Rogers 2002, Vignon 2006). Among middle-aged and elderly people in one study, many of whom were overweight or obese, recreational exercise neither protected against nor increased their risk of developing knee osteoarthritis (Felson 2007). Although elevated BMI increases the risk of knee osteoarthritis progression, the effect of body weight appears to be limited to knees in which moderate malalignment exists, presumably because of the combined focus of load from incorrect alignment and excess mechanical loads from increased weight (Felson 2004).

Regular low and moderate aerobic or resistance activities are recommended for older adults because they are less stressful to joints than more intense workouts (Messier 2000, 2004; Magrans-Courtney 2011). Low-intensity resistance training can be beneficial for muscular fitness in older individuals when high-intensity exercise is contraindicated (Bemben 2000). Engaging in non–weight-bearing activities like cycling and aquatic exercise may help arthritic pain, and activities should include strength and full range-of-movement exercises around painful joints (Vignon 2006). After activities, ice may need to be applied to arthritic joints (particularly knees) for 15–20 min to reduce swelling and help prevent soreness (Wexler 1995). Anti-inflammatory medications like aspirin and ibuprofen may be used to manage exercise-related discomfort (Paoloni 2009, Verkleij 2011).

OSTEOPOROSIS AND BONE FRACTURE CONCERNS

Healthy bones and joints are crucial to mobility and extended youthfulness, as well as living a pain-free life (American College of Sports Medicine 1995). Slow bone demineralization occurs throughout adulthood starting around the age of 25 years. Once a critical minimal bone density is reached, these thinner bones experience a greater incidence of fractures, especially of the hip, wrist, or spine, and hip fracture risk in particular is elevated in diabetic individuals (Vestergaard 2007, Khazai 2009). Whereas bone loss occurs over many years, osteoporosis may not be detected until fractures are blatant or postural changes are well advanced. Repeated, undetected compression fractures in the vertebrae of the spine can lead to stooped posture and backaches, both of which are common in older women (and some men). Hip fractures resulting from this disease can be immensely debilitating, often signaling the start of a downward trend of reduced strength and a lower quality of life.

Causes. Osteoporosis risk is increased by small frame size; female sex; age; hereditary factors; Caucasian or Asian race; early menopause; prolonged immobilization; low levels of estrogen or testosterone; excess thyroid hormones (e.g., overactive thyroid gland); cigarette smoking; excessive alcohol consumption; extended steroid use (e.g., prednisone); physical inactivity; and inadequate intake of calcium, magnesium, and vitamin D (Kanis 2005, Khazai 2009). After menopause, women lose bone at an average rate of 2–3% per year, while men of a similar age are losing only 0.4% annually (Borer 2005). The most visible sign of this loss is a gradual shortening in overall height. Bed rest results in a profound decline in bone mass and is best avoided or minimized, if possible (American College of Sports Medicine 1995). Even mild to moderate renal dysfunction (common in individuals with diabetes) increases risk of osteoporosis in both women and men and likely should indicate the need for osteoporosis screening (Jassal 2007, Ishani 2008, Jamal 2010).

Prevention and management. Some largely effective strategies to prevent and limit potential bone problems include consuming adequate calcium, magnesium, and vitamin D, engaging in regular weight-bearing exercises, avoiding phosphorus-filled sodas, moderating protein intake, and possibly using hormone replacement therapies. Physical activity participation stimulates increases in bone diameter throughout the life span, which reduces the risk of fractures by mechanically counteracting the thinning of bones and increased bone porosity (Borer 2005). Moderate physical activity in people with osteoporosis can reduce the risk of falls and fractures, decrease pain, and improve fitness and overall quality of life. It also may stimulate bone gain and decrease bone loss (Prior 1996). Moderate levels of activity, including walking, are associated with substantially lower risk of hip fracture in postmenopausal women (Feskanich 2002).

In a recent review of exercise training effects on bone mass in older individuals, it was reported that walking only provides a modest increase in the loads on the skeleton above gravity and may be less effective in osteoporosis prevention, whereas strength exercise is a more powerful stimulus to improve and maintain bone mass during aging. Moreover, multicomponent exercise programs that include strength, aerobic, high impact, or weight-bearing training, as well as whole-body vibration alone or in combination with exercise, may help increase or at least prevent decline in bone mass with aging, especially in postmenopausal women (Gomez-Cabello 2012). Weight-bearing exercise in general, and resistance exercise in particular, should be recommended, along with exercise targeted to improve balance, mobility, and posture to reduce the likelihood of falling (Guadalupe-Grau 2009).

Diabetes-specific risk of fractures. A serious complication of diabetes is the increase in fracture risk observed in both type 1 diabetes (T1D) and T2D, which have unique and overlapping mechanisms of bone loss. Although T1D is associated with reduced bone mineral density because of suppressed bone formation, this usually is not seen in T2D (McCabe 2011). In fact, individuals with T2D have a higher bone mineral density compared with the general population, yet they remain unprotected from fractures, possibly due to alterations in bone geometry (Gorman 2011). People with T1D have a greater risk of fractures and a lower bone mineral density compared with the general population (Khazai 2009).

Hyperglycemia, present in both types of diabetes, alters bone matrix proteins through nonenzymatic glycation, which can decrease bone toughness and increase fracture risk even in the absence of bone loss (McCabe 2011). Diabetes is associated with increased inflammation and altered adipokine and calcitrophic hormone levels, which further contribute to bone pathophysiology. Potential contributors to the suppression of bone formation in T1D include increased marrow adiposity, hyperlipidemia, reduced insulin signaling, hyperglycemia, inflammation, altered adipokine and endocrine factors, increased cell death, and altered metabolism (McCabe 2007). Recently, studies have shown an association between advanced glycation endproducts (AGEs) and increased fracture risk in diabetic individuals. Thus, poor glycemic control and chronic hyperglycemia likely have a direct detrimental effect on bone quality. In addition, increased fracture risk in diabetes has been associated with peripheral and autonomic neuropathy, recurrent hypoglycemic events, vitamin D deficiency, and thiazolidinedione use (Khazai 2009).

IMPACT AND PREVENTION OF FALLS

Falling down occasionally is inevitable at any age, and engaging in physical activity increases the risk of falls. Most falls, however, occur indoors during normal activities (Kent 2006). The negative impact of falling down is undeniable (Siracuse 2012). About 95% of all hip fractures result from falls and are the major cause of hospital emergency room visits and admissions for injuries in older individuals (Kent 2006). It is still unclear whether osteoporosis or falls are more important in fractures; it may depend on the region prone to fracture and the individual's health status (Kemmler 2011). Older individuals with diabetes have an increased fracture rate, suggesting that assessment of fall risk factors and exercise prescription for falls prevention is critical (Gorman 2011).

Fear of falling, which may cause individuals to choose to become less active and socially oriented, can lead to social isolation, depression, and impaired activities of daily living (ADL) from further declines in strength (Zijlstra 2007). Although falls are less common among adults in their middle years, one in three people >60 years of age falls each year (Muir 2010).

Causes of and risk factors for falling. Aging by itself is associated with a number of physical changes that increase the risk of falling, such as having a more variable gait, slower walking speed, less flexible ankles, and weaker legs (Morrison 2010). Poor balance that can develop over time also can result in increased falls (Muir 2010). Risk is elevated whenever an individual develops a new disease or condition that significantly affects health, even if it only has a temporary effect. Fainting for any reason (e.g., due to a drop in blood pressure after eating, abnormal heart rhythms, anemia, straining while urinating or defecating, and use of certain medications) causes falls. Delirium is its own risk factor, as is dementia. For individuals with Alzheimer's disease, falls risk is increased because of their taking shorter steps, swaying more, and varying their gait from one step to the next. Bunions, calluses, deformed toes, diabetes-related changes to feet (e.g., Charcot foot), or toe amputations can additionally modify gait or inhibit adequate movement and increase the risk of falling. Impaired executive function also can increase falls risk in older individuals without balance issues (Buracchio 2011).

The major risk factors associated with falls are quadriceps muscle weakness, balance problems, gait disorders, sensory loss, dizziness, recent changes in medications, upright posture, having a history of falls, and wearing ill-fitting glasses or bifocals that affect downward vision. In particular, multifocal glasses may impair contrast sensitivity, depth perception, and ability to negotiate obstacles (Lord 2010). Other factors are listed in Table 23.1.

FALLS PREVENTION

Falls prevention is an essential component of any strategy for decreasing fracture risk and injury in old age (Boonen 2008). Many of the potential risks arising from physical changes with aging can be substantially lowered by doing strengthening, balance, and flexibility exercises. Weight-bearing exercise in general, and resistance exercise, in particular, should be recommended, along with exercise targeted to improve balance, mobility, and posture to reduce the likelihood of falling (Guadalupe-Grau 2009). Even home-based interventions and tai chi programs for the elderly may be effective in reducing fear of falling, which may lead to greater physical activity participation (Zijlstra 2007).

In addition, falls risk can be lowered by properly lighting areas where individuals walk (particularly at night), wearing good shoes, correcting vision (e.g., cataract removal, appropriate glasses), controlling incontinence with medications or through other means, and removing floor clutter and throw rugs (Lord 2010). Individuals who are prone to falling may reduce their risk of injury by wearing hip pads to soften their landings and lower the potential for hip fractures.

IMPACT AND MANAGEMENT OF FRAILTY

Frailty generally marks the end of an independent lifestyle for an older population, but luckily it is largely preventable. People who become frail undeniably experience a decline in their mobility (Fried 2001). Weakness may serve as a warn-

Table 23.1 Risk Factors for Falling

- Strength problems (particularly in quadriceps muscles)
- Low blood pressure and orthostatic hypotension (dizziness with standing)
- Atherosclerotic disease (that leads to fainting)
- Poorly fitting glasses or multifocal lenses
- Medications (e.g., certain side effects like dizziness and hypotension)
- Sight problems (poor vision from cataracts, glaucoma, or macular changes)
- Walking on uneven surfaces or with poor lighting
- Unsteady balance or altered gait
- Nocturia (i.e., a frequent need to urinate overnight)
- Foot changes or deformities (e.g., sensory loss, bunions, toe amputations)
- Use of restraints that prevent physical activity
- Excessive alcohol intake
- Impaired executive function
- Delirium
- Prior falls

ing sign of increasing vulnerability in early frailty development, and weight loss and exhaustion may help to identify individuals most at risk for rapid adverse progression (Xue 2008). Frail individuals usually are less socially active, fall down more, are more prone to fractures due to osteoporosis, may become incontinent, and lose much of their quality of life (Hubbard 2011). In fact, falls can be an important marker of frailty, particularly because they frequently play a role in accelerating the loss of health and independence of a frail individual and can lead to decreased activity, depression, social isolation, functional decline, and a diminished quality of life (Xue 2008). Moreover, a fear of falling that keeps individuals from being active only makes their ability to function on any level decline more quickly (Zijlstra 2007). Clinical tests of neuromuscular function are best for prediction of falls in frail older people (Shimada 2009).

Prediction of frailty. Frailty occurs in ~7% of all people >50 years and in more women than men (Hubbard 2011). One of the best predictors of who is going to become frail (and when) is simply how well someone performs basic ADL (Mitnitski 2005, Xue 2008). Furthermore, if individuals come into the hospital (for any reason), and these abilities are intact, they are 82% likely to still be living and doing well 6 months later. If not, they have a less than 50% chance of living another 6 months and are likely to be residing in a nursing home. Thus, performance of basic activities that are required for daily living is a better predictor of frailty than disease (Mitnitski 2005). The only other good predictor is body weight, which is reflective of nutritional status. If they have a BMI <21, most individuals have lost much muscle mass and strength and are more likely to be or become frail.

Causes of frailty. Vision, hearing, memory, sense of smell, appetite, thirst, hormones, muscle mass, and bone minerals are all affected by aging over time, and these slow, physiological changes associated with getting older are the prefrailty that everyone goes through to some extent after the age of 50 years. Frailty is frequently related to loss of muscle mass through sarcopenia, or muscle wasting, and its resulting muscular weakness (Scott 2012). The rate of muscle loss has been estimated to range from 1% to 2% per year past the age of 50 years, as a result of which 25% of people <70 years of age and 40% >80 years of age are sarcopenic (Marzetti 2006).

About half of people with sarcopenia are also obese, making any physical movement challenging for them (Baumgartner 2000, 2004). Obese, inactive, older women are more prone to this cause of frailty, particularly if they have knee or hip pain from osteoarthritis (Scott 2012). Similarly, visceral fat deposition increases the release of certain deleterious cytokines, such as tumor necrosis factor-α, from the excess fat tissue that can contribute to sarcopenic obesity by speeding the loss of muscle mass (Baumgartner 2000). Insulin resistance also leads to T2D, hypertension, elevated blood fats, and heart disease, all of which are associated with frailty (Fried 2001, Xue 2008). When individuals are unable to function in the most basic ways, frailty is present, and it has multiple possible causes (listed in Table 23.2).

Reversal of frailty. Certain causes of frailty are actually reversible. For example, anorexia, lack of exercise, pain, depression, diabetes, delirium, atherosclerosis, sar-

Table 23.2 Potential Causes of Frailty

- Diabetes or metabolic syndrome
- Decline in overall function
- Visual problems
- Nutritional deficiencies
- Polypharmacy (taking too many medications)
- Balance problems
- Anemia (low blood levels of iron and hemoglobin)
- Congestive heart failure
- Osteoporosis (fractures)
- Sarcopenia (muscle loss)
- Decline in endurance
- Pain

copenia, weight loss, low body weight, dehydration, heart disease, stroke, cognitive impairment, and delirium are all part of the frailty cascade, and most are treatable or preventable themselves, although the overabundance of possible causes often can make frailty difficult to completely reverse (Mohandas 2011). Anemia is strongly associated with frailty, and dizziness is associated with standing, falls, mental declines, depression, and advanced kidney disease (Khoshdel 2008). Accordingly, treating anemic people with rEPO (a recombinant form of the body's natural hormone [EPO], which boosts red blood cells) or darbepoetin to reverse anemia also may reduce the risk of frailty (Ritz 2005). Depression can cause symptoms of frailty but often can be reversed with the treatment of depression with increased physical activity (Lysy 2008). Removal of cataracts can decrease risk of frailty as well by increasing ability to engage in physical activity (Tumosa 2008, Obrosova 2010). Natural reductions in hormones, such as testosterone, estrogen, vitamin D, growth hormone, and dehydroepiandrosterone, over time can contribute to symptoms of frailty. Declining testosterone levels in aging men predict muscle mass losses, and its replacement in aging men may be indicated (Ibanez 2008). Even taking too many prescribed medications is a reversible cause of frailty (Clarfield 2010, Gadsby 2012). Older individuals should maintain their calorie, protein, and fluid intakes, along with doing resistance exercise and balance exercises (Winett 2009).

MEDICATION ISSUES AFFECTING OLDER ADULTS

Many elderly adults take multiple medications, some of which are taken to reduce the side effects of other ones (Berlie 2010). Polypharmacy, defined as taking four or more drugs per day, is highly prevalent in older individuals with diabetes (Gadsby 2012). Although not all have an impact during physical activity, they may have other effects that affect the health of these individuals and their overall ability to be active (Caldwell 1987). For example, even statin use (which is widespread among older adults) can double the risk of a myopathic event, such as myalgia and myositis (Nichols 2007). Moreover, use of select diuretics for hypertension management may reduce exercise tolerance and increase hypotension and falls risk in direct proportion to the degree of dehydration induced by them (Caldwell 1987, Leipzig 1999).

As far as commonly prescribed diabetes medications are concerned, fit elderly with life expectancy >10 years should have A1C targets similar to younger adults, whereas in frail elderly people with multiple comorbidities, the goal should be somewhat higher (Chiniwala 2011, Lee 2011). In overweight patients, metformin has been associated with reductions in risk for all-cause mortality and stroke compared with insulin and sulfonylureas. Older individuals, however, who are frail, anorexic, or underweight and those with congestive heart failure (CHF), renal or hepatic insufficiency, or dehydration may not be appropriate candidates for metformin therapy (Neumiller 2009). Metformin use may lead to secondary vitamin B_{12} deficiency, neuropathy symptoms, and increased risk of falls (Berlie 2010). Thiazolidinediones generally should be avoided in CHF and are contraindicated in anyone with more severe heart failure. Their use also has been associated with peripheral edema, as well as with decreases in bone mineral density in women and may worsen falls-related outcomes (Khazai 2009, Berlie 2010).

The substantial risk of hypoglycemia with insulin secretagogues (sulfonylureas in particular) is increased significantly in the elderly (Choudhary 2009), although this risk may be somewhat counterbalanced by their extensive experience in using them (Neumiller 2009). Although pramlintide does not increase hypoglycemia risk in younger adults (Amiel 2005), its effects in older adults, particularly the frail elderly, have not been well studied, and it should be used with caution (Neumiller 2009). Many older individuals with T2D eventually require insulin; however, because of the risk of hypoglycemia and related morbidity, careful use of insulin is required, particularly in geriatric individuals with altered cognitive function at higher risk of severe hypoglycemia (Bremer 2009) or falls (Berlie 2010).

Limited information on dipeptidyl peptidase-4 (DPP-4) inhibitors in the elderly exists, and renal dysfunction will require dose adjustments in all of these medications with the exception of linigliptin in affected individuals (McGill 2012). Exenatide may be beneficial in those with limited mobility who should lose some weight, whereas it is not recommended for frail, underweight adults or for anyone with an abnormally low creatinine clearance (<30 ml/min) (Russell-Jones 2012). Moreover, α-glucosidase inhibitor use in older individuals is associated with gastrointestinal concerns (Neumiller 2009). Overall, a scarcity of data exists regarding the use of pharmacologic agents in older adults with diabetes, and clinical guidance is largely based on data obtained from younger populations, which may or may not be relevant and makes choosing an appropriate drug regimen challenging (Neumiller 2009).

PHYSICAL ACTIVITY PARTICIPATION BY ELDERLY ADULTS

For older adults, recommended intensity of aerobic activity should take into account the older adult's aerobic fitness. In addition, physical activities that maintain or increase flexibility are recommended, along with balance exercises, particularly for older adults at risk of falls. In short, activity should be both preventive and therapeutic and emphasize moderate-intensity aerobic activity, muscle-strengthening activity, reducing sedentary behavior, and risk management (Nelson 2007).

EXERCISE PRESCRIPTION FOR OLDER ADULTS

Elderly adults who have been primarily sedentary may have physical limitations (Nelson 2007). Getting an elderly person to do any kind of physical activity can benefit not only blood glucose control but also muscle tone, flexibility, and mental outlook. For older women, physical activity may help reduce the severity of symptoms associated with menopause and result in better health-related quality-of-life measures (Villaverde-Gutierrez 2006, Daley 2007). Physical activity during weight loss also prevents weight regain in this population (Wang 2008). Yard work and housework are activities many people feel comfortable doing and can be beneficial for maintaining ability to engage in ADL (Blair 1992), but inclusion of resistance work to gain strength and retain muscle mass is also recommended (Nelson 2007, Garber 2011).

Although the exercise guidelines for adults also apply to older adults, some additional guidelines apply only to older adults (Nelson 2007, Physical Activity Guidelines Advisory Committee 2008):

- When older adults cannot do 150 min/week of moderate-intensity aerobic activity because of chronic conditions, they should be as physically active as their abilities and conditions allow.
- Older adults should do exercises that maintain or improve balance, particularly if they are at risk of falling.
- Older adults should determine their level of effort for physical activity relative to their level of fitness.
- Older adults with chronic conditions should understand whether and how their conditions affect their ability to do regular physical activity safely.

Frequency and intensity. Generally, elderly individuals should engage in some physical activity each day (Nelson 2007). Setting goals that this population can reach is the most important strategy. For example, a very sedentary elderly person may only be able to walk for 5 min for 3 days/week and increase that by 1–2 min/week.

Safety considerations. Safety is an issue as well. Safety concerns may preclude someone from walking who has a high risk for falls and subsequent fracture. Options may include using a stationary bicycle, lifting light weights, or exercising while seated. Exercise videos, classes, and routines that can be done from a chair, rather than standing, may be helpful in this population.

Physical activity modifications for older adults. When working with older adults, give special consideration to changes in body composition that may have occurred over the years (e.g., declines in muscle mass and muscle strength, with resultant decreases in basal metabolic rate, activity level, and energy expenditure). Guide-

Table 23.3 Recommended Exercise Rx for Elderly Adults

Mode	Aerobic: Walking, cycling, swimming, rowing, aquatic activities, seated exercises, dancing, conditioning machines, and more
	Resistance: All major muscle groups, using resistance bands, free weights, resistance training machines, isometric exercises, and/or calisthenics (using body weight); include four or five upper-body and four or five lower-body/core exercises
	Flexibility: Include exercises that stretch the major muscle groups in both the upper and the lower body.
	Balance: Simple balance training exercises, such as practice standing on one leg, are important in preventing falls.
Intensity	Aerobic: 40–89% heart rate reserve, or HRR (initial intensity may need to be on the lower end for sedentary, deconditioned, and overweight individuals)
	Resistance: 50/60–80% 1 RM (starting on the low end)
	Both: Perceived exertion of "somewhat hard" to start; 5–7 (on 10-point scale)
Frequency	Aerobic: At least 3 nonconsecutive days/week, but ideally 5–7 days/week, depending on orthopedic or other limitations
	Resistance: A minimum of 2 days per week (preferably 3), with at least 48 h of rest between sessions
Duration	Aerobic: 30 min daily, for a total of at least 150 min/week of moderate-intensity (or possibly higher) activity; start with a minimum of 5–10 min/exercise session; intersperse brief rest periods until a continuous activity for at least 10 min at a time can be achieved, and add 2–5 min/week until desired goal is met
	Resistance: 8–12 repetitions per exercise as a goal, but 10–15 repetitions initially; one to three sets per exercise
Progression	Aerobic: Start out on the "low" side and progress slowly over weeks to months; increase duration and frequency first, intensity last (if at all)
	Resistance: Start with one or two sets of 8–15 repetitions: one set of 10–15 repetitions to fatigue initially, progressing to 8–10 harder repetitions, and finally to two or three sets of 8–10 repetitions), although the presence of orthopedic or other limitations may require staying with higher repetitions and less resistance

Note: 1 RM, one-repetition maximum.

lines for adults with and without diabetes also apply to older adults (ages ≥65 years) (Nelson 2007, Physical Activity Guidelines Advisory Committee 2008, Colberg 2010, Garber 2011). Brisk walking, gardening, yard work, and housework are good examples of recommended moderate-intensity activities that help retain physical function, build strength, and expend calories (Blair 1992).

For older individuals, it is never too late to begin an exercise program and benefit from it. For example, in the Diabetes Prevention Program, the older adults

Table 23.4 Additional Physical Activity Recommendations for Older Adults

Aerobic Activity for Older Adults

- A thorough medical exam is needed before starting an exercise program of moderate or higher intensity
- Recommend that older adults do at least 150 min/week of moderate- to vigorous-intensity aerobic exercise, performed in episodes of at least 10 min, and preferably spread throughout the week
- Instruct individuals to increase exercise duration and frequency before intensity
- Recommend a conservative approach to increasing exercise intensity, and avoid vigorous aerobic activity when starting an exercise program
- For previously sedentary individuals, advise starting at lower levels, progressing slowly, and gradually increasing the duration and frequency to reach the desired fitness level
- Advise older adults that if they cannot do 150 min/week of moderate-intensity aerobic activity because of chronic conditions, they should be as physically active as their abilities and conditions allow
- Recommend aquatic or chair exercises and stationary cycling for individuals with less tolerance for weight-bearing activities, such as those with severe degenerative joint disease or osteoarthritis
- Advise that no matter what its purpose—gardening, walking the dog, taking a dance or exercise class, or bicycling to the store—aerobic activity of all types counts toward meeting recommended levels of physical activity.

who met the activity goal of 150 min/week were found to derive the greatest benefit from exercise in preventing T2D compared with their younger counterparts (Knowler 2002). Table 23.4 summarizes the guidelines for aerobic exercise in older adults. As stated, guidelines for adults ages 18–64 years for aerobic exercise, resistance training, and flexibility exercise also apply to older individuals; however, special considerations may be needed for an older population or one that is symptom or condition limited.

EXERCISING WITH COMORBID HEALTH ISSUES

Assessment of overall health, and identification and prevention of cardiovascular disease risk factors and other diabetes-related health complications are essential components of effective diabetes care (American Diabetes Association 2013). Macrovascular (e.g., coronary, cerebrovascular, and peripheral) and microvascular (peripheral and autonomic nerves, kidney, and eye) diseases are common and constitute the diabetes-related complications that develop and worsen with inadequate blood glucose control (Booth 2006a, 2006b; American Diabetes Association 2013). The onset and progression of vascular and neural complications of diabetes often cause physical limitation and varying levels of disability and are linked with depression and cognitive deficits (Egede 2003, Lustman 2005, Colberg 2008, Lysy 2008, Pan 2010). Thus, the quality of life in those with diabetes can be adversely affected without aggressive management of these health issues. For those who have difficulty managing blood glucose levels, it is prudent to refer them to allied health professionals (e.g., diabetes educator, diabetes nurse, registered dietician) to assist them in improving their diabetes management and care (American Diabetes Association 2013).

Older individuals with chronic health problems respond just as well to exercise training as their younger counterparts, yet many older individuals still choose not to be physically active. One reason may be their health, as the vast majority of individuals >65 years old have some health problem that they may view as a deterrent to exercise. Exercise, however, is beneficial for individuals with most diseases, including diabetes. In addition to improving diabetes-related health, regular exercise lessens the potential impact of most of the other cardiovascular risk factors, including elevated blood lipids (cholesterol and other blood fats), insulin resistance, obesity, and hypertension (Stewart 2002, Kirk 2004, Zoppini 2006, Buse

Table 23.5 Additional Physical Activity Precautions for Older Adults

Comorbid Health Issue	Precautions
Autonomic neuropathy	■ Elevated resting heart rate (HR) and blunted maximal HR ■ Impaired sympathetic or parasympathetic nerves yield abnormal exercise HR, blood pressure, and stroke volume ■ Prone to dehydration and impaired thermoregulation ■ Use of heart rate reserve (HRR) with measured maximal HR or perceived exertion to determine exercise intensity is recommended
Peripheral neuropathy	■ Check feet daily, and minimize participation in exercise that may cause trauma to the feet (e.g., prolonged hiking, jogging, or walking on uneven surfaces) ■ Non–weight-bearing exercises (e.g., cycling, chair exercises, swimming) may be more appropriate in some cases, although reulceration risk not increased by walking if ulcers healed ■ Walking and aquatic exercises are not recommended with unhealed ulcers ■ Keep feet clean and dry and assess condition daily ■ Choose shoes carefully for proper fit ■ Avoid activities requiring a great deal of balance
Nephropathy	■ High blood pressure common ■ Lower intensity of physical activities recommended ■ Avoid exercise that increases blood pressure excessively (e.g., weightlifting, high-intensity aerobic exercise) and refrain from breath holding
Retinopathy	■ With proliferative and severe stages of retinopathy, avoid vigorous, high-intensity activities that involve breath holding (e.g., weightlifting and isometrics) or overhead lifting ■ Avoid activities that lower the head (e.g., yoga, gymnastics) or that jar the head ■ Consult an ophthalmologist for specific restrictions and limitations
Hypertension	■ Avoid heavy weightlifting or breath holding ■ Perform dynamic exercises using large muscle groups, such as walking and cycling at a low to moderate intensity. ■ Follow blood pressure guidelines to keep within safe zone

Comorbid Health Issue	Precautions
Osteoarthritis	■ Individuals should match the type and amount of physical activity to their abilities and the severity of their arthritis ■ Low to moderate activities are recommended, although some individuals may progress to doing more intense ones ■ Start with range-of-motion activities around affected joints and light resistance training ■ Low-impact activities may be better for some individuals ■ Use pain as a guide for intensity and duration of activities ■ Avoid sports with high risk of joint trauma, such as contact sports, racquetball, and others with frequent directional changes
Osteoporosis	■ Individuals should engage in weight-bearing activities and use resistance training to build bone strength ■ Exercise targeted to improve balance, mobility, and posture may reduce the likelihood of falling ■ Avoid activities with a higher risk of falling or potential joint trauma
Falls or falls risk	■ Prevention of falls is critical, particularly with the increased fracture risk seen in all individuals with diabetes ■ Focus on correcting quadriceps muscle weakness, balance out with hamstring and calf exercises as well ■ Avoid exercises dependent on good balance, especially if balance problems are present ■ Wear good shoes and avoid uneven surfaces that can affect balance or cause falls ■ Consider engaging in stationary cycling or aquatic exercises where falls risk is lower ■ Individuals should wear glasses that fit well and adequately correct their vision
Frailty	■ Build endurance with low-intensity aerobic activities ■ Include resistance training of any type or intensity to prevent additional muscle mass loss and to reverse sarcopenia ■ Allow adequate rest between resistance training sessions and consume adequate calories and protein to promote muscle gains ■ Engaging in more daily movement may lead to additional strength and endurance gains
General	■ Carry identification with diabetes information ■ Maintain hydration (drink fluids before, during, and after exercise) ■ Avoid exercise in the heat of the day and in direct sunlight (wear hat and sunscreen when in the sun). ■ Carry rapid-acting carbohydrate sources during all physical activity ■ Get a glucagon kit to treat severe hypoglycemia in insulin users

2007, Coccheri 2007, Kadoglou 2007, Eddy 2008, Look Ahead Research Group 2010, Kones 2011, Maahs 2011). Table 23.5 gives additional precautions needed for older individuals exercising with comorbid health problems.

DAILY MOVEMENT

Exercising most days for just a short time, albeit important, is in many ways less critical than what individuals do during the rest of the day. For elderly adults,

Table 23.6 Strategies to Increase Activities of Daily Living

- Individuals should park their cars at the farthest point away in the lot
- Take the stairs whenever possible
- When sitting, individuals should consciously move their legs and hands (fidget more)
- Get up and move around after every 30 min of a sedentary activity
- Walk the dog instead of just letting it go outside on its own
- Monitor and increase daily steps using a pedometer
- Walk somewhere for fun every day
- Take public transportation whenever possible (to walk more)
- Go dancing once a week (or more)
- Work outside in the garden or yard, or do housework to get moving
- Play with kids or grandchildren
- Be creative in finding ways to move more throughout the day

simply increasing their spontaneous physical activity will bestow innumerable health benefits, including preventing the loss of muscle mass, reductions in mobility, and the onset of frailty (Manini 2009a, 2009b). To be most effective, a formal exercise program lasting 30 min/day needs to be combined with more frequent unplanned activities, the so-called ADL, as shown in Table 23.6.

In a recent study of older adults (ages 70–82 years), for every 287 calories/day they expended doing anything active, they increased their chances of living longer by 68%, even just doing 75 min of activity a day of activities like volunteering, walking at a pace of 2.5 miles per hour, child or adult care, and household chores (Manini 2006). Greater energy expenditure during daily activity may be protective against cognitive impairment in a dose-response manner (Middleton 2011). Despite the importance of being more active in all aspects of living, most people naturally try to do as little as possible. For instance, television watching can contribute to fat weight gain, loss of muscle mass, and development of frailty, whereas simply stepping in place during commercials can significantly increase the energy cost and amount of activity performed during television viewing (Steeves 2012). Independent of exercise levels, sedentary behaviors, especially television watching, are associated with significantly elevated risk of obesity and T2D, whereas even light to moderate activity results in substantially lower risk (Hu 2003).

Case in Point: Wrap-Up

BA has been retired for almost 20 years from his former job as a coal miner in western Pennsylvania, a job that was physically demanding and kept him physically active. In retirement, he started doing significantly less physical activity, and 5 years into it, he developed his diabetes. Since then, he has made an effort to manage his diet more effectively, and he has prevented any additional weight gain in the ensuing years. In fact, recently he suffered from a bad case of the flu that left him 10 lb lighter and feeling a lot weaker.

Exercise Program Goals

Mode of Activity: Given BA's knee arthritis, he should focus on doing a mix of weight-bearing and non–weight-bearing activities, including stationary cycling, seated exercises, and use of conditioning machines that are lower impact (such as cross-trainers and elliptical machines). Varying his choice of activities during the week is also recommended to lower the impact on his affected knee. He can include some walking exercise, using pain as his guide. More importantly, however, BA needs to add in some lower-body resistance training to help strengthen the muscles around knees to prevent pain, along with some upper-body and core exercises to regain some of his lost strength and muscle mass to prevent frailty. Flexibility exercises will be important for him to retain his full range of movement around all his joints. Finally, he should add in some simple balance exercises to prevent falls.

Intensity: BA's exercise intensity should optimally be "somewhat hard" on most days, using knee pain as his guide on any given day. His target heart rate should be in the range of 112 to 117 bpm (40–50% heart rate reserve, or HRR) as he attempts to regain his lost fitness, with a later training goal of closer to 122 bpm (59% of HRR). For him, engaging in lower intensities of activities will be beneficial to manage his knee pain, body weight, and diabetes and should be encouraged. For resistance training, he can start with just one set of lower-intensity work (less resistance and higher repetitions).

Frequency: For optimal diabetes management, BA should attempt to engage in physical activity 5–7 days/week, never letting >2 days pass without any activity. He should start resistance training 2 days/week for the present and add in balance training on 3–5 days/week as well.

Duration: If BA is still feeling weak from his illness, he can engage in shorter bouts of exercise training to start (5–10 min), separated by a rest period and with a goal of training for 20–30 min continuously as he was doing before, for both aerobic and resistance training sessions. He should aim to do 150 min of moderate physical activity spread throughout the week.

Progression: BA should increase the duration of his planned workouts until he reaches 150 min/week of moderate exercise (or possibly more if he is doing lower intensity work), although his real goal at his age should simply be to remain as physically active as possible, regardless of the duration or intensity of his activities. He can either maintain his level of fitness or very slowly progress to adding in some higher-intensity work even if it just involves some faster intervals or a "hill" profile on the stationary cycle, using knee pain as his guide. He should also include different activities (i.e., cross-train) to limit repetitive stress on his knee. In addition, he should progress to doing resistance training 3 days/week, increasing the number of sets he is doing, making his training more moderate (with higher resistance and fewer repetitions), and focusing on strengthening all areas of his body, with a special emphasis on the muscles around his knees. He also can do flexibility exercises with his balance training, both of which he can progress to doing almost daily.

Daily Movement: At his age, BA should be focusing on increasing his ADLs to maintain a minimal functionality that will enable him to continue living at home with his wife (without the need for assisted living or outside care). Standing more, taking more daily steps, and continuing to be physically active will help him accomplish this goal.

Precautions: Exercise-associated hypoglycemia should not be a concern because BA is taking two diabetes medications that do not increase its risk. Before his short illness, BA was engaging in regular mild to moderate physical activity, so he should not be required to have an exercise stress test unless he develops any signs or symptoms of heart disease. He should avoid overworking his knee and causing an increase in pain that would prevent him from being physically active. He should be aware of the development of any symptoms related to peripheral or autonomic neuropathy as those could affect his safe participation in exercise and require some adjustments.

Aging reduces physical function on its own, but the presence of diabetes can be an exacerbation to many of these declines over time. The best defense is prevention or reversal of some of these with regular physical activity participation. Older individuals can exercise safely and effectively when certain modifications are made to accommodate normal changes associated with aging and abnormal ones caused by diabetes and other health comorbidities.

PROFESSIONAL PRACTICE PEARLS

- Aging causes changes in physical function and exercise performance, and diabetes can accelerate those declines in many cases.
- Elderly individuals face other unique challenges related to physical activities, including osteoarthritis, osteoporosis and fracture risk, increased falls risk, and frailty.
- Older individuals are both past their peak for most activities and more prone to developing acute and overuse injuries related to sports and physical activity participation.
- Joints become less flexible with age, and changes in the body's connective tissues combined with arthritis and hyperglycemia put increased stress on joints during physical activity.
- Regular physical activity (i.e., low and moderate aerobic or resistance activities) should be encouraged for individuals with osteoarthritis and may improve joint symptoms.
- Osteoporosis risk is increased by a number of factors, including age, race, early menopause, excess thyroid hormones, cigarette smoking, excessive alcohol consumption, extended steroid use, inadequate micronutrient intake, and physical inactivity.
- Hyperglycemia alters bone matrix proteins through nonenzymatic glycation, which can decrease bone toughness and increase fracture risk even in the absence of bone loss.
- Strength, aerobic, high-impact, or weight-bearing training may help increase or at least prevent decline in bone mass with aging, especially in postmenopausal women.

- Falling down occasionally is inevitable at any age, and engaging in physical activity increases the risk of falls; however, most falls occur indoors during normal activities.
- Aging is associated with a number of physical changes that increase the risk of falling, such as a more variable gait, slower walking speed, less flexible ankles, and weaker legs.
- Physical activity interventions may reduce both falls risk in older individuals and fear of falling, which otherwise frequently leads to greater physical inactivity.
- Frailty generally marks the end of an independent lifestyle for an older population, but luckily it is largely preventable and many of its causes (like anemia) are reversible.
- Anorexia, physical inactivity, pain, depression, diabetes, delirium, atherosclerosis, sarcopenia, weight loss, low body weight, dehydration, heart disease, stroke, cognitive impairment, and delirium contribute to frailty, and most are treatable or preventable.
- Polypharmacy, defined as taking four or more drugs per day, is highly prevalent in older individuals with diabetes and may negatively affect their ability to be physically active.
- Elderly individuals should include aerobic, resistance, flexibility, and balance training as part of their weekly physical activity programs.
- A thorough medical exam is recommended for older individuals before starting an exercise program of moderate or higher intensity.
- If older adults cannot do 150 min of moderate-intensity aerobic activity a week, they should be as physically active as their abilities and conditions allow.
- Resistance training should include a minimum of one set of 8–10 exercises for each major muscle group two to three times a week, progressing up to two or three sets per exercise session.
- Aging individuals will benefit from engaging in a well-rounded stretching program to counteract decreases in flexibility, as well as training to improve balance and agility.
- Older individuals with chronic health problems respond just as well to exercise training, yet many choose not to be physically active due to health comorbidities.
- For elderly adults, simply increasing their spontaneous physical activity will bestow innumerable health benefits, including preventing the onset of frailty.

REFERENCES

Abate M, Schiavone C, Pelotti P, Salini V: Limited joint mobility in diabetes and ageing: recent advances in pathogenesis and therapy. *Int J Immunopathol Pharmacol* 23:997–1003, 2011

Amati F, Dubé JJ, Coen PM, Stefanovic-Racic M, Toledo FG, Goodpaster BH: Physical inactivity and obesity underlie the insulin resistance of aging. *Diabetes Care* 32:1547–1549, 2009

American College of Sports Medicine: American College of Sports Medicine position stand: osteoporosis and exercise. *Med Sci Sports Exerc* 27:i–vii, 1995

American Diabetes Association: Standards of medical care in diabetes—2013. *Diabetes Care* 36 (Suppl. 1):S11–S66, 2013

Amiel SA, Heller SR, Macdonald IA, Schwartz SL, Klaff LJ, Ruggles JA, Weyer C, Kolterman OG, Maggs DG: The effect of pramlintide on hormonal, metabolic or symptomatic responses to insulin-induced hypoglycaemia in patients with type 1 diabetes. *Diabetes Obes Metab* 7:504–516, 2005

Anton MM, Spirduso WW, Tanaka H: Age-related declines in anaerobic muscular performance: weightlifting and powerlifting. *Med Sci Sports Exerc* 36:143–147, 2004

Basta G, Lazzerini G, Massaro M, Simoncini T, Tanganelli P, Fu C, Kislinger T, Stern DM, Schmidt AM, De Caterina R: Advanced glycation end products activate endothelium through signal-transduction receptor RAGE: a mechanism for amplification of inflammatory responses. *Circulation* 105:816–822, 2002

Baumgartner RN: Body composition in healthy aging. *Ann N Y Acad Sci* 904:437–448, 2000

Baumgartner RN, Wayne SJ, Waters DL, Janssen I, Gallagher D, Morley JE: Sarcopenic obesity predicts instrumental activities of daily living disability in the elderly. *Obes Res* 12:1995–2004, 2004

Bemben DA, Fetters NL, Bemben MG, Nabavi N, Koh ET: Musculoskeletal responses to high- and low-intensity resistance training in early postmenopausal women. *Med Sci Sports Exerc* 32:1949–1957, 2000

Berlie HD, Garwood CL: Diabetes medications related to an increased risk of falls and fall-related morbidity in the elderly. *Ann Pharmacother* 44:712–717, 2010

Blair SN, Kohl HW, Gordon NF, Paffenbarger RS Jr: How much physical activity is good for health? *Annu Rev Public Health* 13:99–126, 1992

Boonen S, Dejaeger E, Vanderschueren D, Venken K, Bogaerts A, Verschueren S, Milisen K: Osteoporosis and osteoporotic fracture occurrence and prevention in the elderly: a geriatric perspective. *Best Pract Res Clin Endocrinol Metab* 22:765–785, 2008

Booth GL, Kapral MK, Fung K, Tu JV: Recent trends in cardiovascular complications among men and women with and without diabetes. *Diabetes Care* 29:32–37, 2006a

Booth GL, Kapral MK, Fung K, Tu JV: Relation between age and cardiovascular disease in men and women with diabetes compared with non-diabetic people: a population-based retrospective cohort study. *Lancet* 368:29–36, 2006b

Borer KT: Physical activity in the prevention and amelioration of osteoporosis in women: interaction of mechanical, hormonal and dietary factors. *Sports Med* 35:779–830, 2005

Bremer JP, Jauch-Chara K, Hallschmid M, Schmid S, Schultes B: Hypoglycemia unawareness in older compared with middle-aged patients with type 2 diabetes. *Diabetes Care* 32:1513–1517, 2009

Buracchio TJ, Mattek NC, Dodge HH, Hayes TL, Pavel M, Howieson DB, Kaye JA: Executive function predicts risk of falls in older adults without balance impairment. *BMC Geriatr* 11:74, 2011

Buse JB, Ginsberg HN, Bakris GL, Clark NG, Costa F, Eckel R, Fonseca V, Gerstein HC, Grundy S, Nesto RW, Pignone MP, Plutzky J, Porte D, Redberg R, Stitzel KF, Stone NJ, American Heart Association, American Diabetes Association: Primary prevention of cardiovascular diseases in people with diabetes mellitus: a scientific statement from the American Heart Association and the American Diabetes Association. *Circulation* 115:114–126, 2007

Caldwell JE: Diuretic therapy and exercise performance. *Sports Med* 4:290–304, 1987

Chiniwala N, Jabbour S: Management of diabetes mellitus in the elderly. *Curr Opin Endocrinol Diabetes Obes* 18:148–152, 2011

Choudhary P, Lonnen K, Emery CJ, MacDonald IA, MacLeod KM, Amiel SA, Heller SR: Comparing hormonal and symptomatic responses to experimental hypoglycaemia in insulin- and sulphonylurea-treated type 2 diabetes. *Diabet Med* 26:665–672, 2009

Clarfield AM: Screening in frail older people: an ounce of prevention or a pound of trouble? *J Am Geriatr Soc* 58:2016–2021, 2010

Clevenger CM, Parker Jones P, Tanaka H, Seals DR, DeSouza CA: Decline in insulin action with age in endurance-trained humans. *J Appl Physiol* 93:2105–2111, 2002

Coccheri S: Approaches to prevention of cardiovascular complications and events in diabetes mellitus. *Drugs* 67:997–1026, 2007

Colberg SR, Sigal RJ, Fernhall B, Regensteiner JG, Blissmer BJ, Rubin RR, Chasan-Taber L, Albright AL, Braun B, American College of Sports Medicine, American Diabetes Association: Exercise and type 2 diabetes: the American College of Sports Medicine and the American Diabetes Association: joint position statement. *Diabetes Care* 33:e147–e167, 2010

Colberg SR, Somma CT, Sechrist SR: Physical activity participation may offset some of the negative impact of diabetes on cognitive function. *J Am Med Dir Assoc* 9:434–438, 2008

Cosca DD, Navazio F: Common problems in endurance athletes. *Am Fam Physician* 76:237–244, 2007

Coupland CA, Cliffe SJ, Bassey EJ, Grainge MJ, Hosking DJ, Chilvers CE: Habitual physical activity and bone mineral density in postmenopausal women in England. *Int J Epidemiol* 28:241–246, 1999

Daley A, Macarthur C, Stokes-Lampard H, McManus R, Wilson S, Mutrie N: Exercise participation, body mass index, and health-related quality of life in women of menopausal age. *Br J Gen Pract* 57:130–135, 2007

Eddy DM, Schlessinger L, Heikes K: The metabolic syndrome and cardiovascular risk: implications for clinical practice. *Int J Obes (Lond)* 32 (Suppl. 2):S5–S10, 2008

Egede LE, Zheng D: Independent factors associated with major depressive disorder in a national sample of individuals with diabetes. *Diabetes Care* 26:104–111, 2003

Felson DT, Goggins J, Niu J, Zhang Y, Hunter DJ: The effect of body weight on progression of knee osteoarthritis is dependent on alignment. *Arthritis Rheum* 50:3904–3909, 2004

Felson DT, Niu J, Clancy M, Sack B, Aliabadi P, Zhang Y: Effect of recreational physical activities on the development of knee osteoarthritis in older adults of different weights: the Framingham Study. *Arthritis Rheum* 57:6–12, 2007

Feskanich D, Willett W, Colditz G: Walking and leisure-time activity and risk of hip fracture in postmenopausal women. *JAMA* 288:2300–2306, 2002

Fried LP, Tangen CM, Walston J, Newman AB, Hirsch C, Gottdiener J, Seeman T, Tracy R, Kop WJ, Burke G, McBurnie MA, Cardiovascular Health Study Collaborative Research Group: Frailty in older adults: evidence for a phenotype. *J Gerontol A Biol Sci Med Sci* 56:M146–M156, 2001

Gadsby R, Galloway M, Barker P, Sinclair A: Prescribed medicines for elderly frail people with diabetes resident in nursing homes-issues of polypharmacy and medication costs. *Diabet Med* 29:136–139, 2012

Garber CE, Blissmer B, Deschenes MR, Franklin BA, Lamonte MJ, Lee IM, Nieman DC, Swain DP, American College of Sports Medicine: American College of Sports Medicine position stand. Quantity and quality of exercise for developing and maintaining cardiorespiratory, musculoskeletal, and neuromotor fitness in apparently healthy adults: guidance for prescribing exercise. *Med Sci Sports Exerc* 43:1334–1359, 2011

Gomez-Cabello A, Ara I, Gonzalez-Aguero A, Casajus JA, Vicente-Rodriguez G: Effects of training on bone mass in older adults: a systematic review. *Sports Med* 42:301–325, 2012

Gorman E, Chudyk AM, Madden KM, Ashe MC: Bone health and type 2 diabetes mellitus: a systematic review. *Physiother Can* 63:8–20, 2011

Guadalupe-Grau A, Fuentes T, Guerra B, Calbet JA: Exercise and bone mass in adults. *Sports Med* 39:439–468, 2009

Herriott MT, Colberg SR, Parson HK, Nunnold T, Vinik AI: Effects of 8 weeks of flexibility and resistance training in older adults with type 2 diabetes. *Diabetes Care* 27:2988–2989, 2004

Hollenberg M, Yang J, Haight TJ, Tager IB: Longitudinal changes in aerobic capacity: implications for concepts of aging. *J Gerontol A Biol Sci Med Sci* 61:851–858, 2006

Hoogeboom TJ, den Broeder AA, Swierstra BA, de Bie RA, van den Ende CH: Joint-pain comorbidity, health status, and medication use in hip and knee osteoarthritis: a cross-sectional study. *Arthritis Care Res (Hoboken)* 64:54–58, 2012

Hootman JM, Macera CA, Helmick CG, Blair SN: Influence of physical activity-related joint stress on the risk of self-reported hip/knee osteoarthritis: a new method to quantify physical activity. *Prev Med* 36:636–644, 2003

Hu FB, Li TY, Colditz GA, Willett WC, Manson JE: Television watching and other sedentary behaviors in relation to risk of obesity and type 2 diabetes mellitus in women. *JAMA* 289:1785–1791, 2003

Hubbard RE, Rockwood K: Frailty in older women. *Maturitas* 69:203–207, 2011

Ibanez J, Gorostiaga EM, Alonso AM, Forga L, Arguelles I, Larrion JL, Izquierdo M: Lower muscle strength gains in older men with type 2 diabetes after resistance training. *J Diabetes Complications* 22:112–118, 2008

Ishani A, Paudel M, Taylor BC, Barrett-Connor E, Jamal S, Canales M, Steffes M, Fink HA, Orwoll E, Cummings SR, Ensrud KE, Osteoporotic Fractures in Men Study Group: Renal function and rate of hip bone loss in older men: the Osteoporotic Fractures in Men Study. *Osteoporos Int* 19:1549–1556, 2008

Jamal SA, Swan VJ, Brown JP, Hanley DA, Prior JC, Papaioannou A, Langsetmo L, Josse RG, Canadian Multicentre Osteoporosis Study Research Group: Kidney function and rate of bone loss at the hip and spine: the Canadian Multicentre Osteoporosis Study. *Am J Kidney Dis* 55:291–299, 2010

Jassal SK, von Muhlen D, Barrett-Connor E: Measures of renal function, BMD, bone loss, and osteoporotic fracture in older adults: the Rancho Bernardo study. *J Bone Miner Res* 22:203–210, 2007

Jobe FW, Schwab DM: Golf for the mature athlete. *Clin Sports Med* 10:269–282, 1991

Kadoglou NP, Iliadis F, Angelopoulou N, Perrea D, Ampatzidis G, Liapis CD, Alevizos M: The anti-inflammatory effects of exercise training in patients with type 2 diabetes mellitus. *Eur J Cardiovasc Prev Rehabil* 14:837–843, 2007

Kanis JA, Johnell O, Oden A, Johansson H, De Laet C, Eisman JA, Fujiwara S, Kroger H, McCloskey EV, Mellstrom D, Melton LJ, Pols H, Reeve J, Silman A, Tenenhouse A: Smoking and fracture risk: a meta-analysis. *Osteoporos Int* 16:155–162, 2005

Kemmler W, Stengel S: Exercise and osteoporosis-related fractures: perspectives and recommendations of the sports and exercise scientist. *Phys Sportsmed* 39:142–157, 2011

Kent A, Pearce A: Review of morbidity and mortality associated with falls from heights among patients presenting to a major trauma centre. *Emerg Med Australas* 18:23–30, 2006

Khazai NB, Beck GR Jr, Umpierrez GE: Diabetes and fractures: an overshadowed association. *Curr Opin Endocrinol Diabetes Obes* 16:435–445, 2009

Khoshdel A, Carney S, Gillies A, Mourad A, Jones B, Nanra R, Trevillian P: Potential roles of erythropoietin in the management of anaemia and other complications diabetes. *Diabetes Obes Metab* 10:1–9, 2008

Kirk A, Mutrie N, MacIntyre P, Fisher M: Effects of a 12-month physical activity counselling intervention on glycaemic control and on the status of cardiovascular risk factors in people with type 2 diabetes. *Diabetologia* 47:821–832, 2004

Knobloch K, Yoon U, Vogt PM: Acute and overuse injuries correlated to hours of training in master running athletes. *Foot Ankle Int* 29:671–676, 2008

Knowler WC, Barrett-Connor E, Fowler SE, Hamman RF, Lachin JM, Walker EA, Nathan DM: Reduction in the incidence of type 2 diabetes with lifestyle intervention or metformin. *N Engl J Med* 346:393–403, 2002

Kones R: Primary prevention of coronary heart disease: integration of new data, evolving views, revised goals, and role of rosuvastatin in management. A comprehensive survey. *Drug Des Devel Ther* 5:325–380, 2011

Lee SJ, Eng C: Goals of glycemic control in frail older patients with diabetes. *JAMA* 305:1350–1351, 2011

Leipzig RM, Cumming RG, Tinetti ME: Drugs and falls in older people: a systematic review and meta-analysis: II. Cardiac and analgesic drugs. *J Am Geriatr Soc* 47:40–50, 1999

Look Ahead Research Group, Wing RR: Long-term effects of a lifestyle intervention on weight and cardiovascular risk factors in individuals with type 2 diabetes mellitus: four-year results of the Look AHEAD trial. *Arch Intern Med* 170:1566–1575, 2010

Lord SR, Smith ST, Menant JC: Vision and falls in older people: risk factors and intervention strategies. *Clin Geriatr Med* 26:569–581, 2010

Lustman PJ, Clouse RE: Depression in diabetic patients: the relationship between mood and glycemic control. *J Diabetes Complications* 19:113–122, 2005

Lysy Z, Da Costa D, Dasgupta K: The association of physical activity and depression in type 2 diabetes. *Diabet Med* 25:1133–1141, 2008

Maahs DM, Nadeau K, Snell-Bergeon JK, Schauer I, Bergman B, West NA, Rewers M, Daniels SR, Ogden LG, Hamman RF, Dabelea D: Association of insulin sensitivity to lipids across the lifespan in people with type 1 diabetes. *Diabet Med* 28:148–155, 2011

Magrans-Courtney T, Wilborn C, Rasmussen C, Ferreira M, Greenwood L, Campbell B, Kerksick CM, Nassar E, Li R, Iosia M, Cooke M, Dugan K, Willoughby D, Soliah L, Kreider RB: Effects of diet type and supplementation of glucosamine, chondroitin, and MSM on body composition, functional status, and markers of health in women with knee osteoarthritis initiating a resistance-based exercise and weight loss program. *J Int Soc Sports Nutr* 8:8, 2011

Manini TM, Everhart JE, Anton SD, Schoeller DA, Cummings SR, Mackey DC, Delmonico MJ, Bauer DC, Simonsick EM, Colbert LH, Visser M, Tylavsky F, Newman AB, Harris TB: Activity energy expenditure and change in body composition in late life. *Am J Clin Nutr* 90:1336–1342, 2009a

Manini TM, Everhart JE, Patel KV, Schoeller DA, Colbert LH, Visser M, Tylavsky F, Bauer DC, Goodpaster BH, Harris TB: Daily activity energy expenditure and mortality among older adults. *JAMA* 296:171–179, 2006

Manini TM, Everhart JE, Patel KV, Schoeller DA, Cummings S, Mackey DC, Bauer DC, Simonsick EM, Colbert LH, Visser M, Tylavsky F, Newman AB, Harris TB, Aging Health and Body Composition Study: Activity energy expenditure and mobility limitation in older adults: differential associations by sex. *Am J Epidemiol* 169:1507–1516, 2009b

Marzetti E, Leeuwenburgh C: Skeletal muscle apoptosis, sarcopenia and frailty at old age. *Exp Gerontol* 41:1234–1238, 2006

McCabe LR: Understanding the pathology and mechanisms of type I diabetic bone loss. *J Cell Biochem* 102:1343–1357, 2007

McCabe L, Zhang J, Raehtz S: Understanding the skeletal pathology of type 1 and 2 diabetes mellitus. *Crit Rev Eukaryot Gene Expr* 21:187–206, 2011

McGill JB, Sloan L, Newman J, Patel S, Sauce C, von Eynatten M, Woerle HJ: Long-term efficacy and safety of linagliptin in patients with type 2 diabetes and severe renal impairment: a 1-year, randomized, double-blind, placebo-controlled study. *Diabetes Care* 2012 [Epub ahead of print]

McLennan JG, McLennan JC: Cycling and the older athlete. *Clin Sports Med* 10:291–299, 1991

Messier SP, Loeser RF, Miller GD, Morgan TM, Rejeski WJ, Sevick MA, Ettinger WH Jr, Pahor M, Williamson JD: Exercise and dietary weight loss in overweight and obese older adults with knee osteoarthritis: the Arthritis, Diet, and Activity Promotion Trial. *Arthritis Rheum* 50:1501–1510, 2004

Messier SP, Loeser RF, Mitchell MN, Valle G, Morgan TP, Rejeski WJ, Ettinger WH: Exercise and weight loss in obese older adults with knee osteoarthritis: a preliminary study. *J Am Geriatr Soc* 48:1062–1072, 2000

Michaelsson K, Byberg L, Ahlbom A, Melhus H, Farahmand BY: Risk of severe knee and hip osteoarthritis in relation to level of physical exercise: a prospective cohort study of long-distance skiers in Sweden. *PLoS One* 6:e18339, 2011

Middleton LE, Manini TM, Simonsick EM, Harris TB, Barnes DE, Tylavsky F, Brach JS, Everhart JE, Yaffe K: Activity energy expenditure and incident cognitive impairment in older adults. *Arch Intern Med* 171:1251–1257, 2011

Mitnitski A, Song X, Skoog I, Broe GA, Cox JL, Grunfeld E, Rockwood K: Relative fitness and frailty of elderly men and women in developed countries and their relationship with mortality. *J Am Geriatr Soc* 53:2184–2189, 2005

Mohandas A, Reifsnyder J, Jacobs M, Fox T: Current and future directions in frailty research. *Popul Health Manag* 14:277–283, 2011

Morrison S, Colberg SR, Mariano M, Parson HK, Vinik AI: Balance training reduces falls risk in older individuals with type 2 diabetes. *Diabetes Care* 33:748–750, 2010

Morrison S, Colberg SR, Parson HK, Vinik AI: Relation between risk of falling and postural sway complexity in diabetes. *Gait Posture* 35:662–668, 2012

Muir SW, Berg K, Chesworth B, Klar N, Speechley M: Quantifying the magnitude of risk for balance impairment on falls in community-dwelling older adults: a systematic review and meta-analysis. *J Clin Epidemiol* 63:389–406, 2010

Nelson ME, Rejeski WJ, Blair SN, Duncan PW, Judge JO, King AC, Macera CA, Castaneda-Sceppa C: Physical activity and public health in older adults: recommendation from the American College of Sports Medicine and the American Heart Association. *Med Sci Sports Exerc* 39:1435–1445, 2007

Neumiller JJ, Setter SM: Pharmacologic management of the older patient with type 2 diabetes mellitus. *Am J Geriatr Pharmacother* 7:324–342, 2009

Nichols GA, Koro CE: Does statin therapy initiation increase the risk for myopathy? An observational study of 32,225 diabetic and nondiabetic patients. *Clin Ther* 29:1761–1770, 2007

Obrosova IG, Chung SS, Kador PF: Diabetic cataracts: mechanisms and management. *Diabetes Metab Res Rev* 26:172–180, 2010

Pan A, Lucas M, Sun Q, van Dam RM, Franco OH, Manson JE, Willett WC, Ascherio A, Hu FB: Bidirectional association between depression and type 2 diabetes mellitus in women. *Arch Intern Med* 170:1884–1891, 2010

Paoloni JA, Milne C, Orchard J, Hamilton B: Non-steroidal anti-inflammatory drugs in sports medicine: guidelines for practical but sensible use. *Br J Sports Med* 43:863–865, 2009

Physical Activity Guidelines Advisory Committee: *Physical Activity Guidelines Advisory Committee Report, 2008*. Washington, DC, U.S. Department of Health and Human Services, 2008

Prior JC, Barr SI, Chow R, Faulkner RA: Prevention and management of osteoporosis: consensus statements from the Scientific Advisory Board of the Osteoporosis Society of Canada. 5. Physical activity as therapy for osteoporosis. *CMAJ* 155:940–944, 1996

Richardson AB, Miller JW: Swimming and the older athlete. *Clin Sports Med* 10:301–318, 1991

Ritz E, Haxsen V: Diabetic nephropathy and anaemia. *Eur J Clin Invest* 35 (Suppl. 3):66–74, 2005

Rogers LQ, Macera CA, Hootman JM, Ainsworth BE, Blairi SN: The association between joint stress from physical activity and self-reported osteoarthritis: an analysis of the Cooper Clinic data. *Osteoarthritis Cartilage* 10:617–622, 2002

Russell-Jones D, Cuddihy RM, Hanefeld M, Kumar A, Gonzalez JG, Chan M, Wolka AM, Boardman MK, Duration-4 Study Group: Efficacy and safety of exenatide once weekly versus metformin, pioglitazone, and sitagliptin used as monotherapy in drug-naive patients with type 2 diabetes (DURATION-4): a 26-week double-blind study. *Diabetes Care* 35:252–258, 2012

Scott D, Blizzard L, Fell J, Jones G: Prospective study of self-reported pain, radiographic osteoarthritis, sarcopenia progression, and falls risk in community-dwelling older adults. *Arthritis Care Res (Hoboken)* 64:30–37, 2012

Shimada H, Suzukawa M, Tiedemann A, Kobayashi K, Yoshida H, Suzuki T: Which neuromuscular or cognitive test is the optimal screening tool to predict falls in frail community-dwelling older people? *Gerontology* 55:532–538, 2009

Siracuse JJ, Odell DD, Gondek SP, Odom SR, Kasper EM, Hauser CJ, Moorman DW: Health care and socioeconomic impact of falls in the elderly. *Am J Surg* 203:335–338, 2012

Steeves JA, Thompson DL, Bassett DR Jr: Energy cost of stepping in place while watching television commercials. *Med Sci Sports Exerc* 44:330–335, 2012

Stewart KJ: Exercise training and the cardiovascular consequences of type 2 diabetes and hypertension: plausible mechanisms for improving cardiovascular health. *JAMA* 288:1622–1631, 2002

Thé DJ, Ploutz-Snyder L: Age, body mass, and gender as predictors of masters olympic weightlifting performance. *Med Sci Sports Exerc* 35:1216–1224, 2003

Trappe S: Master athletes. *Int J Sport Nutr Exerc Metab* 11 (Suppl.):S196–S207, 2001

Tumosa N: Eye disease and the older diabetic. *Clin Geriatr Med* 24:515–527, vii, 2008

Verkleij SP, Luijsterburg PA, Bohnen AM, Koes BW, Bierma-Zeinstra SM: NSAIDs vs acetaminophen in knee and hip osteoarthritis: a systematic review regarding heterogeneity influencing the outcomes. *Osteoarthritis Cartilage* 19:921–929, 2011

Verweij LM, van Schoor NM, Deeg DJ, Dekker J, Visser M: Physical activity and incident clinical knee osteoarthritis in older adults. *Arthritis Rheum* 61:152–157, 2009

Vestergaard P: Discrepancies in bone mineral density and fracture risk in patients with type 1 and type 2 diabetes—a meta-analysis. *Osteoporos Int* 18:427–444, 2007

Vignon E, Valat JP, Rossignol M, Avouac B, Rozenberg S, Thoumie P, Avouac J, Nordin M, Hilliquin P: Osteoarthritis of the knee and hip and activity: a systematic international review and synthesis (OASIS). *Joint Bone Spine* 73:442–455, 2006

Villaverde-Gutierrez C, Araujo E, Cruz F, Roa JM, Barbosa W, Ruiz-Villaverde G: Quality of life of rural menopausal women in response to a customized exercise programme. *J Adv Nurs* 54:11–19, 2006

Vleck VE, Bentley DJ, Millet GP, Cochrane T: Triathlon event distance specialization: training and injury effects. *J Strength Cond Res* 24:30–36, 2010

Wang X, Lyles MF, You T, Berry MJ, Rejeski WJ, Nicklas BJ: Weight regain is related to decreases in physical activity during weight loss. *Med Sci Sports Exerc* 40:1781–1788, 2008

Wexler RK: Lower extremity injuries in runners. Helping athletic patients return to form. *Postgrad Med* 98:185–187, 191–193, 1995

Willick SE, Hansen PA: Running and osteoarthritis. *Clin Sports Med* 29:417–428, 2010

Winett RA, Williams DM, Davy BM: Initiating and maintaining resistance training in older adults: a social cognitive theory-based approach. *Br J Sports Med* 43:114–119, 2009

Xue QL, Bandeen-Roche K, Varadhan R, Zhou J, Fried LP: Initial manifestations of frailty criteria and the development of frailty phenotype in the Women's Health and Aging Study II. *J Gerontol A Biol Sci Med Sci* 63:984–990, 2008

Zamparo P, Gatta G, di Prampero PE: The determinants of performance in master swimmers: an analysis of master world records. *Eur J Appl Physiol* 112:3511–3518, 2012

Zijlstra GA, van Haastregt JC, van Rossum E, van Eijk JT, Yardley L, Kempen GI: Interventions to reduce fear of falling in community-living older people: a systematic review. *J Am Geriatr Soc* 55:603–615, 2007

Zoppini G, Targher G, Zamboni C, Venturi C, Cacciatori V, Moghetti P, Muggeo M: Effects of moderate-intensity exercise training on plasma biomarkers of inflammation and endothelial dysfunction in older patients with type 2 diabetes. *Nutr Metab Cardiovasc Dis* 16:543–549, 2006

Chapter 24
Children and Adolescents

Children (ages 5–11 years) and adolescents (ages 12–17 years) face some unique physiological responses to physical activity participation that older individuals do not, such as underdeveloped neuromotor and muscular systems before reaching puberty (Vasudevan 2011). Regardless, it is both possible and recommended that young individuals participate in regular physical training to receive numerous health benefits, including higher peak bone mineral content, improved cardiorespiratory fitness levels, and reversal of early cardiovascular changes with diabetes that raise risk of later events (Khan 2000, Babar 2011). Poor glycemic control likely impairs pulmonary, cardiac, and vascular responses to exercise (Baldi 2010a, 2010b), but usually can be reversed with regular participation in physical activity. With such a long road ahead with diabetes, it is doubly important for diabetic youth to establish an exercise habit early and maintain it throughout their lifetimes to improve their health (Colberg 2009).

Case in Point: Exercise Rx for a Young Boy with T1D

SK is a 12-year-old boy with type 1 diabetes (T1D) since the age of 6 years. He has just recently started a period of accelerated growth and has gained 2 inches in height in the past 3 months. However, he has only reached Tanner stage 2 in pubertal development so far (out of 5 stages). His parents have encouraged him to be as physically active as he can, and they have worked with his endocrinologist to learn how to adjust their son's food intake and insulin doses (he uses an insulin pump) to maintain his blood glucose levels as close to normal as possible.

Resting Measurements

Height: 62 inches
Weight: 95 lb
BMI: 17.4 (normal for a prepubescent boy)
Heart rate: 88 beats per minute (bpm)
Blood pressure: 105/65 mmHg

Fasting Labs

Plasma glucose: variable (45–305 mg/dl, controlled with an insulin pump)
A1C: 7.5%

Medications

Insulin pump (apidra), with several possible basal regimens depending on physical activity levels and bolus injections ranging from 1–5 units for meals, snacks, and corrections

Questions to Consider

1. What type of physical activities should someone SK's age with T1D consider doing?
2. What precautions should SK take, and does he have any exercise limitations?

(Continued on page 454.)

EFFECTS OF PHYSICAL ACTIVITY ON DEVELOPMENT OF YOUTH

Physical activity should be an integral part of diabetes management for youth with any type of diabetes because of the health benefits that can be gained by engaging in a physical fitness plan (Colberg 2009). Because of the physical changes being experienced by children and adolescents during maturation to adulthood, however, some exercise responses may be altered.

MATURATION AND RESPONSES TO PHYSICAL TRAINING

Neuromotor control and muscular development are ongoing in children and adolescents until they finish going through full sexual maturation (i.e., puberty). Some differences that are present in prepubescent youth affect their physical coordination and ability to be physically active (Vasudevan 2011). Even adolescent athletes have reduced anaerobic power compared with adults, likely because of intrinsic properties of muscles undergoing development. Resistance training studies in male adolescents (and, to a lesser extent, female adolescents) have shown that substantial relative strength gains are possible in that age-group (Faigenbaum 2009). Moreover, aerobic trainability in young boys appears to improve markedly during the adolescent years likely because of substantial growth of the cardiorespiratory and musculoskeletal systems; studies in adolescent girls, however, are scarce and inconclusive (Naughton 2000). Intense training does not appear to impair normal growth, development, or maturation, although adolescent athletes who experience rapid growth combined with large increases in training volumes may be vulnerable to overuse injuries (Naughton 2000).

BONE DEVELOPMENT AND PHYSICAL ACTIVITY

Childhood activity is strongly associated with bone mineral accrual that may persist, at least partly, despite reduced adult physical activity, suggesting that physical activity during the most active period of maturity (with respect to longitudinal growth) plays a vital role in reaching an optimal peak bone mass (Khan 2000).

Bone mineral density reaches 90% of its peak by the age of 20 years, but one-quarter of adult bone is accumulated during the 2 years surrounding the peak bone growth velocity (i.e., early puberty), making that time particularly critical for mineralization and capitalizing on the effects of exercise-induced gains. In girls, in particular, early puberty is an opportune time for exercise interventions to positively affect bone health (Mackelvie 2001). It remains unclear what defines an optimal exercise program, although weight-bearing exercise is recommended (Hind 2007). Greater physical activity during childhood and adolescence, therefore, may be able to prevent bone fractures and osteoporosis later in life, which is particularly important in individuals with T1D who generally have lower bone mineral density (Khazai 2009) and for those with type 2 diabetes (T2D) who are more prone to fractures (Gorman 2012).

In contrast, participation in strenuous physical activity may affect the female reproductive system and lead to "athletic amenorrhea," the prevalence of which is 4–20 times higher in female athletes than the general population (Eliakim 2003). As a result, bone demineralization may develop, leading to increased skeletal fragility and fractures. Menstrual abnormalities (amenorrhea) in heavily training female athletes result from suppression of gonadotropin-releasing hormone. Reduced energy availability because of inadequate caloric intake with the level of training is the main cause; the training load should be reduced and caloric intake increased to prevent menstrual abnormalities and deleterious bone effects during critical periods of rapid bone growth (Eliakim 2003).

CARDIORESPIRATORY FITNESS

Peak oxygen consumption increases with age and maturation. Boys, however, have a peak value that is higher than for girls, even when differences in body mass and lean body mass are taken into account (Bertelloni 2006). Body composition is the main predictor for differences in peak oxygen consumption in children ages 8–11 years (with girls having higher body fat) (Dencker 2006). Young athletes of both sexes, however, have higher peak oxygen consumption and better lactate kinetics at the same relative exercise intensity than their untrained peers.

Maximum oxygen uptake generally is considered to be the best single marker for aerobic fitness. Although a positive relationship between daily physical activity and aerobic fitness has been established in adults, the relationship remains less clear in children and adolescents (Dencker 2011). All youth can increase peak values to some extent with exercise training, although levels of habitual physical activity generally do not correlate with aerobic fitness (Armstrong 2011). Moreover, when measured with accelerometers, physical activity of higher intensities undertaken by youth is not more closely related to maximal oxygen consumption than lower intensities (Dencker 2006, 2011).

Most adolescents with T2D have a fitness level that is lower than their peers and youth with T1D (Faulkner 2005, 2010). Some, but not all, youth with T1D have the same aerobic capacity as their similar-age counterparts without diabetes. Poor glycemic control likely impairs pulmonary, cardiac, and vascular responses to exercise (Baldi 2010a, 2010b). Although exercise training in diabetic youth improves their aerobic fitness levels (Seeger 2011), it remains to be seen whether reduced fitness in children with T1D is attributable to lower physical activity levels or to physiological changes resulting from diabetes itself (Williams 2011). In either case, high fitness levels appear to modify the impact that body fatness has on the metabolic syndrome score in children. In general, youth with a lower BMI have lower blood pressure and blood lipid levels, regardless of their fitness level, compared with similar-age youth with a higher BMI, and being heavy and unfit leads to the most adverse metabolic and potential cardiovascular outcomes (Eisenmann 2007a, 2007b). Thus, increasing the fitness level of overweight youth with any type of diabetes could be one method for reducing their risk of obesity-related comorbidities and is highly recommended (DuBose 2007).

OBESITY AND CARDIOVASCULAR CONCERNS

Rates of overweight and obesity in youth and adults have risen sharply during the past 20 years, likely reflective of sedentary lifestyles and dietary changes in combination with genetic predisposition (Skilton 2006). The earliest physical signs of atherosclerosis, the underlying disease process that leads to increased risk of heart disease, myocardial infarction, and stroke, may be present from early childhood when accelerated by the presence of comorbid conditions, such as obesity, diabetes, hypertension, and dyslipidemia. Children and adolescents once were considered to be low risk, but health issues related to sedentary lifestyle, poor diet, and obesity may lead to an earlier need for cardiovascular screening and interventions, especially in youth with both weight issues and diabetes (Short 2009). A substantial proportion of youth with T1D or T2D already exhibit abnormal serum lipids (Kershnar 2006), and glycemic control and lipid levels are independently associated in youth with either types of diabetes (Petitti 2007). Moreover, preadolescent children with T1D have been shown to have some endothelial dysfunction and systemic inflammation, known harbingers of future cardiovascular risk, despite relatively short diabetes duration (Babar 2011).

Early detection of vascular dysfunction is important to identify youth at risk for eventual cardiovascular morbidity and mortality and to initiate interventions to reduce that risk (Trigona 2010). Screening can include noninvasive methods like measurements of endothelial function, arterial compliance, and intima-media thickness. Youth with T1D present early signs of atherosclerosis, as well as low physical activity levels and levels of cardiorespiratory fitness, but their endothelial function can be enhanced by engaging in >60 min of daily moderate- to vigorous-intensity physical activity (Trigona 2010). Regular activity also improves blood pressure, body weight, and risk of health complications (Moy 1993, Laaksonen 2000, Costacou 2007, Herbst 2007, Heyman 2007, Bishop 2009, Conway 2009, Trigona 2010, D'Hooge 2011, Maahs 2011). Therefore, current strategies for prevention of vascular disease should include exercise programs, dietary interventions, and possible pharmacological therapy (Skilton 2006, Short 2009, Landberg 2012).

EXERCISE RESPONSES IN YOUTH WITH DIABETES

CHANGES IN INSULIN ACTION AND DOSAGES

Heavier adolescents with T2D in particular have poorer glycemic control, although regular exercise almost invariably improves it (Faulkner 2005). Physical activity participation by youth with T1D, however, may not necessarily ameliorate blood glucose control without appropriate changes in insulin and carbohydrate intake, and sedentary behavior has been associated with poorer glycemic management in T1D (Eberling 1995, Roberts 2002, Ramalho 2006). Exercise is considered an indispensable component in the treatment of adolescents with T1D in any case as it can improve their glycemic control (Salem 2010). Moreover, children with T1D who exercise more than twice weekly have better A1C levels, particularly when engaging in physical activity for ≥60 min at a time (Aouadi 2011).

Even in postmenarche adolescent girls with T1D, a combination of aerobic and resistance training increases muscle mass and lowers their risk of insulin resistance (Heyman 2007). Insulin resistance in adolescents with T2D is associated with a greater body weight, but for youth with T1D, a resistant state is frequently present without necessarily being closely linked to body weight (Reinehr 2005). Insulin doses, however, are reduced by regular exercise participation because of improvements in insulin action whether or not A1C levels are improved (Trigona 2010, Seeger 2011). Physical activity has been shown to reverse the negative glycemic impact of sedentary pursuits as well (Benevento 2010).

USING SPRINTS TO MAINTAIN GLYCEMIC CONTROL

Many youth with T1D in particular engage in team sports that involve intermittent high-intensity training. Although studies have not been undertaken with that population, young adults with T1D have participated in high-intensity protocols consisting of 4 s sprints done every 2 min during moderate activity to simulate team sport play (Guelfi 2005a). With sprinting included, blood glucose levels decrease less during activities and remain higher following the activity for at least 1 h. The conclusion of such research is that intermittent high-intensity exercise does not increase the risk of early postexercise hypoglycemia in T1D (Guelfi 2005b), likely related to a lesser glycemic decrement during exercise and attenuated blood glucose uptake during exercise and early recovery (Guelfi 2007). Such training also has been shown to enhance muscle oxidative metabolism in young adults with T1D, which may have clinically important health benefits (Harmer 2008). It also may protect against nocturnal hypoglycemia in young athletes with T1D (Iscoe 2011).

Hypoglycemia may be prevented by capitalizing on the adrenergic effects of sprinting. For example, young individuals with T1D who engage in a 10-s maximal sprint at the end of a bout of moderate activity prevent their blood glucose levels from decreasing as much as if they were resting (Bussau 2006). Performing a 10-s sprint immediately before moderate-intensity exercise also prevents blood glucose decrements during early recovery from moderate-intensity exercise (Bussau 2007). One note of caution, however, is that intermittent, high-intensity training may result in a higher incidence of delayed nocturnal hypoglycemia without appropriate regimen changes (Maran 2010).

THERMOREGULATION IN YOUTH DURING PHYSICAL ACTIVITY

Children and adults employ different thermoregulatory strategies, particularly in response to heat. For instance, youth rely more on dry heat exchange given that they have a lesser ability to sweat before reaching puberty, whereas adults lose more heat through evaporative losses (i.e., sweating) (Falk 2011). Along with lower sweating rates, children also exhibit a greater surface-area-to-mass ratio, higher peripheral blood flow in the heat, and greater vasoconstriction in the cold, along with a lower exercise economy and lesser cardiac output at the same workload compared with adults (Rowland 2008). Although youth can acclimatize to exercising in the heat, it usually takes them longer to adapt, which increases their risk of thermal injury during activity in hotter environments. Despite these differences, however, recent studies have not found that maturation stage greatly affects thermal balance or endurance performance during exercise in the heat, and young athletes are not more vulnerable to heat injury than adults under most environment conditions (Rowland 2008). Apparently, their reliance on dry heat dissipation via their larger relative skin surface area enables them to evaporate sweat more efficiently while conserving body water better than adults (Falk 2008). Hence, although exercising in hot conditions raises concerns about proper hydration and heat dissipation, children and adolescents may not have additional worries beyond those faced by older individuals. With diabetes, however, they must focus on managing blood glucose levels to prevent water losses that can occur with hyperglycemia and that could negatively affect their ability to dissipate heat during activities (Manz 2007, Ugale 2012).

Case in Point: Continued

SK has a passion that revolves around playing soccer, which he started doing at the age of 4 years, 2 years before developing T1D. His parents have encouraged him to play as much as he wants to, and up through last year, he was playing on both fall and spring soccer leagues. This year, however, he began playing with a travel soccer team that practices year-round and has harder and more frequent practices, and now he has begun experiencing more problems with his diabetes control. Coupled with his recent growth spurt, he feels like he can never get enough to eat, but intake of large quantities of food makes his insulin dosing more problematic, and he has started experiencing wider swings in his blood glucose levels and more frequent bouts of hypoglycemia.

Additional Questions to Consider

1. What steps can SK take to prevent hypoglycemia associated with physical activity?
2. What should he do to treat hyperglycemia associated with intense activities or consuming too many carbohydrates?

(Continued on page 463.)

MAKING APPROPRIATE EXERCISE-RELATED REGIMEN CHANGES

Youth with any type of diabetes need to learn how to adequately adjust their diet and possibly insulin requirements to maximize performance, maintain glycemic control, and reduce fatigue (Gallen 2011). With an appropriate adjustment of insulin dose and diet, children and adolescents with T1D can effectively and safely participate in a wide variety of competitive events and sports (Koivisto 1992). Youth with T2D may have exercise-related concerns because of their body weight, but they also can participate in a variety of physical activities (American Diabetes Association 2000, Graf 2009, Graves 2010).

General management of blood glucose levels during and after exercise, hypoglycemia prevention and treatment, hyperglycemia and dehydration, and balancing insulin use with physical activity are critical topics associated with exercise prescription for youth with T1D or for youth with T2D taking insulin, as discussed in chapters 11 through 14 of this book.

SELF-MONITORING OF BLOOD GLUCOSE

Blood glucose responses to physical activity depend on duration, intensity, food intake, insulin doses, and more. In all youth, moderate aerobic exercise usually causes blood glucose levels to drop rapidly, whereas higher-intensity activities may cause them to rise. Use of self-monitoring of blood glucose (SMBG) will assist in making appropriate regimen changes to maintain glycemic balance. Some youth with T1D also may use continuous glucose monitoring (CGM) systems to help determine their usual glycemic responses, trends of hypoglycemia and hyperglycemia, and exercise effects (Riddell 2009, Maran 2010, Chu 2011). CGM reduces the incidence and duration of hypoglycemia, but it does so only to a limited extent because it overestimates blood glucose levels in the low range and lags behind real-time values by 15–20 min (Davey 2010), although trends and directional changes can be used to establish better glycemic management (Riddell 2009).

APPROPRIATE CARBOHYDRATE INTAKE

In youth with T1D, carbohydrate intake may be required to prevent hypoglycemia both during and after exercise, depending on the type of activity done, duration, and timing relative to insulin dosing and doses. In one study on adults with T1D, blood glucose levels were reportedly higher during 60 min of moderate treadmill walking when consuming a glucose polymer sports drink and prevented the onset of postexercise hypoglycemia without causing hyperglycemia (Tamis-Jortberg 1996). Ingestion of either whole milk and sports drinks designed for either quick or long-lasting nutrient replenishment may be effective in preventing postexercise hypoglycemia overnight (Hernandez 2000). For youth using an insulin pump and engaging in moderate or vigorous activity without altering basal rates, ingestion of sugary drinks during exercise, reduction of the overnight basal rate, reduction of the predinner insulin bolus, or a bedtime snack may be needed to prevent hypoglycemia (Delvecchio 2009).

To estimate carbohydrate utilization in youth who differ in size and energy expenditure based on the activity, a table of recommended carbohydrate intake for 30 min of activity may be a useful starting point (see Table 24.1) (Chu 2011). These values estimate the amount of additional carbohydrate that may be needed during 30 min of a given sport when peak insulin levels are high and if no reductions in insulin are made in anticipation of the activity. Timing of exercise matters, however, as carbohydrate requirements progressively decrease when 1 h of exer-

Table 24.1. Recommended Carbohydrate Intake (Grams) for Type 1 Diabetic Youth for 30 Minutes of Activity (Based on Body Mass)

	Body Mass lb (kg)		
	44 (20)	88 (40)	132 (60)
Basketball	23	45	68
Cycling			
moderate	7	11	18
heavy	10	18	27
Skating	18	36	54
Running			
moderate	17	30	41
heavy	30	41	55
Soccer	17	32	48
Swimming			
breaststroke	14	27	52
Tennis	11	19	28

cise is performed 1, 2.5, 4, and 5.5 h after a meal preceded by an injection of a standard dose (1 U/kg) of regular insulin (Francescato 2004).

Consuming a high-carbohydrate diet for sport-specific training is not advisable for youth with T1D, at least not without making compensatory insulin changes and achieving adequate glycemic control, as the hyperglycemia that can result may impair postexercise muscle and liver glycogen restoration rather than enhance it (Burke 1999, McKewen 1999, American Dietetic Association 2009). For most youth, intake of at least 40% of calories from carbohydrates, along with adequate protein and total daily calories, is likely to restore glycogen most effectively without causing hyperglycemia (American Dietetic Association 2009).

COMPENSATORY INSULIN ADJUSTMENTS

For children with T1D and those with T2D taking insulin, careful review of insulin dosages, insulin peaks and durations of action, and timing of meals and snacks is critical to avoidance of problems with widely variant blood glucose levels related to physical activity. Frequent SMBG (i.e., before, during, and after exercise) will assist in guiding adjustments in insulin dosing. Because of an increased uptake of glucose into skeletal muscle during exercise, children who are developing a new pattern of regular activity or conditioning may be particularly susceptible to hypoglycemic episodes, during or following exercise or even hours afterward (Ploug 1984). To avoid problems, a decrease in "insulin onboard" during active periods and modifications in food intake may be needed.

Hypoglycemia risk can be lowered by making adjustments to insulin doses and timing of doses both during and following exercise. For example, a 75%

reduction of insulin with a meal taken 2 h before 45 min of moderate running results in more effective blood glucose management during and after activity compared with 0%, 25%, and 50% dose reductions and allows for a lesser intake of food during the next 24 h (West 2010). The types of insulin and insulin regimens used also can affect exercise-related adjustments. Insulin detemir is associated with less hypoglycemia than glargine both during and after exercise (Arutchelvam 2009), although the use of a basal-bolus regimen with insulin lispro for meals and insulin glargine at bedtime by preschool-age children with T1D actually improved overall glycemic control and decreased frequency of severe hypoglycemia (Alemzadeh 2005). For youth on an insulin pump, discontinuing basal insulin during exercise is an effective strategy for reducing hypoglycemia, but the risk of hyperglycemia is increased (Diabetes Research in Children Network Study Group 2006).

Adolescents with T1D on insulin pump therapy have been shown to reduce their risk of severe hypoglycemia by as much as 50%, even while achieving lower A1C levels (Boland 1999). They also have been studied doing moderate- or high-intensity physical activity with their insulin pumps switched on or off (Delvecchio 2009). Their postexercise blood glucose levels were much higher with the pump off and unchanged or lower with the pump on. Thus, it may be advisable to leave the basal rate going during most physical activity, with the understanding that doing so likely will require consumption of carbohydrate during the exercise, a lowered basal rate overnight, a small insulin bolus for dinner, and a possible bedtime snack to prevent hypoglycemia. Exercise increases glycemic variability after a meal, depending on its intensity. Thus, the absolute glucose level after a typical bout of exercise in the fed state should be a good guide to carbohydrate or insulin adjustment on subsequent occasions (Biankin 2003).

A fuller discussion of insulin regimen changes is included in chapter 14. For comprehensive coverage of insulin, food, and exercise regimen changes for youth (and for adults with T1D and other insulin users with T2D), refer to *Diabetic Athlete's Handbook: Your Guide to Peak Performance* (Colberg 2009).

PREVENTION OF HYPOGLYCEMIA

Fear of hypoglycemia is the strongest barrier to regular physical activity in anyone with T1D (Brazeau 2008), and prevention and management of hypoglycemia is fully discussed in chapter 12. Use of education, frequent SMBG, use of rapid-acting and basal insulin analogs, insulin pump therapy, exercise-related insulin modifications, and use of CGM may all reduce its incidence (Realsen 2011). Delayed onset of hypoglycemia, especially overnight during sleep, is common and a major concern for youth with T1D (Tsalikian 2005). In fact, glucose requirements after exercise are biphasic, with additional carbohydrate needed both following afternoon exercise and 7–11 h later, thereby increasing the risk of nocturnal hypoglycemia (McMahon 2007). Youth with T1D and those with T2D who use insulin will need to make adjustments in glycemic management before and after any physical activity to minimize its occurrence (MacDonald 1987, Hernandez 2000, Kalergis 2003, Alemzadeh 2005, Tsalikian 2005, Diabetes Research in Children Network Study Group 2006, McMahon 2007, Tamborlane 2007, Cooperberg 2008, Wilson 2008).

PHYSICAL ACTIVITY PARTICIPATION BY CHILDREN AND ADOLESCENTS

For almost all youth with diabetes, the potential benefits far exceed the potential risks associated with physical activity. Both children and adolescents should be encouraged to be physically active daily as part of play, games, sports, transportation, recreation, physical education, or planned exercise in the context of family, school, and community (e.g., volunteer, employment) activities (Khan 2000, Graf 2009, Agmon 2011, Bailey 2011). In addition, they should be engaging in normal activities associated with daily living (daily movement) to promote a healthy weight, better glycemic management, and prevention of complications (Dencker 2011). For youth with a sedentary lifestyle, participating in physical activity below the recommended levels can provide some health benefits, and it is entirely appropriate to start with smaller amounts of activity and gradually increase duration, frequency, and intensity as a stepping stone to meeting the guidelines.

RESISTANCE TRAINING PROGRAMS

Many groups used to recommend that children and prepubescent adolescents avoid heavy weight training because the epiphyseal growth plates on their bones could be injured and close prematurely. The very rare reports of growth plate fractures in children who trained with weights, however, occurred as a result of inadequate supervision, improper form, or excess weight, and there have been no reports of injuries to growth plates in youth training programs that followed established guidelines. At present, the National Strength and Conditioning Association recognizes that many of the benefits associated with adult resistance training programs are attainable by children and adolescents who follow age-specific resistance training guidelines (Faigenbaum 2009, 2010a). In addition to increasing muscular strength and power, regular participation in a pediatric resistance training program may have a favorable influence on body composition, bone health, and reduction of sports-related injuries (Hind 2007, D'Hooge 2011). Resistance training targeted to improve low fitness levels, poor trunk strength, and deficits in movement mechanics can offer observable health and fitness benefits to young athletes (Faigenbaum 2010b). Pediatric resistance training programs need to be well designed and supervised by qualified professionals, however, who understand the physical and psychosocial uniqueness of children and adolescents, particularly those with diabetes (Faigenbaum 2010b).

Regular participation in a multifaceted resistance training program that begins during the preseason and includes instruction on movement biomechanics may reduce the risk of sports-related injuries in young athletes (Faigenbaum 2010a, 2010b). Children actually have a lower risk of resistance training–related joint sprains and muscle strains than adults. The majority of youth resistance training injuries are the result of accidents (e.g., performing an exercise incorrectly or dropping a weight) that are potentially preventable with increased supervision and stricter safety guidelines (Myer 2009).

EXERCISE PRESCRIPTION FOR CHILDREN AND ADOLESCENTS

Physical activity has a direct impact on weight control, cardiovascular risk factors, bone development, and mental health over a lifetime. A sedentary lifestyle in young people often is seen to lead to negative health consequences in the near term and later in life.

ENGAGING IN AGE-APPROPRIATE ACTIVITIES

Updated guidelines recommend that children and adolescents participate in at least 60 min of moderate-intensity physical activity most days of the week, preferably daily (Haskell 2007, Physical Activity Guidelines Advisory Committee 2008). Children and adolescents, however, should engage in activities that are age-appropriate and cater to their natural patterns of movement, which differ from adults (Physical Activity Guidelines Advisory Committee 2008). Most children's activities are unstructured play that is intermittent in nature, such as during recess and in their free play and games. They often employ basic aerobic and bone-strengthening activities, such as running, hopping, skipping, and jumping, to develop movement patterns and skills, alternating brief periods of moderate- and vigorous-intensity physical activity with similar rest periods. Children also commonly increase muscle strength through unstructured activities that involve lifting or moving their body weight or working against resistance and rarely do or require formal muscle-strengthening programs like lifting weights. They should be encouraged to participate in school physical education classes, recreation leagues, school sports, and active family outings, and parents should be involved in the planning and development of appropriate physical activity programs for their children.

Adolescents begin to develop more adult-like physical activity patterns, with participation in organized sports for longer, sustained periods of time (Physical Activity Guidelines Advisory Committee 2008). Even if brief, any intermittent activity they engage in can count toward meeting the recommended levels of moderate or vigorous intensity. Adolescents may include free play (like skateboarding or Frisbee), structured programs (e.g., sports participation), or both. Structured exercise programs can include aerobic activities, as well as muscle-strengthening activities like lifting weights, working with resistance bands, or using body weight for resistance (e.g., push-ups, pull-ups, and sit-ups). Any muscle-strengthening activities that involve a moderate to high level of effort and work the major muscle groups of the body (legs, hips, back, abdomen, chest, shoulders, and arms) help them reach recommended daily participation.

Mode. Care should be taken to identify safe and age-appropriate options for physical activity, which should evolve as the young individual undergoes normal maturation in coordination, motor skills, social development, and personal interests. They should include a variety of aerobic, muscle-strengthening, and bone-strengthening activities on a weekly basis.

Intensity, frequency, and duration. For youth, the recommendation is for them to engage in ≥60 min of physical activity performed on all days of the

Table 24.2 Recommended Types of Physical Activities for Youth with Diabetes

Children and adolescents should do ≥60 min of physical activity daily consisting of a mix of the following activities. It is important to encourage young people to participate in physical activities that are age-appropriate and enjoyable and that offer variety.

- **Aerobic:** Most of the ≥60 min/day should be either moderate- or vigorous-intensity aerobic physical activity, and should include vigorous-intensity physical activity at least 3 days/week.
- **Muscle-strengthening:** As part of their ≥60 min of daily physical activity, children and adolescents should include muscle-strengthening physical activity on at least 3 days/week.
- **Bone-strengthening:** As part of their ≥60 min of daily physical activity, children and adolescents should include bone-strengthening physical activity on at least 3 days/week.

week that includes moderate- to vigorous-intensity mixed aerobic and anaerobic physical activity, for a total of at least 420 min/week (60 min/day) (Janssen 2007).

Hypoglycemia prevention. The blood glucose changes that occur during physical activity need to be addressed for all youth who use insulin and have a higher risk of hypoglycemia. Lower starting blood glucose levels increased the incidence of hypoglycemia during physical activities (Diabetes Research in Children Network Study Group 2006). Hypoglycemia occurred in 86% of youth doing a 75-min physical activity session with starting blood glucose values <120 mg/dl, in 13% starting glucose between 120 and 180 mg/dl, and in 6% starting at 180 mg/dl or higher, and a 15-g carbohydrate snack frequently was insufficient to successfully treat a hypoglycemic event (Diabetes Research in Children Network Study Group 2006). This study reinforces the necessity of beginning at a target blood glucose level and consuming a sufficient amount of carbohydrate to decrease the risk of experiencing a hypoglycemic episode during (and following) physical activity. In addition, insulin reductions may be necessary to prevent hypoglycemia during longer-duration exercise (West 2010). It also is important to teach parents of young exercisers with diabetes not to overreact to postexercise hyperglycemia, which is usually only transient and may need reduced or no insulin to treat effectively for several hours afterward (Delvecchio 2009).

Assigned responsibilities. Responsibility for diabetes care decisions also evolves with the maturity of youth, with adolescents (and some children) taking on more of the responsibility for diabetes management and seeking independence from parental supervision. Parents and their children should work together to clearly assign the diabetes care tasks to be performed and distribution of these responsibilities.

Special concerns. Athletes with diabetes may be even more prone to repetitive-use, soft-tissue injuries that can be avoided with a modified training schedule, especially

Table 24.3 Recommended Exercise Rx for Children and Adolescents

Mode	Aerobic: Aerobic activities are those in which youth rhythmically move their large muscles by doing things like running, hopping, skipping, jumping rope, swimming, dancing, and bicycling that increase cardiorespiratory fitness. In addition, young children often do activities in short bursts, which may not technically be aerobic activities
	Muscle-strengthening: These activities can be unstructured and part of play, such as playing on playground equipment, climbing trees, and playing tug-of-war; structured examples include lifting weights or working with resistance bands
	Bone-strengthening: Activities that produce a force on the bones that promotes bone growth and strength, commonly produced by impact with the ground; examples include running, jumping rope, basketball, tennis, and hopscotch, many of which can also be considered aerobic and/or muscle-strengthening
Intensity	Aerobic: 40–89% heart rate reserve, or HRR (initial intensity may be lower for sedentary, unfit, and overweight youth); moderate- or vigorous-intensity aerobic physical activity, but include a vigorous-intensity physical activity at least 3 days/week
	All Activities: Perceived exertion of "somewhat hard" to "hard," or 5–8 (on 10-point scale), at least intermittently
Frequency	Aerobic: Ideally 7 days/week (daily), as part of an exercise routine with muscle- and bone-strengthening activities on some days
	Muscle-Strengthening: Include this type of activity at least 3 days/week
	Bone-Strengthening: Include this type of activity at least 3 days/week
Duration	Aerobic: Most of the 60 min/day or more of activity should be either moderate- or vigorous-intensity aerobic physical activity
	Muscle-Strengthening: Include as part of the 60 min/day or more of activity (on at least 3 days)
	Bone-Strengthening: Include as part of the 60 min/day or more of activity (on at least 3 days)
Progression	Start slowly if unfit, overweight, or primarily sedentary, and progress to doing longer-duration activity more days per week until meeting minimum requirements; increase total amount of vigorous activity last to avoid injuries; vary activities as well to promote adherence and enjoyment

for youth that participate in sports year-round (Yeung 2001, Craig 2008). Furthermore, disordered eating behaviors are prevalent among teens and young adults, and this behavior has been reported in adolescents with diabetes as well (Meltzer 2001, Ackard 2008). Insulin omission and misuse (presumably to control body weight) have been reported in both adolescent girls and boys (Quinn 2003, Ackard 2008, Olmsted 2008). Likewise, exercise patterns can become compulsive in this age-group in an attempt to control both blood glucose levels and body weight with excessive physical activity.

EXERCISING WITH AN INSULIN PUMP

Insulin pump (continuous subcutaneous insulin infusion) therapy became more widely accepted for youth with T1D in the mid-1990s after the availability of the first rapid-acting insulin analog, insulin lispro. Pediatric endocrinologists previously were cautious about pump use in children, particularly as a result of the threefold increase in severe hypoglycemia reported among intensively treated patients in the Diabetes Control and Complications Trial (DCCT) (DCCT Research Group 1997). Of these, two-thirds used an insulin pump at some time, and all used regular insulin. With advances in insulin development and in pump features, however, the fear of severe hypoglycemia associated with intensive diabetes management has diminished (Maahs 2010). In fact, in contrast to the increase in severe hypoglycemic events after the DCCT results were released, the introduction of rapid-acting insulins for pump use has not resulted in an increase in the number of severe hypoglycemic episodes despite further improvements in A1C values (Chase 2001). Modern pump use in children and adolescents with T1D likely also lowers their overall risk for episodes of hypoglycemia of any severity (Boland 1999, Kordonouri 2011).

Pump use allows for modulation of basal insulin doses, along with the use of temporary basal rates. During exercise, pumps can have basal rates unchanged, reduced, or turned off, or the pump can be removed completely (Admon 2005, Delvecchio 2009). Discontinuing basal insulin during exercise is an effective strategy for reducing hypoglycemia, but the risk of hyperglycemia is increased (Diabetes Research in Children Network Study Group 2006). Pump discontinuation usually is not recommended for longer than 1 h, but it has been studied during moderate exercise for up to 3 h. The length of time without basal insulin administration results in increased plasma levels of fatty acids and ketone bodies. A correction bolus will rapidly raise plasma insulin levels, but it may take at least 90 min to normalize blood glucose levels and ketones (Jankovec 2011). Youth are able to administer multiple daily basal rates that account for recent physical activity and other factors with ease while wearing an insulin pump. Additional correction boluses can be given without the need for another needle prick.

Table 24.4 Advantages and Disadvantages of Insulin Pump Use

Advantages	Disadvantages
Improved blood sugar control	Have to remember to give insulin boluses
Insulin availability and convenience	with food intake
Use of multiple basal rates	Rapid onset of ketoacidosis if insulin
Use of temporary basal rates	delivery suspended too long or blocked
Ease of administering multiple boluses	(e.g., bad infusion site)
Reduction of hypoglycemia	Psychological factors
Flexibility and freedom	Expense
Control of postmeal blood sugar	Weight gain with tighter control
Ease of adjusting insulin doses with	Skin infections (infusion set placement)
exercise	Insulin unavailability and instability
Ease of adjusting insulin doses with travel	Infusion site locations and set changes
	Physical and logistical considerations

Case in Point: Wrap-Up

SK's parents have found that his practices can be managed effectively when he eats dinner 45 min before starting his usual 90-min soccer practices in the evenings, assuming that he cuts his insulin lispro bolus for dinner back by 20–25% for what he usually eats. During practices, he removes his insulin pump and checks his blood glucose if he starts to feel hypoglycemic. At bedtime, he eats a large snack (usually cereal and some protein) and takes a smaller bolus than usual for it. Depending on his bedtime blood glucose (lower or higher than 150 mg/dl), he may need to reduce his overnight basal rates or eat a bit extra. Despite this routine, however, he and his parents are finding it hard to keep his blood glucose levels stable overnight with his new year-round schedule and harder practices, and they are all weary from having to wake up at 2:00 A.M. every day to test SK's blood glucose levels.

Exercise Program Goals

Mode of Activity: SK's soccer practices include a mix of aerobic, muscle-strengthening, and bone-strengthening activities by the time his coach has them do some conditioning drills (including jumping jacks), ball drills, game play, and abdominal and upper-body work (i.e., curls, planks, and push-ups). His goal will be to increase his fitness level so that he can play not only one tournament game, but also two games in a day without getting excessively tired during the second one.

Intensity: Almost all SK's soccer practices include a mix of moderate and intense activities, including intermittent high-intensity work.

Frequency: SK will be meeting the recommendation of daily physical activity, given that he has soccer practice 5 days/week and games on one or both days of the weekends. He also has physical activity classes that he is required to take in school, and they are active in that class most days, which adds to his daily physical activity.

Duration: SK should be getting at least 1 h/day of physical activity, and with his travel soccer schedule, he is exceeding that amount on most days of the week. On his "rest" days, he should attempt to minimally break up his sitting time during the days by walking around and doing activities of daily living (or free play).

Progression: With his tough schedule, SK should be careful with progressing to doing any more intense activities than he already is. He may be more prone to developing overuse injuries with diabetes, and an injury that sidelines him would have a sizeable impact on his blood glucose management and should be avoided. He should use the down time between seasonal play (the few weeks when practices are reduced several times a year) to engage in alternative activities like cycling or swimming.

Regimen Changes: SK will need to plan ahead for soccer practices and games, especially those occurring within 1–2 h after meals, and lower his rapid-acting insulin doses to compensate. After longer practices or intense games, he will need to be particularly vigilant about moderating his postexercise meal insulin boluses and overnight basal rates, along with consuming an appropriate (balanced) bedtime snack to prevent hypoglycemia and provide extra calories. During exercise sessions, he should always have a rapid-acting carbohydrate source, like glucose tablets or gels, readily available to treat low blood glucose levels, as well as additional snacks that can provide extra carbohydrates (like granola bars). Finally, given that play during games can be less predictable and more intense, he should plan on supplementing with carbohydrates as needed during games based on SMBG results rather than adjusting insulin doses until later, although he may take off his pump during play and reconnect it during breaks to prevent hyperglycemia. Any boluses he gives for correction of elevated blood glucose levels either during or following activities should be reduced significantly (likely by ≥50%). SK's parents may consider having him use a CGM system, especially at night, to alert him to hypoglycemia then and to establish patterns and trends at other times of day.

Possible Precautions: SK's parents should ask his health-care provider to prescribe a glucagon pen as a treatment for severe hypoglycemia. SK should keep it with him at all times, and both his parents and soccer coaches should be instructed on its use.

Youth with diabetes can participate in recommended amounts of physical activity. Activities should include a mix of aerobic training, muscle-strengthening activities, and bone-strengthening activities. Children should focus more on free play and other physical activities, although adolescents may start engaging in competitive sports and resistance training and experience more adult-like responses to training. Although maintaining glycemic control can be challenging at time, the benefits to be gained from being physically activity far outweigh the possible risks for youth of all ages who have either T1D or T2D.

PROFESSIONAL PRACTICE PEARLS

- Children (ages 5–11 years) and adolescents (ages 12–17 years) face some unique physiological responses to physical activity participation that older individuals do not.
- Regular physical activity participation during longitudinal growth in youth plays a vital role in reaching an optimal peak bone mass.
- Youth with any type of diabetes may have lower cardiorespiratory fitness, and poor glycemic control likely impairs pulmonary, cardiac, and vascular responses to exercise.
- Most youth with T2D have lower fitness levels, whereas some, but not all, individuals with T1D have the same aerobic capacity as similar-age people without diabetes.
- Increasing the fitness level of overweight youth with any type of diabetes may reduce their risk of obesity-related comorbidities and is highly recommended.
- Early detection of vascular dysfunction is important to identify youth at risk for eventual cardiovascular morbidity and mortality and to initiate interventions to reduce that risk.

■ Youth with any type of diabetes need to adjust their diet and possibly insulin doses to maximize exercise performance, maintain glycemic control, and reduce fatigue.

■ Moderate exercise usually causes a decline in blood glucose levels; conversely, high-intensity training can maintain more stable levels or possibly result in hyperglycemia.

■ Appropriate diabetes regimen changes using frequent monitoring must be made if improved blood glucose management is an expected outcome of regular physical activity.

■ Regimen changes to manage glycemic balance with physical activity likely will involve greater food intake, changes in insulin doses and timing, or both.

■ Hypoglycemia risk can be lowered by engaging in a 10 s maximal sprint immediately before or at the end of a bout of moderate activity or by intermittent sprints during moderate activities (such as during most team sport play).

■ Many of the benefits associated with adult resistance training programs are attainable by children and adolescents who follow age-specific resistance training guidelines.

■ All youth should engage in at least ≥60 min/day of physical activity 7 days/week, including aerobic, muscle-strengthening, and bone-strengthening activities.

■ Youth should include vigorous-intensity activities at least 3 days/week and activities that strengthen muscles and bone at least 3 days/week.

■ Children and adolescents should start out slowly if deconditioned, but they all should progress to engaging in vigorous activity at least three times weekly.

■ Youth should vary activities, but it is possible for them to meet the recommended levels of physical activity by doing free play, structured programs, or both.

REFERENCES

Ackard DM, Vik N, Neumark-Sztainer D, Schmitz KH, Hannan P, Jacobs DR Jr.: Disordered eating and body dissatisfaction in adolescents with type 1 diabetes and a population-based comparison sample: comparative prevalence and clinical implications. *Pediatr Diabetes* 9 (4 Pt 1):312–319, 2008

Admon G, Weinstein Y, Falk B, Weintrob N, Benzaquen H, Ofan R, Fayman G, Zigel L, Constantini N, Phillip M: Exercise with and without an insulin pump among children and adolescents with type 1 diabetes mellitus. *Pediatrics* 116:e348–355, 2005

Agmon M, Perry CK, Phelan E, Demiris G, Nguyen HQ: A pilot study of Wii Fit exergames to improve balance in older adults. *J Geriatr Phys Ther* 34:161–167, 2011

Alemzadeh R, Berhe T, Wyatt DT: Flexible insulin therapy with glargine insulin improved glycemic control and reduced severe hypoglycemia among preschool-aged children with type 1 diabetes mellitus. *Pediatrics* 115:1320–1324, 2005

American Diabetes Association: Type 2 diabetes in children and adolescents. *Diabetes Care* 23:381–389, 2000

American Dietetic Association, Dietitians of Canada, American College of Sports Medicine, Rodriguez NR, Di Marco NM, Langley S: American College of Sports Medicine position stand. Nutrition and athletic performance. *Med Sci Sports Exerc* 41:709–731, 2009

Aouadi R, Khalifa R, Aouidet A, Ben Mansour A, Ben Rayana M, Mdini F, Bahri S, Stratton G: Aerobic training programs and glycemic control in diabetic children in relation to exercise frequency. *J Sports Med Phys Fitness* 51:393–400, 2011

Armstrong N, Tomkinson G, Ekelund U: Aerobic fitness and its relationship to sport, exercise training and habitual physical activity during youth. *Br J Sports Med* 45:849–858, 2011

Arutchelvam V, Heise T, Dellweg S, Elbroend B, Minns I, Home PD: Plasma glucose and hypoglycaemia following exercise in people with type 1 diabetes: a comparison of three basal insulins. *Diabet Med* 26:1027–1032, 2009

Babar GS, Zidan H, Widlansky ME, Das E, Hoffmann RG, Daoud M, Alemzadeh R: Impaired endothelial function in preadolescent children with type 1 diabetes. *Diabetes Care* 34:681–685, 2011

Bailey BW, McInnis K: Energy cost of exergaming: a comparison of the energy cost of 6 forms of exergaming. *Arch Pediatr Adolesc Med* 165:597–602, 2011

Baldi JC, Cassuto NA, Foxx-Lupo WT, Wheatley CM, Snyder EM: Glycemic status affects cardiopulmonary exercise response in athletes with type I diabetes. *Med Sci Sports Exerc* 42:1454–1459, 2010a

Baldi JC, Hofman PL: Does careful glycemic control improve aerobic capacity in subjects with type 1 diabetes? *Exercise & Sport Sciences Reviews* 38:161–167, 2010b

Benevento D, Bizzarri C, Pitocco D, Crino A, Moretti C, Spera S, Tubili C, Costanza F, Maurizi A, Cipolloni L, Cappa M, Pozzilli P, IMDIAB Group: Computer use, free time activities and metabolic control in patients with type 1 diabetes. *Diabetes Res Clin Pract* 88:e32–34, 2010

Bertelloni S, Ruggeri S, Baroncelli GI: Effects of sports training in adolescence on growth, puberty and bone health. *Gynecol Endocrinol* 22:605–612, 2006

Biankin SA, Jenkins AB, Campbell LV, Choi KL, Forrest QG, Chisholm DJ: Target-seeking behavior of plasma glucose with exercise in type 1 diabetes. *Diabetes Care* 26:297–301, 2003

Bishop FK, Maahs DM, Snell-Bergeon JK, Ogden LG, Kinney GL, Rewers M: Lifestyle risk factors for atherosclerosis in adults with type 1 diabetes. *Diab Vasc Dis Res* 6:269–275, 2009

Boland EA, Grey M, Oesterle A, Fredrickson L, Tamborlane WV: Continuous subcutaneous insulin infusion. A new way to lower risk of severe hypoglycemia, improve metabolic control, and enhance coping in adolescents with type 1 diabetes. *Diabetes Care* 22:1779–1784, 1999

Brazeau AS, Rabasa-Lhoret R, Strychar I, Mircescu H: Barriers to physical activity among patients with type 1 diabetes. *Diabetes Care* 31:2108–2109, 2008

Burke LM, Hawley JA: Carbohydrate and exercise. *Curr Opin Clin Nutr Metab Care* 2:515–520, 1999

Bussau VA, Ferreira LD, Jones TW, Fournier PA: The 10-s maximal sprint: a novel approach to counter an exercise-mediated fall in glycemia in individuals with type 1 diabetes. *Diabetes Care* 29:601–606, 2006

Bussau VA, Ferreira LD, Jones TW, Fournier PA: A 10-s sprint performed prior to moderate-intensity exercise prevents early post-exercise fall in glycaemia in individuals with type 1 diabetes. *Diabetologia* 50:1815–1818, 2007

Chase HP, Lockspeiser T, Peery B, Shepherd M, MacKenzie T, Anderson J, Garg SK: The impact of the Diabetes Control and Complications Trial and Humalog insulin on glycohemoglobin levels and severe hypoglycemia in type 1 diabetes. *Diabetes Care* 24:430–434, 2001

Chu L, Hamilton J, Riddell MC: Clinical management of the physically active patient with type 1 diabetes. *Phys Sportsmed* 39:64–77, 2011

Colberg SR: *Diabetic Athlete's Handbook.* Champaign, IL, Human Kinetics, 2009

Conway B, Miller RG, Costacou T, Fried L, Kelsey S, Evans RW, Orchard TJ: Adiposity and mortality in type 1 diabetes. *Int J Obes (Lond)* 33:796–805, 2009

Cooperberg BA, Breckenridge SM, Arbelaez AM, Cryer PE: Terbutaline and the prevention of nocturnal hypoglycemia in type 1 diabetes. *Diabetes Care* 31:2271–2272, 2008

Costacou T, Edmundowicz D, Prince C, Conway B, Orchard TJ: Progression of coronary artery calcium in type 1 diabetes mellitus. *Am J Cardiol* 100:1543–1547, 2007

Craig ME, Duffin AC, Gallego PH, Lam A, Cusumano J, Hing S, Donaghue KC: Plantar fascia thickness, a measure of tissue glycation, predicts the development of complications in adolescents with type 1 diabetes. *Diabetes Care* 31:1201–1206, 2008

D'Hooge R, Hellinckx T, Van Laethem C, Stegen S, De Schepper J, Van Aken S, Dewolf D, Calders P: Influence of combined aerobic and resistance training on metabolic control, cardiovascular fitness and quality of life in adolescents with type 1 diabetes: a randomized controlled trial. *Clin Rehabil* 25:349–359, 2011

Davey RJ, Jones TW, Fournier PA: Effect of short-term use of a continuous glucose monitoring system with a real-time glucose display and a low glucose alarm on incidence and duration of hypoglycemia in a home setting in type 1 diabetes mellitus. *J Diabetes Sci Technol* 4:1457–1464, 2010

Delvecchio M, Zecchino C, Salzano G, Faienza MF, Cavallo L, De Luca F, Lombardo F: Effects of moderate-severe exercise on blood glucose in type 1 diabetic adolescents treated with insulin pump or glargine insulin. *J Endocrinol Invest* 32:519–524, 2009

Dencker M, Andersen LB: Accelerometer-measured daily physical activity related to aerobic fitness in children and adolescents. *J Sports Sci* 29:887–895, 2011

Dencker M, Thorsson O, Karlsson MK, Linden C, Svensson J, Wollmer P, Andersen LB: Daily physical activity and its relation to aerobic fitness in children aged 8–11 years. *Eur J Appl Physiol* 96:587–592, 2006

Diabetes Control and Complications Trial Research Group: Hypoglycemia in the Diabetes Control and Complications Trial. *Diabetes* 46:271–286, 1997

Diabetes Research in Children Network Study Group, Tsalikian E, Kollman C, Tamborlane WB, Beck RW, Fiallo-Scharer R, Fox L, Janz KF, Ruedy KJ, Wilson D, Xing D, Weinzimer SA: Prevention of hypoglycemia during exercise in children with type 1 diabetes by suspending basal insulin. *Diabetes Care* 29:2200–2204, 2006

DuBose KD, Eisenmann JC, Donnelly JE: Aerobic fitness attenuates the metabolic syndrome score in normal-weight, at-risk-for-overweight, and overweight children. *Pediatrics* 120:e1262–1268, 2007

Ebeling P, Tuominen JA, Bourey R, Koranyi L, Koivisto VA: Athletes with IDDM exhibit impaired metabolic control and increased lipid utilization with no increase in insulin sensitivity. *Diabetes* 44:471–477, 1995

Eisenmann JC, Welk GJ, Ihmels M, Dollman J: Fatness, fitness, and cardiovascular disease risk factors in children and adolescents. *Med Sci Sports Exerc* 39:1251–1256, 2007a

Eisenmann JC, Welk GJ, Wickel EE, Blair SN: Combined influence of cardiorespiratory fitness and body mass index on cardiovascular disease risk factors among 8-18 year old youth: The Aerobics Center Longitudinal Study. *Int J Pediatr Obes* 2:66–72, 2007b

Eliakim A, Beyth Y: Exercise training, menstrual irregularities and bone development in children and adolescents. *J Pediatr Adolesc Gynecol* 16:201–206, 2003

Faigenbaum AD, Kraemer WJ, Blimkie CJ, Jeffreys I, Micheli LJ, Nitka M, Rowland TW: Youth resistance training: updated position statement paper from the national strength and conditioning association. *J Strength Cond Res* 23 (5 Suppl.):S60–S79, 2009

Faigenbaum AD, Myer GD: Pediatric resistance training: benefits, concerns, and program design considerations. *Curr Sports Med Rep* 9:161–168, 2010a

Faigenbaum AD, Myer GD: Resistance training among young athletes: safety, efficacy and injury prevention effects. *Br J Sports Med* 44:56–63, 2010b

Falk B, Dotan R: Children's thermoregulation during exercise in the heat: a revisit. *Appl Physiol Nutr Metab* 33:420–427, 2008

Falk B, Dotan R: Temperature regulation and elite young athletes. *Med Sport Sci* 56:126–149, 2011

Faulkner MS: Cardiovascular fitness and quality of life in adolescents with type 1 or type 2 diabetes. *J Spec Pediatr Nurs* 15:307–316, 2010

Faulkner MS, Quinn L, Rimmer JH, Rich BH: Cardiovascular endurance and heart rate variability in adolescents with type 1 or type 2 diabetes. *Biol Res Nurs* 7:16–29, 2005

Francescato MP, Geat M, Fusi S, Stupar G, Noacco C, Cattin L: Carbohydrate requirement and insulin concentration during moderate exercise in type 1 diabetic patients. *Metabolism* 53:1126–1130, 2004

Gallen IW, Hume C, Lumb A: Fueling the athlete with type 1 diabetes. *Diabetes Obes Metab* 13:130–136, 2011

Gorman E, Chudyk AM, Madden KM, Ashe MC: Bone health and type 2 diabetes mellitus: a systematic review. *Physiother Can* 63:8–20, 2012

Graf DL, Pratt LV, Hester CN, Short KR: Playing active video games increases energy expenditure in children. *Pediatrics* 124:534–540, 2009

Graves LE, Ridgers ND, Williams K, Stratton G, Atkinson G, Cable NT: The physiological cost and enjoyment of Wii Fit in adolescents, young adults, and older adults. *J Phys Act Health* 7:393–401, 2010

Guelfi KJ, Jones TW, Fournier PA: The decline in blood glucose levels is less with intermittent high-intensity compared with moderate exercise in individuals with type 1 diabetes. *Diabetes Care* 28:1289–1294, 2005a

Guelfi KJ, Jones TW, Fournier PA: Intermittent high-intensity exercise does not increase the risk of early postexercise hypoglycemia in individuals with type 1 diabetes. *Diabetes Care* 28:416–418, 2005b

Guelfi KJ, Ratnam N, Smythe GA, Jones TW, Fournier PA: Effect of intermittent high-intensity compared with continuous moderate exercise on glucose production and utilization in individuals with type 1 diabetes. *Am J Physiol Endocrinol Metab* 292:E865–870, 2007

Harmer AR, Chisholm DJ, McKenna MJ, Hunter SK, Ruell PA, Naylor JM, Maxwell LJ, Flack JR: Sprint training increases muscle oxidative metabolism during high-intensity exercise in patients with type 1 diabetes. *Diabetes Care* 31:2097–2102, 2008

Haskell WL, Lee IM, Pate RR, Powell KE, Blair SN, Franklin BA, Macera CA, Heath GW, Thompson PD, Bauman A: Physical activity and public health: updated recommendation for adults from the American College of Sports

Medicine and the American Heart Association. *Med Sci Sports Exerc* 39:1423–1434, 2007

Herbst A, Kordonouri O, Schwab KO, Schmidt F, Holl RW, DPV Initiative of the German Working Group for Pediatric Diabetology Germany: Impact of physical activity on cardiovascular risk factors in children with type 1 diabetes: a multicenter study of 23,251 patients. *Diabetes Care* 30:2098–2100, 2007

Hernandez JM, Moccia T, Fluckey JD, Ulbrecht JS, Farrell PA: Fluid snacks to help persons with type 1 diabetes avoid late onset postexercise hypoglycemia. *Med Sci Sports Exerc* 32:904–910, 2000

Heyman E, Toutain C, Delamarche P, Berthon P, Briard D, Youssef H, Dekerdanet M, Gratas-Delamarche A: Exercise training and cardiovascular risk factors in type 1 diabetic adolescent girls. *Pediatr Exerc Sci* 19:408–419, 2007

Hind K, Burrows M: Weight-bearing exercise and bone mineral accrual in children and adolescents: a review of controlled trials. *Bone* 40:14–27, 2007

Iscoe KE, Riddell MC: Continuous moderate-intensity exercise with or without intermittent high-intensity work: effects on acute and late glycaemia in athletes with type 1 diabetes mellitus. *Diabet Med* 28:824–832, 2011

Jankovec Z, Krcma M, Gruberova J, Komorousova J, Tomesova J, Zourek M, Rusavy Z: Influence of physical activity on metabolic state within a 3-h interruption of continuous subcutaneous insulin infusion in patients with type 1 diabetes. *Diabetes Technol Ther* 13:1234–1239, 2011

Janssen I: Physical activity guidelines for children and youth. *Can J Public Health* 98 (Suppl. 2):S109–S121, 2007

Kalergis M, Schiffrin A, Gougeon R, Jones PJ, Yale JF: Impact of bedtime snack composition on prevention of nocturnal hypoglycemia in adults with type 1 diabetes undergoing intensive insulin management using lispro insulin before meals: a randomized, placebo-controlled, crossover trial. *Diabetes Care* 26:9–15, 2003

Kershnar AK, Daniels SR, Imperatore G, Palla SL, Petitti DB, Pettitt DJ, Marcovina S, Dolan LM, Hamman RF, Liese AD, Pihoker C, Rodriguez BL: Lipid abnormalities are prevalent in youth with type 1 and type 2 diabetes: the SEARCH for Diabetes in Youth Study. *J Pediatr* 149:314–319, 2006

Khan K, McKay HA, Haapasalo H, Bennell KL, Forwood MR, Kannus P, Wark JD: Does childhood and adolescence provide a unique opportunity for exercise to strengthen the skeleton? *J Sci Med Sport* 3:150–164, 2000

Khazai NB, Beck GR Jr, Umpierrez GE: Diabetes and fractures: an overshadowed association. *Curr Opin Endocrinol Diabetes Obes* 16:435–445, 2009

Koivisto VA, Sane T, Fyhrquist F, Pelkonen R: Fuel and fluid homeostasis during long-term exercise in healthy subjects and type I diabetic patients. *Diabetes Care* 15:1736–1741, 1992

Kordonouri O, Hartmann R, Danne T: Treatment of type 1 diabetes in children and adolescents using modern insulin pumps. *Diabetes Res Clin Pract* 93 (Suppl. 1):S118–S124, 2011

Laaksonen DE, Atalay M, Niskanen LK, Mustonen J, Sen CK, Lakka TA, Uusitupa MI: Aerobic exercise and the lipid profile in type 1 diabetic men: a randomized controlled trial. *Med Sci Sports Exerc* 32:1541–1548, 2000

Landberg R, Naidoo N, van Dam RM: Diet and endothelial function: from individual components to dietary patterns. *Curr Opin Lipidol* 23:147–155, 2012

Maahs DM, Horton LA, Chase HP: The use of insulin pumps in youth with type 1 diabetes. *Diabetes Technol Ther* 12 (Suppl. 1):S59–S65, 2010

Maahs DM, Nadeau K, Snell-Bergeon JK, Schauer I, Bergman B, West NA, Rewers M, Daniels SR, Ogden LG, Hamman RF, Dabelea D: Association of insulin sensitivity to lipids across the lifespan in people with type 1 diabetes. *Diabet Med* 28:148–155, 2011

MacDonald MJ: Postexercise late-onset hypoglycemia in insulin-dependent diabetic patients. *Diabetes Care* 10:584–588, 1987

Mackelvie KJ, McKay HA, Khan KM, Crocker PR: A school-based exercise intervention augments bone mineral accrual in early pubertal girls. *J Pediatr* 139:501–508, 2001

Manz F: Hydration and disease. *J Am Coll Nutr* 26 (5 Suppl.):535S–541S, 2007

Maran A, Pavan P, Bonsembiante B, Brugin E, Ermolao A, Avogaro A, Zaccaria M: Continuous glucose monitoring reveals delayed nocturnal hypoglycemia after intermittent high-intensity exercise in nontrained patients with type 1 diabetes. *Diabetes Technol Ther* 12:763–768, 2010

McKewen MW, Rehrer NJ, Cox C, Mann J: Glycaemic control, muscle glycogen and exercise performance in IDDM athletes on diets of varying carbohydrate content. *Int J Sports Med* 20:349–353, 1999

McMahon SK, Ferreira LD, Ratnam N, Davey RJ, Youngs LM, Davis EA, Fournier PA, Jones TW: Glucose requirements to maintain euglycemia after moderate-intensity afternoon exercise in adolescents with type 1 diabetes are increased in a biphasic manner. *J Clin Endocrinol Metab* 92:963–968, 2007

Meltzer LJ, Johnson SB, Prine JM, Banks RA, Desrosiers PM, Silverstein JH: Disordered eating, body mass, and glycemic control in adolescents with type 1 diabetes. *Diabetes Care* 24:678–682, 2001

Moy CS, Songer TJ, LaPorte RE, Dorman JS, Kriska AM, Orchard TJ, Becker DJ, Drash AL: Insulin-dependent diabetes mellitus, physical activity, and death. *Am J Epidemiol* 137:74–81, 1993

Myer GD, Quatman CE, Khoury J, Wall EJ, Hewett TE: Youth versus adult "weightlifting" injuries presenting to United States emergency rooms: accidental versus nonaccidental injury mechanisms. *J Strength Cond Res* 23:2054–2060, 2009

Naughton G, Farpour-Lambert NJ, Carlson J, Bradney M, Van Praagh E: Physiological issues surrounding the performance of adolescent athletes. *Sports Med* 30:309–325, 2000

Olmsted MP, Colton PA, Daneman D, Rydall AC, Rodin GM: Prediction of the onset of disturbed eating behavior in adolescent girls with type 1 diabetes. *Diabetes Care* 31:1978–1982, 2008

Petitti DB, Imperatore G, Palla SL, Daniels SR, Dolan LM, Kershnar AK, Marcovina S, Pettitt DJ, Pihoker C, Search for Diabetes in Youth Study Group: Serum lipids and glucose control: the SEARCH for Diabetes in Youth study. *Arch Pediatr Adolesc Med* 161:159–165, 2007

Physical Activity Guidelines Advisory Committee: Physical Activity Guidelines Advisory Committee Report, 2008. Washington, DC, U.S. Department of Health and Human Services, 2008

Ploug T, Galbo H, Richter EA: Increased muscle glucose uptake during contractions: no need for insulin. *Am J Physiol* 247 (6 Pt 1):E726–731, 1984

Quinn M, Ficociello LH, Rosner B: Change in glycemic control predicts change in weight in adolescent boys with type 1 diabetes. *Pediatr Diabetes* 4:162–167, 2003

Ramalho AC, de Lourdes Lima M, Nunes F, Cambui Z, Barbosa C, Andrade A, Viana A, Martins M, Abrantes V, Aragao C, Temistocles M: The effect of resistance versus aerobic training on metabolic control in patients with type-1 diabetes mellitus. *Diabetes Res Clin Pract* 72:271–276, 2006

Realsen JM, Chase HP: Recent advances in the prevention of hypoglycemia in type 1 diabetes. *Diabetes Technol Ther* 13:1177–1186, 2011

Reinehr T, Holl RW, Roth CL, Wiesel T, Stachow R, Wabitsch M, Andler W, DPV-Wiss Study Group: Insulin resistance in children and adolescents with type 1 diabetes mellitus: relation to obesity. *Pediatr Diabetes* 6:5–12, 2005

Riddell M, Perkins BA: Exercise and glucose metabolism in persons with diabetes mellitus: perspectives on the role for continuous glucose monitoring. *J Diabetes Sci Technol* 3:914–923, 2009

Roberts L, Jones TW, Fournier PA: Exercise training and glycemic control in adolescents with poorly controlled type 1 diabetes mellitus. *J Pediatr Endocrinol Metab* 15:621–627, 2002

Rowland T: Thermoregulation during exercise in the heat in children: old concepts revisited. *J Appl Physiol* 105:718–724, 2008

Salem MA, Aboelasrar MA, Elbarbary NS, Elhilaly RA, Refaat YM: Is exercise a therapeutic tool for improvement of cardiovascular risk factors in adolescents with type 1 diabetes mellitus? A randomised controlled trial. *Diabetol Metab Syndr* 2:47, 2010

Seeger JP, Thijssen DH, Noordam K, Cranen ME, Hopman MT, Nijhuis-van der Sanden MW: Exercise training improves physical fitness and vascular function in children with type 1 diabetes. *Diabetes Obes Metab* 13:382–384, 2011

Short KR, Blackett PR, Gardner AW, Copeland KC: Vascular health in children and adolescents: effects of obesity and diabetes. *Vasc Health Risk Manag* 5:973–990, 2009

Skilton MR, Celermajer DS: Endothelial dysfunction and arterial abnormalities in childhood obesity. *Int J Obes (Lond)* 30:1041–1049, 2006

Tamborlane WV: Triple jeopardy: nocturnal hypoglycemia after exercise in the young with diabetes. *J Clin Endocrinol Metab* 92:815–816, 2007

Tamis-Jortberg B, Downs DA Jr, Colten ME: Effects of a glucose polymer sports drink on blood glucose, insulin, and performance in subjects with diabetes. *Diabetes Educ* 22:471–487, 1996

Trigona B, Aggoun Y, Maggio A, Martin XE, Marchand LM, Beghetti M, Farpour-Lambert NJ: Preclinical noninvasive markers of atherosclerosis in children and adolescents with type 1 diabetes are influenced by physical activity. *J Pediatr* 157:533–539, 2010

Tsalikian E, Mauras N, Beck RW, Tamborlane WV, Janz KF, Chase HP, Wysocki T, Weinzimer SA, Buckingham BA, Kollman C, Xing D, Ruedy KJ, Diabetes Research in Children Network DirecNet Study Group: Impact of exercise on overnight glycemic control in children with type 1 diabetes mellitus. *J Pediatr* 147:528–534, 2005

Ugale J, Mata A, Meert KL, Sarnaik AP: Measured degree of dehydration in children and adolescents with type 1 diabetic ketoacidosis. *Pediatr Crit Care Med* 13:e103–107, 2012

Vasudevan EV, Torres-Oviedo G, Morton SM, Yang JF, Bastian AJ: Younger is not always better: development of locomotor adaptation from childhood to adulthood. *J Neurosci* 31:3055–3065, 2011

West DJ, Morton RD, Bain SC, Stephens JW, Bracken RM: Blood glucose responses to reductions in pre-exercise rapid-acting insulin for 24 h after running in individuals with type 1 diabetes. *J Sports Sci* 28:781–788, 2010

Williams BK, Guelfi KJ, Jones TW, Davis EA: Lower cardiorespiratory fitness in children with type 1 diabetes. *Diabet Med* 28:1005–1007, 2011

Wilson D, Chase HP, Kollman C, Xing D, Caswell K, Tansey M, Fox L, Weinzimer S, Beck R, Ruedy K, Tamborlane W, Diabetes Research in Children Network Study Group: Low-fat vs. high-fat bedtime snacks in children and adolescents with type 1 diabetes. *Pediatr Diabetes* 9 (4 Pt 1):320–325, 2008

Yeung EW, Yeung SS: Interventions for preventing lower limb soft-tissue injuries in runners. *Cochrane Database Syst Rev*:CD001256, 2001

Chapter 25

Behavior Change and Adoption of an Active Lifestyle

L earning to overcome barriers that interfere with a more physically active lifestyle is a critical part of effective diabetes self-management, especially when health complications like neuropathy, nephropathy, and retinopathy make being active more challenging (Johansen 2005, Costello 2011). Certain physical movements also may pose safety issues, and not all individuals are capable of participating in or willing to start a fitness program, regardless of the health benefits they can achieve (Miller 2009, Costello 2011). Supervised physical activity participation frequently is recommended and encouraged during the initial phases of an exercise program to aid in monitoring signs and symptoms, exercise responses, and blood glucose levels (Lavie 1993, 1996; Ibanez 2005; Winett 2009; Negri 2010).

Efforts to promote physical activity should focus on developing self-efficacy and fostering social support from family, friends, and health-care and fitness professionals (McAuley 2000, Aljasem 2001, Collins 2010, King 2010, Luszczynska 2011, Plotnikoff 2011). Encouraging mild or moderate activities may be most beneficial to adoption and maintenance of regular participation in individuals with type 2 diabetes (T2D) (Shinji 2007, Song 2009, Negri 2010). In individuals with type 1 diabetes (T1D), addressing the fear of hypoglycemia associated with physical activity is likely important to promoting their participation as well (Dubé 2006, Brazeau 2008, Realsen 2011).

Case in Point: Overcoming Barriers to Physical Activity Participation

JB is a 74-year-old woman with T2D for 4 years. Before her diagnosis, she used to work daily doing a job that required continual standing and arm movement, and she walked around her small town with her husband every morning, getting in ~1–2 miles. Five years ago, however, her husband died from cancer, leaving her on her own, and she injured her arm preventing a fall during icy weather. Although she is now retired and living in an assisted living facility, she finds that her energy levels are low, and she has every reason in the book not to be active. She has gained all of the weight back (~30 lb) that she lost in the year after her husband died, and now her knee is bothering her when she walks as well. She takes a number of medications, including ones for osteoporosis, blood pressure, high cholesterol, and diabetes management (metformin). She also takes an antiseizure medication to prevent problems from a small, benign tumor growing in the frontal lobe of her brain.

Resting Measurements

Height: 62 inches
Weight: 165 lb
BMI: 30.2 (obese)
Heart rate: 85 beats per minute (bpm)
Blood pressure: 132/88 mmHg (on medication)

Fasting Labs

Plasma glucose: 145 mg/dl (controlled with metformin)
A1C: 7.2%
Total cholesterol: 188 mg/dl
Triglycerides: 135 mg/dl
High-density lipoprotein cholesterol: 42 mg/dl
Low-density lipoprotein cholesterol: 119 mg/dl

Questions to Consider

1. What are JB's barriers to physical activity participation?
2. How can these barriers be addressed to remove them?
3. What other strategies can help motivate JB to be more regularly active?

(Continued on page 484.)

ADOPTION AND MAINTENANCE OF PHYSICAL ACTIVITY

The majority of U.S. adults with T2D or at highest risk for developing it do not engage in regular physical activity, and their rate of participation is significantly below national norms (Morrato 2007). It is apparent that additional strategies are needed to increase the adoption and maintenance of physical activity. Lifestyle interventions may have some efficacy in promoting physical activity behavior and can benefit health. For example, in individuals with T1D, behavior change interventions improve glycemic control (Conn 2008).

LIFESTYLE INTERVENTIONS

Large-scale trials like the DPP (Diabetes Prevention Program) and Look AHEAD (Action for Health in Diabetes) have been successful lifestyle interventions that help promote physical activity with goal-setting, self-monitoring, frequent contact, and stepped-care protocols (Wadden 2006, Delahanty 2008, Eakin 2008), but such programs require extensive access to resources, staff, and space (Jacobs-van der Bruggen 2007, 2009). These large studies also have been multifactorial, targeting a number of behaviors that include physical activity as well as diet and weight loss or management (Malpass 2009). Physical activity interventions that address weight management are highly relevant to most individuals with T2D and many with T1D (Donnelly 2009). Effective short-term interventions have successfully used print (Dutton 2008), phone (Clark 2004, Kirk 2004, Sacco

2009), in-person (Keyserling 2002, Jackson 2007), or Internet (Glasgow 2005, Liebreich 2009) delivery of programs and education, although their long-term effectiveness has not been assessed (Muller-Riemenschneider 2008).

Affective responses to exercise may be important predictors of adoption and maintenance, and encouraging activity at intensities below the ventilatory threshold may be most beneficial (Williams 2008a, 2008b; Lind 2008). Many individuals with T2D prefer walking as an aerobic activity (Mier 2007), and they may be able to effectively utilize pedometer-based interventions to increase physical activity (Tudor-Locke 2004, Bravata 2007, Ogilvie 2007). Current research on the role of sedentary behaviors in metabolic risk suggests that future interventions also may incorporate strategies that decrease sitting time and extended sedentary periods (Healy 2008a, 2008b).

BARRIERS TO EXERCISE PARTICIPATION

Barriers have been shown to greatly reduce exercise participation, and many potential barriers exist, obesity being just one of them. For example, in women enrolled in a physical activity promotion trial, obese women reported a greater number of barriers compared with normal and overweight women (Napolitano 2011). The larger women's barriers to physical activity included feeling too overweight, being self-conscious, having minor aches and pains, and lacking self-discipline. Given that the obese women with high barriers participated in 70 min/week less exercise, it can be concluded that such barriers have detrimental effects on their attempts to change physical activity behaviors. Barriers for African American women also are affected by body weight, with obese women being less likely to have no barriers to exercise participation compared with normal weight or overweight women (Genkinger 2006). For these obese African American women, their most frequent barrier was "lack of motivation" to participate.

Other research has elucidated what keeps many older individuals from being more physically active (Costello 2011). In individuals age ≥60 years, sedentary adults apparently have much lower fitness expectations for becoming an "active" older adult, along with more perceived barriers to regular participation. They require individual tailoring of an exercise program, but they are intimidated by fitness facilities and concerned about slowing others down in a group exercise setting. Inactive older people also described physical activity as needing to be purposeful and fun. Most important, most inactive individuals already perceived themselves to be physically active as their perception was grounded in their social context (such as an assisted living facility). Although both active and inactive elders share some barriers to regular participation, physically active individuals are more capable of developing strategies to overcome them (Costello 2011).

Strategies to improve self-care behaviors in diabetes should focus on improving the individual's perception of their control in overcoming barriers with regard to diabetes management. For instance, in diabetic individuals who use insulin, fear of hypoglycemia associated with physical activity has been reported to be the strongest barrier to regular physical activity participation (Dubé 2006, Brazeau 2008, Realsen 2011), and they must be informed and supported in hypoglycemia management for them to overcome this barrier (Brazeau 2008, Realsen 2011).

FACTORS INFLUENCING PHYSICAL ACTIVITY PARTICIPATION

Greater effort needs to be focused on the promotion of regular exercise among individuals with and at risk for developing T2D and gestational diabetes mellitus (GDM) in particular because lifestyle choices largely influence their onset, although health behavior change interventions benefit glycemic control in T1D as well (Conn 2008). The central determining factors influencing activity across the life span in all individuals, with and without diabetes, are generally self-efficacy (i.e., having confidence in one's ability to be active), enjoyment of physical activity, lack of perceived barriers to being physically active, positive beliefs concerning the benefits of physical activity, support from others to continue exercising, and cultural beliefs and practices. Behaviorally based exercise interventions, the use of behavior change strategies, supervision by an experienced fitness instructor, and exercise that is pleasant and enjoyable can improve adoption and adherence to prescribed exercise programs (Garber 2011). The availability of facilities, pleasant places to walk, and economical exercise options (i.e., the built environment) also may be important predictors of regular physical activity participation.

SELF-EFFICACY

Beliefs about self-efficacy influence health behaviors. Individuals tend to pursue tasks they feel competent to perform and avoid those in which they feel incompetent. Self-efficacy may be enhanced by developing realistic activity goals that an individual is likely to attain (thereby promoting feelings of mastery); progressing programs slowly using small, incremental steps; observing others in a similar situation succeeding at being physically active in an exercise class or by watching a video; rehearsing or practicing intended exercise behaviors; and getting regular, supportive feedback from others about their participation and progress (McAuley 2000, Aljasem 2001, Gleeson-Kreig 2006, Dutton 2009, King 2010, Luszczynska 2011, Naik 2011, Plotnikoff 2011).

One of the most consistent predictors of greater levels of physical activity—both aerobic and resistance training—has been higher levels of self-efficacy, which reflect confidence in the ability to exercise (McAuley 2000, Aljasem 2001, Delahanty 2006, Dutton 2009, Luszczynska 2011, Plotnikoff 2011). For individuals with T1D, confidence in the ability to avoid hypoglycemia related to activity is an important determinant in their participation (Realsen 2011), while use of newer continuous glucose monitoring (CGM) technologies may increase exercise compliance in individuals with either T1D or T2D (Cauza 2005a, 2005b; Allen 2008; Maran 2010; Adolfsson 2011). In individuals with T2D in particular, interventions should focus on enhancing self-efficacy, problem solving, and social–environmental support to improve self-management (which includes exercise, dietary, and medication behaviors) (King 2010). Even when diabetes-related complications are present, self-efficacy remains important as a mediator for behavior change and has been associated with walking ability and adherence to walking therapy in individuals with diabetes and peripheral artery disease (Collins 2010).

GOAL SETTING

When planning to increase physical activity participation by overcoming potential obstacles or problems, individuals also must set realistic and practical goals (Luszczynska 2011, Naik 2011). Goals that are too vague, too ambitious, or too distant do not provide enough self-motivation to maintain long-term interest (i.e., they should be short-term goals). Health-care and fitness professionals should encourage individuals with diabetes to specifically plan their exercise participation, track their goals to help see their progress, and identify potential barriers (Lubans 2012). Individuals should set appropriate physical activity goals that are SMART (Specific, Measurable, Attainable, Realistic, and Time-frame specific), as shown in Table 25.1.

Table 25.1 Effective Goal Setting Using SMART Goals

Specific: Set goals that are as precise as possible when identifying details of frequency, duration, intensity, and type of activity

Measurable: Make goals that can be quantified so that individuals can accurately track, measure, and identify progress

Attainable: Set goals that are challenging, but reachable, to increase confidence and the likelihood of setting even more challenging goals in the future

Realistic: Evaluate how likely individuals are to attain their chosen goals in a given situation and modify them, as needed, to be more realistic

Time-frame specific: Set short-term goals that provide more immediate feedback, such as setting ones for just the next week

SOCIAL SUPPORT

Although social support has been associated with greater levels of physical activity (Mier 2007, Gleeson-Kreig 2008, Penn 2008), social dynamics also have been linked to the spread of obesity (Gorin 2008, Bahr 2009). Fortunately, these social dynamics may be exploited to increase the effects of interventions beyond the target individual and potentially can help spread exercise behavior among close individuals. In one study, active overweight women were more likely to identify social reasons for participating in physical activity, whereas inactive participants perceived that their laziness prevented their participation (Jewson 2008).

Likewise, counseling delivered by professionals also may be a meaningful and effective source of support (Armit 2009). On average, physician advice or referral related to exercise occurred at 18% of office visits by diabetic individuals, 73% of whom reported receiving advice at some point to exercise more (Morrato 2006). Clearly such advice has not led to widespread adoption of increased physical activity, and such advice from health-care or fitness professionals appears to be associated with lower A1C values only when combined with dietary advice, but not when given alone (Umpierre 2011).

Even peer mentoring may enhance diabetes management and adoption of healthier lifestyle habits. In a recent study, peer mentorship improved glucose control in African American veterans with diabetes and consistently poor control (Long 2012). Social support to can also empower parents of young children newly diagnosed with T1D (Sullivan-Bolyai 2010). There has been unprecedented growth in diabetes-related social media and online support groups in the past decade, which may provide yet another effective avenue for lasting physical activity behavior change (Chomutare 2011).

SUPERVISION OF TRAINING

Overweight adults with T2D experienced significant improvement in health-related quality of life by enrolling in a weight-management program that yielded significant weight loss, improved physical fitness, and reduced physical symptoms (Williamson 2009). However, exercise interventions showing the greatest impact on glycemic control have all involved supervision of exercise sessions by qualified exercise trainers (Mourier 1997, Castaneda 2002, Dunstan 2002, Sigal 2007, Negri 2010). When supervision is absent, both compliance and glycemic control decrease (Negri 2010).

In the 1-year Italian Diabetes and Exercise Study, for example, all participants with T2D received high-quality exercise counseling that substantially increased self-reported physical activity (Balducci 2008). The intervention group also received supervised, facility-based combined aerobic and resistance exercise training twice weekly, resulting in greater improvements in overall blood glucose control, blood pressure, and body composition. A review of 20 resistance training studies on T2D (Gordon 2009) also found that supervised training of varying volume, frequency, and intensity improved blood glucose control and insulin sensitivity, but that when supervision was removed, both compliance and glycemic control decreased. Diabetic individuals engaging in supervised training gain benefits exceeding those of exercise counseling and increased physical activity undertaken alone (Umpierre 2011).

CULTURAL PRACTICES AND HEALTH BELIEFS

Health-care and fitness professionals must be aware of the cultural practices and beliefs that may influence the adoption of physical activity. Activities should not offend or ignore the cultural beliefs of the individual, and suggestions to help tailor a suitable exercise prescription should be culturally appropriate (Pentecost 2011). By way of example, in one program focusing on Puerto Ricans living in the U.S., these individuals were taught in a culturally appropriate way how inactivity increases the risk for diabetes-related health complications, what the benefits of exercising for people with diabetes are, and how lifestyle activity (e.g., house or yard work, walking a pet, or walking around town to complete errands) can serve as an alternative to traditional, regimented exercise (Osborn 2010). Similarly, dance and music are a vital part of tradition and celebration for many ethnically diverse groups, including Native, Hispanic, and African Americans, while Asian and Middle Eastern groups may have other cultural traditions like yoga, tai chi, and dance that can be part of an exercise routine to manage diabetes and body weight (Garber 2011). In African American women, religion and spirituality have been found to be associated with their glycemic control (Newlin 2008).

USING STAGE-MATCHED INTERVENTIONS TO PROMOTE BEHAVIOR CHANGE

The transtheoretical model of behavior change uses progressive stages of readiness and can be used to tailor exercise interventions in individuals with diabetes and body-weight issues (Marcus 1992, 1994; Tuah 2011). Stage-matched interventions are widely accepted by health-care practitioners and other professionals in assisting individuals trying to make permanent lifestyle changes, including participation in regular exercise (Clark 2004, Kim 2004, Wadden 2011). The stages are listed in Table 25.2, and stage-matched strategies for working with individuals to help them overcome physical activity and exercise barriers are discussed further in the section that follows.

Table 25.2 Stages of Behavior Change Related to Exercise Participation

1. **Precontemplation:** Not regularly active and has no intention of being active in the next 6 months
2. **Contemplation:** Not regularly active but thinking about starting in the next 6 months
3. **Preparation:** Doing some activity but not enough to meet current guidelines for regular physical activity participation
4. **Action:** Has become regularly physically active within the last 6 months
5. **Maintenance:** Has maintained regular physical activity for ≥6 months

STAGE 1: PRECONTEMPLATION

The goal at the precontemplation stage is for individuals to begin thinking about participating in more physical activity.

- Build trust with the individual and provide information as needed
- Emphasize the individual's autonomy in decisions to be more active
- Encourage the individual to think about personally relevant benefits
- Address the individual's specific barriers and encourage him or her to come up with possible solutions to these barriers
- Use appropriate goal-setting activities focused on getting the individual to think about being more active, such as reading a pamphlet on the benefits of exercise
- Discuss pros and cons of physical activity
- Suggest that the individual write down benefits, barriers, reasons to be active, and reasons not to be active

STAGE 2: CONTEMPLATION

The goal at the contemplation stage is for individuals to begin taking steps to be more active and to think about setting physical activity goals.

- Continue to use strategies from the precontemplation stage
- Discuss the individual's personal preferences for physical activity
- Provide support and validation to the individual
- Encourage the individual to think about what has been personally successful in the past regarding physical activity or examples of family and friends who have been successful
- Suggest that the individual use a reinforcement program that provides positive rewards when goals are achieved
- Encourage the individual to identify other people to use for support
- Offer information on physical activity and exercise, emphasizing social, psychological, and general health benefits

STAGE 3: PREPARATION

The goal at the preparation stage is for individuals to increase physical activity to recommended levels.

- Continue to use strategies from precontemplation and contemplation stages
- Praise preparation taken to increase physical activity
- Assist the individual in setting goals to gradually increase physical activity levels
- Encourage individuals to track progress with a physical activity log that details activity type, amount, duration, and frequency
- Suggest that the individual join an exercise class or club as doing so is often helpful at this stage

STAGE 4: ACTION

The goal at the action stage is for individuals to begin making physical activity a regular part of their lives.

- Continue to use strategies from the first three stages
- Praise all efforts of the individual
- Work with the individual to develop a specific plan for tracking progress and setting short-term physical activity goals
- Suggest the individual try new activities or train for an upcoming exercise event (such as walking or a bicycle race)
- Encourage the individual to begin to anticipate barriers
- Limit suggestions for additional changes to one or two at most

STAGE 5: MAINTENANCE

The goal at the maintenance stage is for individuals to prepare for possible setbacks and find ways to continue to increase enjoyment with the personalized physical activity program.

- Use strategies from the action stage
- Continue to praise all efforts of the individual
- Assist the individual in finding ways to avoid boredom, such as varying exercise routines
- Promote relapse prevention strategies and distinguish between a lapse (slight slip) and a relapse (return to former behavior patterns) by having the individual identify potential high-risk situations and develop a plan to deal with them
- Encourage the individual to reflect on the benefits personally achieved with regular physical activity
- Keep in mind that most people are not successful with their first attempt at increasing and maintaining new levels of physical activity

When working through these stages, keep in mind that some individuals may need three or four attempts before physical activity becomes a long-term habit. Individuals will progress through the stages as they learn from past attempts and successes and try different methods for increasing activity. The more an individual takes action to become more physically active, the better his or her chances of progressing forward. The role of the fitness or health-care provider is to support the individual in all stages and apply appropriate intervention strategies as needed.

USING MOTIVATIONAL INTERVIEWING

Motivational interviewing is an individual-centered directive method of communication for enhancing intrinsic motivation to change by exploring and resolving

Table 25.3 Strategies for Motivational Interviewing

A key tool of motivational interviewing is the use of rulers to explore importance and raise confidence regarding the individual's exercise behaviors.

- Start by asking the individual to rate on a 10-point scale how important it is and how confident he or she is about a particular activity behavior, such as walking three times a week for 15 min
- After the individual chooses a number on the 10-point scale, ask why that specific number was chosen instead of a lower number
- Obtain permission from the individual before providing information or offering advice; the individual may give permission by asking for advice; or both ask permission to give advice and preface advice with permission to disagree or disregard
- Use strategic feedback, reflections, and questions to help the individual recognize his or her own internalized discrepancies with regard to remaining inactive
- Use decisional balance scales to help the individual weigh the pros and cons of being more active to remaining inactive or less active
- Emphasize the individual's autonomy and freedom to choose not to be physically active
- Encourage the individual's acceptance of responsibility for change and consequences of not changing activity habits

ambivalence (Miller 2009, Dellasega 2012). This technique can be used with individuals to help increase motivational readiness to make positive behavior changes related to physical activity. Patient perceptions of standard care are often negative, which may be improved or made more positive with effective use of motivational interviewing. For instance, in lower-income groups, motivational interviewing was found to be most effective when it used themes: nonjudgmental accountability, being heard and responded to as a person, encouragement and empowerment, collaborative action planning and goal setting, and coaching rather than critiquing (Dellasega 2012). Key strategies that professionals can use with individuals experiencing ambivalence with physical activity participation are listed in Table 25.3 (Miller 2009, Dellasega 2012).

Case in Point: Wrap-Up

JB has a large number of perceived exercise barriers, more now than ever. For starters, she admits that she thought she could walk around her assisted living facility for exercise, but once she moved in there, she found that she does not like to do that because the other residents watch her walk by and that makes her uncomfortable. Although they do have a small exercise room there, she also does not feel that comfortable exercising in a group. She never has done much physical activity other than walking, so she really does not know what else to do. Although she does have a car and could go out, she seldom leaves the facility and, therefore, gets very little daily movement other than walking to get to the cafeteria for meals. She does not even do her own laundry or cleaning anymore, making her more sedentary than she has ever been before in her life. After expressing these concerns to the facility's health-care team, JB sits down with one of them who makes the following suggestions for her to overcome her barriers to being more physically active:

1. *Get more daily movement.* The best way to start being active is by simply doing more daily movement by taking more steps and standing up more, even while you are watching television. Walk in place during commercials while watching your favorite shows. Go out and do something active with your family and friends. Do stretches in your living room. Stand up when you have conversations with others (in person or on the phone) rather than always sitting down. Everyday activities you do on your own like gardening and household chores can get you moving and help burn calories.

2. *Do not worry if you are too shy to exercise in a group.* Choose an activity you can do on your own, such as following along with an aerobics class on television or doing exercise videos or other home-based activities. Try walking in place, doing stretching, or using cans of food or water bottles for weights, or buy some inexpensive resistance bands to use. After a while, try a group fitness class that you can take with a friend.

3. *Pick joint-friendly activities to limit pain.* Try seated exercises or other low-impact exercises that may be less painful. Many chair exercises can be found online, along with videos for those exercises and chair dancing. You may need to find out where in your community you can get inexpensive access to aquatic exercise (classes, water walking, and swimming laps), stationary bikes, or other

joint-friendly workout machines. Keep in mind that moderate amounts of walking likely will reduce the pain in your knees rather than necessarily making it worse.

4. ***Seek out alternative activities that are nearby.*** Look for inexpensive resources in your community like programs in senior centers, park and recreation programs, walking trails, school running tracks, or other wellness programs. Find something you enjoy doing. Try different activities on different days. Exercise with someone else to keep you company.

5. ***Even if you have failed at fitness programs before, try again.*** You will need to set reasonable goals, pick a fitness program that will meet those goals, and progress appropriately. Do not try to do too much too soon; rather, start out slowly and build your participation the same way.

Changing behaviors to include regular physical activity is an important aspect of getting people with diabetes physically active for a lifetime. Doing so may involve addressing barriers to participation and devising strategies to overcome them. In particular, self-efficacy is an important factor in physical activity behavior change. Setting appropriate, specific, and realistic exercise goals can help. With all the health benefits to be gained from physical activity participation, all individuals with diabetes need to be encouraged to make, and assisted in achieving, this critical behavior change.

PROFESSIONAL PRACTICE PEARLS

- Learning to overcome barriers that interfere with a more physically active lifestyle is a critical part of effective diabetes self-management.
- Efforts to promote physical activity should focus on developing self-efficacy and fostering social support from family, friends, and health-care and fitness professionals.
- Encouraging mild or moderate activities may be most beneficial to adoption and maintenance of regular participation in individuals with T2D.
- In individuals with T1D and those with T2D using insulin, addressing the fear of hypoglycemia associated with physical activity is important to promote participation.
- Barriers have been shown to greatly reduce exercise participation, and a great number of potential barriers exist, including obesity.
- The primary factors influencing activity are self-efficacy, enjoyment, lack of perceived barriers, positive beliefs, support from others, and cultural beliefs and practices.
- A consistent predictor of greater levels of physical activity is higher levels of self-efficacy, which reflect confidence in the ability to exercise.
- When planning to increase physical activity participation by overcoming potential obstacles or problems, individuals must set realistic and practical (i.e., SMART) goals.
- Social support has been associated with greater levels of physical activity and can be used to promote adoption of behavior change.

- Diabetic individuals may benefit from participating in supervised exercise training, particularly when starting a new program.
- Cultural practices and beliefs may influence the adoption of physical activity and such nuances should be taken into account when choosing programs.
- A model with progressive stages of readiness can be used to tailor exercise interventions in individuals with diabetes and body-weight issues.
- Motivational interviewing can be used with individuals to help increase their readiness to make positive behavior changes related to physical activity.

REFERENCES

Adolfsson P, Nilsson S, Lindblad B: Continuous glucose monitoring system during physical exercise in adolescents with type 1 diabetes. *Acta Paediatr* 100:1603–1609, 2011

Aljasem LI, Peyrot M, Wissow L, Rubin RR: The impact of barriers and self-efficacy on self-care behaviors in type 2 diabetes. *Diabetes Educ* 27:393–404, 2001

Allen NA, Fain JA, Braun B, Chipkin SR: Continuous glucose monitoring counseling improves physical activity behaviors of individuals with type 2 diabetes: A randomized clinical trial. *Diabetes Res Clin Pract* 80:371–379, 2008

Armit CM, Brown WJ, Marshall AL, Ritchie CB, Trost SG, Green A, Bauman AE: Randomized trial of three strategies to promote physical activity in general practice. *Preventive Medicine* 48:156–163, 2009

Bahr DB, Browning RC, Wyatt HR, Hill JO: Exploiting social networks to mitigate the obesity epidemic. *Obesity* 17:723–738, 2009

Balducci S, Zanuso S, Fernando F, Nicolucci A, Cardelli P, Cavallo S, Fallucca S, Alessi E, Pugliese G, Fallucca F: The Italian Diabetes and Exercise Study. *Diabetes* 57 (Suppl. 1):A306–A307, 2008

Bravata DM, Smith-Spangler C, Sundaram V, Gienger AL, Lin N, Lewis R, Stave CD, Olkin I, Sirard JR: Using pedometers to increase physical activity and improve health: a systematic review. *JAMA* 298:2296–2304, 2007

Brazeau AS, Rabasa-Lhoret R, Strychar I, Mircescu H: Barriers to physical activity among patients with type 1 diabetes. *Diabetes Care* 31:2108–2109, 2008

Castaneda C, Layne JE, Munoz-Orians L, Gordon PL, Walsmith J, Foldvari M, Roubenoff R, Tucker KL, Nelson ME: A randomized controlled trial of resistance exercise training to improve glycemic control in older adults with type 2 diabetes. *Diabetes Care* 25:2335–2341, 2002

Cauza E, Hanusch-Enserer U, Strasser B, Kostner K, Dunky A, Haber P: Strength and endurance training lead to different post exercise glucose profiles in diabetic participants using a continuous subcutaneous glucose monitoring system. *Eur J Clin Invest* 35:745–751, 2005a

Cauza E, Hanusch-Enserer U, Strasser B, Ludvik B, Kostner K, Dunky A, Haber P: Continuous glucose monitoring in diabetic long distance runners. *Int J Sports Med* 26:774–780, 2005b

Chomutare T, Arsand E, Hartvigsen G: Mobile peer support in diabetes. *Stud Health Technol Inform* 169:48–52, 2011

Clark M, Hampson SE, Avery L, Simpson R: Effects of a tailored lifestyle self-management intervention in patients with type 2 diabetes. *Br J Health Psychol* 9 (Pt 3):365–379, 2004

Collins TC, Lunos S, Ahluwalia JS: Self-efficacy is associated with walking ability in persons with diabetes mellitus and peripheral arterial disease. *Vasc Med* 15:189–195, 2010

Conn VS, Hafdahl AR, Lemaster JW, Ruppar TM, Cochran JE, Nielsen PJ: Meta-analysis of health behavior change interventions in type 1 diabetes. *Am J Health Behav* 32:315–329, 2008

Costello E, Kafchinski M, Vrazel J, Sullivan P: Motivators, barriers, and beliefs regarding physical activity in an older adult population. *J Geriatr Phys Ther* 34:138–147, 2011

Delahanty LM, Conroy MB, Nathan DM: Psychological predictors of physical activity in the diabetes prevention program. *J Am Diet Assoc* 106:698–705, 2006

Delahanty LM, Nathan DM: Implications of the diabetes prevention program and Look AHEAD clinical trials for lifestyle interventions. *J Am Diet Assoc* 108 (4 Suppl. 1):S66–S72, 2008

Dellasega C, Anel-Tiangco RM, Gabbay RA: How patients with type 2 diabetes mellitus respond to motivational interviewing. *Diabetes Res Clin Pract* 95:37–41, 2012

Donnelly JE, Blair SN, Jakicic JM, Manore MM, Rankin JW, Smith BK: American College of Sports Medicine position stand. Appropriate physical activity intervention strategies for weight loss and prevention of weight regain for adults. *Med Sci Sports Exerc* 41:459–471, 2009

Dubé MC, Valois P, Prud'homme D, Weisnagel SJ, Lavoie C: Physical activity barriers in diabetes: development and validation of a new scale. *Diabetes Res Clin Pract* 72:20–27, 2006.

Dunstan DW, Daly RM, Owen N, Jolley D, De Courten M, Shaw J, Zimmet P: High-intensity resistance training improves glycemic control in older patients with type 2 diabetes. *Diabetes Care* 25:1729–1736, 2002

Dutton GR, Provost BC, Tan F, Smith D: A tailored print-based physical activity intervention for patients with type 2 diabetes. *Prev Med* 47:409–411, 2008

Dutton GR, Tan F, Provost BC, Sorenson JL, Allen B, Smith D: Relationship between self-efficacy and physical activity among patients with type 2 diabetes. *J Behav Med* 32:270–277, 2009

Eakin EG, Reeves MM, Lawler SP, Oldenburg B, Del Mar C, Wilkie K, Spencer A, Battistutta D, Graves N: The Logan Healthy Living Program: a cluster randomized trial of a telephone-delivered physical activity and dietary behavior intervention for primary care patients with type 2 diabetes or hypertension from a socially disadvantaged community—rationale, design and recruitment. *Contemporary Clinical Trials* 29:439–454, 2008

Garber CE, Blissmer B, Deschenes MR, Franklin BA, Lamonte MJ, Lee IM, Nieman DC, Swain DP, American College of Sports Medicine: American College of Sports Medicine position stand. Quantity and quality of exercise for developing and maintaining cardiorespiratory, musculoskeletal, and neuromotor fitness in apparently healthy adults: guidance for prescribing exercise. *Med Sci Sports Exerc* 43:1334–1359, 2011

Genkinger JM, Jehn ML, Sapun M, Mabry I, Young DR: Does weight status influence perceptions of physical activity barriers among African-American women? *Ethn Dis* 16:78–84, 2006

Glasgow RE, Nutting PA, King DK, Nelson CC, Cutter G, Gaglio B, Rahm AK, Whitesides H: Randomized effectiveness trial of a computer-assisted intervention to improve diabetes care. *Diabetes Care* 28:33–39, 2005

Gleeson-Kreig J: Social support and physical activity in type 2 diabetes: a social-ecologic approach. *Diabetes Educator* 34:1037–1044, 2008

Gleeson-Kreig JM: Self-monitoring of physical activity: effects on self-efficacy and behavior in people with type 2 diabetes. *Diabetes Educ* 32:69–77, 2006

Gleeson-Kreig J, Bernal H, Woolley S: The role of social support in the self-management of diabetes mellitus among a Hispanic population. *Public Health Nurs* 19:215–222, 2002

Gordon BA, Benson AC, Bird SR, Fraser SF: Resistance training improves metabolic health in type 2 diabetes: a systematic review. *Diabetes Res Clin Pract* 83:157–175, 2009

Gorin AA, Wing RR, Fava JL, Jakicic JM, Jeffery R, West DS, Brelje K, Dilillo VG: Weight loss treatment influences untreated spouses and the home environment: evidence of a ripple effect. *Int J Obes* 32:1678–1684, 2008

Healy GN, Dunstan DW, Salmon J, Cerin E, Shaw JE, Zimmet PZ, Owen N: Breaks in sedentary time: beneficial associations with metabolic risk. *Diabetes Care* 31:661–666, 2008a

Healy GN, Wijndaele K, Dunstan DW, Shaw JE, Salmon J, Zimmet PZ, Owen N: Objectively measured sedentary time, physical activity, and metabolic risk: the Australian Diabetes, Obesity and Lifestyle Study (AusDiab). *Diabetes Care* 31:369–371, 2008b

Ibanez J, Izquierdo M, Arguelles I, Forga L, Larrion JL, Garcia-Unciti M, Idoate F, Gorostiaga EM: Twice-weekly progressive resistance training decreases abdominal fat and improves insulin sensitivity in older men with type 2 diabetes. *Diabetes Care* 28:662–667, 2005

Jackson R, Asimakopoulou K, Scammell A: Assessment of the transtheoretical model as used by dietitians in promoting physical activity in people with type 2 diabetes. *J Hum Nutr Diet* 20:27–36, 2007

Jacobs-van der Bruggen MA, Bos G, Bemelmans WJ, Hoogenveen RT, Vijgen SM, Baan CA: Lifestyle interventions are cost-effective in people with different levels of diabetes risk: results from a modeling study. *Diabetes Care* 30:128–134, 2007

Jacobs-van der Bruggen MA, van Baal PH, Hoogenveen RT, Feenstra TL, Briggs AH, Lawson K, Feskens EJ, Baan CA: Cost-effectiveness of lifestyle modification in diabetic patients. *Diabetes Care* 32:1453–1458, 2009

Jewson E, Spittle M, Casey M: A preliminary analysis of barriers, intentions, and attitudes towards moderate physical activity in women who are overweight. *J Sci Med Sport* 11:558–561, 2008

Johansen KL: Exercise and chronic kidney disease: current recommendations. *Sports Med* 35:485–499, 2005

Keyserling TC, Samuel-Hodge CD, Ammerman AS, Ainsworth BE, Henriquez-Roldan CF, Elasy TA, Skelly AH, Johnston LF, Bangdiwala SI: A randomized trial of an intervention to improve self-care behaviors of African-American women with type 2 diabetes: impact on physical activity. *Diabetes Care* 25:1576–1583, 2002

Kim CJ, Hwang AR, Yoo JS: The impact of a stage-matched intervention to promote exercise behavior in participants with type 2 diabetes. *Int J Nurs Stud* 41:833–841, 2004

King DK, Glasgow RE, Toobert DJ, Strycker LA, Estabrooks PA, Osuna D, Faber AJ: Self-efficacy, problem solving, and social-environmental support are associated with diabetes self-management behaviors. *Diabetes Care* 33:751–753, 2010

Kirk A, Mutrie N, MacIntyre P, Fisher M: Effects of a 12-month physical activity counselling intervention on glycaemic control and on the status of cardiovascular risk factors in people with type 2 diabetes. *Diabetologia* 47:821–832, 2004

Lavie CJ, Milani RV: Effects of cardiac rehabilitation and exercise training in obese patients with coronary artery disease. *Chest* 109:52–56, 1996

Lavie CJ, Milani RV, Littman AB: Benefits of cardiac rehabilitation and exercise training in secondary coronary prevention in the elderly. *J Am Coll Cardiol* 22:678–683, 1993

Liebreich T, Plotnikoff RC, Courneya KS, Boulé N: Diabetes NetPLAY: A physical activity website and linked email counselling randomized intervention for individuals with type 2 diabetes. *Int J Behav Nutr Phys Act* 6:18, 2009

Lind E, Ekkekakis P, Vazou S: The affective impact of exercise intensity that slightly exceeds the preferred level: "pain" for no additional "gain." *J Health Psychol* 13:464–468, 2008

Long JA, Jahnle EC, Richardson DM, Loewenstein G, Volpp KG: Peer mentoring and financial incentives to improve glucose control in African American veterans: a randomized trial. *Ann Intern Med* 156:416–424, 2012

Lubans DR, Plotnikoff RC, Jung M, Eves N, Sigal R: Testing mediator variables in a resistance training intervention for obese adults with type 2 diabetes. *Psychol Health* 27:1388–1404, 2012

Luszczynska A, Schwarzer R, Lippke S, Mazurkiewicz M: Self-efficacy as a moderator of the planning-behaviour relationship in interventions designed to promote physical activity. *Psychol Health* 26:151–166, 2011

Malpass A, Andrews R, Turner KM: Patients with type 2 diabetes experiences of making multiple lifestyle changes: a qualitative study. *Patient Educ Couns* 74:258–263, 2009

Maran A, Pavan P, Bonsembiante B, Brugin E, Ermolao A, Avogaro A, Zaccaria M: Continuous glucose monitoring reveals delayed nocturnal hypoglycemia after intermittent high-intensity exercise in nontrained patients with type 1 diabetes. *Diabetes Technol Ther* 12:763–768, 2010

Marcus BH, Selby VC, Niaura RS, Rossi JS: Self-efficacy and the stages of exercise behavior change. *Res Q Exerc Sport* 63:60–66, 1992

Marcus BH, Simkin LR: The transtheoretical model: applications to exercise behavior. *Med Sci Sports Exerc* 26:1400–1404, 1994

McAuley E, Blissmer B: Self-efficacy determinants and consequences of physical activity. *Exercise & Sport Sciences Reviews* 28:85–88, 2000

Mier N, Medina AA, Ory MG: Mexican Americans with type 2 diabetes: perspectives on definitions, motivators, and programs of physical activity. *Preventing Chronic Disease* 4:A24, 2007

Miller ST, Marolen KN, Beech BM: Perceptions of physical activity and motivational interviewing among rural African-American women with type 2 diabetes. *Womens Health Issues* 20:43–49, 2009

Morrato EH, Hill JO, Wyatt HR, Ghushchyan V, Sullivan PW: Are health care professionals advising patients with diabetes or at risk for developing diabetes to exercise more? *Diabetes Care* 29:543–548, 2006

Morrato EH, Hill JO, Wyatt HR, Ghushchyan V, Sullivan PW: Physical activity in U.S. adults with diabetes and at risk for developing diabetes, 2003. *Diabetes Care* 30:203–209, 2007

Mourier A, Gautier JF, De Kerviler E, Bigard AX, Villette JM, Garnier JP, Duvallet A, Guezennec CY, Cathelineau G: Mobilization of visceral adipose tissue related to the improvement in insulin sensitivity in response to physical training in NIDDM. Effects of branched-chain amino acid supplements. *Diabetes Care* 20:385–391, 1997

Muller-Riemenschneider F, Reinhold T, Nocon M, Willich SN: Long-term effectiveness of interventions promoting physical activity: a systematic review. *Prev Med* 47:354–368, 2008

Naik AD, Palmer N, Petersen NJ, Street RL Jr, Rao R, Suarez-Almazor M, Haidet P: Comparative effectiveness of goal setting in diabetes mellitus group clinics: randomized clinical trial. *Arch Intern Med* 171:453–459, 2011

Napolitano MA, Papandonatos GD, Borradaile KE, Whiteley JA, Marcus BH: Effects of weight status and barriers on physical activity adoption among previously inactive women. *Obesity (Silver Spring)* 19:2183–2189, 2011

Negri C, Bacchi E, Morgante S, Soave D, Marques A, Menghini E, Muggeo M, Bonora E, Moghetti P: Supervised walking groups to increase physical activity in type 2 diabetic patients. *Diabetes Care* 33:2333–2335, 2010

Newlin K, Melkus GD, Tappen R, Chyun D, Koenig HG: Relationships of religion and spirituality to glycemic control in Black women with type 2 diabetes. *Nurs Res* 57:331–339, 2008

Ogilvie D, Foster CE, Rothnie H, Cavill N, Hamilton V, Fitzsimons CF, Mutrie N, Scottish Physical Activity Research Collaboration: Interventions to promote walking: systematic review [see comment]. *BMJ* 334:1204, 2007

Osborn CY, Amico KR, Cruz N, O'Connell AA, Perez-Escamilla R, Kalichman SC, Wolf SA, Fisher JD: A brief culturally tailored intervention for Puerto Ricans with type 2 diabetes. *Health Educ Behav* 37:849–862, 2010

Penn L, Moffatt SM, White M: Participants' perspective on maintaining behaviour change: a qualitative study within the European Diabetes Prevention Study. *BMC Public Health* 8:235, 2008

Pentecost C, Taket A: Understanding exercise uptake and adherence for people with chronic conditions: a new model demonstrating the importance of exercise identity, benefits of attending and support. *Health Educ Res* 26:908–922, 2011

Plotnikoff RC, Trinh L, Courneya KS, Karunamuni N, Sigal RJ: Predictors of physical activity in adults with type 2 diabetes. *Am J Health Behav* 35:359–370, 2011

Realsen JM, Chase HP: Recent advances in the prevention of hypoglycemia in type 1 diabetes. *Diabetes Technol Ther* 13:1177–1186, 2011

Sacco WP, Malone JI, Morrison AD, Friedman A, Wells K: Effect of a brief, regular telephone intervention by paraprofessionals for type 2 diabetes. *J Behav Med* 32:349–359, 2009

Shinji S, Shigeru M, Ryusei U, Mitsuru M, Shigehiro K: Adherence to a home-based exercise program and incidence of cardiovascular disease in type 2 diabetes patients. *Int J Sports Med* 28:877–879, 2007

Sigal RJ, Kenny GP, Boulé NG, Wells GA, Prud'homme D, Fortier M, Reid RD, Tulloch H, Coyle D, Phillips P, Jennings A, Jaffey J: Effects of aerobic training, resistance training, or both on glycemic control in type 2 diabetes: a randomized trial. *Annals of Internal Medicine* 147:357–369, 2007

Song R, Ahn S, Roberts BL, Lee EO, Ahn YH: Adhering to a tai chi program to improve glucose control and quality of life for individuals with type 2 diabetes. *J Altern Complement Med* 15:627–632, 2009

Sullivan-Bolyai S, Bova C, Leung K, Trudeau A, Lee M, Gruppuso P: Social Support to Empower Parents (STEP): an intervention for parents of young children newly diagnosed with type 1 diabetes. *Diabetes Educ* 36:88–97, 2010

Tuah NA, Amiel C, Qureshi S, Car J, Kaur B, Majeed A: Transtheoretical model for dietary and physical exercise modification in weight loss management for overweight and obese adults. *Cochrane Database Syst Rev*:CD008066, 2011

Tudor-Locke C, Bell RC, Myers AM, Harris SB, Ecclestone NA, Lauzon N, Rodger NW: Controlled outcome evaluation of the First Step Program: a daily physical activity intervention for individuals with type II diabetes. *Int J Obes Relat Metab Disord* 28:113–119, 2004

Umpierre D, Ribeiro PA, Kramer CK, Leitao CB, Zucatti AT, Azevedo MJ, Gross JL, Ribeiro JP, Schaan BD: Physical activity advice only or structured exercise training and association with HbA1c levels in type 2 diabetes: a systematic review and meta-analysis. *JAMA* 305:1790–1799, 2011

Wadden TA, Neiberg RH, Wing RR, Clark JM, Delahanty LM, Hill JO, Krakoff J, Otto A, Ryan DH, Vitolins MZ, Look Ahead Research Group: Four-year weight losses in the Look AHEAD study: factors associated with long-term success. *Obesity (Silver Spring)* 19:1987–1998, 2011

Wadden TA, West DS, Delahanty L, Jakicic J, Rejeski J, Williamson D, Berkowitz RI, Kelley DE, Tomchee C, Hill JO, Kumanyika S: The Look AHEAD study: a description of the lifestyle intervention and the evidence supporting it. *Obesity* 14:737–752, 2006

Williams DM: Exercise, affect, and adherence: an integrated model and a case for self-paced exercise. *Journal of Sport & Exercise Psychology* 30:471–496, 2008a

Williams DM, Dunsiger S, Ciccolo JT, Lewis BA, Albrecht AE, Marcus BH: Acute affective response to a moderate-intensity exercise stimulus predicts physical activity participation 6 and 12 months later. *Psychol Sport Exerc* 9:231–245, 2008b

Williamson DA, Rejeski J, Lang W, Van Dorsten B, Fabricatore AN, Toledo K, Look Ahead Research Group: Impact of a weight management program on health-related quality of life in overweight adults with type 2 diabetes. *Arch Intern Med* 169:163–171, 2009

Winett RA, Williams DM, Davy BM: Initiating and maintaining resistance training in older adults: a social cognitive theory-based approach. *Br J Sports Med* 43:114–119, 2009

Appendix A

Generic and Brand Names of Current U.S. Diabetes Medications

Mechanism of Action	Generic Name(s)	Brand Name(s)
Enhance insulin effects		
Biguanide	Metformin Metformin SR or XR	Glucophage, Fortamet, Glumetza, Riomet Glucophage XR
Thiazolidinediones or glitazones	Rosiglitazone Pioglitazone	Avandia (restricted in U.S.) Actos
α-Glucosidase inhibitors	Acarbose Miglitol	Precose Glyset
Augment insulin supply		
Sulfonylureas	Tolbutamide Chlorpropamide Tolazamide Glipizide, Glipizide ER Glyburide Glimepiride	Orinase Diabinese Tolinase Glucotrol, Glucotrol XL DiaBeta, Micronase, Glynase Amaryl
Glinides	Repaglinide Nateglinide	Prandin Starlix
Modify hormonal systems		
Amylinomimetic	Pramlintide	Symlin
Incretin mimetics	Exenatide Exenatide Extended-Release Liraglutide	Byetta Bydureon Victoza
Dipeptidyl peptidase IV Inhibitors (DPP-4)	Sitagliptin Saxagliptin Linagliptin	Januvia Onglyza Tradjenta
Exogenous insulins		
Rapid-acting analogs	Lispro Aspart Glulisine	Humalog Novolog Apidra
Short-acting analogs	Regular	Humulin R, Novolin R, Actrapid
Intermediate-acting analogs	Isophane	Humulin N, Novolin N
Long-acting analogs	Glargine Detemir	Lantus Levemir
Ultra–long-acting analogs	Degludec Degludec, plus Aspart (70/30)	Tresiba Ryzodeg

Appendix B
Physical Activity Tools for Professionals

ONLINE RESOURCES

American Association of Diabetes Educators. Available at www.aadenet.org.

American College of Sports Medicine: Position stand on exercise and type 2 diabetes mellitus, 2010. Available at www.acsm.org/access-public-information/position-stands.

American Diabetes Association. Available at www.diabetes.org.

Centers for Disease Control and Prevention, National Center for Chronic Disease Prevention and Health Promotion. Available at www.cdc.gov/diabetes/index.htm.

National Institute of Diabetes and Digestive and Kidney Diseases. Available at www2.niddk.nih.gov.

SUGGESTED READINGS

American College of Sports Medicine, Durstine JL, Moore G, Painter P: *ACSM's Exercise Management for Persons with Chronic Diseases and Disabilities*. 3rd ed. Champaign, IL, Human Kinetics, 2009

American College of Sports Medicine: *ACSM's Guidelines for Exercise Testing and Prescription*. 9th ed. Baltimore, MD, Williams & Wilkins, 2013

American College of Sports Medicine: *ACSM's Resource Manual for Exercise Testing and Prescription*. 7th ed. Baltimore, MD, Williams & Wilkins, 2013

American College of Sports Medicine, American Diabetes Association: Exercise and type 2 diabetes: American College of Sports Medicine and the American Diabetes Association: joint position statement. *Med Sci Sports Exerc* 42:2282–2303, 2010

American Diabetes Association: Physical activity/exercise and diabetes. *Diabetes Care* 27 (Suppl. 1):S58–S62, 2004

Colberg SR: *Diabetic Athlete's Handbook: Your Guide to Peak Performance*. Champaign, IL, Human Kinetics, 2009

Colberg SR: *The 7 Step Diabetes Fitness Plan: Living Well and Being Fit with Diabetes, No Matter Your Weight.* New York, Marlowe & Company, 2007

Colberg SR, Sigal RJ, Fernhall B, et al.: Exercise and type 2 diabetes: the American College of Sports Medicine and the American Diabetes Association: joint position statement. *Diabetes Care* 33:e147–167, 2010

Garber CE, Blissmer B, Deschenes MR, Franklin BA, Lamonte MJ, Lee IM, Nieman DC, Swain DP, American College of Sports Medicine: American College of Sports Medicine position stand. Quantity and quality of exercise for developing and maintaining cardiorespiratory, musculoskeletal, and neuromotor fitness in apparently healthy adults: guidance for prescribing exercise. *Med Sci Sports Exerc* 43:1334–1359, 2011

Haskell WL, Lee IM, Pate RR, et al.: Physical activity and public health: updated recommendation for adults from the American College of Sports Medicine and the American Heart Association. *Med Sci Sports Exerc* 39:1423–1434, 2007

Hayes C: *The "I Hate to Exercise" Book for People with Diabetes.* 2nd ed. Alexandria, VA, American Diabetes Association, 2006

Miller WR, Rollnick S: *Motivational Interviewing: Preparing People for Change.* 2nd ed. New York, Guilford Press, 2002

Nelson ME, Rejeski WJ, Blair SN, et al.: Physical activity and public health in older adults: recommendation from the American College of Sports Medicine and the American Heart Association. *Med Sci Sports Exerc* 39:1435–1445, 2007

Physical Activity Guidelines Advisory Committee: Physical Activity Guidelines Advisory Committee Report, 2008. Washington, DC, U.S. Department of Health and Human Services, 2008

Sigal RJ, Kenny GP, Wasserman DH, Castaneda-Sceppa C: Physical activity/exercise and type 2 diabetes. *Diabetes Care* 27:2518–2539, 2004

Sigal RJ, Kenny GP, Wasserman DH, Castaneda-Sceppa C, White RD: Physical activity/exercise and type 2 diabetes: a consensus statement from the American Diabetes Association. *Diabetes Care* 29:1433–1438, 2006

Index